AGGRESSION AND ANTISOCIAL BEHAVIOR IN CHILDREN AND ADOLESCENTS

Aggression and Antisocial Behavior in Children and Adolescents

Research and Treatment

DANIEL F. CONNOR

Foreword by Russell A. Barkley

THE GUILFORD PRESS
New York   London

© 2002 The Guilford Press
A Division of Guilford Publications, Inc.
72 Spring Street, New York, NY 10012
www.guilford.com

Printed in the United States of America

This book is printed on acid-free paper.

Last digit is print number: 9 8 7 6 5 4 3 2 1

Library of Congress Cataloging-in-Publication Data

Connor, Daniel F.
   Aggression and antisocial behavior in children and adolescents :
research and treatment / Daniel F. Connor ; foreword by Russell A.
Barkley.
       p. cm.
Includes bibliographical references and index.
   ISBN 1-57230-738-2 (alk. paper)
   1. Aggressiveness in children. 2. Conduct disorders in children. 3.
Violence in children. 4. Oppositional defiant disorder in
children—Treatment. I. Title.
   RJ506.A35 C665 2002
   155.4′18232—dc21
                                              2002003552

To Sara, Charlotte, and David
for life and meaning

About the Author

Daniel F. Connor, MD, is currently an Associate Professor of Psychiatry in the Division of Child and Adolescent Psychiatry at the University of Massachusetts Medical School in Worcester, Massachusetts. He is also Director of Pediatric Psychopharmacology at the University of Massachusetts Memorial Health Care. A clinician and clinical researcher in child and adolescent psychiatry, Dr. Connor is certified by the American Board of Psychiatry and Neurology in the specialty of Psychiatry and the subspecialty of Child and Adolescent Psychiatry. As a practicing clinician, Dr. Connor evaluates and treats a wide variety of youth with serious emotional and behavioral disturbances, most of whom have troubles with excessive, inappropriate, and maladaptive aggression and related problems.

An active clinical investigator, Dr. Connor has authored numerous scientific articles and book chapters on aggression, pediatric psychopharmacology, attention-deficit/hyperactivity disorder (ADHD), and disruptive behavior disorders. As Director of the Pediatric Psychopharmacology Clinical Trials Program at the University of Massachusetts Medical School, he participates in many multisite clinical drug trials developing new therapies for children and adolescents with ADHD and disruptive behavior disorders.

Foreword

The field of maladaptive aggression in children and adolescents is not one for the faint of heart. The literature is voluminous, the definitions too many to count, the research prolific, and the complexities labyrinthine. Approaching this vast storehouse of knowledge, one feels what an average person would sense being placed in a wrestling ring with a rhinoceros: How on earth is one to take hold of it, much less bring it down in some meaningful way? So formidable is the task that few have ventured to do so. This book was written by one of those few—a sturdy, persistent, insightful, yet incisive and generally optimistic soul who believes that a comprehensive understanding of maladaptive aggression can be brought within our grasp. It now has been done by Daniel F. Connor, my colleague, friend, and collaborator at the University of Massachusetts Medical School for many years. When he first approached me concerning his decision to write a book on this topic, I was admittedly skeptical that he could ever see it through to completion, given the monstrous amount of information the topic comprised. The field of child psychopathology should be immeasurably grateful to him for doing so. There are few topics of greater importance than this one, in view of the extraordinary social costs associated with aggression, and few books have dealt with this topic with such sensitivity, breadth, and scope.

Dr. Connor was just the right man for the job. A hugely energetic, good-natured, and intelligent child psychiatrist and psychopharmacologist, he has dealt with entities that are even more recalcitrant than this field of knowledge; perhaps this fact accounts for his undaunted zeal. He is just the right person to wrestle with the topic of childhood aggression, to be undismayed by the challenges so posed, and to bring it down to the mat of our level of understanding. We are all made the better for his courage and adventurousness in doing so, for he has produced a stunningly comprehensive, yet easily comprehensible summary of what is known about aggression in young people. The reference section alone is worth the price of the book. To have at one's disposal the most recent, far-flung, and important citations on the topic is a worthy outcome by itself. Yet the book's contents are far more important than a compendium would suggest, given the added value one obtains through Dr. Connor's interpretations, insights, and innovative conclusions.

From sociology, anthropology, evolutionary biology, psychopathology, epidemiology, and neuropsychology, to psychosocial interventions and psychopharmacology, Dr. Connor has spared no perspective in his relentless search for information on the nature, course, outcome, etiology, and management of youthful aggression and antisocial behavior. This is scientific scholarship at its best, distilling out of the seemingly limitless quantity of information on this topic what one needs to know to be truly educated about it. As the philosopher/scientist David Deutsch (1997) wrote in *The Fabric of Reality*, his treatise on scientific knowledge, one does not have to know every detail of science to be a truly informed person. What one needs to know instead are the great scientific theories, their principles, and their implications, to which all extant scientific knowledge has pointed and from which all that is to come will likely flow. In similar, albeit smaller-scale fashion, Dr. Connor takes us through the major perspectives and findings on aggression and shows us their principles and implications; as a result, the reader becomes a truly educated person on the topic.

Throughout it all, Dr. Connor has stuck close to the scientific literature, critically prodding its weaknesses while acclaiming its strengths. Avoiding mere reductionistic and fashionable clichés that would attribute this significant social and clinical problem merely to low childhood self-esteem, father-absent families, or violent television/video games (convenient yet simplistic targets all), Dr. Connor demonstrates the numerous factors contributing to aggression, spanning every level of the biopsychosocial framework. Dr. Connor tells us what our science has to say about maladaptive aggression—how complex the problem actually is; how manifold its impact is on both the affected youth and society; and, just as important, what this complexity and this impact may mean for clinical interventions and prevention efforts directed at the problem. Yet he also just as sagely tells us what we still do not know and what is yet to be done. From definitions to prevalences to comorbidities to outcomes to treatments, the reader is treated to a veritable continent of information. But this one comes with a wise, well-prepared guide to show us not just the way through it, but the why of it. No matter how much the reader may know about childhood aggression, there are new insights here along with new results from recent studies to make it well worth the journey, even for seasoned veterans.

Dr. Connor undertook an awesome task several years ago when he began this work, and it is an awesome book that has resulted from the many hundreds of hours he has spent in its completion. Thank you, Dan, for doing so, and thank you, dear reader, for having the uncommonly good sense to acquire this text. As the 18th-century philosopher Caleb C. Colton once said, "There are three difficulties in authorship: —to write anything worth publishing—to find honest [people] to publish it—and to get sensible [people] to read it." Dr. Connor has seen to the first two of these tasks with great success; your challenge as its sensible consumer is to complete the triad. You undoubtedly will be much the wiser for having done so.

RUSSELL A. BARKLEY, PhD
Professor of Psychiatry and Neurology
University of Massachusetts Medical School

Preface

Many fine books have been written on the subject of aggression and related behaviors in children and adolescents. Many of these books approach the subject from a discipline-specific point of view: Some emphasize criminology in their approach to the problem of youth violence; others take a behavioral or a psychobiological approach to the subject; still others approach this subject from a highly academic perspective, emphasizing theoretical approaches.

The purpose of this book is to bring together in one place empirically based information from many different scientific fields on what is presently known about aggression and related behaviors in children and adolescents. In essence, then, the book is a multidisciplinary review of the subject. A further purpose of this book is to facilitate research into these behaviors by collecting into one volume the present state of the research. It is always easier to know where to go if you know where you have been.

There are many people whom I wish to thank for their support and encouragement in the writing of this book, and for critical comments that improved it. First, I would like to thank Sara N. B. Connor for her encouragement throughout the duration of this project. Dr. Richard H. Melloni, Jr., provided critical commentary and much-needed support. Dr. Yvon Delville aided me in the drawing of several figures depicting neurobiological systems. Ann Dahl, LICSW, Professor Robert Dahl, Dr. Russell Barkley, and Dr. Thomas Grisso each provided invaluable commentary on sections of the manuscript. Jean Foran supplied much-needed administrative help. I would like to thank Seymour Weingarten, Editor-in-Chief of The Guilford Press, for support of this project. Finally, my gratitude to two anonymous reviewers whose careful reading of the manuscript and subsequent commentary greatly improved the book's content and organization.

DANIEL F. CONNOR

Contents

❖ CHAPTER 1

Definitions and Subtyping of Aggressive Behavior

A ggression and related behaviors in children and adolescents are central issues in our time. From public school shootings and similar instances of "children killing other children," to concern about rising rates of youth crime and delinquency in the community, to the relationship between unrecognized and untreated mental illness and violence in youngsters, there are many worries and much debate about excessive, inappropriate aggression in young people in our society. Dispute continues over the role of violent mass media presentations in the etiology of youth violence. There is also dissent over the relative importance of psychosocial versus neurobiological causation in the development of maladaptive aggression in juveniles. Many times this debate has been acrimonious, with sharp disagreements and polarized positions over the important causes of youth aggression and the best approaches to its prevention and treatment.

Aggression in youth is not a new concern. Over the past 80 years, much research has been completed examining early-onset aggressive/antisocial behaviors from multiple perspectives. The vast majority of this research has been conducted in the field of psychology, including experimental, social, personality, and clinical psychology. The other major field conducting research into such behaviors in juveniles is the discipline of criminal justice. The fields of sociology and anthropology have also made contributions. Psychiatry, as the branch of medicine that deals with human behavior, mood, cognition, and mental illness, has long been concerned with the problem of human aggression and violence. For much of the past century, however, psychiatry's approach to this problem was through psychoanalysis. The failure of psychoanalysts to use empirical methods and to scientifically test and validate their theories has led to a turning away from these approaches in psychiatry. More recently, theo-

ries from neurobiology, neuropharmacology, developmental psychopathology, and integrated biosocial approaches to aggression, which are testable via
experimental methods, have helped move the field forward. The path into the
future will emphasize integrated theories about the interaction of biology with
maladaptive rearing environments over the course of individual development,
to facilitate understanding of the etiology of early-onset aggression in children
and adolescents.

Aggression and related behaviors in the young are complex, heterogeneous conditions with diverse etiologies and consequences. In efforts to understand these behaviors, knowledge from many different scientific disciplines
must be tapped in order to provide an overall picture of what we presently
know about the aggressive child or adolescent. In the chapters that follow,
psychobiological, personality, and psychosocial issues and their complicated
interactions across development are presented, in order to facilitate a greater
understanding of this important problem.

ISSUES RELATED TO TERMINOLOGY AND DEFINITIONS

Perhaps the complexity inherent in understanding the problem of aggression
in youth is best captured by the myriad definitions and terms used to describe
these youngsters. Terms such as "aggressive," "violent," "conduct-disordered,"
"oppositional," "psychopathic," "underaroused," "delinquent," and "antisocial" have all been used by different disciplines to describe youth with persistent and frequent aggressive behavior. The multiple systems that serve these
youngsters, including school, juvenile justice, and mental health systems, and
the multiple professional disciplines that study these youngsters all have developed their own specific languages to describe children and adolescents with
difficult behaviors. This myriad of terms may be quite confusing to the reader
seeking a basic definition of aggression in youth.

Some fundamental conceptual issues need to be discussed at the outset.
First, given that aggression is a heterogeneous condition, no single term is adequate to capture all the variegated and diverse presentations of such behavior
in youth. This fact alone will result in multiple definitions of this behavior.
Second, "aggression," "violence," "conduct disorder," "delinquency," and
"antisocial behavior" all share some referents, but each has its own specific
definition that distinguishes it from the others. Finally, as noted above, different disciplines (e.g., mental health, juvenile justice, sociology, education) all
approach the problem of antisocial youth differently. Different disciplines
have different theoretical orientations and use different specialized terminology to describe and characterize aggressive youngsters. For example, within
the field of mental health, there are at least two approaches to deviancy: statistical and clinical diagnostic/medical. The implications of different approaches
may be confusing. Behaviors may be statistically meaningful for an individual
as compared to age and gender population norms (the statistical approach),
but may not be sufficient to meet diagnostic criteria for a psychiatric disorder

(the medical/diagnostic approach). At the same time, they may be troublesome enough to require clinical referral. The implications of different approaches may conflict, as when an individual accused of committing a crime also has a diagnosable psychiatric condition. A medical diagnosis has implications for one's responsibility and thus culpability under the law. In other words, is such an individual psychiatrically ill or criminally responsible?

These definitions greatly influence the manner in which professionals in various disciplines understand, conceptualize, research, and intervene with aggressive youngsters. A historic problem has been the traditional lack of "crosstalk" between researchers and treatment staff members across the many professions involved with aggressive juveniles. As a result, individual disciplines are denied relevant findings from other fields of study that might influence a more complete understanding of violent youth. For example, the growing "get tough on crime" movement popularized by politicians and law enforcement officials tends to conceptualize violence among youngsters as criminal, identifies these children as early-starter criminals, and increasingly prescribes adult penalties (such as lengthy incarceration) to young children who commit crimes of violence. This is reflected in the fact that more and more states are making it easier to transfer youngsters accused of violent crimes from juvenile court to adult court, where they are subject to adult sentencing guidelines. This conceptualization minimizes research findings from the fields of clinical mental health and behavioral sciences, which emphasize the importance of family, rearing environment, developmental, psychosocial, psychobiological, and psychopathological considerations in the understanding of and intervention with these children and adolescents. Thus how we define these youth has a great impact on their lives.

In the chapters that follow, findings from multiple disciplines and different areas of research are brought together in order to facilitate a more complete understanding of early-onset aggression and related behaviors. Since how we define aggressive behavior is so important in how we conceptualize these children and adolescents, the book begins with a discussion of various definitions of child aggression, delinquency, and antisocial behavior. In this chapter, a general definition of aggression is followed by a discussion of the importance of distinguishing adaptive from maladaptive aggression. Definitions from the perspectives of juvenile justice, clinical diagnostic/medical settings, psychometrics, and personality/social psychology are next presented. Various ways of subtyping aggressive behavior, as approaches to the problem of heterogeneity in terminology, follow. The chapter concludes with a brief discussion of the limitations of current definitions and subtypes of aggression.

A GENERAL DEFINITION OF AGGRESSION

What is basically meant by the terms "aggression" and "aggressive"? *Webster's Ninth New Collegiate Dictionary* (1989) defines these terms as follows:

Aggression (n). 1. a forceful action or procedure (as an unprovoked attack) esp. when intended to dominate or master. 2. the practice of making unprovoked attacks or encroachments. 3. hostile, injurious, or destructive behavior esp. when caused by frustration.

Aggressive (adj.). 1a. tending toward or practicing aggression. b. marked by combative readiness: militant. 2a. marked by driving forceful energy or initiative: enterprising. b. marked by obtrusive energy: self-assertive. Syn.: militant, self-assertive, pushing. Aggressive implies a disposition to dominate, often in disregard of others' rights or in determined and energetic pursuit of one's ends. (p. 64)

Aggression, then, is a heterogeneous and very broad category of behavior. It is distinguished from "violence," which is defined as a physical force exerted so as to cause damage, abuse, or injury. Violence may be caused by either animate or inanimate physical forces, but aggression requires a living agent. A hurricane may be violent, but only animals, primates, and human beings can be aggressive.

ADAPTIVE AND MALADAPTIVE AGGRESSION

For the purposes of this book it is important to distinguish "appropriate" or "adaptive" aggression from "excessive," "inappropriate," or "maladaptive" aggression. This book is concerned only with the second type of aggression. The distinction is important, since the focus of research efforts and the types of interventions directed at the problem may be different, depending on the type of aggression. For example, adaptive aggression may not necessarily require mental health research or treatment, or criminal justice intervention; other family, social service, political, and/or economic interventions may be more appropriate. Failing to recognize adaptive aggression and incorrectly identifying it as maladaptive aggression may have serious consequences for a child or adolescent.

For example, adaptive aggression often occurs in the service of ensuring the integrity or survival of the individual. Consider an adolescent who runs away from home to escape an abusive situation with his or her parents, steals food from a store in order to eat while "on the street," and repeatedly fights other individuals who may attempt to steal his or her possessions. This teenager fulfills enough symptoms to meet psychiatric diagnostic criteria for conduct disorder, a mental disorder. But are these behaviors really a core syndrome of psychopathology in the individual, or are these behaviors adaptive and in the service of survival? Although the teen is clearly breaking the law and violating societal rules and norms, this type of aggression is not necessarily an expression of individual psychopathology. At this level, general conceptions of aggression, and existing diagnostic categories describing aggressive youth as maladaptive, dysfunctional, or pathological, may begin to break down. A distinction between adaptive and maladaptive aggression is needed to clarify when aggression occurs because of individual psychopathology and when it occurs in the service of environmental adaptation. Not distinguishing between adaptive and maladaptive aggression may obscure important decisions concerning intervention, and confuse important distinctions in etiology and prognosis for aggressive youth. Some conceptions of psychopathology have been offered that may help distinguish adaptive from maladaptive aggression.

Maladaptive Aggression as Harmful Dysfunction

In his critique of the conceptual validity of mental disorders as defined by the *Diagnostic and Statistical Manual of Mental Disorders* (DSM), Wakefield (1992a, 1992b, 1997) has introduced the concept of "harmful dysfunction." For a condition to be considered a disorder, it must have two elements. First, the condition must cause negative consequences for the individual possessing it. Second, the condition must represent some dysfunction in the natural action of an internal mechanism; that is the mechanism is *not* performing in the manner it was designed to function, across the range of environments for which it was meant, as determined by natural selection (i.e., evolution) (Wakefield, 1992). Internal mechanisms can be biological, psychological, cognitive, or emotional. This concept of disorder not only has a social value criterion (e.g., negative consequences for the individual as generally defined by society), but a factual criterion as well (the disordered mechanism).

Wakefield's definition is particularly useful when applied to aggression. Adaptive aggression is the behavioral expression of intact internal mechanisms (biological, psychological, cognitive, emotional) serving their natural function as designed by evolutionary biology, and utilized across a range of environments, in the service of competition for desired but scarce resources and/or in defense of the individual or group to ensure physical intactness and survival, without incurring large negative consequences as defined by a given society at a given time in history. Maladaptive aggression meets two criteria: First, maladaptive aggression is not in the service of individual or group competition for resources or defense within the context of the rules of a given society; second, maladaptive aggression is an expression of a disordered internal mechanism, such as a neuropsychiatric illness. The first, a social value criterion, may change as societies change. The second, a factual criterion, should remain stable. Like mental disorders in general, maladaptive aggression lies on the boundary between the constructed social world and the given natural world.

Thus aggression is not necessarily a mental disorder per se or an expression of psychopathology. In certain contexts and environments, aggressive behavior is very adaptive. However, a subset of aggressive behavior as described above may be quite maladaptive. This type of aggression is the focus of this book. Maladaptive aggression requires recognition in clinical treatment settings; provides a justification for possible psychosocial, environmental, biomedical, and/or neuropsychiatric treatment intervention; and requires further research. Moreover, maladaptive aggression needs to be recognized in juvenile justice settings, so that incarcerated youth who have violated the law can receive needed mental health services.

Characteristics of Maladaptive Aggression

What are some of the descriptive characteristics of maladaptive aggression? Research on aggression and brain dysfunction in nonhuman primates provides some clues. Kraemer and Clarke (1996) studied infant rhesus monkeys randomly assigned to one of two rearing conditions: mother-reared or peer-reared. Being raised in the absence of a biological mother from early infancy appeared to constitute a major stress for the peer-raised monkeys. At approximately 6–7 months of age, mother-reared and peer-reared monkeys were placed in social groups, and their adaptive social behavior (including aggression) was observed and measured. Although all the monkeys demonstrated aggression, the peer-raised monkeys demonstrated many characteristics of unusual aggression as observed within their social milieu. Their attacks on other monkeys were generally less coupled to a definable social context than those of the mother-reared monkeys; that is, attacks were less predictable from social cues in the environment. Their aggression also generally occurred more frequently over time, was more repetitive, lasted longer, did not terminate appropriately, and was of greater severity than aggression demonstrated by the mother-raised monkeys. For peer-raised monkeys, aggression seemed less likely to occur in the service of social goals, such as attaining or retaining increased status within the troop, than aggression expressed by the mother-reared monkeys.

These same qualities of unusual aggression can be found in some humans. These characteristics include aggression that appears to occur independently of a usual, definable social context; aggression that occurs in the absence of antecedent social cues; aggression that is out of proportion to its apparent causes in intensity, frequency, duration, and/or severity; and aggression that does not terminate appropriately. Maladaptive aggression appears to be unregulated, disinhibited aggression. When this type of aggression occurs, has negative consequences for the individual, and appears to result from the inability of internal mechanisms to function as they were designed (usually the central nervous system or CNS) across the range of environments in which they were meant to function by natural selection, a disorder of maladaptive aggression exists. This disorder then can become an important target for research, intervention, and treatment, including the possibility of biomedical interventions.

Many other types of aggression exist today between individuals or groups of people in society. In response to a variety of real and/or perceived threats such as dangerous neighborhoods, increased fear, or increased competition for scarce resources, aggressive acts between individuals or groups of individuals may erupt. In contrast to the previous discussion, these acts probably reflect intact neural mechanisms. Although aggression in these circumstances may bring very real negative consequences to the individuals, the community, and society, this aggressive behavior reflects functioning internal CNS mechanisms working as natural selection designed them to work. Therefore, this type of aggression can probably be considered adaptive for an individual according to evolutionary biology, although it may cause great harm to the individual and social problems for the community. This type of aggression should be the focus of political, economic, social, community, and/or educational interventions, rather than biomedical intervention.

DEFINITIONS OF AGGRESSION FROM DIFFERENT PROFESSIONAL PERSPECTIVES

Definitions from Juvenile Justice

Criminal justice definitions of aggressive youth emphasize the terms "antisocial behavior," "criminality," and "delinquency." These are further discussed in Chapter 2. "Antisocial behavior" is any act that violates the rules and laws of society—an act that is illegal, no matter what the age of the perpetrator. Examples include homicide, theft, assault, burglary, and larceny. Individuals who commit antisocial acts may or may not be caught and adjudicated by the authorities. As such, antisocial behavior encompasses a broad definition of illegal acts, many of which may go unreported. "Criminality" and "delinquency" are subsets of antisocial behavior. "Criminality" generally refers to serious offenses and antisocial acts committed by an adult. For "delinquency," many definitions exist. Juvenile justice definitions of delinquency generally refer to both serious criminal acts and less serious offenses and antisocial acts committed by a minor. Note, however, that both criminality and delinquency involve illegal acts. Their definitions vary by age of the perpetrator and the fact that delinquency encompasses both less serious as well as more serious crimes. These juvenile justice definitions tend to narrowly emphasize the specific unlawful acts perpetrated by individuals (Steiner & Cauffman, 1998).

"Status offenses" are acts committed by a minor that would be legal if committed by an adult. These acts come to the attention of the court because of the offender's young age and a request, generally by parents, for court intervention because of the youth's "ungovernable" behavior. Examples include underage drinking, breaking curfew, and school truancy. Status offenses are not crimes, are not adjudicated in criminal court, and are generally processed in family court.

Clinical Diagnostic/Medical Definitions

Clinical mental health definitions of aggressive and antisocial youth often refer to "conduct disorder" (CD). In the current psychiatric diagnostic nomenclature, CD is present when a person under 18 years old demonstrates a constellation of symptoms, including aggression, deceitfulness, rule violations, and property destruction, in which the basic rights of others and major age-appropriate societal norms or rules are violated (American Psychiatric Association [APA], 1994). The emphasis is not on narrow judicial definitions of specific unlawful acts committed by an individual. Rather, it is on a putative psychopathological syndrome in which enough antisocial acts accumulate over time to meet chronicity and intensity criteria for the conclusion that behaviors are driven by some inner deficit in the person—a deficit that operates independently of his or her environment (Rogers, Johansen, Chang, & Salekin, 1997; Steiner & Cauffman, 1998). Although the psychiatric diagnosis of CD emphasizes aggressive behaviors toward others, other antisocial behaviors are also included in this disorder. Moreover, many aggressive youth meet criteria for both CD and another psychiatric diagnosis—attention-deficit/hyperactivity disorder (ADHD), which is characterized by age-inappropriate attention span deficits, impulsivity, and motor overactivity. Youngsters with both CD and ADHD are at risk for an early onset of aggressive behaviors, persistence of aggression over time, and extremely poor outcomes over the course of development. Because their behavior is so disturbing to others around them, these psychiatric diagnoses (along with a milder variant of CD called oppositional defiant disorder, or ODD) are sometimes called the "disruptive behavior disorders." The relationships between aggression and these disorders, and between aggression and other psychiatric illnesses, are more fully discussed in Chapter 4.

Psychometrically Based Definitions

Psychologists employing statistical approaches have identified empirical syndromes of child behavior problems derived from descriptions of child and adolescent problems in clinical case records, from consultation with mental health professionals, and from parent and teacher rating scales of children's problem behaviors at home and in the classroom (Achenbach & Edelbrock, 1978; McConaughy, 1992). It is important to note that these syndromes are not equivalent to psychiatric diagnoses. Individual behavior items are subjected to multivariate statistical analyses (such as principal-components analysis, factor analysis, and cluster analysis) to empirically derive syndromes of child and adolescent problem behaviors from a myriad of individual descriptive items. Multiple studies report two broad child behavior syndromes emerging from these multivariate analyses: "externalizing" and "internalizing" syndromes (Achenbach & Edelbrock, 1978; Naglieri, LeBuffe, & Pfeiffer, 1994). An externalizing syndrome represents undercontrolled child and adolescent behavior. Included in this syndrome are impulsive, hyperactive, aggressive, and delinquent behaviors. The internalizing syndrome represents overcontrolled behaviors and includes anxiety, fearfulness, depression, and social withdrawal. These behavior syndromes are distributed continuously throughout the population, and some youth will have internalizing and/or externalizing behavior of sufficient severity and frequency to identify them as abnormal compared to age- and gender-matched comparison groups. Youth with aggressive behavior, or those who carry a psychiatric diagnosis of CD, are often identified as having an externalizing behavior disorder, based upon parent and teacher ratings of their demeanor. Although "externalizing behavior" is not synonymous with "delinquency" or "CD," it captures many of the same problems. Rating scales that assess the externalizing syndrome are discussed in Chapter 10.

Definitions from Personality and Social Psychology

"Psychopathic personality" and "psychopathy" are closely related terms used to describe a subset of individuals with chronic serious criminality and recidivistic antisocial behavior. The psychiatric diagnosis of antisocial personality disorder (ASPD), which is coded on Axis II of the DSM-IV under personality disorders, is closely related to the concept of psychopathy. The essential feature of ASPD is a pervasive pattern of disregard for, and violation of, the rights of others that begins in childhood or early adolescence and continues into adulthood (APA, 1994; see Chapter 4). Because ASPD is a categorical psychiatric diagnosis, individuals either meet diagnostic criteria and are assigned the diagnosis, or they do not.

The concept of psychopathy expands beyond the diagnosis of ASPD to include deviant personality traits as well as antisocial behaviors. These traits are continuously distributed within the population, so that individuals may have none, some, or many of these traits. There is no discrete criterion threshold for having or not having psychopathic personality traits, as there is for the psychiatric diagnosis of ASPD. These personality traits include (but are not limited to) lying, insincerity, manipulation of others, superficial charm, callous disregard of others, unreliability, lack of remorse, poor insight, antisocial acts, and failure to learn from experience (Cleckley, 1950; Hare, 1980). Persons with these personality traits may be intermittently aggressive. This terminology has generally been reserved for adults. However, research is beginning to examine psychopathic traits in children (Frick, 1998) and adolescents (Myers, Burket, & Harris, 1995). Psychopathy is discussed again in Chapter 4.

SUBTYPES OF AGGRESSION

Since aggression is so heterogeneous a phenomenon and encompasses such a wide variety of behaviors and definitions, attempts have been made to subtype aggression into more homogeneous categories. This research is motivated by the realization that aggression is one of the most common and costly behaviors confronting juvenile justice personnel and mental health clinicians who treat referred children and adolescents. Given the many different terms and definitions describing aggressive youth, subtyping aggression offers the hope of creating a common classification that may facilitate communication across the many disciplines involved with these juveniles. Classifying aggression into more homogeneous categories may also lead to more specific psychosocial and pharmacological treatment modalities. Aggression subtypes are empirically derived from statistical techniques such as factor analysis, and are attempts to classify the broad behavioral domain of aggression into more coherent groupings. As such, this classification is evidence-based as opposed to theory-based. Because current research supporting various subtypes of aggression in children and adolescents is so widely scattered in the psychology and psychiatry literature, individual studies examining the validity of the various aggression subtypes are discussed in this section, in order to have a comprehensive discussion of this subject in one place.

Overt and Covert Aggression

The distinction between "overt" and "covert" forms of aggression has been a focus of psychometric research for many years (Quay, 1986a, 1986b). Currently, this dimensional subtype of aggression has the most empirical research evidence to support its validity. Overt aggression is defined as an openly confrontational act of physical aggression. Examples include physical fighting, bullying others, using weapons in hostile acts, and open defiance of rules and authority figures. Covert aggression is defined as any hidden, furtive, clandestine act of aggression. Examples include behaviors such as stealing, fire setting, truancy, and running away from home. Oppositional defiant behavior appears to lie on the midpoint of the overt–covert continuum.

Empirical support for this division comes from several sources. Loeber and Schmaling (1985), examining 28 studies found in 22 reports of child and adolescent psychopathology, performed a meta-analysis to empirically determine underlying dimensions of juvenile aggressive behavior. These studies reported data on 11,603 children and adolescents aged 2–18 years. Using the statistical technique of multidimensional scaling, they determined that antisocial behavior in youth, as rated by parents or clinician observers, could be conceptualized as unidimensional and bipolar. The two poles of behavior revealed by this analysis were overtly confrontive antisocial behaviors and furtive, covert acts (see Figure 1.1).

In another study, parent ratings of child and adolescent conduct problems were analyzed to determine underlying dimensions of antisocial behavior (Achenbach, Conners, Quay, Verhulst, & Howell, 1989). This study utilized factor analysis of parent behavior ratings for 8,194 American and Dutch children and adolescents aged 6–16 years. Consistent with the results of Loeber and Schmaling (1985), two conduct problem factors emerged from this analysis. One factor, labeled "aggressive," included overtly confrontational behaviors (e.g., defiance of authority figures, bullying, and physical fighting). The second

Overt Aggression

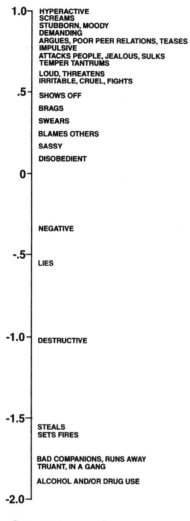

Covert Aggression

FIGURE 1.1. Overt and covert antisocial behaviors in one dimension. From Loeber and Schmaling (1985). Copyright 1985 by Kluwer Academic/Plenum Publishers. Reprinted by permission.

factor was labeled "delinquent" and included covertly aggressive behaviors, substance abuse, and having delinquent companions. (Note, however, that this definition of delinquency [from Achenbach et al.] was ascertained from rating scales of general child and adolescent psychopathology. The juvenile justice definition of delinquency and the definition of this term from rating scales of general child and adolescent psychopathology discuss it in different contexts, and so the definitions for this term vary.) The results from these factors provided some independent confirmation for the overt–covert dimension of aggressive behavior. More recently, additional support for this dimension has been found. In a study of children with ADHD and antisocial behaviors, stealing and property destruction formed a valid dimension of covert aggression that was distinguishable from more overt forms of aggression (Hinshaw, Simmel, & Heller, 1995). These studies support the internal validity of the overt–covert dimension of aggression in children and adolescents.

The overt–covert continuum has also received external validation. Research on family management practices and parent–child interaction patterns has revealed associations with more covert forms of aggressive behavior and delinquency. In a study of preadolescent boys, disruptions in parental monitoring of their children's whereabouts, the kind of companions they kept, or the types of activities they engaged in, coupled with a lack of consistent parent-administered discipline for rule breaking acts, were associated with increased risk for delinquent behavior (Patterson & Stouthamer-Loeber, 1984). Similarly, negative mother–child interaction patterns have been found to be associated with covert forms of aggressive behaviors in boys with ADHD (Hinshaw et al., 1995). In a twin study of genetic influences on dimensions of child and adolescent behavior, evidence for greater heritability of aggressive behavior (more overt) as compared to delinquent behavior (more covert) was found (Edelbrock, Rende, Plomin, & Thompson, 1995). Some investigations into the neurochemistry and dimensions of aggressive and delinquent behavior have also supported differences between overt and covert forms of aggression. Undersocialized boys with high scores on overt aggressive dimensions of behavior had lower levels of peripheral dopamine-beta-hydroxylase, an enzyme important in catecholamine metabolism and anxiety, compared to boys without overtly aggressive behaviors (Gabel, Stadler, Bjorn, Shindledecker, & Bowden, 1993b). In another study, peripheral measures of serotonin metabolism were found to be lower in boys who scored high on dimensions of overtly aggressive and hostile behavior than in boys with covert delinquency or no aggressive behavior (Birmaher et al., 1990). Finally, in a 6-year longitudinal study, the behavioral dimension of aggression as measured by the Child Behavior Checklist—a well-validated parent-completed rating scale of child psychopathology (Achenbach & Edelbrock, 1983)—proved to be a more stable trait over time than the dimension of delinquency (Achenbach, Howell, McConaughy, & Stanger, 1995b). Taken together, these studies begin to provide some external validation for the distinctiveness of the overt–covert dimension of aggressive behavior in children and adolescents.

One study has provided some modifications to, and provided additional empirical support for, the overt–covert dimension. In a meta-analysis of disruptive child behavior, Frick et al. (1993) studied 60 factor analyses published in 44 reports of 28,401 children and adolescents aged 2–18 years. In this study, a second independent dimension emerged from the factor analysis; this dimension is called "destructive–nondestructive." When crossed with the overt–covert dimension, four quadrants of aggressive behaviors are empirically identified (see Figure 1.2). Quadrant A is composed mainly of property violations, which are consistent with the covertly aggressive behaviors contained in the DSM-IV (APA, 1994) diagnosis of CD. Quadrant B contains mostly aggressive behaviors directed against people and is consistent with the overtly aggressive behaviors contained in the DSM-IV diagnosis of CD. Quadrant C contains status violations, which are also found in the DSM-IV symp-

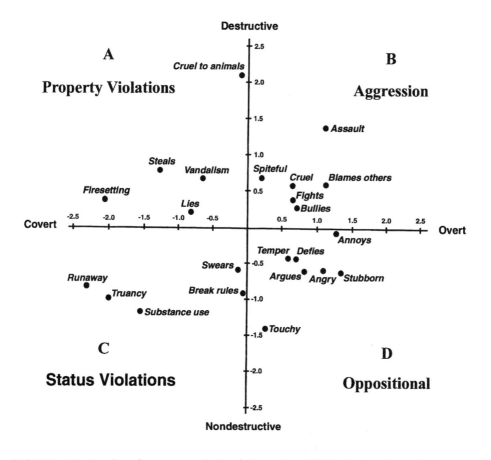

FIGURE 1.2. Results of a meta-analysis of disruptive child behavior. From Frick et al. (1993). Copyright 1993 by Elsevier Science. Reprinted by permission.

tom list for CD. (As noted earlier, these are behaviors that are legal for adults, but are illegal for children because of their minor status in the eyes of the law.) Quadrant D is composed mainly of oppositional defiant behaviors, which are found in the separate DSM-IV diagnosis of ODD. Thus this meta-analysis provides support for the distinct diagnoses of CD or ODD in the categorical DSM-IV psychiatric diagnostic system, and it identifies orthogonal dimensions that permit a finer-grained analysis of the domain of antisocial and aggressive behaviors in youth.

In psychiatrically referred youth evaluated in clinical settings, the focus has largely been on the overt pole of the overt–covert continuum. This is because aggressive behaviors such as physical assault, verbal threats of harm to others, self-injurious behaviors, and malicious destruction of property can be highly dramatic, costly, and demanding of treatment in the clinical setting. The study of these behaviors in clinical treatment settings has been facilitated by several observer-completed aggression rating scales that have empirical support for their reliability and validity with psychiatric patients (Kay, Wolkenfeld, & Murrill, 1988; Sorgi, Ratey, Knoedler, Markert, & Reichman, 1991; Yudofsky, Silver, Jackson, Endicott, & Williams, 1986). These rating scales measure the frequency and severity of several categories of aggressive behavior, including physical assault, verbal threats of violence, self-injurious behaviors, and property destruction (see Chapter 10).

Categories of overt aggression have been examined empirically in a study of children and adolescents referred to a residential treatment setting. When youth exhibiting high versus low rates of physical assault were compared, several differences were found in a cross-sectional study design. The children and adolescents with high rates of assaultive behavior were found to have significantly higher frequencies of verbal threats to others, self-injurious behaviors, and property destruction; a greater number of lifetime out-of-home placements; and a greater frequency of physical abuse in their developmental histories (Connor, Melloni, & Harrison, 1998). These data provide some preliminary evidence for differences between youngsters with high versus low overt categorical aggression in treatment settings.

Although not all studies agree (see Frick et al., 1993, for discussion), there is much empirical evidence to support the distinction between overt and covert dimensions of aggression. These dimensions have been found in statistical analyses evaluating conduct problems in over 36,000 children and adolescents, both clinically referred and in community samples. External validity as demonstrated by differing longitudinal outcomes, biochemical measures, parent management techniques, and heritability has provided additional support for this distinction. In more severely disturbed youth with a multiplicity of symptoms and problems seen in psychiatrically referred settings, these dimensions probably overlap, and distinctions may be obscured. Nevertheless, the finding that there are distinct patterns of aggressive behavior in youth should facilitate further research defining this continuum and exploring differential therapeutics, prevention strategies, and interventions.

Reactive and Proactive Aggression

The distinction between "reactive" and "proactive" forms of aggression arises out of a long tradition in aggression research that emphasizes two broad types of aggressive behavior as occurring in both animals and humans. One type of aggression arises in response to frustration in goal-directed behavior, and has been termed the "frustration–aggression" model (Dollard, Doob, Miller, Mowrer, & Sears, 1939). This model holds that aggression is a hostile, angry reaction to perceived frustration. The goal of this type of aggression is to defend oneself against a perceived threat or to inflict harm on a source of frustration. The precipitants and instigators of aggression are emphasized in this model, such as threat, goal blocking, frustrated expectations, population overcrowding, and even hot environmental temperatures (Berkowitz, 1993). Physiologically and behaviorally, this type of aggression is characterized by intense CNS autonomic arousal, irritability, fear or anger responses, frenzied, unplanned attacks on the object of frustration, and defensive posturing in the face of threat (Dodge, 1991). The other major type of aggression is termed "instrumental" or "predatory" aggression (Hartup, 1974). In this type of aggression, the goal is to obtain a desired reward or outcome (e.g., food, territory, social dominance, object acquisition). Physiologically and behaviorally, this type of aggression appears quite distinct. There is little CNS arousal, irritability, anger, or fear (see Chapters 6 and 7). Instrumental aggression is highly organized, patterned, and directed toward the promise of reward. In humans, instrumental aggression is described in the social learning theories of Bandura (1973). In this model, aggression is a learned phenomenon reinforced by social role modeling and positive outcomes for aggressive behaviors in social settings.

Reactive aggression has its theoretical roots in the frustration–aggression model, and proactive aggression has its theoretical roots in social learning theory. Reactive aggression is an angry, defensive response to threat, frustration, or provocation, and proactive aggression is a deliberate, coercive behavior controlled by external reinforcements and used as a means of obtaining a desired goal (Crick & Dodge, 1996). Research on this continuum of aggression has been facilitated by the development of rating instruments that reliably and validly identify groups of children and adolescents with reactive versus proactive aggression as assessed by teachers in community school classrooms and in play groups, and by evaluators of adjudicated adolescents (K. Brown, Atkins, Osborne, & Milnamow, 1996; Dodge & Coie, 1987; Smithmyer, Hubbard, & Simons, 2000; Waschbusch, Willoughby, & Pelham, 1998). The three items assessed in the Reactive Aggression subscale of Dodge and Coie's (1987) Proactive–Reactive Aggression Scale, and the three items assessed in the Proactive Aggression subscale, appear in Table 1.1.

Research on reactive and proactive aggression has largely focused on assessing elementary school children in community settings who are not clinically referred. This research has investigated social cognition and social information processing in children with reactive, proactive, combined, and no aggression.

TABLE 1.1. Reactive and Proactive Aggression Items

Reactive Aggression

1. When this child has been teased or threatened, he or she gets angry easily and strikes back.
2. This child always claims that other children are to blame in a fight and feels that they started the trouble.
3. When a peer accidentally hurts this child (such as by bumping into him or her), this child assumes that the peer meant to do it, and then overreacts with anger and fighting.

Proactive Aggression

1. This child gets other kids to gang up on a peer that he or she does not like.
2. This child uses physical force (or threatens to use force) in order to dominate other kids.
3. This child threatens or bullies others in order to get his or her own way.

Note. Data from Dodge and Coie (1987).

According to social information-processing models, children's social behavior is a function of sequential steps of processing, including encoding of social cues, interpretation of cues, clarification of goals, response accessing, response evaluation, and behavioral enactment (see Table 1.2) (Crick & Dodge, 1996; Dodge, 1986). This model has been used to explore social information-processing biases and deficits in children who exhibit reactive and proactive aggression. Children with reactive aggression to social stimuli demonstrate a number of such biases and deficits at an early stage. They exhibit a hostile bias in their attributions of peers' intentions in provocative or ambiguous social situations, are hyper-vigilant to hostile social cues, have a hostile attributional bias to minor social cues, and demonstrate unwarranted fear responses that lead to overreactive, defensive aggressive responses (Dodge, 1991; Crick & Dodge, 1996). Children with proactive aggression demonstrate social information-processing biases at a later stage. These children have significantly more positive expectations of aggressive behavior than children with reactive aggression do. They also evaluate themselves as skilled in responding to others with aggression (Matthys, Cuperus, & Van Engeland, 1999), which easily leads to the use of aggression to obtain objects from others or to establish social dominance over others (see Table 1.2) (Dodge, 1991; Smithmyer et al., 2000).

Proactive and reactive aggression have received much support for their internal and external validity. High internal consistencies have been reported for rating scales assessing proactive and reactive aggression (K. Brown et al., 1996; Price & Dodge, 1989; Waschbusch et al., 1998). In terms of external validity, research investigating the social correlates of these aggressive subtypes has found reactive aggression to be significantly associated with peer rejection, whereas proactive aggression may receive favorable evaluations from peers as to the outcome of aggressive behaviors, especially in boys under the age of 9 (Dodge, 1991; Dodge & Coie, 1987). Reactive aggression is correlated with peer victimization, whereas proactive aggression correlates with so-

TABLE 1.2. Social Information Processing in Reactive and Proactive Aggression

Cognitive processing stages (to a social cue)	Social information-processing biases and deficits	Aggressive subtype[a]	
		Reactive	Proactive
1. Encoding	Failure to attend to relevant or alternative social cues/ hypervigilance to hostile cues	+	–
2. Interpretation	Misinterpretation of other's hostile intent/hostile attributional bias to minor social cues	+	–
3. Goal clarification			
4. Response accessing	Response repertoire limited to aggressive problem-solving strategies	+	–
5. Response evaluation	Expectation of positive outcomes from aggressive behavior/self-evaluation = easy to respond to others with aggression	–	+
6. Behavioral enactment		+	+

Note. Data from Crick and Dodge (1996), Dodge (1986), and Dodge and Coie (1987).
[a] +, more frequently; –, less frequently.

cial dominance (Schwartz, Dodge, et al., 1998). As compared to proactive aggression, reactive aggression has been found to begin earlier in life and to be more highly associated with early developmental experiences of harsh parental discipline, physical abuse, social problems, family instability, exposure to violence, and early neuropsychiatric problems (including impulsivity and inattention). In contrast, proactive aggression may have its origins in social learning during the elementary school years (Dodge, Lochman, Harnish, Bates, & Pettit, 1997). Reactive aggression is significantly correlated with overall functional impairment in the school-age years, as compared to proactive aggression (Waschbusch et al., 1998).

Differences in predictive validity that support the distinction between proactive and reactive aggression have also been found. In a study assessing a community sample of 742 boys first evaluated at 12 years of age and reassessed at age 15, proactive aggression predicted delinquency and disruptive behavior disorders at outcome. Reactive aggression did not predict later disruptive behaviors in adolescence (Vitaro, Gendreau, Tremblay, & Oligny, 1998). In another longitudinal study, Pulkkinen (1996) found males assessed as exhibiting proactive aggression at age 14 years to be significantly more prone to externalizing behaviors (aggression, antisocial behaviors) and criminality during adulthood, as compared to males assessed as exhibiting reactive aggression in adolescence and followed into adulthood. Evidence to support the predictive validity of reactive and proactive aggression thus extends from childhood to adolescence and from adolescence to adulthood.

In summary, there is growing research evidence to support the distinction between reactive and proactive aggression. These subtypes of aggressive behavior have currently been investigated in over 4,000 children and adolescents. External validity showing differences in social information processing, social behaviors, functional impairment, neuropsychiatric symptoms, and longitudinal outcomes have been found. External validation with specific neurochemical markers and heritability is presently lacking, however. Unlike the distinction between overt and covert forms of aggressive behavior, the dimension of reactive and proactive aggression does suggest more specific treatment interventions (Dodge, 1991). To the extent that youth with reactive aggression are impulsive, inattentive, and sensitive to hostile attributional biases and distortions, social problem-solving skills training may prove effective (Spivak & Shure, 1974). Pharmacology to down-regulate impulsivity and anxiety, and to up-regulate attention span, may also help decrease aggression in these youngsters. Given their vulnerability to intense displays of aggression, anger control training may be useful for children who display reactive aggression (Lochman & Curry, 1986). Since proactive aggression appears largely learned, contingent upon social modeling and reinforcement in the environment, strategies focusing on parent education and nonaggressive parent management practices may be important for this subtype of aggression (Patterson, 1982).

There presently exist several limitations in research investigating proactive and reactive aggression. First, most such research has been conducted on elementary school children assessed in the classroom by teachers or in contrived play group situations in which researchers observe children's aggressive interactions. If the reactive–proactive dimension is to be used as a measure of more generalized externalizing behavior problems, not just as a measure of elementary-school-age children's social-cognitive style, peer adjustment, or classroom behavioral adjustment, then this dimension of aggression needs to be investigated with a broader range of measures and in more diverse settings. Some work on this issue is occurring. Support for the distinction between reactive and proactive aggression has been found in a small sample of boys clinically referred for violent behavior and in incarcerated adolescents (Dodge et al., 1997; Smithmyer et al., 2000). More research is needed to determine whether these subtypes are valid in psychiatrically referred youth or in youth referred to juvenile justice settings. Second, the majority of children studied using this dimension have been 6–12 years of age; more research with adolescents is needed. Lastly, most research has been conducted with boys. Investigations of aggressive girls are needed to ascertain possible gender differences in these subtypes.

Instrumental and Hostile Aggression

A prominent model for subtyping aggression distinguishes "instrumental" from "hostile" aggression. As defined by Feshbach (1970), instrumental aggression provides some reward or advantage to the aggressor that is unrelated to the victim's discomfort. Hostile aggression is intended to inflict injury or pain upon a victim, with little intention of advantage to the aggressor. This model has largely been investigated in children and adults who are not clinically referred. Research has provided only mixed support for the independence of these two aggressive responses.

One problem is that the responses of instrumental and hostile aggression may overlap. Many aggressive episodes contain elements of both constructs (Hartup & de Wit, 1974). This problem has arisen in investigations of children's social perceptions of instrumental and hostile aggression. In a study of children, insults (hostile aggression) and goal blocking (instrumental aggression) led to highly similar attitudes and social perceptions (Rule, 1974). Another study found similar results: Willis and Foster (1990) found that instrumental and hostile aggression were evaluated equally negatively by child peers. These studies suggest that social peer perceptions and attitudes do not support the differentiation of instrumental and hostile aggression as separate subtypes of aggression.

Other studies suggest that a different domain—that of children's behavior—does discriminate between hostile and instrumental aggression. Hartup (1974) investigated instrumental (object-oriented) and hostile (person-oriented) aggression in the peer interactions of preschoolers and elementary school children. Instrumental aggression decreased with age, and hostile aggression increased with age. Gender differences were also apparent, in that boys demonstrated more hostile aggression than girls. There were no gender differences in the use of instrumental aggression in this sample. These results were generally supported by the work of Hoving, Wallace, and LaForme (1979), who found that older children exhibited higher rates of both instrumental and hostile aggression than younger children, and that boys were more aggressive than girls. More recent work further supports the distinction of instrumental and hostile aggression in studies of clinically referred children and early adolescents. In two studies of boys aged 8–14 years clinically referred with disruptive behavior disorders (ADHD, ODD, CD), support for the distinction between instrumental and hostile aggression was found on a laboratory task assessing aggression in a competitive game (Atkins & Stoff, 1993; Atkins, Stoff, Osborne, & Brown, 1993). These studies reported an association between impulsivity and hostile (but not instrumental) aggression, further supporting a distinction between the two subtypes.

In summary, some evidence does exist that instrumental aggression can be distinguished from hostile aggression, especially in the domain of children's behavior. Support for the validity of these two types of aggressive response is not found when social peer perception is investigated. Many fewer children and adolescents have been studied in regard to the instrumental–hostile aggression distinction than in regard to the overt–covert and reactive–proactive continuums. Investigations of instrumental and hostile aggression have largely focused on children in community samples, and few clinically referred children have been studied. The utility of this distinction for clarifying aggression in the clinical setting thus remains unresolved. However, the reported correlation of impulsivity (found in many psychiatric diagnoses) and hostile aggression is interesting and deserving of further study in children and adolescents referred for mental health services.

Predatory and Affective Aggression

The descriptive characteristics of "predatory" and "affective" aggression are very similar to those of reactive and proactive aggression. A distinction lies in the conceptual origin of these two dimensions of aggression. The theoretical roots of reactive and proactive aggression lie in social-psychological research on aggressive responding in humans. The theoretical roots of predatory and affective aggression lie in neurobiological research on aggression in animals.

There is evidence that the different types of aggression exhibited by animals can be broadly subdivided into predatory and affective aggression (Eichelman, 1987; Moyer, 1976). These two subdivisions in animal models have been shown to have differing behavioral characteristics and outcomes. For example, predatory aggression is a motivated, goal-oriented behavior that is executed with planning by the animal, with good motor control, and with low autonomic nervous system (ANS) arousal. In contrast, affective aggression is reactive to a threat. This threat may be directed to the animal, its young, or its territory. The goal is defense. This type of aggression is accompanied by unplanned attack, poor modulation of motor control, and high ANS arousal. The distinction in aggression classification is further supported by differing neurochemical substrates that mediate the two types of behavior. In some animal models, cholinergic stimulation induces predatory aggression. Dopamine has been found to facilitate affective aggression. Gamma-aminobutyric acid has been found to inhibit affective aggression, and serotonin inhibits both affective and predatory aggression (Eichelman, 1987).

Based on this classification, researchers are beginning to explore the utility of similarly classifying aggression in children and adolescents who are psychiatrically referred with high rates of aggressive behaviors. In a study of psychiatrically hospitalized children and adolescents, predatory and affective aggressive behaviors were investigated (Vitiello, Behar, Hunt, Stoff, & Ricciuti, 1990). A Predatory–Affective Aggression Questionnaire was developed by cluster analysis of a wide variety of aggressive behaviors documented in these subjects. The items forming the two subscales of this questionnaire appear in Table 1.3; it can be seen that these items assess different behaviors than the items that assess reactive and proactive aggression (compare Table 1.1). The items for predatory aggression attempt to define a pattern of aggressive behavior that is planned, goal-directed toward a reward, and self-controlled. The affective items define a pattern of behavior that is impulsive, unplanned, poorly coordinated, and not driven by contingent reward (Vitiello et al., 1990). In a study of 73 children and adolescents with a history of aggressive behavior admitted to a psychiatric hospital or a day treatment facility, the internal consistency of this rating scale was good (Cronbach's alpha = .73) (Vitiello et al., 1990). Affective aggression signif-

TABLE 1.3. Predatory and Affective Aggression Items

Predatory Aggression
1. Hides aggressive acts
2. Can control own behavior when aggressive
3. Very careful to protect self from injury when aggressive
4. Plans aggressive acts
5. Steals

Affective Aggression
1. Damages own property
2. Completely out of control when aggressive
3. Exposes self to injury and physical harm when aggressive
4. Aggression does not seem to have a purpose
5. Aggression is unplanned, occurs out of the blue

Note. Data from Vitiello, Behar, Hunt, Stoff, and Ricciuti (1990).

icantly correlated with lower verbal intelligence (IQ) and more treatment with psychiatric medication. Predatory aggression correlated with a history of alcohol and "street drug" abuse in this sample (Vitiello et al., 1990). In a small pilot study, these two types of aggressive behavior were differentially correlated with treatment response to psychiatric medication. Psychiatrically referred children who were rated by staff as exhibiting predominantly affective aggression had a significantly better response to lithium than children who exhibited mostly predatory types of aggression (Malone et al., 1998). Although preliminary, this study suggests that the predatory–affective distinction may be useful in assessing medication treatment response for aggression in psychiatrically referred children and adolescents.

The distinction between predatory and affective forms of aggression also receives support from a recent neuroimaging study assessing brain functioning in affective, impulsive violence versus planned, predatory violence. Glucose metabolism (a measure of brain neuronal activity) was assessed via positron emission tomography (PET) in 15 adults convicted of murder whose killings were predatory in nature, 9 adult murderers whose crimes were affective in nature, and 41 adult control subjects. The affective group, relative to comparison subjects, had lower prefrontal neuronal functioning. The predatory group had intact prefrontal cortical functioning relative to controls, but higher subcortical neuronal activity. Results support the hypothesis that those who commit emotional, unplanned, and impulsive murders are less able to regulate, inhibit, and control aggressive impulses generated from subcortical structures due to deficient prefrontal (inhibitory) regulation. Those who commit predatory murders demonstrate excessive aggressive behavior as a result of disproportionate subcortical activity, but have sufficiently intact prefrontal inhibitory functioning to regulate emotional functioning to allow planning of the aggressive act (Raine, Meloy, et al., 1998).

In summary, work on validating a predatory–affective aggression dimension in clinically referred children and adolescents has just begun. A scale assessing these subtypes shows acceptable internal validity and partial external validation with variables including psychiatric history, substance abuse history, verbal IQ, and response to medication. Preliminary research on adults convicted of murder supports different neuroanatomical substrates for these two types of aggressive behavior. To date, only a small number of psychiatrically referred aggressive children and adolescents have been studied. Further external validation with neurochemical correlates, treatment response, variables assessing social information processing, and longitudinal outcomes is needed. This subtype also requires validation in samples of aggressive but not clinically referred youth. Finally, investigation to ascertain gender differences in this subtype of aggression in both clinically referred and community samples of girls and boys is needed.

Offensive and Defensive Aggression

A concept that is conceptually closely related to proactive–reactive and predatory–affective aggression is the dimension of "offensive" and "defensive" aggression. This dimension of aggressive behavior arises out of neurobiological research on animal models of aggression. Offensive aggression is defined as unprovoked attack on another. In the animal world, this type of attack generally arises out of challenge over obtaining a scarce resource. Defensive aggression is provoked in response to a threatening situation. This prototype is well studied in preclinical models of aggression (Blanchard & Blanchard, 1984).

The applicability of offensive and defensive aggression to human aggression remains largely theoretical. It has been suggested that unprovoked bullying or insulting of another, accompanied by the emotion of anger or rage, is a model for human offensive aggression. Defending oneself in the face of a threat, accompanied by the emotion of fear, may be a model for human defensive aggression (Blanchard & Blanchard, 1984). However, the distinction between offensive and defensive aggression in humans largely lacks empirical support. One review has concluded that most of human aggression is defensive aggression in reaction to a real or perceived threat (Albert, Walsh, & Jonik, 1993).

In one of the only empirical tests of the offensive–defensive paradigm, 196 boys and 173 girls, with an average age of 8.3 years, were studied in second-grade classrooms in Finland (Pulkkinen, 1987). Offensive aggression was defined as unprovoked verbal or physical attack on another child. Defensive aggression was defined as angry reaction to an irritation. Behavioral characteristics were studied via peer nominations of aggressive behavior and teacher rating scales. It was assumed that aggressive and nonaggressive patterns of behavior in an annoying, irritating interpersonal situation could be characterized in terms of two orthogonal (independent) dimensions, which the author labeled Social Activity–Social Passivity and Strong Control of Behavior–Weak Control of Behavior. Results did not support the independence of offensive and defensive aggression within this two-dimensional framework. All the variables for aggression were found in one quadrant of the framework, labeled Social Activity and Weak Control of Behavior. Thus, although the distinction between offensive and defensive subtypes of aggression has much research support in preclinical aggression models, it presently lacks support in human aggression research.

Relational Aggression

Gender differences in the quality and quantity of aggression are well documented. Investigations consistently demonstrate elevated rates of verbal aggression, physical aggression, and violent crime in boys as compared to girls (Hinshaw & Anderson, 1996). These findings have been interpreted as an overall lack of aggression in girls' peer interactions. However, an alternative explanation is that the forms of aggression assessed in this research are more salient for boys than for girls, rather than that an actual gender difference exists in levels of overall aggressiveness (Crick & Grotpeter, 1995).

In recent years, more attention has been focused on gender differences in the expression of aggression. These investigations have focused on unique forms of aggression that may have been overlooked in past research, and may more specifically pertain to girls. One such type of aggression has been labeled "relational" aggression (Crick & Grotpeter, 1995; Crick & Werner, 1998) or "indirect" aggression (Hood, 1996). This research hypothesizes that when children act aggressively toward peers, they do so in ways that best thwart or damage the goals valued by their respective gender peer groups. Boys tend to value the instrumental use of aggression in the service of obtaining rewards or peer dominance. Overt forms of aggression, such as physical fighting or verbal threats, are consistent with these goals. Since girls are more likely than boys to focus on relational issues during social interactions, their aggressive behaviors are more focused on these themes. Aggressive behavior among girls as assessed in community samples takes the form of harming another child's friendships or feelings of inclusion by the peer group. Examples include angrily excluding another girl from a play group, purposefully withdrawing friendship to reject another, spreading rumors about a child in order to hurt her, having friends retaliate indirectly toward a peer who has made one angry, or tattling on a rival.

When this subtype of aggression is investigated in nonreferred community samples of children, the often-cited male predominance in aggressive behavior begins to disappear. Relational aggression appears at higher rates in females than in males (Bjorkqvist, Osterman, & Kaukiainen, 1992). In females assessed at puberty, girls were as aggressive as boys in their interactions with parents, and their aggressive behavior was not related to age or to visible stage of pubertal development (Inoff-Germain et al., 1988). A developmental shift in the expression of girls' aggression may occur between the ages of 8 and 14 years, with decreasing amounts of overt aggression and increasing frequency of relational forms of aggression (Cairns & Cairns, 1986; Hood, 1996). (For further discussion, see Chapter 9.)

Support for the validity of this subtype of aggression has been found in several investigations. A study of 491 third- through fifth-grade elementary school students used a peer nomination instrument to assess relational aggression and overt aggression, and a self-report instrument to assess psychological and social adjustment (Crick & Grotpeter, 1995). A factor analysis of responses yielded related but separate factors for overt and relational types of aggression. Boys were mostly included in the overtly aggressive group, and girls in the relationally aggressive group. On measures of psychological and social adjustment, girls with relational aggression were found to be more disliked and more lonely than girls who were not relationally aggressive. In a follow-up study relational aggression was found to be significantly associated with girls' anger and intent to harm others—key components in any definition of aggressive behavior (Crick, Bigbee, & Howes, 1996).

Taken together, these results support the validity of a relational form of aggression that is distinct from overt aggression and that is more characteristic of girls in nonreferred community settings than boys. These studies also support the idea that the degree of aggression in girls has been underestimated in previous research, largely because forms of aggression relevant to girls' normative peer groups have not been assessed (Crick & Grotpeter, 1995). Further research needs to investigate whether relational types of aggression in girls who evidence signs of psychological and social maladjustment in community settings predict any specific response to treatment interventions. In addition, this subtype of aggression has not yet been investigated in females who are clinically referred to psychiatric treatment, exhibit high levels of aggression, and meet criteria for a psychiatric diagnosis. It remains unclear whether this subtype will also be relevant for seriously emotionally disturbed girls, and, if so, whether it can predict specific responses to treatment in the clinical setting.

Summary of the Research on Subtypes

One approach to the heterogeneity inherent in aggressive behavior and in the terminology used to describe it is to begin to subtype aggression into more homogeneous groups. Efforts to subtype aggression in youth may prove fruitful in facilitating a greater understanding of this pervasive and problematic form of behavior. Subtyping may also prove important in constructing more specific prevention, remedial, and treatment planning for children and adolescents who demonstrate excessive and maladaptive forms of aggression, violence, and antisocial behavior. Many of the subtypes reviewed above have growing evidence to support their internal and external validity. The research to date on these subtypes is summarized in Table 1.4. An estimate of their present external and internal validity is also provided.

Much more research into subtyping aggression needs to be accomplished. For example, many of the subtypes with strongest support have been validated in community samples of children. These include reactive–proactive aggression (mostly in boys) and relational aggression (in girls). It remains to be seen whether these subtypes are also relevant for clinically referred youth with seri-

TABLE 1.4. Subtypes of Aggression in Children and Adolescents

Subtypes	Subjects studied	Internal validation[a]	External validation[a]
Overt–covert	>35,000 children and adolescents, 2 to 18 yo,[b] clinic-referred and community, boys > girls	++++	+++
Reactive–proactive	>4,000 children and adolescents, 6 to 15 yo, community >> clinic-referred, boys >> girls	++++	+++
Instrumental–hostile	>300 children and adolescents, 3 to 14 yo, community >> clinic-referred, boys >> girls	++	++
Predatory–affective	84 children and adolescents, 9 to 18 yo, all referred, boys >> girls	+	+
Offensive–defensive	196 boys, 173 girls, 8 yo, all community/no clinic-referred	–	–
Relational or indirect	>1,000 8 to 14 yo, all community/ no clinic-referred, girls > boys	+++	++

Note. [a]Evidence: ++++, very strong; +++, strong; ++, moderate; +, weak; –, none.
[b]yo, years old.

ous emotional disturbances and psychiatric diagnoses. Many of the subtypes with the strongest support for validity, such as the overt–covert dimension, have not yet been informative in suggesting subtype-specific forms of treatment that predict efficacy in diminishing aggression for that particular subtype. Only the proactive–reactive dimension (in community samples) and the predatory–affective dimension (in psychiatrically hospitalized youth) suggest specific interventions. Respectively, these include social problem-solving skills training and anger control training for youth with reactive aggression, and psychopharmacological interventions for psychiatrically referred youth with affective aggression. Research investigating subtyping aggression in clinic-referred or juvenile-justice-referred youth lags far behind studies subtyping aggression in community samples, despite the overwhelming prevalence of aggression as a cause of referral to these settings. Finally, research is beginning to suggest gender-specific subtype differences, as shown in relational aggression patterns in community-assessed elementary school girls. Clearly, much more research on subtyping of aggression in children and adolescents is needed.

LIMITATIONS OF CURRENT CONCEPTS OF AGGRESSION

As noted throughout this chapter, the present definitions of aggression and related behaviors in youth do have certain limitations. One important difficulty is that current concepts and definitions of such behaviors often ignore the environmental context in which the behaviors occur. Aggressive behavior can be adaptive or maladaptive, given the context in which it occurs. The fact that an individual engages in aggressive behavior does not automatically mean that this behavior is pathological or maladaptive. To state the obvious, aggressive behavior may be very adaptive in the service of survival if an individual is assaulted on an urban street at night and self-defense is required. But this same behavior is maladaptive if it occurs without provocation in a child's classroom at school. Lack of attention to the environmental contexts in which aggression occurs is a shortcoming of current definitional concepts.

A second limitation is the lack of developmental considerations in these concepts. Current concepts assume that similar criteria may be applied to children and to adolescents. This may be acceptable for criminal justice definitions, which have a narrow emphasis on the specific illegal acts committed by adjudicated individuals. These acts violate the laws of society, no matter what the age or developmental level of the child or adolescent who perpetrates them. However, it is more unclear whether other concepts of aggression and antisocial behavior are similar in young children and in adolescents. For example, the symptoms of CD tend to vary with age as an individual develops increased physical strength, cognitive abilities, and sexual maturity (APA, 1994). Less severe behaviors, such as lying, bullying, and shoplifting, tend to emerge first in development. These are followed by more serious antisocial behaviors, such as rape or theft while confronting a victim (e.g., mugging), which tend to emerge only later in adolescence. These developmental trends may be meaningful in assessing the severity of a youngster's disorder, prognosis over the course of life, and treatment; yet they are obscured by the diagnosis of CD itself.

Another potential problem is the overlap between aggression turned outward on others and aggression turned inward on the self. Often definitions of aggression do not include the possibility of self-injurious behavior. It is not at all clear that these are separate phenomena. Deliberate self-harm or parasuicidal behavior, without intent to die, can be a common symptom in some individuals with certain psychiatric conditions such as mood or psychotic disorders. Self-injury can also be correlated with outward expressions of aggression. For example, in a population of 51 seriously emotionally disturbed children and adolescents residing in a residential treatment center, moderate and statistically significant correlations were found between the aggressive behaviors of physical assault, verbal threats of violence, explosive property destruction, and self-injury. Of the children and adolescents who committed self-injurious acts, all were also found to be assaultive toward others (Connor, Melloni, & Harrison, 1998). Although other studies have identified referred children and adolescents with self-injurious behavior without other-directed aggression (Pfeffer, Plutchik, & Mizruchi, 1983b), this study suggests the possibility that self-injury is part of the spectrum of aggression in some clinically referred patients; it thus raises the possibility that self-injurious behavior may require inclusion in definitions of aggression occurring in some psychiatric illnesses.

CHAPTER SUMMARY

This chapter first provides a general definition of aggression, and distinguishes between adaptive and maladaptive aggression. It next discusses definitions of aggression, conduct problems, and antisocial behaviors found in juvenile justice, diagnostic/medical settings, psychometric approaches, and personality/social psychology. Current research supporting the validity of subtypes of aggression as a means of decreasing the heterogeneity inherent in the aggression domain is then reviewed. Clear definitions of aggression are important. Definitional confusion and vagueness hamper research, confuse public policy debate, confound treatment, and can harm individuals.

One of the challenges for the future is to distinguish maladaptive aggression more clearly from adaptive types of aggression found in individuals and in society. Definitions of adaptive and maladaptive aggression based on principles from evolutionary biology may help clarify subtypes of aggression that can be responsive to differential biosocial treatments; this is an important arena of future aggression research. The delineation of possible CNS mechanisms that are dysfunctional and may underlie vulnerability to maladaptive aggression, such as might be found in certain psychiatric disorders, is important. This type of maladaptive aggression may be helped by biomedical treatment. Adaptive aggression, when socially harmful, may require multimodal, cross-disciplinary family, psychosocial, political, economic, educational, and/or community interventions. The clarification of maladaptive aggression versus adaptive aggression is also important in order to distinguish more clearly among subtypes of aggression; these might entail differences in risk factors, etiology, longitudinal prognosis, and effectiveness of social, economic, criminal justice, and clinical interventions.

The current terms and concepts used in various fields to describe aggressive youth are not identical and are partially separable, but they also overlap and correlate with one another. In the chapters that follow, a broad definition of aggression and related behaviors in youth is adopted. Concepts including "delinquency, "antisocial behavior," "aggression," "CD," "conduct problems," and "externalizing behavior disorders" are often discussed together. This is not meant to imply that these concepts are identical, and distinctions are made where possible. Research does not yet support precise definitions and distinct subtypes of aggressive behaviors in children and adolescents. As a result, this book's concept of aggression and related behaviors in youth is a wide-ranging one that includes the various concepts discussed above. Although this is not an ideal situation, research does not presently allow more explicit distinctions to be made.

CHAPTER 2

Prevalence of Aggression, Antisocial Behaviors, and Suicide

Over the past 50 years, rates of maladaptive aggression and antisocial behaviors have increased in frequency and severity among children and adolescents in the United States. Although most youth are not seriously aggressive or antisocial, the rates of these behaviors are nevertheless alarming. The consequences of youth violence and related activities presently pose a major public health problem for society. The identification, containment, referral, assessment, and treatment of aggressive young people are challenges for many community institutions, including schools, juvenile justice authorities, and clinical mental health resources. After a peak in the late 1980s and early 1990s, rates of aggression and antisocial behaviors among young people are falling as the new century begins, but they remain at historically high levels.

This chapter discusses the prevalence of excessive, inappropriate aggressive behaviors in children and adolescents. Because some degree of aggression is generally very common and part of normal development, especially in young children, normal developmental aspects of aggression are first discussed. A discussion of the prevalence of maladaptive aggression, antisocial behaviors, and suicide follows. This discussion first draws on community epidemiological data describing the prevalence of conduct disorder (CD), and then presents information from youth public opinion surveys ascertaining self-reported fears and concerns about aggression and violence. Juvenile justice statistics on rates of both victimization and offenses are next considered. Teenage suicide rates are then examined, since suicide can be viewed as the ultimate act of aggression against the self and since violent behavior increases the risk of suicide (Conner et al., 2001). Finally, how rates of juvenile aggression and suicide have affected referrals to clinical child and adolescent mental health treatment is discussed.

In Chapter 1, an attempt has been made to highlight the importance of careful definitions of aggression and to distinguish between adaptive and maladaptive aggression. This chapter defines the topic more broadly. Since little research using homogeneous definitions of aggression has been completed, by necessity this chapter mixes "aggression" with "violence," "delinquency," "crime," and "disruptive problem behavior."

ADAPTIVE AGGRESSION IN NORMAL CHILDHOOD DEVELOPMENT

Aggression is a normal and highly frequent behavior in young developing children. Healthy aspects of aggression facilitate competence in social assertiveness, competition in games, and success in meeting daily challenges. Infants can recognize facial configurations associated with the expression of anger in adults at 3 months of age (Izard et al., 1995). Almost all children display aggressive behavior to some degree during development. Across most cultures, boys are consistently found to be more aggressive than girls. The frequency of aggressive behavior in infants and young children has been examined by researchers studying social conflict. Observational studies (Holmberg, 1977) indicate that approximately 50% of the social interchanges between children 12–18 months of age in a nursery school setting can be viewed as disruptive or conflictual. By age 2½ years, the proportion of conflicted social interchanges decreases to 20%. Almost all of the disruptive behavior in these children is directed toward peers, with very little directed toward adult caregivers. Early interpersonal conflicts serve as a training ground for infants to develop and learn effective social strategies for assertiveness, ownership of objects, and resolution of social conflict. These are important lessons for children to learn if they are to participate effectively in the greater social milieu as they grow older (Hay & Ross, 1982). As such, this type of aggression fits the definition of adaptive aggression.

The forms that aggressive behavior takes also change across development. There is a tendency for physical forms of aggression such as hitting to decrease, and verbally mediated forms of aggression to increase, between 2 and 4 years of age (Goodenough, 1931). In addition, the social purpose or goal of aggression seems to change with age. Children younger than 6 years engage in much aggressive behavior for the purpose of obtaining objects, territory, or privileges from others. This is called "instrumental" aggression (Rule, 1974). Slightly older children, aged 6–7 years, increasingly engage in person-oriented aggression ("hostile" aggression) designed as retaliation toward another child for presumed intentional frustration in a goal-directed activity, an insult, or other threats to one's self-esteem (Hartup, 1974). Over the preschool and early elementary school years, there appears to be a decrease in instrumental aggression and an increase in person-directed, hostile, retaliatory aggression (Parke & Slaby, 1983). At the same time, there is an overall decrease in the frequency and intensity of both kinds of aggression; verbally mediated interpersonal skills increase as children channel aggressive impulses and drives into more socially acceptable activities, such as sports, social, and academic achievement.

The precipitants or triggers of aggression also appear to change with development. Anger outbursts in infancy are usually elicited by physical discomfort or the need for attention, whereas "habit training" in toileting, hygiene, and feeding commonly causes outbursts in toddlers (Goodenough, 1931). Conflicts among peers over the possession of objects are also common from 18 to 65 months of age (Dawe, 1934; Hartup, 1974). As children grow older, insults and negative social comparisons (e.g., ridicule, tattling, criticism) become increasingly likely to elicit verbally mediated retaliatory aggression, but relatively unlikely to elicit physical attack (Parke & Slaby, 1983). As development proceeds into adolescence and young adulthood, overt aggression, defined as open confrontation with the environment (e.g., temper tantrums, physical fighting) tends to decline; covert or hidden aggression (e.g., breaking the rules, not telling the truth, cheating, stealing) becomes more common (Loeber, 1990). In adolescence, with the onset of sexual maturity, conflicts to establish or maintain social dominance may be important, especially for males.

Table 2.1 shows these general trends in the developmental aspects of normative aggression. Although hardly scientific, specific, or precise, these broad trends in development can help us begin to recognize which children may be at risk for developing more maladaptive forms of aggression. For example, the preschool child who largely directs aggression toward adults in an out-of-home environment such as a nursery school does not fit what is presently known about the normative aspects of aggression. The school-age child who frequently and repetitively initiates physical attacks on others, rather than beginning to modulate overt aggressive behavior with words, may also be deviating from a normative developmental trajectory. The elementary school child who continues to use physical aggression to obtain possessions from others is another example. These children may be at risk for the development of maladaptive aggression as they grow older. Knowledge about the normative de-

TABLE 2.1. Childhood Age Trends in the Developmental Aspects of Normative Aggression

	Age	
Aspect of aggression	Younger	Older
% time spent in social conflict	High	Low
Form of aggression	Physical	Verbal
Type of aggression	Overt confrontation	Covert and hidden
Goal of aggression	Instrumental (obtaining possessions)	Hostile (self-esteem maintenance)
Triggers	Environmental demands	Social threats

velopmental aspects of childhood aggression can help parents, teachers, and health care providers identify children who might benefit from further evaluation of their aggression at a young age, when treatment for maladaptive behavior may be more effective than later in development (Loeber & Hay, 1997).

PREVALENCE OF MALADAPTIVE AGGRESSION IN COMMUNITY SAMPLES

Conduct Disorder

Since the psychiatric diagnosis of CD contains criteria for many varied acts of maladaptive aggression, prevalence surveys of CD can give a rough estimate of the prevalence of maladaptive aggression among youth living in the community in different countries. As noted in Chapter 1, CD is a disturbance of behavior lasting at least 6 months in which basic rights of others and/or major age-appropriate norms and rules of society are repeatedly violated (American Psychiatric Association [APA], 1994). Overt physical aggression, such as fighting and fighting with weapons, occurs commonly in this condition. Covert, hidden forms of aggression, such as stealing, fire setting, lying, and vandalism, are also frequent among youth meeting diagnostic criteria for this diagnosis. Seven of the 15 criteria used to make the diagnosis of CD in its current form (APA, 1994) code for various aspects of physical aggression. Standardization of the diagnostic criteria for CD has enabled epidemiological studies to determine the prevalence of this diagnosis in different societies.

A summary of these community-based studies is presented in Table 2.2. As can be seen, prevalence rates vary by sampling time frame and range from 0.9% to 20%, with the higher prevalence rates generally reflecting longer sampling times. These rates suggest that maladaptive aggression as ascertained by a diagnosis of CD is not rare among the youth of many different countries. In general, this disorder is less prevalent in prepubertal children than in adolescents. Boys have higher prevalence rates than girls in the prepubertal age range; however, the rate of CD rises for female adolescents and can approach the prevalence for males in the adolescent age range (Kashani et al., 1987). The peak ages for CD-like behavior in boys are 10–13 years. For girls, such behavior peaks at age 16 (Bauermeister, Canino, & Bird, 1994). These findings suggest sex-related differences in the prevalence rates of aggressive behavior that vary as a function of age. Thus, both age and gender are important factors to consider in documenting community prevalence rates for children and adolescents with CD.

Youth Attitudes, Fears, and Concerns about Violence

Public opinion surveys suggest that for many adolescents, issues of aggression, violence, and safety in their schools and neighborhoods are matters of daily concern. A survey of teenagers' attitudes completed in 1996 included a ques-

TABLE 2.2. Estimated Prevalence of CD in Cross-Sectional Studies from the General Population

Study	Age (yr)	Time frame (mo)	Dx. criteria	Prevalence (%)
Ontario, Canada[a]				
Overall	4–16	Past 6	DSM-III	5.5
Preadolescent				
Girls	4–11			1.8
Boys	4–11			6.5
Adolescent				
Girls	12–16			4.1
Boys	12–16			10.4
Puerto Rico[b]	4–16	Past 6	DSM-III	1.5
Pittsburgh, PA[c]	7–11	Past 12	DSM-III	2.6
Dunedin, New Zealand[d]	11	Past 12	DSM-III	3.4
New York, NY[e]	9–18	Past 6	DSM-III-R	
Preadolescent				
Girls	9–12			0.0
Boys	9–12			8.0
Adolescent				
Girls	13–18			3.0
Boys	13–18			9.0
Columbia, MO[f]				
Overall	14–16	Current	DSM-III	8.7
Girls	14–16			8.0
Boys	14–16			9.3
Mannheim, Germany[g]				
Overall	8	Past 6	ICD-9	0.9
Girls	8			0.0
Boys	8			1.9
Zuid-Holland, the Netherlands[h]	4–16	Past 12–96	DSM-III-R	20.0
MECA[i] (United States)				
Overall	9–17	Past 6	DSM-III-R	5.8
Girls				1.5
Boys				4.3
MECA[j] (United States)				
Overall	9–17	Past 6	DSM-III-R	8.0

[a] Offord et al. (1992).
[b] Bird et al. (1988).
[c] Costello et al. (1988).
[d] Anderson et al. (1987).
[e] Cohen et al. (1987).
[f] Kashani et al. (1987).
[g] Esser et al. (1990).
[h] Velhurst et al. (1993).
[i] Lahey et al. (1996, 1998). MECA, Methods for the Epidemiology of Child and Adolescent Mental Disorders.
[j] Shaffer, Fisher, et al. (1996).

tion about the most important problem facing the United States today and in the future; responses revealed that the issue most frequently endorsed by adolescents was "violence and crime." Adolescents also endorsed "violence and crime" as the third most important issue today facing America's youth (after "drugs" and "peer pressure") (Maguire & Pastore, 1997, p. 115). The percentage of high school seniors who reported worrying "sometimes or often" about violence and crime rose from 79.4% in 1986 to 90.1% in 1996, before falling slightly to 84.4% in 1998 (Maguire & Pastore, 1999, p. 148). Many adolescents also report safety concerns in their activities of everyday life. In 1995, 42% of teenagers reported feeling "only sometimes" or "never" safe in the area around school, and 28% reported safety concerns while inside their school building. Although 61% of teenagers reported never feeling unsafe in any situation, 28% reported avoiding at least one public place because of safety concerns (Young Women's Christian Association [YWCA], 1996). Public opinion surveys assessing youth attitudes therefore indicate that many teenagers have fears and concerns about violence and aggression.

JUVENILE JUSTICE STUDIES AND STATISTICS

Among other sources of information on prevalence rates of maladaptive aggression for children and adolescents living in the community are criminal justice statistics, particularly annual crime indices. The federal government keeps statistics on certain offenses called "index offenses." These offenses consist of the following eight felonies: willful homicide, forcible rape, robbery, burglary, aggravated assault, larceny over $50, motor vehicle theft, and arson. The Federal Bureau of Investigation combines statistics on these eight felonies into its annual "crime index." (Note that this index does not include drug-related offenses.) These offenses are much more serious crimes than the general idea of delinquency denotes.

Since the annual crime index includes statistics on the ages of crime victims and offenders, statistics on juvenile crime may be ascertained. Rates of youth victimization; youth offending for delinquency; youth offending for violent crime, such as murder, non-negligent manslaughter, and aggravated assault; and arrest rates in individuals under age 18 can be identified. These statistics have been kept for many years, and rates of change over time can be studied. Since only those offenses or events that come to the attention of authorities or result in the arrest of a perpetrator are counted in these statistics, they probably represent underestimations of the true offense and victimization prevalence rates for youth. This may be more true for less serious delinquent offenses and less true for more serious criminal offenses.

Self-Report Delinquency Methodology

The problem of underdetection of youth crime and delinquency as a result of relying on official arrest statistics has led to alternative methods of detecting child and adolescent offenses. One such method is "self-report delinquency methodology" (Loeber, Green, Lahey, & Stouthamer-Loeber, 1991). Instead of relying on official statistics, investigators ask youngsters, their parents, and their teachers directly about the youth's problem behaviors. Self-report studies usually aim to record nonpersonal crimes, victimless acts of delinquency, and covert acts of aggression, which official crime statistics often underestimate. The procedure followed in such research is to give respondents a standard list of specified delinquent activities. These can be presented as interview questions or as a self-report questionnaire. Often the information gathered from multiple informants (youngsters, parents, and teachers) is combined into a best-estimate evaluation (Hart, Lahey, Loeber, & Hanson, 1994). Evidence of validity for such an approach to estimating rates of antisocial behaviors among teenagers has emerged (Hart et al., 1994; Junger-Tas, 1992).

Self-report delinquency methodology is largely used with psychiatrically referred children and adolescents. Thus it cannot directly provide population-wide estimates of antisocial behavior prevalence rates. However, these methods represent a systematic approach to ascertaining the frequency of such events that are not covered by official crime indices. Findings on the nature of adolescent crime from self-report studies indicate that self-report data generally portray less serious offending overall, with the majority of undetected offending by young people being theft-related. Self-report studies suggest higher levels of delinquency among the juvenile population than would be anticipated on the basis of official statistics. These studies also suggest higher rates of delinquency among women than official statistics suggest (Rutter, Giller, & Hagell, 1998).

The remainder of this section discusses juvenile justice statistics about the prevalence of aggressive and violent acts involving youngsters that have come to the attention of authorities in the community. Again, it is important to keep in mind that use of official statistics probably underestimates the true population prevalence of adolescent antisocial behaviors.

Youth Victim Statistics: Nonfatal Personal Violence

Important information about the prevalence of maladaptive aggression comes from statistics on violent victimization of youth. Crimes of violence against one's person (other than murder or non-negligent manslaughter, which are considered later) include aggravated and simple assault, robbery, sexual assault, and attempted/threatened violence. Overall, between 10% and 11% of adolescents reported some crime of violence against them in 1997 (Bureau of Justice Statistics, 2000). Although the majority of youth have never been victims of such crimes, an appreciable number of teenagers have reported being assaulted, robbed, or threatened with violence. Figure 2.1 graphically depicts these victimization rates for 1997.

Personal violence in schools has become a particular concern in recent years. Figure 2.2 illustrates rates of in-school violent victimization in grades 8

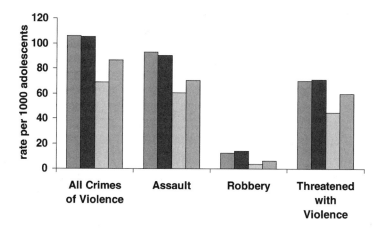

FIGURE 2.1. Estimated rates of violent personal victimization per 1,000 adolescents for the year 1997. Columns from left to right: males aged 12–15 years, males aged 16–19 years, females aged 12–15 years, and females aged 16–19 years. Data from Bureau of Justice Statistics (2000).

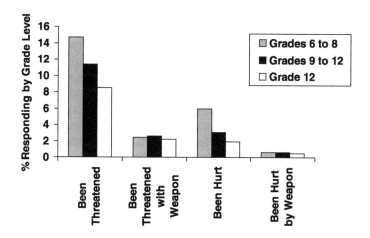

FIGURE 2.2. Students reporting violent victimization experiences at school by grade level for the 1997–1998 academic year. Data from Pride, Inc. (1999).

through 12 for the 1997–1998 academic year. These data suggest that younger teenagers and preadolescents in grades 6–8 are victimized in school more often than older high school students are (Pride, Inc., 1999). Although rates of school violence appear much lower than rates of violence in the community as a whole, students' reports of being injured by violence and of being exposed to other students with weapons while attending school are nonetheless disturbing. Rates of high school seniors reporting being threatened with a weapon at least once in school during the past 12 months have remained stable at about 9% to 11% in the years between 1984 and 1998 (Maguire & Pastore, 1999, p. 195). Although threats with weapons in high school may have remained constant over time, recent years have witnessed horrific school shootings in multiple locations across the United States, where students have murdered and wounded multiple classmates and teachers on school grounds. (Again, for further discussion of murder rates, see below.) This suggests the possibility of rare, episodic, and hard-to-predict, yet escalating, violence potential occurring at school. Although it is difficult to ascertain precise trends over time from these statistics, they do suggest that over the past 15 years violent aggression may directly harm about 10% of adolescents in the United States per year.

Youth Offender Statistics: Weapons Carrying and Fighting

Figure 2.3 reports statistics on the selected offenses of weapons carrying and physical fighting for high school students for 1997, taken from survey data (Maguire & Pastore, 1999, p. 229). From 16% to 20% of students in the 9th through 12th grades reported carrying a gun, knife, or club one or more times in the 30 days preceding the survey. Of these teenagers, from 5% to 8% re-

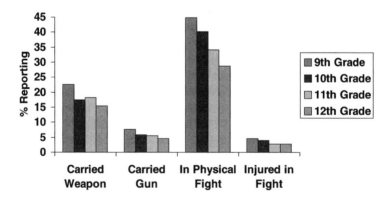

FIGURE 2.3. High school students reporting carrying weapons or fighting one or more times in the past 30 days, 1997. Data from Maguire and Pastore (1999, p. 229).

ported carrying a gun during this time period. From one-third to one-half reported physically fighting, but fewer than 5% reported injury in a fight. For all categories, males reported more activity than females. Similar to the violence rates reported above, these data suggest that younger teenagers (9th grade) engage more frequently in these selected acts, and that the frequency drops toward the end of high school. This is consistent with the peak ages for CD-like behavior being 10–13 years for males in community epidemiological surveys of antisocial activity in children and adolescents (Lahey et al., 1998).

Youth Victim Statistics: Murder and Non-Negligent Manslaughter

The most catastrophic form of maladaptive aggression in society is taking the life of another. Victimization rates for murder and non-negligent manslaughter rise with age during the developing years. When 21-year trends are compared, children less than 13 years of age have a risk of death by violence of about 2 per 100,000 children. Rates of violent death increase greater than twofold in the early adolescent years (ages 14–17), and they rise again almost threefold for young adults aged 18–24 years (Figure 2.4) (Maguire & Pastore, 1999, p. 294). The data reveal that rates of murder and non-negligent manslaughter victimization have remained constant for youth under age 13 over the past two decades. Examining temporal trends over the past 21 years, Figure 2.4 illustrates a precipitous rise in death rates for teenagers and young adults beginning in the late 1980s and early 1990s. This spike in victimization rates began to decline in the last half of the 1990s, but remains elevated compared to rates in the 1970s.

It is also important to appreciate that although the murder and non-negli-

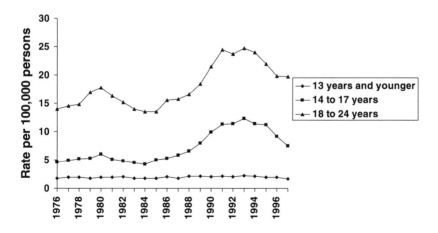

FIGURE 2.4. Developmental and temporal trends in rates of youth murder and non-negligent manslaughter victimization, by child and adolescent age group. Data from Maguire and Pastore (1999, p. 294).

gent manslaughter victimization rates for children 13 years and younger are small, they are not zero (Figure 2.4). Children are being murdered in the United States. However, victimization rates rise steeply with adolescence and have increased over the last two decades in adolescents and young adults, while remaining stable in younger children.

Youth Offender Statistics: Murder and Non-Negligent Manslaughter

Youth offender rates for murder and non-negligent manslaughter are illustrated in Figure 2.5. Although isolated cases occur and are widely reported in the mass media, children aged 13 years or younger rarely commit murder in the United States. Rates for this age group have remained constant throughout the past 21 years. By early to middle adolescence, murder and manslaughter rates rise 10-fold for youths aged 14–17 years in the population. By late adolescence and early adulthood, the rates more than double yet again (Maguire & Pastore, 1999, p. 296). In terms of temporal trends, the late 1980s and 1990s witnessed a rise in murder rates among adolescents and young adults in the United States. This trend has since reversed itself, but rates remain much higher than they were two decades ago.

The rise in juvenile murder and non-negligent manslaughter offender rates appears to be largely accounted for by a rise in black male teenage and young adult violence (Figure 2.6); rates of these offenses among white male adolescents and young adults have risen much more slowly (Maguire & Pastore, 1999, p. 295). Rates for black females have declined over the same time period and rates for white females have remained low and fairly constant (Figure 2.7) (Maguire & Pastore, 1999, p. 295).

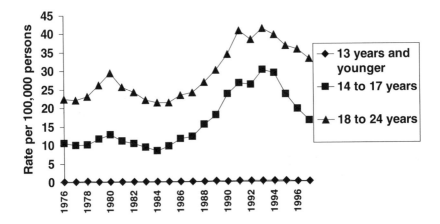

FIGURE 2.5. Developmental and temporal trends in rates of youth committing murder and non-negligent manslaughter, by child and adolescent age group. Data from Maguire and Pastore (1999, p. 296).

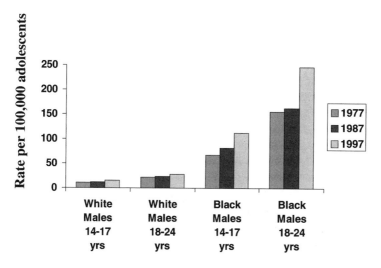

FIGURE 2.6. Rates of murder and non-negligent manslaughter offenses for 14- to 17-year-old and 18- to 24-year-old males by race. Data from Maguire and Pastore (1999, p. 295).

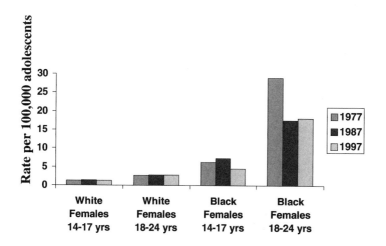

FIGURE 2.7. Rates of murder and non-negligent manslaughter offenses for 14- to 17-year-old and 18- to 24-year old females by race. Data from Maguire and Pastore (1999, p. 295).

The seriousness of adolescent violence is also reflected in a 150% rise in arrest rates for teenagers less than 18 years of age for murder/non-negligent manslaughter over the decade spanning 1985 to 1994 (Federal Bureau of Investigation, 1994). During this same period, teenage arrests for violent crime in general increased 75%. Toward the end of the 1990s, arrest rates have fallen from these high levels, yet remain elevated compared to arrest rates of four to five decades ago.

Summary of the Juvenile Justice Data

In summary, the juvenile justice statistics ascertaining offense and victimization rates for violence-related behaviors all support the conclusion that such behaviors are far too common in the daily lives of many preadolescents and teenagers. Some of these behaviors directly result in death and injury. Although other behaviors may not lead to physical injuries, they are strongly associated with risk for injury, exposure to intimidation and threats, and perceptions of fear and vulnerability (Brener, Simon, Krug, & Lowry, 1999). These behaviors are also extremely costly to society. To give just one example, across all child, adolescent, and adult age groups in the United States for the year 1997, gunshots caused 31,636 fatal injuries and 100,000 nonfatal injuries (Cook, Lawrence, Ludwig, & Miller, 1999). The estimated cost of medically treating such injuries was estimated at $2.3 billion in 1994 dollars (Cook et al., 1999).

Toward the end of the 1990s, rates of violence-related behaviors among high school students began to fall. From 1991 to 1997, the incidence of adolescents' carrying weapons decreased 31%, and the incidence of physical fighting declined 16% (Brener et al., 1999). From 1993 to 1997, the percentage of students who carried a gun in the preceding 30 days fell 25% (Brener et al., 1999). Although these data show that some progress is being made in reducing the threat of violent maladaptive aggression to youth in America, rates of homicide, nonfatal but violent victimization, and perpetration of violence among the young remain at historically high levels.

PREVALENCE OF YOUTH SUICIDE

Rates of suicide (maladaptive aggression turned toward the self) have also been documented for youth and contribute further to our understanding of overall maladaptive aggression in this population. Since suicide rates are largely determined from coroner death certificate data completed at autopsy, these official rates may represent an underestimation of the true rate of adolescent suicide. The adolescent suicide rate has quadrupled since 1950 (from 2.5 to 11.2 per 100,000) and currently represents 12% of the mortality of this age group (Birmaher et al., 1996; Brent, Perper, & Allman, 1987; Lewinsohn,

Klein, & Seeley, 1993). Developmental trends in youth suicide rates since 1980 are presented in Figure 2.8. The rate of suicide in late adolescence (15–19 years of age) is more than eight times the rate of suicide in early adolescence (10–14 years of age) (Maguire & Pastore, 1999, p. 299). For both age groups, suicide rates peaked in the mid- to late 1980s. Although suicide rates seem to have begun decreasing in the mid-1990s for 15- to 19-year-old teenagers, they remain at historically high levels. Lower rates (but still elevated over levels found in the 1970s) have remained generally steady for the younger group of preteenagers and early adolescents over this same time period, with no sign of falling.

Gender trends in the suicide rate since 1950 for male and female late adolescents (ages 15–19 years) are illustrated in Figure 2.9. There has been a precipitous rise in late adolescent male mortality from suicide, beginning in the 1950s and continuing every decade until 1990. Rates for males have since slowly declined, but remain at historically high levels (Maguire & Pastore, 1999, p. 300). Although the rate of death by suicide for late adolescent females is much lower, it has also crept upward over the past 40 years, and shows no sign of falling (Maguire & Pastore, 1999, p. 300).

As noted above, official suicide rates may underrepresent the actual prevalence of suicide for youth. For example, fatal accidents involving a single motor vehicle may represent suicides, but may not be reported as such. In addition, the official rates are only for death by suicide (completed suicide) and do not reflect the prevalence of attempted suicide or suicidal ideation, both of which occur commonly in the adolescent age range. In 1995, 8.7% of high school seniors surveyed reported attempting suicide, and an additional 17.7% had made a suicide plan in the 12 months prior to being surveyed (Centers for Disease Control and Prevention, 1996b).

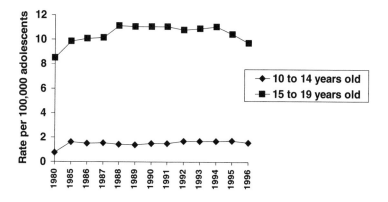

FIGURE 2.8. Developmental and temporal trends in rates of adolescent suicide. Data from Maguire and Pastore (1999, p. 299).

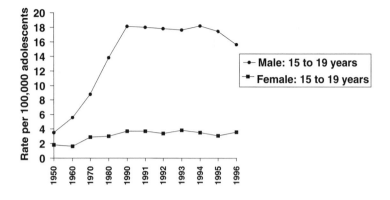

FIGURE 2.9. Developmental trends since 1950 in suicide rates for 15- to 19-year-old adolescents, by gender. Data from Maguire and Pastore (1999, p. 300).

PREVALENCE OF MALADAPTIVE AGGRESSION IN PSYCHIATRICALLY REFERRED SAMPLES

Rising community rates of serious youth aggression are reflected in rising rates of referrals of children and adolescents with aggressive, antisocial, or suicidal behaviors to mental health treatment settings. As such, the evaluation, management, and treatment of aggression are rapidly becoming the major clinical challenges facing pediatric mental health professionals.

There currently exist no national representative surveys of pediatric mental health treatment settings that give us information on rates of aggression in clinically referred youth. Rates must be inferred from research studies across individual settings. As such, this information is more fragmented and incomplete than the data on CD in the community and the juvenile justice statistics cited above. However, enough data are available to suggest that the prevalence of aggression in child and adolescent mental health treatment settings is quite high.

Table 2.3 presents data on the prevalence of aggressive behaviors/CD in children and adolescents admitted to inpatient, outpatient, and residential mental health treatment settings reported in the scientific literature over the past two decades. (In these studies "aggression" is usually defined as physical assault, threats of harm toward another, or explosive anger outbursts that result in property destruction.) It can be seen that aggressive behavior is frequent in these settings, occurring in between 25% and 90% of patients treated, depending on the site in which the research is completed and the gender of the sample population. These prevalence rates are from 10 to 100 times higher than rates of CD and aggression occurring in community-based samples of nonreferred children and adolescents. Prevalence rates for aggressive

TABLE 2.3. Prevalence of Aggressive Behaviors/CD in Cross-Sectional Studies from Psychiatrically Referred Populations

Study	Age	Sample size	Time frame (mo)	Prevalence (%)
Pfeffer et al. (1983a)				
Overall	6–12	103 I/O[a]	Past 6	67
Girls		19		26
Boys		84		62
Pfeffer et al. (1987)				
Overall	6–12	101 O	Past 6	46
Overall	6–12	102 I	Past 6	59
Delga et al. (1989)				
Overall	15	75 I	Lifetime	33
Girls		33		39
Boys		42		69
Garrison et al. (1990)	5–15	99 I	Past 12	76
Gabel and Shindledecker (1991)				
Overall	4–18	348 I	Past 12	38
Girls		123		20
Boys		225		48
Fritsch et al. (1992)	10–18	145 I	Lifetime	50
Connor, Ozbayrak, Kusiak, et al. (1997)	5–19	83	Lifetime	90
Lahey et al. (1998)				
Overall	4–17	440 I/O/R[b]	Past 12	29
Girls				25
Boys				29

[a]I/O, inpatients/outpatients.
[b]R, residential treatment patients.

behavior in psychiatrically referred youth are high for both boys and girls. In some studies, rates of female aggression are equal to the rates for male aggression (Lahey et al., 1998). These data support the idea that the identification, assessment, containment, and treatment of maladaptive aggression and associated disruptive behaviors are important tasks facing child and adolescent mental health clinicians in both ambulatory and institutional treatment settings.

Similarly, suicidal behaviors are very common in child and adolescent psychiatric treatment settings. Table 2.4 presents some data reported in five studies over the past two decades. (In these reports, "suicidal behaviors" include suicidal ideas, suicidal threats, and suicide attempts—but not death by completed suicide, which largely occurs outside treatment settings.) The rates of these behaviors vary between 17% and 61% of patients in these studies,

TABLE 2.4. Prevalence of Suicidal Behaviors in Cross-Sectional Studies
from Psychiatrically Referred Populations

Study	Age	Sample size	Time frame (mo)	Prevalence (%)
Pfeffer et al. (1983b)				
Overall	6–12	102 I/O	Past 6	58
Girls				42
Boys				61
Delga et al. (1989)				
Overall	15	75 I	Lifetime	17
Girls		33		33
Boys		42		45
Gabel and Shindledecker (1991)	4–18	348 I	Past 12	49
Fritsch et al. (1992)	10–18	145 I	Lifetime	43
Connor, Ozbayrak, Kusiak, et al. (1997)	5–19	83 R	Lifetime	35

Note. Abbreviations as in Table 2.3.

and suggest that aggression turned inward is another problem commonly faced by professionals treating referred youth in clinical settings.

CHAPTER SUMMARY

This chapter first reviews the normal developmental course of aggressive behavior in infants and toddlers, and then presents prevalence data on attitudinal concerns about and rates of maladaptive aggressive behavior among children and adolescents. Data from studies of CD in the community, youth attitude surveys, juvenile justice statistics, and clinical mental health studies are reviewed. Developmentally, conflictual behavior between toddlers and preschool children is a common and normal part of early social life. Physical aggression over the possession of objects and territory decreases as children mature. Verbal aggression strategies begin to replace physical fighting with entry into elementary school. However, for a not insignificant number of children and adolescents, maladaptive aggression continues as they mature. Prevalence rates for maladaptive aggression are reviewed from a number of perspectives. The prevalence of CD varies between 1.5% and 20% (depending on the time frame of the study) of nonreferred 4- to 18-year-olds as assessed in different communities in Europe and North America. In the United States, rates of delinquency and aggravated assault are rising for adolescents aged 14 and older, as assessed over the past 30 years. Youth murder and manslaughter offender and victimization rates peaked in the 1990s. These rates are slowly falling as the 21st century begins, yet remain at historically high levels. Suicide rates have risen dramatically for both female and male adolescents in the years since World War II. All these rising societal rates of outwardly and inwardly directed aggression are also reflected in the high prevalence rates found for aggressive and suicidal behavior in psychiatrically referred children and adolescents. The current rates of maladaptive aggression in children and adolescents, with resultant injury and death, constitute a serious public health issue for the United States (Brener et al., 1999). Presently, the identification, assessment, containment, referral, and clinical treatment of aggressive children and adolescents are among the greatest challenges today facing professionals working in juvenile justice, educational, psychiatric, and mental health treatment settings.

Aggression: Stability, Impairment, and Desistance

It has been known for some time that maladaptive aggression and related behaviors can be quite stable over time and development for certain children. During the past two decades, a number of research studies have followed children and adolescents classified as exhibiting aggression or diagnosed with conduct disorder (CD) as they grow up. Most of these investigations have focused on males, but females have also been studied. We now have some data on adolescent and young adult outcomes of children who were assessed as highly aggressive early in their development. For some individuals, these studies show that early-onset aggression can be greatly impairing as children grow older, with increased rates of school failure, interpersonal relationship difficulties, continued legal offending, long periods of unemployment as adults, increased mental health problems, and increased rates of adverse general health care outcomes.

These longitudinal studies also point out that though most adults with clinically significant antisocial behavior in adulthood also had CD as children and adolescents, many children and adolescents with CD change their behavior and do *not* become antisocial as adults. These youth stop on the developmental pathway that leads to an antisocial adult lifestyle. Current research is attempting to better understand the factors that are associated with childhood-onset CD's persistence into adulthood, as well as desistance before adult antisocial patterns are established.

This chapter reviews research on the stability of maladaptive aggression and CD-like behaviors, both in clinically referred youth and in nonreferred youth residing in the community. First, some methodological issues are discussed. Next, stability is addressed from a developmental perspective, from the preschool years to adulthood; differences between male and female stability rates are also noted. Although research on children with early-onset inappropriate aggression has begun to reveal subtypes that may explain persistence and desistance, studies indicate that aggressive children are at risk for a variety of impaired outcomes across multiple domains of functioning in life. Finally, a discussion of desistance from aggression and factors that may be related to discontinuities in the stability of such behaviors is presented.

METHODOLOGICAL ISSUES

In general, the stability of a constellation of behaviors such as CD is examined in studies that assess subjects over time as they grow older. These so-called "longitudinal" studies begin by first assessing subjects at baseline, which is often called "Time 1." Subjects are then reassessed at fixed time intervals over a number of years at "Time 2," "Time 3," and so on. In the best-designed studies, a control or comparison group of subjects who do not have the behaviors in question at Time 1 are also assessed at fixed time intervals over a number of years. How the behaviors being studied change over time with growth and development from the first assessment to later assessments, compared to the behavior of the control group, can then be examined. Factors that are associated with either continuation or desistance of the behaviors can also be studied in comparison to the control group. Longitudinal studies take a long time and are very expensive to complete; however, they do provide the most useful data.

A less powerful methodology is called a "cross-sectional" study. Such a study examines children and/or adolescents in an identified population at a single point in time, and compares children with the behaviors to be studied with children who do not have these behaviors. Cross-sectional studies can suggest factors that are associated with the behaviors, but cannot provide information about causal relationships between variables or developmental changes over time.

Aggressive or CD-like behaviors are measured in a variety of ways. Some studies ask parents or teachers to complete rating scales coding their observations of behaviors in the population to be studied. Other studies utilize self-report measures, in which subjects document their own behaviors. Still others use peer nomination surveys, in which peers (generally in the neighborhood or classroom) are asked to indicate the most aggressive child they know; these children then become the study subjects. Still other studies use official arrest records to identify aggressive subjects. Finally, children and adolescents meeting psychiatric diagnostic criteria for CD can be identified in a population and followed over time. As can be seen, there are many different methods for measuring aggression and CD. Each has its advantages and disadvantages. The best-designed studies utilize more than one measure in their assessments, use multiple raters and observers of the subjects' problem behaviors, and have a longitudinal component.

The stability of these problem behaviors over time is often expressed in terms of a "stability coefficient." This is a statistical correlation that compares the rank ordering of individuals on the basis of the studied behaviors at Time 1 with the rank ordering at Time 2. Stability coefficients, like all statistical correlations, can range between 0 (not correlated at all) and 1.00 (completely correlated). High stability coefficients indicate that the rank ordering of individuals expressing the target behaviors at Time 1 is similar to that at Time 2 (Loeber & Stouthamer-Loeber, 1998). A second method of measuring the stability of aggressive behaviors is to report the percentages of children in a study sample who have such behaviors at first assessment and then continue to manifest symptoms of aggression over time. A third approach is to report the percentage of aggressive children as first assessed at baseline who then demonstrate impairment in various outcome domains later in development, such as interpersonal relationship difficulties, employment problems, academic underfunctioning, or arrest rates.

STABILITY OF AGGRESSION AND RELATED BEHAVIORS IN COMMUNITY SAMPLES

Preschool to Childhood

Relatively few studies have examined the stability of aggressive, CD-like, and hyperactive behaviors (externalizing behavioral problems) from the preschool to the school-age period. However, evidence suggests that the stability of these behaviors during the preschool period is quite high and comparable with that found during childhood and adolescence (Campbell, 1991). In a longitudinal study, 46 parent-referred 3-year-old toddlers with externalizing behavior problems and 22 same-age toddlers without such problems were followed and systematically reassessed at age 6 years. Staff observations and parent ratings were used as outcome measures. Results showed that aggression scores at age 3 were predictive of aggression scores at ages 4 and 6 (stability coefficients of .77 and .51, respectively). At 3, 4, and 6 years of age, aggression and hyperactivity were highly intercorrelated. Mothers who experienced their preschoolers as hyperactive and distractible were also more likely to be concerned about aggressive behavior. These behaviors were also most likely to persist in this study when they were also associated with more family disruption and a negative mother–child relationship (Campbell, Breaux, Ewing, & Szumowski, 1986; Campbell & Ewing, 1990).

In another study, 185 children aged 4 years from a London borough were systematically assessed for early-onset behavioral and psychiatric problems (Richman, Stevenson, & Graham, 1982). The children were reassessed 5 years later. Results showed that 61% of the children identified as problematic at age 3 years still demonstrated considerable behavioral difficulties at ages 8–9 years.

These studies suggest that for some toddlers and preschoolers, identifiable behavior problems and aggression persist across the developmental transition to the elementary school years. For these children, the idea that they "will just grow out of" their difficulties does not seem to be true. Accurate and early identification of these "at-risk" youngsters is very important as a first step in early intervention efforts, to prevent the possible crystallization of an antisocial lifestyle as the children mature.

Childhood to Adolescence

A number of studies have assessed the stability of aggression, delinquency, and CD from childhood to adolescence. These studies have been completed in a number of different countries, including Canada, the United States, the Netherlands, and New Zealand; they are presented in Table 3.1.

TABLE 3.1. Stability of Aggressive and CD-Like Behaviors from Childhood to Adolescence in Community Samples

Study	n	Age at T1	Duration (yr)	Outcome
Offord et al. (1992)	881	4–12	4	44.8% of children with CD dx. at T1 had CD at T2.
Stanger et al. (1992)	2,479	4–16	3	Aggression at T1 predicted 51% of the variance in aggression at T2.
Verhulst and van der Ende (1992)	936	4–11	6	32% of aggressive and delinquent children at T1 were aggressive and delinquent at T2.
McGee et al. (1992)	976	11	4	81% of children with CD dx. at T1 had CD at T2.
Fischer et al. (1993)[a]	169	4–12	8	Stability coefficient for aggression = .33, for delinquency = .55.
Lochman and Wayland (1994)	114	11	4	Stability coefficient for CD = .53.
Lahey, Loeber, et al. (1995)	171	7–12	4	50% of boys were rediagnosed with CD at 1-, 2-, or 3-year follow-up.
MacDonald and Achenbach (1999)	2,479	4–16	6	30% of males and 18% of females had signs of CD at 6-year outcome.
Hofstra et al. (2000)	1,615	4–11	14	Stability coefficients: Delinquent behavior for males = .20, for females = .10; aggressive behavior for males = .33, for females = .37.

[a] Sample of children with attention-deficit/hyperactivity disorder.

The outcomes of children who were found to have aggression and related behaviors at initial assessment have been reported in various ways in these studies. Some investigations have reported the percentage of youth in the study sample continuing to demonstrate these behaviors at follow-up (Time 2) assessment. Others have reported how much of the difference in aggressive behaviors in the study sample at Time 2 can be uniquely and solely attributed to aggression at baseline (Time 1) assessment. This is called the "variance" and is expressed as a percentage. Still other studies have reported correlations between aggressive behaviors at the two assessment times. This is a stability coefficient.

Regardless of the method of assessment, inspection of Table 3.1 reveals fairly high rates of stability over the developmental period encompassing childhood to adolescence. From 32% to 81% of children assessed as meeting criteria for CD in childhood continued to meet these criteria as adolescents. Across these studies, stability coefficients ranged between .33 and .53, depending on the specific behaviors being followed and the types of information (parent report, teacher report, child self-report, direct observation) utilized in the study design. Indeed, an appreciable amount of the difference in aggression at follow-up can be explained by aggression at baseline. Taken together, these studies suggest that various forms of maladaptive aggression can persist into the teenage years for many children who demonstrate early-onset aggression in the school-age years.

Childhood/Adolescence to Young Adulthood

A number of studies have followed children or adolescents into young adulthood to assess the stability of aggressive and antisocial behavior. Huesmann, Eron, Lefkowitz, and Walder (1984) followed several hundred children from New York State and found that peer-nominated aggression at age 8 years significantly predicted self-reported aggression and legal convictions for males at age 30 years. Table 3.2 lists some of the more recent studies assessing stability of aggression and antisocial behaviors from childhood and adolescence into young adulthood; these studies have been carried out in Great Britain, Holland, and the United States. As they do between childhood and adolescence, the various forms of maladaptive aggression studied demonstrate considerable stability from childhood and adolescence into young adulthood for nonreferred samples assessed in the community, especially for males.

Similar continuities appear to exist when clinically referred young people are evaluated in mental health settings. In an investigation of the stability and predictive strength of behavioral problems in a referred sample, 1,652 children and adolescents aged 4–18 years were assessed at baseline and then again 6 years later (Visser, van der Ende, Koot, & Verhulst, 1999). The behaviors assessed at Time 1 were correlated with the same behaviors assessed at Time 2. For delinquent behaviors, stabilities averaged .51 for parent reports and .57 for teacher reports. For aggressive behaviors, stabilities averaged .61 for par-

TABLE 3.2. Stability of Aggressive and CD-Like Behaviors from Childhood/
Adolescence to Young Adulthood in Community Samples

Study	*n*	Age at T1	Duration (yr)	Outcome
Farrington (1991)	411	8	24	49% of the most aggressive males at ages 8–10 years were still the most aggressive at age 32 years.
Zoccolillo et al. (1992)	254	Childhood	Avg. 26 yo at T2	40% of males and 35% of females meet criteria for adult ASPD.
Achenbach et al. (1995)	749	13–16	6	Aggression at T1 predicted 37% of the variance in aggression at T2.
Ferdinand and Verhulst (1995)	459	13–16	8	Stability coefficient for externalizing behavior for males = .30, for females = .17.
Hofstra et al. (2000)	1,615	4–16	14	Stability coefficients: aggression for males = .25, for females = .53; delinquency for males = .30, for females = .30.

ent reports and .53 for teacher reports. These findings indicate a high continuity of aggressive and antisocial behaviors over time in mental-health-referred young people, as well as for nonreferred aggressive youth assessed in the community.

Finally, in a definitive analysis, Olweus (1979) reviewed 16 studies published between 1935 and 1978 reporting on the stability of aggressive behavior in males. Subjects were from 2 to 18 years of age, and aggression was longitudinally assessed from 6 months to 21 years. The average length of follow-up was 5.7 years for older subjects and 1.5 years for younger subjects. Olweus (1979) found stability coefficients for aggressive behavior in males to be quite high (.81 for three studies using direct observation and .79 for studies using teacher ratings of aggressive behavior). This degree of longitudinal stability is similar to the stability typically found for intelligence (IQ) testing. Olweus concluded that aggression in males is quite stable over time and that marked individual differences in habitual aggression manifest themselves early in life, certainly by the age of 3 years.

GENDER AND STABILITY

Aggression in females has been studied much less frequently than aggression in males. Early research suggested differences in the stability of aggressive behavior across gender. Kagan and Moss (1962) found considerable stability for male aggression between childhood and adolescence, and between childhood and adulthood; less stability for female aggression between childhood and adolescence; and limited stability for female aggression from childhood to adulthood. However, these findings were not replicated. In another analysis evaluating six studies reporting on the stability of aggressive behavior in comparable male and female subjects up to age 19 years, Olweus (1982) found almost the same stability for females as for males. In these studies the average age of subjects was 7 years, and they were followed for intervals ranging from 6 months to 10 years. The average follow-up time was 2.8 years. The average stability coefficient for males was .497 and for females was .439, a relatively small difference.

However, subsequent research evaluating gender differences in aggression over time has continued to show possible differences in the developmental paths for male and females. In a 6-year study testing different developmental continuities and paths from adolescent psychiatric syndromes to young adult syndromes, different predictors for female aggression than for male aggression were found (Achenbach, Howell, McConaughy, & Stanger, 1995b). Male aggression in young adulthood was predicted by adolescent aggression, poor social competence, and stressful experiences. Female aggression in young adulthood was predicted by more diverse and varied adolescent difficulties, including somatic and withdrawn problems. To give another example, a longitudinal follow-up study of children initially assessed at age 11 years and reassessed at age 15 years found significant continuity of aggressive behavior for boys but not for girls (McGee, Feehan, Williams, & Anderson, 1992). These studies support possible gender differences in the continuity of aggression for male and female adolescents.

In short, there appears to be some evidence for stability of aggressive behavior in girls between childhood and adolescence. However, by mid-adolescence and young adulthood, the levels of female aggression appear less closely related to levels of aggression in childhood than for males. Developmental continuities, stability, and predictors of aggressive and related behaviors in females remain understudied and constitute an important area for further research. Chapter 9 of this book discusses the existing literature in females in more detail.

STABILITY-BASED SUBTYPES OF AGGRESSION

Subsequent research into the stability of aggression over time has revealed the possibility of subtypes of aggression with different longitudinal stabilities. These investigations suggest individual differences in the stability of aggression and antisocial behaviors. Moffitt (1993a) has noted that although many children and adolescents behave antisocially, this behavior is temporary and situational for most. Time-limited aggression and CD-like behavior may be particularly common for adolescents. When this behavior begins in adolescence and is dependent on contextual cues in the environment (e.g., peer influences), it may cease when the adolescent matures into the responsibilities and privileges of young adulthood (Moffitt, 1993a). Only a small subset of aggressive youth (generally males) display a persistent, stable pattern of aggression and antisocial behavior over time as they grow into adulthood.

This stable and persistent pattern is often characterized by an early onset of aggressive behavior (by 8 years of age), in contrast to the later-developing, time-limited adolescent-onset behavior pattern. This early-onset subtype of aggression may account for large stability coefficients in samples followed longitudinally. For example, in a New Zealand study of 1,037 children followed prospectively every 2 years from age 3 until age 15, only 5% of the boys were persistently aggressive at all time points assessed in the study. This 5% accounted for 68% of the overall stability for aggressive behavior in this sample (Henry, Moffitt, Robins, Earls, & Silva, 1993). In another study of 1,721 Australian toddlers initially assessed at ages 2–3 years and reassessed every 18 months, Kingston and Prior (1995) found that only 3% were persistently aggressive at all time points evaluated.

Indeed, evidence is emerging that a small group of children with early-onset aggression (generally males) display high rates of aggression across time and in diverse situations. In Patterson's (1982) study, of the 5% of boys evaluated as most aggressive in the third grade, 39% of them ranked above the sample median for aggression 10 years later. It is well known that of adults with antisocial personality disorder (ASPD) and aggression, almost all had CD and aggression as children. However, only about 33% of children with CD go on to develop ASPD as adults (Robins, 1978). Most youth with CD eventually stop their disordered behavior. Early-onset aggression may define a subset of all childhood aggression that persists and is stable over time, and that constitutes a risk for particularly poor outcomes.

This type of aggressive behavior has many characteristics that suggest a psychopathological syndrome (Moffitt, 1993a). First, it is statistically uncommon (occurring in about 5% of males), which is consistent with the statistical definition of an abnormality. Second, it demonstrates stability across time and biological maturation. Third, the expression of aggression occurs in many different environments (home, school, community) and does not seem to be mediated by a specific environmental setting. Fourth, the aggression is of sufficient severity and frequency to be highly maladaptive and to cause much impairment for the individual child. Finally, early-onset and persistent aggression may have a biological basis in subtle dysfunctions of the central nervous system (Moffitt, 1993b). As such, this type of aggression may fit the definition of maladaptive aggression defined from an evolutionary biology perspective, as described in Chapter 1. This subtyping is only partially reflected in the *Diagnostic and Statistical Manual of Mental Disorders*, fourth edition (American Psychiatric Association, 1994) as CD, childhood-onset type (onset occurring before age 10 years).

However, research also supports the idea that other subtypes of serious aggression may exist. Not all violently aggressive adults have a history of serious childhood aggression that is chronic and persistent from an early age in life. Some individuals who go on to commit serious aggressive acts in later life demonstrate a gradual, cumulative progression from a difficult temperament in infancy and oppositional behavior in early childhood, to bullying behaviors and physical fighting in the school-age years, to more serious violence during adolescence and the young adult years (Loeber, 1990). For these individuals, aggressive behavior proceeds in a stepwise fashion, slowly progressing from minor forms of aggression and annoyance in early childhood to violence in the later years. This research suggests a cumulative, progressive, orderly, and nonrandom development of aggression for some individuals. This subtype—a "cumulative" as opposed to an "early-onset" subtype—suggests learned behavior as opposed to a psychopathological syndrome. Aggression becomes more varied, frequent, and serious, and expresses itself in more situations, as the individual learns that violence will result in rewards (social status in a peer group, material goods, etc.) and is contingently reinforced for this behavior as development unfolds.

In summary, childhood aggression and related behaviors show substantial rates of stability over time. Stability has been demonstrated from preschool to childhood, from school age to adolescence, and into young adulthood, especially for males. However, subsets may be identifiable. Stability may vary by gender and by age at onset of aggressive behavior. These subsets may be important and yield different longitudinal outcomes, prognoses, etiologies, and possibly treatment interventions. Early-onset and persistent aggression in males may be a form of psychopathology, whereas cumulative, progressive aggression may represent learning and environmental reinforcement.

IMPAIRED LONGITUDINAL OUTCOMES OF AGGRESSIVE CHILDREN

Children who express early-onset, persistent aggression and related behaviors are at high risk for a broad variety of negative outcomes and impaired functioning in a number of areas of life as they grow older. Research has investigated several problematic domains of functioning, including behavior problems, academic underachievement, poor employment histories, maladaptive interpersonal functioning, negative mental health outcomes, and adverse general health care outcomes (including premature mortality from unnatural causes).

Behavior Problems

Problematic behavioral outcomes at an older age in children who were first identified as excessively and inappropriately aggressive when young include school and academic difficulties, police contacts, and continued aggressive behavior or arrest for legal offenses. Outcome information is now available about problematic behaviors from several studies. Huesmann et al. (1984)

found that peer-nominated aggression at age 8 years predicted self-reported aggression and legal convictions for males at age 30 years. This finding has been replicated. Farrington (1991) followed over 400 male children from the ages of 8 to 32 years. He also found that aggressive behavior in childhood significantly predicted self-reported legal offenses and continued aggressive behavior in adulthood. Lundy, Pfohl, and Kuperman (1993) followed 170 preadolescent children admitted to a psychiatric hospital for a variety of difficulties. They reported that a history of assaultive behavior in childhood predicted adult imprisonment at 7- to 20-year follow-up. In an outcome study of children with CD, Zoccolillo, Pickles, Quinton, and Rutter (1992) found that 40% of males and 35% of females met criteria for ASPD as adults, compared with 4% of male controls without childhood CD and 0% of female controls. Although most children who display aggressive and antisocial behaviors in childhood do not continue to do so as adults, these studies support the idea that early-onset childhood aggression may have a significantly negative impact on adult behavioral functioning, with the data more robust for males.

Academic and Occupational Underachievement

Many, but not all, studies have documented impairment in academic achievement for aggressive children. In a previously mentioned study of 1,721 Australian children assessed every 18 months, persistently aggressive children evaluated for academic skills were found to have lower reading ability and poorer adaptive functioning in the school setting at age 8 years, compared with nonaggressive children (Kingston & Prior, 1995). Many studies have reported that aggressive children have poorer reading and academic skills; however, not all research supports this finding. Offord et al. (1992), in their longitudinal follow-up of a community sample of 881 youth in Canada, found that the school performance of children with CD was not significantly different from that of control students. However, the extant literature generally supports the finding that children with early-onset and persistent aggression appear to function less well in school and to have poorer overall academic skills than comparison children. They are at risk for academic deficiencies, lower academic achievement, school behavior problems, early dropout, grade repetition, and specific skill deficits (Kazdin, 1994, 1996; MacDonald & Achenbach, 1999).

The employment histories of adults who are identified as highly aggressive as children also reveal functional impairments. In Farrington's (1991) study, early aggression identified by the third grade predicted long periods of unemployment at age 32 years for males. Although early-onset aggression was not found to predict low job status or low take-home pay in this study, it did significantly predict not being a homeowner by age 32 years. This may reflect a more transient lifestyle or lower socioeconomic status in adults identified as aggressive in early childhood.

Poor Interpersonal Relationships and Social Skills

Aggressive youth are likely to demonstrate poor interpersonal relationship skills. They evince diminished social skills with both peers and adults, and show higher levels of peer rejection at all ages (Kazdin, 1994). Farrington (1991) found that early aggression identified in males at ages 12–14 years significantly predicted marital conflict and physical assault on a wife at age 32 years. Interestingly, it did not predict divorce.

Deficits in social skills may be related in part to the cognitive and attributional biases that have been found in aggressive youth. These children appear to have deficits and distortions in cognitive problem-solving skills, a predisposition to attribute hostile intent to others where none exists, and easily aroused resentment and suspiciousness (Dodge & Newman, 1981; Dodge & Frame, 1982; Kazdin, 1994). Youth with early-onset and persistent aggression have been found to be at risk for subtle neurological deficits, such as impulsive responding, difficulty inhibiting inappropriate responses, sustained attentional deficits, and poorer verbal functioning (Moffitt, 1993b). These information-processing vulnerabilities and subtle neuropsychological impairments may make use (let alone mastery) of verbally mediated methods of conflict resolution difficult for these children; this may increase their risk for more physical means of reducing anger, frustration, or other strong emotions, leading to high rates of peer rejection.

Negative Mental Health Outcomes

Children who demonstrate early-onset and persistent aggression are at risk for a variety of negative mental health outcomes. These include higher rates of substance use disorders (SUDs, discussed separately below), suicidal behaviors, and mental health service utilization, as well as a greater number of other psychiatric diagnoses than young people who do not have early serious aggression.

A 7-year longitudinal study reported the mental health problems of 177 boys first assessed when they were 7–12 years old (Loeber, Green, Lahey, & Kalb, 2000). These boys were classified as children who early in life engaged in persistent physical fighting with others. Over the course of the study, some boys stopped fighting and others persisted. These two groups were compared at outcome. The boys who persisted in fighting differed from the children who desisted from fighting by having higher rates of psychiatric hospitalization, lower IQ scores, more mothers with ASPD, a greater number of psychiatric diagnoses at outcome, and more impairment in daily life functioning. These results suggest that children with early-onset aggression are at risk for poor mental health outcomes as they grow older (Loeber et al., 2000).

It is unlikely that aggression directly causes psychiatric disorder. Rather, persistent aggression, poor impulse control, and irritability may be associated symptoms of an underlying psychiatric disorder (Connor & Steingard, 1996).

In addition to CD, other common psychiatric disorders that may be associated with early-onset aggression include attention-deficit/hyperactivity disorder, mood disorders such as depression or bipolar disorder, psychotic disorders, and/or disorders of fear conditioning such as posttraumatic stress disorder. Clinical recognition of an underlying psychiatric disorder in the aggressive child is important for specific treatment interventions that may diminish aggression as an associated symptom of the psychiatric diagnosis (Connor & Steingard, 1996).

Substance Use Disorders

A growing body of scientific literature is beginning to document relationships between early-onset, persistent, inappropriate aggression and later SUDs in adolescence and young adulthood (Brook, Whiteman, Finch, & Cohen, 1996; Bukstein, 1996). These relationships may take several forms. First, substance abuse or dependence may cause or influence aggressive behavior. The pharmacological effects of alcohol and other misused substances (cocaine, phencyclidine) are known to increase the likelihood of subsequent aggressive behavior when consumed or during substance withdrawal, through direct effects on the brain producing stimulation or depression, enhancing irritability, and/or reducing impulse control. In addition, individuals with SUDs often find themselves in environments where aggression and violence are more likely to occur. Second, early-onset aggression may influence the subsequent development of SUDs. Early-onset aggression is known to predict a growing variety of antisocial acts if it persists over time as the child grows older. Not just physical fighting, but theft, vandalism, school truancy, and drug and alcohol misuse blossom and become more frequent and varied as the aggressive child enters adolescence. There exists empirical support for the influence of child aggression on subsequent SUDs. For example, in a 20-year longitudinal study, early childhood aggression had an adverse effect on the development of young adult drug use (Brook et al., 1996). Mediating variables included weak attachments to parents in childhood (Brook, Whiteman, & Finch, 1993) and intrapsychic distress and unconventionality during adolescence (Brook, Whiteman, Finch, & Cohen, 1995). Finally, substance misuse and aggression may not be directly related, but each may be part of a larger syndrome of antisocial behavior (Bukstein, 1996).

Negative General Health Care Outcomes

There also exists evidence that children with aggression and related behaviors are vulnerable to a wide variety of negative general health care outcomes. In a study of factors associated with health care utilization (primary care office visits and emergency room visits), 510 children aged 2–5 years were studied. Children with externalizing behavior disorders—defined as excessive hyperactivity, aggression, attention deficits, oppositional and defiant behavior, and temper difficulties—had significantly more visits to their primary care physicians than children without such disorders (Lavigne et al., 1998). In female adolescents, severe CD predicts early pregnancy (Booth & Zhang, 1996).

Other research suggests the possibility of a more ominous outcome, including premature mortality from unnatural death. In adolescents who were psychiatrically treated for anxiety and depression accompanied by a suicide attempt, high levels of aggression were significantly associated with multiple, repeated suicide attempts (recidivism) as opposed to no or a single suicide attempt (Stein, Apter, Ratzoni, Har-Even, & Avidan, 1998). In combination with mood disorders and substance abuse, CD predicted completed suicide in a case–control, psychological autopsy study of teenage suicides (Shaffer, Gould, et al., 1996). The mortality rate and aggressiveness in a cohort of 2,364 former patients referred to a Stockholm, Sweden, child guidance mental health clinic were studied during a 30-year follow-up period. During this period, 106 of the sample died; this frequency was significantly higher than the calculated mortality rate of the general population. Aggressive behavior was overrepresented in the initial contacts with the child guidance clinic among those who died (de Chateau, 1990). Finally, a 50-year longitudinal study followed 1,000 delinquent and nondelinquent boys from age 14 until age 65 (Laub & Vaillant, 2000). Over the lifespan, delinquent individuals had early mortality rates from unnatural causes (accidents, violence, and SUDs) at more than twice the rate of nondelinquent subjects.

These data suggest that early mortality from unnatural causes, increased primary health care utilization, and other negative health care consequences may be outcomes experienced by children identified as having significant aggressive behavior problems in childhood. Additional research attempting to replicate these findings is needed. Interventions to reduce childhood aggression may reduce overall health care costs in society; this is a particularly important possibility, given current economic and political pressures to reduce health care utilization and costs through managed care initiatives.

DISCONTINUATION AND DESISTANCE FROM AGGRESSION

The substantial stabilities for aggression cited in this chapter can give the impression of high continuity and little change over time. However, this is not supported by the scientific literature. Although aggression is very stable for some individuals, all of the studies reviewed in this chapter suggest that a certain proportion of children and adolescents with early-onset aggressive problems do desist from aggression over time. The stability coefficients found in these research reports are never 1.00, and the proportion of aggressive individuals evaluated at Time 1 is never 100% when evaluated at Time 2. For some children, aggressive behaviors fade away with development.

For example, a study of boys in a community sample evaluated from kindergarten through age 12 years found a decrease in physical fighting in 12%.

These boys fought in kindergarten, but desisted by ages 10 through 12 years. In contrast, fighting remained stable for 8% of the boys, with high frequencies of aggression at all time points evaluated (Haapasalo & Trembly, 1994). In the Kingston and Prior (1995) study, cited earlier, about 25% of the children desisted from aggression when followed from ages 2 to 8 years. Desistance from physical aggression continues to occur during adolescence and young adulthood. A community study of inner-city boys studied in Pittsburgh, Pennsylvania, found that by age 15 years the prevalence of physical fighting in the study sample started to decrease. This trend continued at least through age 17 (Loeber & Hay, 1997).

Critical periods of development for diminishing aggressive behavior may be concentrated in the transitions from preschool to the elementary school years and from late adolescence to the young adult years (Loeber & Hay, 1997). These critical periods are important to recognize, because treatment interventions focused during these times may produce discontinuities in the stability of aggression. However, a comparison of stability coefficients across different studies suggests that the magnitude of the stability coefficients for aggression increases by early adolescence (Loeber, 1982). Thus the longer aggressive behavior continues, the harder it may be to change. This suggests the possibility that interventions during earlier critical periods of development may have proportionally greater treatment effects than interventions at later critical periods. Population changes in the rate of desistance or discontinuity of aggression with age remain poorly studied and are an important area for further research.

What are some possible explanations for desistance? The first possibility is measurement error in research. Correlation coefficients may be poor indicators of the actual degree of stability, continuity, and change in aggressive behavior (Loeber & Stouthamer-Loeber, 1998). Remember that a stability coefficient simply measures the degree to which the rank ordering of individuals on the basis of their aggressive behavior at Time 1 is similar to that at Time 2. Correlations can be high, but the absolute prevalence, frequency, variety, and seriousness of the aggressive behavior may change with time. Correlation coefficients tell us nothing about these changes, and the differences may be quite meaningful for an individual. It may be more useful to know the probabilities that highly aggressive individuals will persist in aggression or desist over time and with development, as well as the probabilities that individuals with low levels of aggression will escalate their behavior to become more aggressive over time. As such, measurements of the severity and frequency of aggression that are comparable over time may be most useful (Loeber & Stouthamer-Loeber, 1998).

Another potential source of error is the measurement of "false-positive" outcomes. Aggression is an episodic and intermittent behavior; it does not occur constantly throughout the day, every day of the year. In a longitudinal study of aggressive behavior, some individuals will not be aggressive when assessed at Time 2. Does this mean they have desisted from aggression, or does it mean they have temporarily stopped displaying aggression coincidentally at the time of measurement, only to display it again at another point in time? These false-positive errors in the prediction of stability are often counted as evidence for desistance (Loeber & Hay, 1997). Only long-term, longitudinal studies that track aggressive individuals over the entire course of their development can give us information about the true rates of desistance. Such studies are enormously (often prohibitively) expensive to undertake and require many decades to complete.

Subtypes of aggression may also help explain desistance. In the early-onset subtype, aggression may persist and have less probability of desistance than aggression first beginning in later life. In the cumulative subtype, early intervention may interrupt stability and lead to increased desistance, as contrasted with interventions delivered later in the course of aggression.

Furthermore, desistance may vary as a function of gender. In the preschool years, girls may "outgrow" aggression more quickly than boys. Gender differences in the rates of desistance from aggression across different periods of development (preschool, school age, adolescence, young adulthood) have been little studied, and a great deal of further research is necessary in this area.

Finally, desistance from aggressive and antisocial behavior may vary with the frequency, variety, and seriousness of the behavior. The stability of such behavior is closely linked to its severity. For males, aggression and CD-like behaviors that are more severe, more frequently displayed, displayed in more variegated ways, and displayed in a greater variety of environments (community, home, school) appear to be more stable over time (Loeber, 1988; Moffitt, 1993a). However, the corollary is not true: Isolated but severe incidents of these behaviors do not imply a lack of stability. These acts may consistently recur, but at a low frequency. Further research remains needed to ascertain whether the relationships between stability and severity of antisocial behavior applies specifically to aggression or to a variety of CD-like behaviors in general.

CHAPTER SUMMARY

This chapter has explored questions concerning stability, impairment, and desistance in referred and nonreferred community samples of aggressive and antisocial children and adolescents. A complicated picture is beginning to emerge. Aggression and related behaviors can be highly stable across development for some, but not most, individuals. Especially when stable, these behaviors are associated with poor longitudinal outcomes across a variety of domains, increase the cost of health care, result in higher probabilities of early mortality, and cause a great deal of daily functional impairment. Some of these individuals demonstrate an early onset of aggression, are males, and engage frequently in a variety of serious aggressive behaviors in a wide assortment of settings, accounting for a large amount of the stability of these behaviors in study populations. Others demonstrate a cumulative, nonrandom, and stepwise progression from minor to more serious antisocial and aggressive behaviors over time.

Early recognition of these subtypes is clinically very important. Different interventions may be required, depending on the subtype. For example, early-onset, persistent aggression may be a form of psychopathology (maladaptive aggression) and require psychiatric intervention—including, but not limited to, the possibility of pharmacological intervention to treat associated psychiatric syndromes and/or psychobiological symptoms such as impulsivity, hyperactivity, irritability, affective instability, and sustained attention deficits. The cumulative subtype may represent a learned and adaptational response to the environment (adaptive aggression); as such, it may require multimodal economic (e.g., parenting and family supports, early child intervention), political, educational, and psychosocial interventions, but not necessarily medication treatment. Further research examining rates of desistance from aggression and how these relate to gender, critical periods in development, neurobiological variables, and psychosocial variables offers the hope of further clarifying which aggressive children or adolescents are most at risk for continuing their behavior into adulthood, which ones have a high probability of desistance, and when critical periods for interventions may occur that offer the greatest possibility of disrupting aggression stabilities in at-risk children.

◈ CHAPTER 4

The Relationship between Categorical Psychiatric Diagnosis and Aggression

Although many youth who are clinically referred to mental health centers are not aggressive, certain psychiatric diagnoses do increase vulnerability to impulsive aggression. Indeed, aggression and related behaviors are among the most common reasons for psychiatric referral of children and adolescents to mental health settings. The purpose of this chapter is to describe relationships between these behaviors and several categorical psychiatric diagnoses frequently found in clinically referred children and adolescents with such behaviors. This chapter does not exhaustively review existing diagnostic systems; rather, it focuses on those psychiatric disorders that have a robust relationship to aggressive behaviors in children and adolescents.

Psychiatric disorders are presently diagnosed according to the criteria set forth in the American Psychiatric Association's (APA's) *Diagnostic and Statistical Manual of Mental Disorders*, currently in its fourth edition (DSM-IV; APA, 1994). The World Health Organization (WHO) classifies psychiatric illness according to the *International Classification of Diseases* (or, to give its full title, the *International Statistical Classification of Diseases and Related Health Problems*), currently in its 10th revision (ICD-10; WHO, 1992). Most clinicians evaluate psychiatric diagnoses in children, adolescents, and adults by using the criterion sets listed in one of these two classifications. The most recent versions of each have increasingly emphasized greater convergence between the two nosologies, although some differences remain (Andrews, Slade, & Peters, 1999; Hinshaw & Anderson, 1996; Tripp, Luk, Schaughency, & Singh, 1999). Both diagnostic systems utilize a categorical approach to diagnosis. That is, if a certain number of criteria are present (as defined by both inclusionary and exclusionary items) and cause impairment to the individual in his or her daily life, a discrete disorder is said to be present that is distinct from other disorders. In contrast, dimensional systems of classification conceive of disorders as existing on a continuum in the population, without a discrete "cutoff" identifying them as present or absent.

At present there is no unified, overarching theory of aggression in psychiatric disorders that allows a single classification system to explain all the variegated presentations of aggressive behavior. Classification systems do exist for aggressive/agonistic behavioral patterns in ethology (Moyer, 1968), but they do not translate easily into the much more complicated, multifaceted presentations of aggressive behaviors in humans. As a result, research into and rational clinical treatment of aggressive behavior in psychiatric disorders have been hampered.

Especially in people clinically referred to mental health treatment settings, one possible way of classifying some aggressive behaviors is to identify any possible association with known psychiatric disorders that already have operational diagnostic criteria. An aggressive behavior occurring within the context of an identifiable psychiatric disorder may then be considered a symptom of the underlying disorder, much as fever is considered a symptom of an underlying infectious illness, or as pain is of an injury. Since modern psychiatric and psychological research is beginning to identify more specific treatments for some (but not all) psychiatric diagnoses, rational treatment of these underlying disorders has a better chance of ameliorating aggression in this context than do nonspecific treatments aimed only at the symptom of aggression. This method of classifying aggressive behaviors thus has the advantage of suggesting more focused and specific possible treatments.

Of course, this approach will not apply to aggressive behavior that occurs independently of an identifiable psychiatric illness. The vast majority of aggressive acts are displayed by people without psychiatric disorders, and most people who suffer from psychiatric disorders are not violent or otherwise aggressive. However, evidence suggests that a not insignificant amount of aggressive behavior occurring in institutions such as psychiatric treatment facilities and in the community may be associated with an underlying psychiatric condition that may or may not be recognized at the time the aggressive behavior occurs (Brennan, Mednick, & Hodgins, 2000; Tiihonen, Isohanni, Rasanen, Koiranen, & Moring, 1997; APA, 1998). Research is also beginning to suggest that some specific types of psychiatric disorders are associated with a greater risk of aggressive behavior, both within psychiatric treatment settings and in the community, compared to other psychiatric disorders (APA, 1997; Arseneault, Moffitt, Caspi, Taylor, & Silva, 2000; Connor, Melloni, & Harrison, 1998; Mulvey, 1994, Swanson, Holzer, Ganju, & Jono, 1990; Taylor & Gunn, 1999).

A descriptive review of the most important categorical psychiatric diagnoses or groups of diagnoses commonly found in clinically referred youth with aggressive behavior is presented in this chapter. These include the disruptive behavior disorders, mood disorders, substance use disorders (SUDs), personality disorders, psychopathy (not a formal psychiatric diagnosis, but important in any discussion of aggression), psychotic disorders, and posttraumatic stress disorder (PTSD). Although ICD-10 criteria (WHO, 1992) are mentioned, the discussion emphasizes the DSM-IV diagnostic criteria (APA, 1994). Description, prevalence, subtypes (where found), and the relationship of each diagnosis to aggression and related behaviors are discussed, with an emphasis on children and adolescents.

DISRUPTIVE BEHAVIORAL DISORDERS

The disruptive behavior disorders encompass three separate but overlapping diagnoses: conduct disorder (CD), oppositional defiant disorder (ODD), and attention-deficit/hyperactivity disorder (ADHD). (DSM-IV [APA, 1994] actually now refers to these three disorders as the "attention-deficit and disruptive behavior disorders," but they continue to be generally known by the shorter term.) These disorders are commonly diagnosed in youth referred to mental health treatment settings and juvenile justice settings. The behavioral symptoms associated with these diagnoses are easily observed by adults in a youngster's environment, and commonly cause distress for those responsible for taking care of the child or adolescent, as well as the youth him- or herself.

Conduct Disorder

Description and Prevalence

The essential characteristic of CD is a persistent behavior pattern in which the basic rights of others or major age-appropriate societal norms or rules are repeatedly violated, beginning in childhood or adolescence. These behaviors fall into four main groupings: aggressive behavior that either threatens or actually causes harm to others; nonaggressive property destruction; covert aggressive behaviors of deceitfulness or theft; and rule violations (APA, 1994). For a diagnosis of CD to be made, at least three criterion behaviors must be present during the past 12 months, with one behavior present in the last 6 months. The DSM-IV criteria have been found to have internal consistency, test–retest reliability, and validity (Lahey, Applegate, Barkley, et al., 1994).

The disturbance in behavior must also cause impairment to the child or adolescent in social, occupational, or academic functioning. The behavior pattern is usually present in a variety of settings, such as home, school, and/or the community. With the exception of requiring that the criteria for adult antisocial personality disorder (ASPD) are not present if the individual is aged 18 years or more, there are no exclusionary criteria. Youth with any diagnosable neuropsychiatric illness (such as depression, an organic condition such as a seizure disorder or head trauma, or schizophrenia) can be additionally diagnosed with CD if their behavior over the past year meets inclusionary and exclusionary criteria.

Youth with CD often have many problematic associated features that are not specifically part of the diagnostic criteria but can cause additional impairment. They may express little empathy and little concern for the emotions, well-being, wishes, and concerns of others. A group of children exhibiting many psychopathic traits, such as callousness toward others and a lack of emotionality, has been identified in clinically referred samples (Christian, Frick, Hill, Tyler, & Frazier, 1997). These more psychopathic traits seem to designate a unique group of youngsters who show a very severe pattern of antisocial behavior, corresponding closely to conceptualizations of adult psychopathy (Cleckley, 1976). Poor frustration tolerance, impulsive responding, irritability, temper outbursts, and reckless behavior without regard to their own safety or the well-being of others are other frequent associated features. CD is also often associated with an early onset of sexual behavior, use of illicit substances and alcohol, and involvement in dangerous activities.

The overall prevalence rates of CD for both boys and girls combined, estimated from seven recent cross-sectional studies in the general population, vary between 0.9% and 8.7% (Bauermeister, Canino, & Bird, 1994). This is somewhat less than the overall prevalence rates of 2% to 16% for CD given in DSM-IV (APA, 1994). Prevalence rates vary, depending on the nature of the population sampled, the time frame of sampling (6 vs. 12 months), gender, urban versus rural residence, and method of ascertainment (cross-sectional vs. longitudinal study design). Males generally have higher prevalence rates than females. In the review of Bauermeister et al. (1994), cross-sectional prevalence rates vary between 1.5% and 10.4% for males and between 0% and 8.0% for females.

Subtypes

Childhood-Onset versus Adolescent-Onset CD. At present, two subtypes of CD are recognized by DSM-IV. In the childhood-onset type, one criterion behavior is present prior to the age of 10 years. In the adolescent-onset type, all the constituent behaviors for diagnosis begin after 10 years of age. Although it has been known for some time that age at onset of antisocial behavior has important implications, the current DSM-IV subtyping largely reflects the work of Moffitt (1993a, 1993b). She has presented evidence that a relatively small group of children (generally boys) with onset of aggressive and antisocial behaviors in childhood (as contrasted with onset in adolescence) display many features suggestive of chronic psychopathology and neuropsychiatric disease. They display neuropsychological deficits; comorbid sustained attentional deficits; failure to inhibit impulsive responding; chronic learning failure and academic underachievement; more violent antisocial behaviors; aggressive and antisocial behaviors that are generally committed alone and not part of a larger social group, such as a gang; a family history characterized by antisocial activities; and a higher risk for a more persistent and chronic course of antisocial activity across development. In epidemiological samples, this early-onset group accounts for a disproportionate amount of illegal activities, despite constituting a tiny fraction of the total population of youngsters.

In contrast, youth with adolescent-onset CD (who generally include girls as well as boys) express less violence in their antisocial activities, and generally desist from such behaviors when they achieve economic, psychological, and educational levels of adult independence in society (Moffitt, 1993a). Although not all studies agree (see Sanford et al., 1999), subsequent research into the validity of the DSM-IV subtypes of CD has generally supported this developmental division into a childhood-onset and an adolescent-onset type. Research finds a steep decline in aggressive behavior (but not nonaggressive antisocial behaviors) when CD begins at around 10 years (Lahey et al., 1998). Youths with earlier ages of onset engage in more conduct problems, especially physical aggression, than youths with later ages of onset (Lahey, Goodman, et al., 1999). The early-onset, persistent subtype of CD is characteristic of about 5% of males in the population (Moffitt, 1993a; Robins, 1985).

Undersocialized Aggressive and Socialized Delinquent CD. Another method of subtyping CD in children is based on whether a child belongs to a deviant social group and commits antisocial acts as part of such a group, or whether the child is not capable of forming social attachments and tends to commit antisocial acts alone. Although this dimension of CD is no longer formally recognized in DSM-IV, a distinction between undersocialized and socialized forms of aggression and conduct problems has emerged in over 50 years of empirical research investigating problem behaviors in youth. These studies used multivariate statistical methods to factor-analyze problem behaviors in large numbers of youth, both those in the community and those who were clinically referred for mental health or special educational services. In almost all of these investigations, these two dimensions of conduct problem behaviors in youth were repeatedly identified (see Quay, 1986a, for a review). These two syndromes have been labeled "undersocialized aggressive" and "socialized delinquent" (Quay, 1993).

The principal characteristics of undersocialized aggressive CD are physical violence, fighting, bullying and intentionally intimidating others, disruptiveness, exploitativeness, and impaired social relationships with both peers and adults. Youth with undersocialized forms of CD appear to have an impairment in their ability to form social bonds with others. They generally commit violent and antisocial acts alone, and not as part of a larger social group such as a gang. In contrast, socialized delinquent CD is exhibited by youth who are also aggressive, but commit antisocial acts largely as part of a social group. The socialized syndrome involves truancy from school and home, furtive group stealing, group drug and alcohol use, cheating, and having "bad" companions. Social relationships with adults and authority figures may be disturbed, but close relations with and loyalty toward peers of the same behavioral persuasion are maintained. Youth with undersocialized aggressive CD are generally highly aggressive, whereas youth with socialized delinquent CD engage more frequently in nonaggressive antisocial behavior (Frick, 1998).

This method of subtyping has been found to have several important clinical implications. Compared to youth with socialized delinquent CD, those with unsocialized aggressive CD tend to exhibit more neuropsychological deficits in such domains as attribution, self-regulation, moral development, empathy, and impulse control. For example, children and adolescents with undersocialized aggressive CD infer greater hostility on the part of others, exhibit a diminished capacity to inhibit responding and verbally self-regulate behavior, demonstrate lower levels of moral reasoning, show less empathy toward others, and have less skill in understanding the perspective of others than youth with the socialized delinquent syndrome. They are also more impulsive and more easily bored, and do not as easily learn to change their behavior in response to negative consequences. Compared to youth with socialized delinquent CD, they have poorer peer relations, are more treatment-resistant when placed in juvenile corrections programs or mental health treatment settings, and have a poorer long-term prognosis (see Quay, 1986b).

Despite the promise of this subtyping, confusion has arisen over the core features that distinguish undersocialized aggressive CD from socialized delinquent CD. It remains unclear whether the principal emphasis should be placed on a capacity for social attachment (e.g., a youngster has loyal friends or no friends), on the context in which antisocial acts are committed (e.g., antisocial acts are committed as part of a group or alone), or on the frequency and intensity of physical aggression (youth with undersocialized aggressive CD are more aggressive than those with socialized delinquent CD). Because aggression is easier to define and because aggression may be the principal component that leads to a poor outcome in this group, DSM-III-R (APA, 1987) focused on distinguishing children with CD who demonstrated aggressive behavior from those that did not. The undersocialized aggressive form of CD defined in DSM-III (APA, 1980) was changed to solitary aggressive CD and socialized delinquent CD was changed to the group type of CD in DSM-III-R (APA, 1987), to emphasize this distinction. As noted above, in the current DSM-IV classification the emphasis is now on distinguishing between childhood-onset and adolescent-onset CD.

The Relationship between CD and Aggression

CD is the prototypic categorical childhood psychiatric diagnosis associated with aggressive and related behaviors. In the DSM-IV criteria for diagnosis, 7 out of 15 behaviors involve direct aggression toward others. In the ICD-10 criteria for diagnosis, 7 out of 23 behaviors describe aggression directed toward others. Support for the relationship of CD to aggression is found in studies examining the adult outcomes of children and adolescents diagnosed with

CD. Although most youth who meet criteria for CD in childhood or adolescence do not progress to a pattern of persistent aggression and antisocial behavior such as ASPD in adulthood, the likelihood of such outcomes is much greater for children diagnosed with CD than for children who do not meet criteria for this disorder. (As noted above, this is especially true of the childhood-onset subtype.) Studies have shown that between 25% and 40% of youth with CD will eventually meet criteria for ASPD as adults (Robins, 1966; Zoccolillo, Pickles, Quinton, & Rutter, 1992).

Oppositional Defiant Disorder

Description and Prevalence

The essential feature of ODD (APA, 1994) is a recurring pattern of defiant, disobedient, negativistic, and hostile behavior toward authority figures that is clearly more frequent, intense, and persistent across the child's or adolescent's development than is typically observed in individuals of similar age and developmental level. Diagnosis requires that symptoms be present for at least 6 months and cause impairment in the youth's social, academic, or occupational functioning. The diagnosis is not made if ODD symptoms occur only during the course of a psychotic or mood disorder. In these cases, the symptoms of ODD are felt to be part of the underlying disorder. In addition, the diagnosis of ODD is not given if symptoms occur within the context of CD or ASPD (in individuals over age 18 years). In these cases, the more serious diagnosis takes precedence.

Associated features include low self-esteem, mood lability, low frustration tolerance, swearing, and the possibility of early-onset alcohol and substance experimentation and misuse. Commonly, conflicts between the youth and parents occur at home; conflict can also occur with familiar adults and peers at school and in the community. Because the symptoms of ODD are normal in preschoolers and adolescents, the diagnosis is only given when symptoms are more intense, more frequent, and cause more impairment than in children and adolescents of comparable age. The onset of a clinically recognizable disorder (as contrasted to normal developmental oppositional symptoms) is usually evident by age 8 years.

Prevalence rates vary by the characteristics of the sample studied (clinical vs. community) and study design. Rates between 2% and 16% have been reported (APA, 1994).

The Relationship between ODD and Aggression

The direct relationship between ODD and aggressive behavior is generally weak (August, Realmuto, Joyce, & Hektner, 1999). In youth who meet diagnostic criteria for ODD, conflicts are usually verbal and do not escalate to physical aggression. However, rather than being directly related, ODD may be importantly related in a more indirect manner to the risk of developing aggressive behavior. Most children who meet diagnostic criteria for ODD do not develop CD at a later age. However, in those who do develop CD, the onset of symptomatic ODD generally occurs earlier in development than the onset of CD symptoms (August et al., 1999; Loeber, Lahey, & Thomas, 1991). In youth with CD, ODD symptoms predict later CD symptoms, such as CD symptoms predict ASPD in adults (Lahey, Applegate, Barkley, et al., 1994). In other words, ODD and CD seem to be strongly and developmentally related. Studies thus suggest that the onset of ODD symptoms may be a possible first step toward a life course characterized by the emergence of more serious antisocial and violent acts for some (but not all) children (August et al., 1999; Loeber, 1990).

Similarly, ODD symptoms in adolescence have been found to be distinct from CD symptoms. Independently of CD, adolescent ODD symptoms have been shown to be a distinct antecedent of adult antisocial outcome (Langbehn, Cadoret, Yates, Troughton, & Stewart, 1998). These results likewise suggest that although ODD is not strongly and directly related to aggressive behavior in youth, it may have important developmental implications for the possibility of later aggressive outcomes for some, but not all, children with ODD.

Attention-Deficit/Hyperactivity Disorder

Description and Prevalence

ADHD is presently thought to contain two major symptom domains: (1) inattention (sustained attentional deficits), and (2) hyperactive–impulsive behavior (disinhibition) (Barkley, 1996; McBurnett et al., 1999). The essential feature of ADHD is a persisting pattern of inattention and/or hyperactivity-impulsivity that is more severe and frequent than is typically seen in individuals at a comparable stage of development (APA, 1994). Some symptoms must be present before the age of 7 years and must clearly interfere with developmentally appropriate social, academic, or occupational functioning. Symptoms must cause interference in two or more settings, such as home, school, community, or work. ADHD is not diagnosed if the symptoms occur only in the context of a pervasive developmental disorder (e.g., autistic disorder) or a psychotic disorder (e.g., schizophrenia), and if they are not better accounted for by another psychiatric disorder (such as a mood, anxiety, dissociative, or personality disorder).

The symptom of inattention is displayed by individuals with ADHD relative to normal individuals of the same age and gender. "Attention" is a multidimensional neuropsychological construct that can refer to alertness, arousal, selectivity, sustained attention, distractibility, or span of apprehension (Barkley, 1998). Persons who meet criteria for ADHD have been found to have their greatest attentional difficulties with sustaining their attention to tasks, especially if the tasks are not immediately reinforcing; these problems are also referred to as deficits in persistence of effort or vigilance. These deficits are not apparent when the task is immediately reinforcing to the child, such as playing a video game or watching a movie. However, when effort is required to sustain attention, such as in completing homework assignments, music lessons, reading, or multistep assignments that require organizational skills, the problems with inattention become obvious in comparison with individuals who do not suffer from ADHD (Barkley, 1996, 1998). Those with ADHD are more disorganized, distracted, and forgetful, and more often fail to finish assignments or chores, than others of the same age and developmental level. Deficits in sustained attention are strongly correlated with academic and occupational underachievement, but not necessarily with negative later life outcomes such as violence, other aggression, or antisocial behaviors (Barkley, 1996; Fischer, Barkley, Fletcher, & Smallish, 1993a; McBurnett et al., 1999).

The symptoms of hyperactivity–impulsivity include difficulties with squirming, fidgetiness, staying seated when required, constant motion, disturbing others when playing, talking excessively, interrupting others' activities, and difficulties awaiting one's turn when required to do so. Individuals meeting criteria for ADHD often express their impulsivity by rushing into things without stopping to think of the consequences of their actions, being constantly in motion, and having difficulty resisting temptations and delaying gratification. In children who go on to meet criteria for ADHD, hyperactive–impulsive symptoms often emerge first in development, by about 3–4 years of age. In the school years, difficulties with sustained attention and task persistence become problematic at about 5–7 years of age (Barkley, 1996). These children have difficulty inhibiting their behavior, and the symptoms of hyperactivity–impulsivity are seen as neuropsychological symptoms of behavioral disinhibition (Barkley, 1998). Childhood symptoms of hyperactivity-impulsivity are strongly related to increased risk for adolescent and adult negative outcomes, including aggression, CD, and adult ASPD (Babinski, Hartsough, & Lambert, 1999; Barkley, 1996; Fischer, Barkley, Fletcher, & Smallish, 1993b; McBurnett et al., 1999; Weiss & Hechtman, 1993).

The associated features of ADHD are considerable, though they vary according to the individual's age and developmental stage. In childhood, low frustration tolerance, temper outbursts, mood lability, stubbornness, parent–child conflicts, social skill difficulties, peer rejection, and low self-esteem may occur. As a child with ADHD grows older, poor academic and eventual vocational underachievement may become problematic. Individuals meeting criteria for ADHD have increased risks for the development of ODD and CD. They are also at increased risk for developing mood and anxiety disorders. Intellectual development may be somewhat lower as well; this may be caused by an interaction between the symptom domain of hyperactivity–impulsivity and diminished Verbal IQ in children with ADHD, accounting for 3% to 10% of the variance in IQ found between persons with ADHD and normal controls (Barkley, 1996; Hinshaw, 1992).

The prevalence of ADHD as defined by the DSM or ICD has been studied in a number of different countries, including the United States (as well as Puerto Rico), New Zealand, Germany, India, China, Brazil, and the Netherlands. Prevalence rates vary as a function of age sampled, gender, and methodological design (e.g., parent report, self-report). All prevalence studies to date have utilized earlier versions of DSM (DSM-III or DSM-III-R; APA, 1980, 1987) or ICD (ICD-9; WHO, 1978) rather than the current DSM-IV and ICD-10. These studies indicate that the prevalence of ADHD ranges from 1.4% to 13.3% (Barkley, 1998; Szatmari, 1992). Prevalence is higher for males than for females; male-to-female ratios range from 2.5:1 to 5.6:1 (Szatmari, 1992). Prevalence is also affected by age and development, with adolescent samples having a generally lower prevalence rate than child samples. Finally, these data indicate that children and adolescents meeting diagnostic criteria for ADHD can be found throughout the world, since ADHD has been identified in every country in which it has been studied.

Subtypes

ADHD-Combined Type, and ADHD, Predominantly Hyperactive–Impulsive Type. Currently, three subtypes of ADHD are recognized in the DSM-IV. Research suggests that ADHD, combined type (ADHD-C), and ADHD, predominantly hyperactive–impulsive type (ADHD-PHI), may actually be different developmental stages of the same type of ADHD. ADHD-PHI is commonly found in preschoolers with ADHD, and ADHD-C is found in school-age children with the disorder. This is the progression that one would expect developmentally if hyperactive–impulsive symptoms precede sustained attention deficits in ADHD (Barkley, 1998; Loeber, Green, Lahey, Christ, & Frick, 1992). ADHD, predominantly inattentive type (ADHD-PI), is the third subtype found in DSM-IV. There appears to be qualitative differences between the ADHD-PI type on the one hand, and the ADHD-C and ADHD-PHI types on the other. Research is beginning to suggest that ADHD-PI may be a distinct disorder from ADHD. For example, the impairments in attention may differ in ADHD-PI. Whereas ADHD-C and ADHD-PHI are associated more closely with problems in sustained attention, persistence of effort, vigilance, and difficulties with distractibility, ADHD-PI seems to be more strongly associated with focused/selective attention and sluggish information processing (Barkley, 1998).

Outcomes also differ across these subtypes. The central problem of disinhibition in the ADHD-C and ADHD-PHI combined and hyperactive-impulsive subtypes predicts negative outcomes in adolescence and adulthood, including increased problems with aggression, antisocial behavior, social skill deficits, poorer occupational functioning, and persistence of ADHD symptoms (Barkley, 1996, 1998). As noted above, deficits in sustained attention (i.e., ADHD-PI) appear to predict only academic difficulties, such as problems completing homework (Lahey, Applegate, McBurnett, et al., 1994; McBurnett et al., 1999). At present, it is unclear whether ADHD-PI is actually a subtype of ADHD or constitutes a separate disorder.

Comorbid ADHD and CD. Although it is not presently recognized in the DSM-IV as a subtype of ADHD, some researchers and clinicians consider the combination of ADHD and CD to be a distinct ADHD subtype. The combination is recognized in ICD-10 as hyperkinetic CD, which combines symptoms of CD and ADHD into one diagnosis. Although the two syndromes are partially separable, studies document much overlap between attention deficits/hyperactivity and conduct problems/aggression (Hinshaw, 1987). Children meeting diagnostic criteria for ADHD often meet diagnostic criteria for CD, and vice versa (Biederman, Newcorn, & Sprich, 1991; Pliszka, 1998). When clinic-referred children with ADHD are studied, up to 50% meet criteria for both disorders (Stewart, Cummings, Singer, & deBlois, 1981). In nonreferred community samples, up to 30% of children with ADHD exhibit this comorbidity (Szatmari, Boyle, & Offord, 1989). Children, especially boys, exhibiting both ADHD and aggressive CD appear to be at the highest risk for aggression, continuing antisocial behavior, and antisocial adult outcomes.

Support for the idea of increased risk as a result of ADHD-CD comorbidity has been suggested by a number of longitudinal outcome studies. For example, Moffitt (1990a) followed a birth cohort of 435 boys for 13 years. At age 13, four groups were defined on the basis of self-reported delinquency and other antisocial behavior, as well as a professional diagnosis of DSM-III attention deficit disorder (ADD): "ADD + delinquent," "ADD only," "delinquent only," and "nondisordered." The comorbid group (ADD + delinquent) consistently fared the worst, with antisocial behavior that began before school age, escalated at school entry, and persisted into adolescence. In another example, Fischer et al. (1993a) followed 123 hyperactive children prospectively for 8 years. Results indicated that hyperactive children with significant aggressive behavior had a much greater risk of poor outcomes in many spheres of activity, including oppositional defiant and antisocial behavior. In a 4-year longitudinal study, increased rates of SUDs, mood disorders, and family conflict were found in boys with the combination of ADHD and CD (Biederman, Mick, Faraone, & Burback, 2001). Because their prognosis is distinct from that of youth with ADHD alone or CD alone, many consider the combination of ADHD-CD a distinct ADHD subtype that predicts poor outcome (Mannuzza, Gittelman-Klein, Bessler, Malloy, & LaPadula, 1993).

The Relationship between ADHD and Aggression

ADHD has an important relationship to aggression, antisocial behavior, and antisocial outcomes. For example, ADHD is a risk factor for antisocial maladjustment in adolescence and adulthood. Several longitudinal studies have now followed children diagnosed in the elementary school years with ADHD for periods of 4–14 years. All of these studies have found, in comparison with normal controls (youth without ADHD and without other psychopathology), a higher rate of externalizing behavior disorders and an increased risk for aggressive behavior, delinquency, and other antisocial behavior (August, Stewart, & Holmes, 1983; Barkley, Fischer, Edelbrock, & Smallish, 1990; Hechtman, Weiss, & Perlman, 1984; Mannuzza, Klein, & Addalli, 1991; Taylor, Chadwick, Heptinstall, & Danckaerts, 1996).

Although it is clear that ADHD and aggression can be related, the nature of the relationship and the developmental mechanisms that confer increased risk are not yet clear. For instance, given that ADHD and CD are often diagnosed in the same child and that early-onset CD increases risk for continued aggressive/antisocial behaviors, this increased risk may be a function of the comorbidity between these two diagnoses. As noted above, the overlap between ADHD and CD is well above the rates that would be expected by chance. However, despite some evidence supporting a distinct subtype of ADHD-CD, other research has found it to be unlikely that ADHD and CD are in reality only one disorder for which different labels are applied. Indeed, although they may partially overlap and have high rates of comorbidity (Hinshaw, 1987), studies have supported the distinctiveness of these two diagnoses (Schachar & Tannock, 1995). Thus the relationship between ADHD and aggression may be explained by high rates of comorbidity with CD.

Second, increased risk for aggressive behavior in ADHD may be related to the specific symptom domain of hyperactivity–impulsivity in ADHD. Taylor et al. (1996) have presented evidence from a 9-year follow-up study of 112 hyperactive children originally assessed at ages 6–7 and reassessed at ages 16–18. They argue for the primacy of early-onset hyperactivity and not early-onset CD as the major developmental risk factor for poor outcomes in children with ADHD. In their sample, hyperactivity in the primary school years was a risk factor for later development, including poor peer relationships, violent and disruptive behaviors, a lack of involvement in socially constructive activities, and poor academic achievement. The risk attaching to hyperactivity could not be accounted for solely by the extent to which it was initially associated with symptoms of CD; in this study, hyperactivity without conduct problems in childhood was also a risk factor for antisocial outcome in adolescence. Taylor et al. (1996) concluded that much of the risk of conduct problems stems from the fact that many children who have CD exhibit hyperactivity as well. A developmental model was postulated in which early-onset and pervasive hyperactivity is a risk factor for the eventual development of CD, which then predicts negative adolescent and adult outcomes, including increased risk for aggression.

Subsequent longitudinal research has supported the finding that the ADHD symptom domain of childhood hyperactivity–impulsivity is a risk factor for later antisocial behaviors. In a 26-year longitudinal study, childhood hyperactivity–impulsivity, but not inattention, predicted criminal activity in adulthood (Babinski et al., 1999). Further support for this position is found in other studies that have found a sizable overlap between hyperactive and CD-like behaviors (Sandberg, Rutter, & Taylor, 1978) and between aggressive CD and hyperactivity (Stewart et al., 1981). An example is the study of Prinz, Connor, and Wilson (1981), who evaluated 109 hyperactive and aggressive children aged 6–8 years. Overall, whereas 32% of the hyperactive group were aggressive, 92% of the aggressive group were hyperactive. This study further underscores the possible importance of a relationship between aggression and hyperactivity–impulsivity. Thus the relationship between ADHD and aggression may also be explained by the correlation of the specific ADHD symptom domain of hyperactivity–impulsivity with increased risk for conduct problems and aggressive behaviors.

The relationship between aggression and hyperactivity is complicated, however, and has been the subject of much debate. Not all research supports the primacy of hyperactivity–impulsivity in predicting aggressive outcomes. In their study of children with ADHD, Milich and Loney (1979) found that the initial level of childhood aggression was more predictive of outcome than the initial level of hyperactivity. Others have argued that the behavioral symptoms of aggression and hyperactivity are both symptoms of CD, which itself increases risk for poor developmental outcomes (Sandberg et al., 1978). This position is currently reflected in the ICD-10 criteria for hyperkinetic CD, which combines hyperactive and conduct symptoms in a single diagnosis. Still others have argued that the behavioral symptom of aggression constitutes a secondary symptom of hyperactivity with a different etiology, developmental course, and outcome (Loney & Milich, 1982).

Finally, increased risk for aggressive behavior in ADHD may also be related to the ADHD symptom of inattention. In general, sustained attention deficits and lack of task persistence predict academic underachievement, such as failure to complete homework assignments (Lahey, Applegate, McBurnett, et al., 1994), and not aggressive/antisocial behaviors. However, a few studies have reported that concentration problems are associated with increased risk of aggression, especially in boys. In an epidemiologically defined sample of 1,084 urban first-grade children assessed in the classroom, concentration problems (although not necessarily the psychiatric diagnosis of ADHD) predicted increased aggressive problems in the classroom (Rebok, Hawkins, Krener, Mayer, & Kellam, 1996). In a longitudinal study, attentional problems predicted increased risk for delinquent and other antisocial behavior over a 3-year follow-up period (Stanger, Achenbach, & McConaughy, 1993). Although there may exist a relationship between inattention and aggression, the cumulative evidence is much weaker than that for the relationship between hyperactivity–impulsivity and aggressive behavior.

Summary of the Disruptive Behavior Disorders

The disruptive behavior disorders as identified by the criteria in DSM-IV and ICD-10 have a strong relationship to aggression and related behaviors in children and adolescents who carry these psychiatric diagnoses. At present, this relationship has been studied much more extensively in males than in females. Childhood-onset, aggressive CD, and the symptom domain of hyperactivity–impulsivity in ADHD, appear to be significant risk factors for continued aggression and antisocial outcomes (especially in males). Risk is especially high for children who carry both the diagnosis of CD and the diagnosis of ADHD-PHI or ADHD-C. The ADHD symptom domain of sustained attention deficits carries less risk for aggression. In addition, ODD carries substantially less risk for antisocial outcome; most children with ODD do not develop severe antisocial behavior. In some children however, it may represent the first step in a developmental progression to the more serious diagnosis of CD.

Research is beginning to suggest that one possible developmental mechanism mediating the relationship between the disruptive behavior disorders and aggressive and antisocial outcomes may be deficits in the neuropsychological dimension of behavioral inhibition. As defined here, "behavioral inhibition" means inhibitory processes usually mediated by mechanisms in the prefrontal cortex. When these neurobiological mechanisms do not function optimally (as is thought to be the case in the disruptive behavioral disorders), this dysfunction may manifest itself as early hyperactive and impulsive behavior, and a lack of self-control and inhibition of action in environments that are stimulating, rewarding, or reinforcing of antisocial activity. Impulsivity and early-onset hyperactivity may serve to increase risk for aggressive and antisocial behaviors through a variety of person–environment interactions. An inability to control one's behavior, and a deficit in the capacity to inhibit action and think of consequences—in combination with social risk factors, such as family dysfunction, criminogenic environments, or criminal opportunity—increase risk for such behaviors. Early-onset aggressive behavior is thus highly associated with continuing aggression as development progresses.

As noted above, the capacity for behavioral inhibition is thought to be mediated by intact neurobiological functioning of an area of the brain known as the prefrontal cortex (a component of the frontal lobes) and its extensive connections (Benton, 1991). Whereas data are strongest for behavioral inhibition deficits in ADHD (Barkley, 1997a), these deficits have also been found in CD independently of ADHD (Oosterlaan, Logan, & Sergeant, 1998; White et al., 1994), although not all studies agree (Pennington & Ozonoff, 1996). The study of the developmental mechanisms underlying the connections among early-onset impulsivity–hyperactivity, behavioral disinhibition, and later aggressive/antisocial outcomes is a rich area for multidisciplinary research and collaboration across the disciplines of behavioral science, experimental psychology, sociology, developmental neurobiology, psychiatry, noninvasive radiology, and juvenile justice.

MOOD DISORDERS

The mood disorders encompass several distinct yet overlapping categorical diagnoses. These include major depressive disorder (MDD), dysthymic disorder (DD), and manic–depressive illness (MDI, otherwise known as bipolar disorder).

Major Depressive Disorder

Description and Prevalence

MDD has been increasingly studied over the past 20 years. This research has established that MDD in children and adolescents is a valid psychiatric disorder that can be reliably diagnosed by clinicians, is common in youth, and is a recurrent disorder that often runs in families (American Academy of Child and Adolescent Psychiatry [AACAP], 1998a; Birmaher et al., 1996; Kovacs, Feinberg, Crouse-Novak, Paulauskas, & Finkelstein, 1984; Mc-Cracken, 1992; Puig-Antich et al., 1989). A general consensus has emerged that MDD in children and adolescents is phenomenologically similar to MDD in adults (Kovacs, 1996). Criteria used to diagnose adults with this disorder can therefore also be used to diagnose youth with depression. Furthermore, depressed prepubertal children do not substantially differ in their presentation or clinical symptoms from depressed adolescents (Mitchell, McCauley, Burke, & Moss, 1988; Ryan et al., 1987).

Some age-related developmental differences in symptom presentation should be noted, however. Irritability, hostility, aggression, and anger may be more prevalent in youth diagnosed with MDD than in adults (Biederman & Spencer, 1999; Knox, King, Hanna, Logan, & Ghaziuddin, 2000). For example, in their study of a community sample of depression in adolescent girls, Goodyear and Cooper (1993) reported that 80% of depressed 11- to 16-year-old girls were irritable. Ryan et al. (1987) found that 87% of their depressed children and adolescents reported irritability. Younger children with depression may be less able to report their subjective internal feeling state in words, perhaps because of cognitive immaturity. As such, they may be more likely to act out dysphoric feelings behaviorally. Depressed prepubertal children also appear to have fewer neurovegetative symptoms than depressed adults. Compared to depressed adults, youth suffering from depression have been found to have more guilt, lower self-esteem, and more unexplained somatic complaints (e.g., stomachaches and headaches). Although depressed prepubertal children have been found to have suicidal ideation and to make multiple suicide attempts, the lethality of their attempts is less than that for depressed adolescents and adults (Mitchell et al., 1988).

Interpersonal and family relationships are often severely impaired during an episode of MDD. For example, Puig-Antich et al. (1985) found that, compared to neurotic children, depressed children had relationships with their mothers, fathers, and siblings that were characterized by more irritable, hostile, and angry feelings. Depression in children and adolescents is associated with an increased risk for suicidal ideation, suicide attempts, and completed suicide. An increased risk for various SUDs has also been found for depressed youth (Kandel & Davies, 1986). Moreover, childhood and adolescent-onset depression is characterized by increased risk for homicidal ideation in later adolescence and adulthood (Birmaher et al., 1996).

MDD with onset in childhood or adolescence rarely occurs in the absence of other diagnosable psychiatric disorders. In youth with MDD, up to 90%

also meet criteria for at least one other psychiatric diagnosis. Two or more comorbid diagnoses are found in 20% to 50% of youngsters with depression (AACAP, 1998a; Angold & Costello, 1992; Kovacs, 1996). Anxiety disorders and comorbidity with chronic low-grade depression or DD are most common (Birmaher et al., 1996).

The natural course of depression has been studied in children and adolescents, and MDD has been found to be a remitting but relapsing disorder with increased risk for recurrence after an initial episode. Clinical and epidemiological studies in children and adolescents have found that the mean length of an episode of MDD is approximately 7–9 months (see Birmaher et al., 1996; Kovacs, Feinberg, Crouse-Novak, Paulauskas, & Finkelstein, 1984). Although the majority of MDD episodes will remit by 2 years after onset in 90% of cases (Kovacs, Feinberg, Crouse-Novak, Paulauskas, & Finkelstein, 1984; Kovacs, Feinberg, Crouse-Novak, Paulauskas, Pollack, & Finkelstein, 1984), the cumulative probability of recurrence is 40% by 2 years and rises to 70% by 5 years (see AACAP, 1998a; Birmaher et al., 1996). Childhood-onset depression can persist into adolescence and increase risk for recurrent depression into adulthood (Harrington, Fudge, Rutter, Pickles, & Hill, 1990; Weissman, Wolk, et al., 1999).

Prevalence of MDD varies by age. Children of elementary school age report low rates, but rates rise with adolescence to approach those of adults. Population studies report prevalence rates of MDD ranging between 0.4% and 2.5% in children, and between 0.4% and 8.3% in adolescents (for reviews, see Birmaher et al., 1996; Fleming & Offord, 1990; Hammen & Rudolph, 1996). Prevalence rates also vary by gender, with higher rates reported in female than in male adolescents. For example, Cohen et al. (1993) reported a prevalence rate of 7.6% in 14- to 16-year-old girls compared with 1.6% in boys of the same age, with a peak in the gender differences in these rates at age 14 years. In the prepubertal age range, the male-to-female ratio for MDD is about 1:1 (Birmaher et al., 1996).

Investigations of clinic-referred and community samples of adults and children with MDD have reported a secular increase in this disorder. This means that individuals born in the latter half of the 20th century appear to be at greater risk for developing MDD, and for doing so at younger ages of onset, than persons born in the early part of the century (Gershon, Hamovit, Gurnoff, & Nurnberger, 1987; Kovacs & Gatsonis, 1994). The reasons for this secular increase are presently unclear.

Subtypes and Comorbidity

MDD and CD. Much research links MDD and CD in clinically referred youth (Puig-Antich, 1982), although the co-occurrence of these two disorders is not an officially recognized subtype of depression. Children with depression frequently meet criteria for CD (Biederman, Faraone, Mick, & Lelon, 1995; Weissman, Wolk, et al., 1999), and children with CD frequently meet criteria for MDD (Biederman et al., 2001; Riggs, Baker, Mikulich, Young, &

Crowley, 1995; Zoccolillo, 1992). This type of comorbidity appears to be characterized by high amounts of irritability, antisocial behaviors, and physical aggression. For example, in a study of psychiatric disorders in youth admitted to a juvenile detention center for a variety of legal offenses, 42% were found to suffer from depression (Pliszka, Sherman, Barrow, & Irick, 2000). In Puig-Antich's sample (1982) of 43 prepubertal boys with MDD, 37% were comorbid for CD. Of the boys with both diagnoses, 75% had histories of physical aggression. Which disorder comes first in development, and is thus the primary disorder, is unclear. Some research documents the onset of comorbid conditions such as CD before the onset of MDD (Biederman et al., 1995, 2001); other studies report the onset of MDD before CD (Puig-Antich, 1982).

In addition to being comorbid conditions, MDD and CD may represent a distinct subtype of depression. Odds of developing ASPD in adulthood are increased in youngsters who suffer from depression (Kasen et al., 2001). These children and adolescents have been found to have depression characterized by increased severity, worse short-term outcome, fewer recurrences of depression, a lower familial aggregation of mood disorders, a higher incidence of adult criminality and other antisocial behavior, and the possibility of increased risk for SUDs, compared to depression not comorbid with CD (see Birmaher et al., 1996; Puig-Antich et al., 1989; Marmorstein & Iacono, 2001; Riggs et al., 1995).

MDD and ADHD. Similarly, there exist high rates of comorbidity between ADHD and MDD in clinically referred children and adolescents (Biederman et al., 1991, 1995). The presence of both disorders can increase the risk of impulsivity, irritability, and aggression. The most well-done studies show prevalence rates of 9% to 38% for depression in children with ADHD (Pliszka, 1998). Depressive symptoms generally have a developmental onset after ADHD symptoms (Biederman et al., 1995).

Psychotic Depression. MDD with psychotic features is a depressive subtype found in DSM-IV. Psychotic depression is characterized by the development of associated delusions and hallucinations. Before puberty, psychotic depression appears to be manifested mostly in auditory hallucinations. With cognitive growth and development, adolescent psychotic depression can be characterized by both hallucinations and delusions. The psychotic subtype of MDD is characterized by more severe depression, poorer prognosis, increased risk of bipolar outcome, and treatment resistance to antidepressant monotherapy (Strober, Lampert, Schmidt, & Morrel, 1993).

MDD and Risk for Bipolar Outcome. Relevant to a discussion of the relationships between mood disorders and aggression is the elevated risk for MDI (bipolar disorder) in children and adolescents diagnosed with early-onset MDD. Aggression, assaultiveness, irritability, and hostility can be prominent symptoms of bipolar disorder. Youths with MDD may convert (switch) to bipolar illness more frequently than do depressed adults (Kovacs, 1996). Follow-up studies have found that 20% to 40% of adolescents with MDD develop bipolar illness within a period of 5 years after their first index episode of depression (Geller, Fox, & Clark, 1994; Strober et al., 1993). Clinical characteristics associated with an increased risk of developing bipolar disorder in adolescence and adulthood include early-onset MDD; depression characterized by rapid onset, psychotic features, or psychomotor retardation; a multigenerational family history of mood disorders; and the development of mania upon exposure to antidepressant medication for the treatment of depression (Geller et al., 1994; Strober & Carlson, 1982).

Dysthymic Disorder

Description

The clinical characteristics of DD include a persistent and long-term change in mood that is generally less intense than in MDD, but is often more chronic over the course of development. The ICD-10 criteria are similar but require the presence of at least 2 years of dysthymic symptoms, whereas DSM-IV requires only 1 year of symptoms for children and adolescents. DD has been recognized as a valid psychiatric disorder that is related to, but distinct from, MDD (Kovacs, Akiskal, Gatsonis, & Parrone, 1994). It often precedes the onset of an MDD episode (Kovacs, Feinberg, Crouse-Novak, Paulauskas, Pollak, & Finkelstein, 1984). DD can have a very early age of onset and has been identified in preschool children (Kashani, Allan, Beck, Bledsoe, & Reid, 1997).

Childhood DD has a protracted course and lasts much longer than an episode of MDD. The mean episode duration of DD is approximately 3–4 years. Early-onset DD is a potent risk factor for the eventual development of MDD in youth and typically precedes the onset of an MDD episode in children and adolescents. It has been found that the overwhelming majority of youth with DD will eventually develop MDD, with the first depressive episode generally occurring 2–3 years after the onset of DD. Of youth meeting criteria for DD, 11% will develop MDD within 1 year of the onset of DD. The simultaneous occurrence of DD and MDD is called "double depression." Double depression is associated with a high degree of psychiatric and psychosocial morbidity. The increased risk for recurrence of depression in dysthymic youth suggests that DD may be one of the gateways to the development of recurrent mood disorder (Kovacs, Akiskal, et al., 1994; Kovacs, Feinberg, Crouse-Novak, Paulauskas, & Finkelstein, 1984; Kovacs, Feinberg, Crouse-Novak, Paulauskas, Pollock, & Finkelstein, 1984).

Comorbidity

Like MDD, DD is associated with a high prevalence of comorbid psychiatric conditions. About 70% of youth with DD have double depression (see above).

CD and ADHD are reported in 24% to 31% of juveniles with DD. Approximately 15% meet criteria for two or more psychiatric disorders (see Birmaher et al., 1996). Kovacs, Akiskal, et al. (1994) reported that bipolar disorder developed in 13% of their sample with DD. No secular increase in DD, unlike MDD, has been found.

The Relationship between MDD, DD, and Aggression

There appears to exist a substantial relationship between MDD and DD in children and adolescents on the one hand, and increased risk for aggression and related behaviors on the other. This relationship has been found both in clinically referred depressed youth (Knox et al., 2000) and in adolescents incarcerated in juvenile justice settings (Pliszka et al., 2000).

The relationship may be mediated in several ways. Resentment, anger, hostility, and irritability are commonly associated with depressive disorders. An increased risk for aggression in early-onset depressive disorders may be mediated in part by these emotions. Depressed children and adolescents may be less able to control the expression of anger and hostility than depressed adults. Because of their cognitive and developmental immaturity, they may have a more difficult time suppressing anger and resentment. As such, there may exist an increased risk for the behavioral expression of these emotions in depressed youth. Evidence for this comes from several sources. Blumberg and Izard (1985) found that maladaptive expressions of anger, aggressive behavior, and denial of angry feelings were correlated with childhood-onset depression. Another study investigated anger expression styles in depressed and matched nondepressed children admitted to a child inpatient psychiatry unit. Depressed children reported significantly more difficulty maintaining cognitive control over their anger than matched nondepressed children did. Family factors across the two groups of depressed and nondepressed children were not found to affect this finding (Kashani, Dahlmeier, Borduin, Soltys, & Reid, 1995). Depressed children in this study were found to have levels of anger expression equivalent to those of children with CD. This study provides support for the idea that depressed children do not suppress their anger as has been found for depressed adults (Riley, Treiber, & Woods, 1989).

A relationship between depression, irritability, and hostility, and the maladaptive behavioral expression of aggression, has been found to begin early in life. In a study of clinically referred children aged 2–6 years, aggressive behavior involving physical assault was found in 100% of children meeting criteria for DD (Kashani et al., 1997).

Next, the relationship of aggression and related behaviors to depressive disorders may be mediated by comorbidity. As discussed above, CD and ADHD co-occur with depressive disorders at rates that far exceed chance levels (Zoccolillo, 1992). This appears true for both males and females. Both CD and ADHD are highly associated with aggressive and antisocial behaviors, especially when these two disorders co-occur. When hyperactivity, impulsive responding, a lack of behavioral inhibition, irritability, hostility, and anger are comorbid with depression, they may create a potent behavioral and emotional mix that can explode into aggression with minimal environmental provocation.

Finally, MDD comorbid with CD symptoms, anger attacks, and physical aggression may constitute a distinct and identifiable subtype of depression. Significant distinctions in phenomenology, family history, and outcome have been found when youth with comorbid MDD and CD have been compared to youth suffering from MDD without CD comorbidity (Biederman et al., 1995; Puig-Antich et al., 1989; Riggs et al., 1995). Support for the possibility of aggressive subtypes in depression also comes from studies of adults with depression. In a series of depressed adult outpatients, 44% reported anger attacks associated with signs of autonomic nervous system (ANS) overarousal and a rapid crescendo of overwhelming anger (Fava et al., 1993). Neuroendocrine studies showed this irritable, explosive, depressed subgroup to possess signs of greater central nervous system (CNS) serotonin (5-HT) dysregulation, compared to the depressed group without anger attacks (Rosenbaum et al., 1993). These findings are consistent with a hypothesis (van Praag, 1986) that disturbances in CNS 5-HT functioning form a common etiology for dysregulation of mood and affect and dysregulation of aggressive behavior.

Manic–Depressive Illness (Bipolar Disorder)

Description and Prevalence

MDI (also known as bipolar disorder) is a disturbance of affect regulation characterized by abnormal mood and mental excitement usually causing a marked change in a youth's baseline level of functioning (AACAP, 1997a). Abnormalities in mood alternate between depression and manic excitement. The change in the youngster's level of daily functioning is severe enough to be generally observable by others in his or her environment. Children and adolescents are currently diagnosed with MDI according to the same criteria used for adults. (DSM-IV actually defines several types of bipolar disorders, rather than MDI per se; see "Types and Comorbidity," below.)

Manic symptoms can include elation, irritability, increased energy with hyperactivity, racing thoughts, pressured rapid speech, a decreased need for sleep, an increased involvement in pleasurable activities (e.g., adolescents' spending more money than they can afford or engaging in conspicuous sexual indiscretions), and psychotic symptoms. Some developmental differences in symptom presentation should be noted. Children with MDI who are under 9 years of age may have more irritability, hostility, extreme aggression, and emotional lability than youth with later-onset MDI. They may also have less grandiosity and fewer delusions. Discrete manic and depressive episodes may be more difficult to identify in preadolescents with MDI; these children may present to clinicians with a more chronic, continuous, and nonepisodic course.

Impulsivity, hyperactivity, concentration deficits, unmanageable temper tantrums, explosive anger, prolonged aggressive episodes, affective lability, and agitation may be predominant symptoms in younger children with MDI. It remains controversial whether MDI can be found in prepubertal children, and, if so, what it looks like. Historically, few children have been diagnosed with MDI (Anthony & Scott, 1960; Kraepelin, 1921). More recently, Goodwin and Jamison (1990) found that only 3 of 898 (0.3%) adults with MDI reported onset before age 10 years. However, recent research has begun to question the view that a clinical syndrome resembling MDI is rare in children (Biederman, Faraone, Chu, & Wozniak, 1999). For example, in a sample of 79 children aged 6–12 with depression, Geller et al. (1994) reported that MDI developed in 25 juveniles (32%). This research suggests the possibility that MDI in youth, especially in those less than 12 years of age, may be underrecognized and consequently underdiagnosed by mental health clinicians. Underdiagnosis may occur because of developmental differences in symptom presentation; comorbidity and symptomatic overlap with more common childhood psychiatric disorders, such as CD or ADHD; natural course of illness; and phenomenology that might make childhood-onset MDI appear different from the classic manic–depressive syndrome described in the literature. A low base rate of MDI among prepubertal children, compared to the frequency of such conditions as ADHD or CD, might also lead to clinical underrecognition (Biederman, Faraone, Chu, et al., 1999; Bowring & Kovacs, 1992).

There exists more agreement among researchers and clinicians that classic MDI occurs in the adolescent years and closely resembles symptoms found in bipolar adults. When adults with diagnosed MDI are questioned about the age of onset of their illness, 25% reported that their symptoms began between the ages of 15 and 19 years (Joyce, 1984). The symptom presentation, natural course of illness, phenomenology, and comorbidity of adolescent-onset MDI appear more similar to the classical symptoms described for adults. Discrete episodes of manic excitement alternating with periods of depression can be more readily identified. Psychotic symptoms may be predominant in adolescent MDI, leading to a frequent misdiagnosis of schizophrenia. Manic symptoms may be characterized by more paranoia, grandiose delusions, and euphoria in older adolescent-onset patients.

In comparison to adult-onset bipolar illness, child and adolescent MDI may be characterized by more mixed states in which both depression and manic symptoms appear concurrently instead of alternating. "Rapid cycling," defined as four or more discrete mood episodes of mania or depression occurring per year, may also be more common in child and adolescent MDI. These types of MDI have been associated with increased resistance to standard pharmacological treatments and a poorer prognosis than classic MDI (AACAP, 1997a; Carlson, 1990; Fristad, Weller, & Weller, 1992; Geller & Luby, 1997; Lewinsohn, Klein, & Seeley, 1995; Varanka, Weller, Weller, & Fristad, 1988; Weller, Weller, & Fristad, 1995; Wozniak et al., 1995).

In adults with MDI, the natural course of the disorder is characterized by episodic recurrences of mania and depression and by a variable course. The majority of adults with MDI will have multiple episodes, usually 10 or more in untreated patients over their lifetimes. Mood episodes tend to come more frequently over time, until the cycle length stabilizes after the fourth or fifth episode (Goodwin & Jamison, 1990). Adolescents with MDI also appear to have an episodic course, with the majority experiencing two or more discrete mood episodes and a relapsing course (Strober et al., 1995). MDI beginning in the prepubertal years may have a more continuous, nonepisodic presentation, without clearly defined mood episodes and with little interepisode improvement in daily functioning (Geller & Luby, 1997).

Compared to adolescents who have never been mentally ill, those with MDI have significantly more suicide attempts, more school failure, and poorer overall global functioning. Adolescents with MDI have been found to be as aggressive as adults with MDI, and to have more police contact and encounters with legal authorities than adults with MDI (McElroy, Strakowski, West, Keck, & McConville, 1997; McGlashan, 1988). In a small sample of psychiatrically hospitalized children diagnosed with MDI, 50% to 60% demonstrated interpersonal difficulties because of hostile, threatening, labile, and irritable moods (Varanka et al., 1988). Adolescents with MDI are at increased risk for completed suicide (Brent, Perper, et al., 1994). In a 5-year naturalistic follow-up of 54 adolescents with bipolar disorder, 20% were found to have made at least one medically serious suicide attempt (Strober et al., 1995). Psychotic symptoms are common in children and adolescents with MDI and contribute to poor global functioning (McElroy et al., 1997; McGlashan, 1988; Varanka et al., 1988). Risk for various SUDs is also an associated feature of adolescent-onset MDI (Geller & Luby, 1997).

The prevalence of juvenile MDI has been studied. In an epidemiological study of a representative community sample of 1,709 adolescents aged 14–19 years, 16 cases of MDI were identified (Lewinsohn et al., 1995). In youth the peak onset of MDI occurs in middle to late adolescence, between 15 and 19 years of age (AACAP, 1997a).

As is the case for MDD, a secular trend for MDI has been identified. Earlier age of onset of MDI in those born in the latter half of the 20th century has been reported (Rice et al., 1987). Rate of onset rises with age, and incidence appears to increase after puberty. Of adults with MDI, 0.5% reported onset between ages 5 and 9 years (see Weller et al., 1995), 7.5% reported onset between ages 10 and 14 years (Loranger & Levine, 1978), and 25% reported age of onset between 15 and 19 years (Joyce, 1984).

Types and Comorbidity

Bipolar I, Bipolar II, and Cyclothymic Disorders. Several types (not subtypes) of bipolar disorders are recognized in DSM-IV and can occur in children and adolescents. Bipolar I disorder is diagnosed when the patient experiences at least one full manic episode severe enough to require psychiatric hospitalization or is accompanied by psychotic symptoms; this DSM-IV diagnosis most closely resembles classic MDI. Patients with bipolar II disorder have had one or more episodes of both major depression and hypomania. A hypomanic episode is accompanied by at least three or more symptoms of a manic episode, but without psychotic symptoms or severity requiring hospitalization (APA, 1994). Bipolar II disorder may be especially common in adolescents with MDI residing in the community (not clinically referred) (Lewinsohn et al., 1995). Cyclothymic disorder (APA, 1994) describes a period of 1 year or more in which there are numerous depressive and hypomanic symptoms that do not meet full criteria for either a major depressive episode or a manic episode, but that do interfere with daily functioning.

MDI and CD. Childhood- and adolescent-onset MDI is highly comorbid with several other psychiatric conditions. Behaviors and symptoms meeting diagnostic criteria for CD frequently co-occur with early-onset MDI (Biederman, Faraone, Chu, et al., 1999). Youngsters with MDI may evidence frequent and serious antisocial behavior, violence, prolonged aggressive outbursts, temper tantrums, irritability, and disruptive behavior. In the midst of a manic decompensation, these children and adolescents may come to the attention of police and be arrested. Between 22% and 69% of prepubertal children meeting criteria for MDI will also meet criteria for CD, either within a mood episode or over the course of development into adulthood (Geller et al., 1995; Kovacs & Pollock, 1995). Those children with both MDI and CD have more police contacts than children with MDI but without CD (Kovacs & Pollock, 1995). In the adolescent years, between 22% and 42% of teenagers with MDI also satisfy diagnostic criteria for CD (Geller & Luby, 1997; Kutcher, Marton, & Kornblum, 1989). The reverse also appears to be true: In one study of adolescents admitted to an inpatient psychiatric unit for CD, significantly more of these also met diagnostic criteria for MDI than patients admitted to the unit without CD (Arredondo & Butler, 1994).

MDI and ADHD. The phenomenological overlap between symptoms of ADHD and MDI is extensive. This often makes it difficult to distinguish the two disorders clinically. Accurate identification is important, because pharmacological treatments for ADHD are different from those for MDI (AACAP, 1997a). In a small sample of adolescents with MDI admitted to a psychiatric hospital, 8 of 14 patients (57%) also met diagnostic criteria for ADHD (West, McElroy, Strakowski, Keck, & McConville, 1995). In this study, symptoms of ADHD were found to antedate the onset of MDI by about 6 years. Adolescents with both ADHD and MDI were found to have a more severe illness and a more variable presentation of MDI symptoms. These authors concluded that ADHD symptoms were common in adolescents psychiatrically hospitalized for mania.

The relationship between ADHD symptoms and MDI in prepubertal children is much less clear and highly controversial. In a study of 43 children aged

12 years or younger referred to an outpatient psychopharmacology clinic and meeting diagnostic criteria for MDI, 98% also met diagnostic criteria for ADHD (Woznick et al., 1995). The clinical presentation of these children was irritable. They also exhibited frequent violent, explosive aggressive behaviors; high rates of psychotic symptoms; mood instability; and a chronic, nonepisodic course. Given the high prevalence rates of ADHD in the general child and adolescent population, if it can be shown that there is great symptomatic overlap with prepubertal MDI, one possible conclusion is that prepubertal MDI is not as rare a disorder as historically thought: Early-onset ADHD may signal a very early onset of MDI in some children (Faraone et al., 1997). This conclusion is highly controversial and not entirely supported by the available evidence, however.

One method of disentangling the relationship between prepubertal ADHD and prepubertal MDI is to follow these children longitudinally over time as they grow into adulthood. If elevated rates of MDI are found in adolescence and adulthood for children diagnosed with ADHD in the elementary school years, the possibility exists that MDI may not be rare in the prepubertal years. To date, most of the longitudinal studies that have followed children with ADHD into adolescence and adulthood do not report elevated rates of MDI at outcome; instead, they report elevation of risk for continuing ADHD (Barkley, 1998). In contrast, studies that have followed 6- to 12-year-old prepubertal children and postpubertal adolescents diagnosed with depression over time report elevated rates of MDI at outcome (Geller et al., 1994; Strober et al., 1995). Furthermore, clinically ascertained juvenile depressions appear to be related to the various types of bipolar disorders and not to ADHD (Akiskal, 1995). Thus these investigations suggest that mood disorders and ADHD "breed true" when ascertained longitudinally, and that childhood ADHD does not substantially increase the risk for a bipolar outcome later in life. These studies also cast some doubt on the conclusion that ADHD in childhood may signal a very early onset of MDI for some children. As noted above, however, this is a thorny issue; much more research is required to clarify the phenomenology, risk factors, prevalence, and indeed the very existence of prepubertal MDI.

MDI and SUDs. High rates of comorbid SUDs have been reported for adolescents with MDI and in the families of patients with MDI (Geller, 1997; Winokur et al., 1996). Comorbid MDI and SUDs have been correlated with a higher risk for suicide in adolescents and young adults (Rich, Sherman, & Fowler, 1990).

The Relationship between MDI and Aggression

It does seem clear that a relationship exists between MDI and aggression. Indeed, youth suffering from MDI can demonstrate intense, protracted aggressive/antisocial behaviors that may meet diagnostic criteria for CD and involve them with police (Biederman, Faraone, Chu, et al., 1999). As with MDD and

DD, the relationship between MDI and aggression may be mediated by symptom phenomenology and/or comorbidity with externalizing behavioral disorders.

In summary, childhood- and adolescent-onset MDI appears characterized by less euphoria and more hostility and irritability than adult-onset MDI. Emotional lability, psychotic misperceptions of environmental stimuli, and impulsivity markedly increase the risk for aggressive interpersonal encounters, as well as for poor judgment leading to antisocial behaviors. Comorbidity with CD and symptom overlap with ADHD appear to increase severity of illness, encounters with police, and behavioral disinhibition, leading to an increased possibility of impulsive, explosive aggression. Clinical underrecognition of a possible syndrome of juvenile mania may be prevalent and contribute to difficulties in treating children and adolescents with CD and ADHD who are also severely aggressive and suffer from marked affective lability and psychotic symptoms.

SUBSTANCE USE DISORDERS

During recent years, increasing attention has been devoted to investigating the relationship between aggression and related behaviors in children and adolescents on the one hand, and the use of illicit drugs and alcohol on the other. This research has examined both the longitudinal relationships between early-onset aggression in childhood and later adolescent and young adult drug and alcohol use, as well as the cross-sectional relationships between substance use and concurrent aggression and antisocial behaviors in both clinic-referred and community samples. Concern about these relationships has been fueled by a growing awareness of the prevalence of SUDs in youth, especially in the adolescent population (Aarons, Brown, Hough, Garland, & Wood, 2001; Randall, Henggeler, Pickrel, & Brondino, 1999; Reinherz, Giaconia, Carmola Hauf, Wasserman, & Paradis, 2000).

Description and Prevalence

Rather than a definition utilizing multiple, different, or specific types of drug or alcohol addiction diagnoses, a general definition of SUDs is adopted in this section for the purposes of discussion and clarity. SUDs as described here encompass both abuse and dependence, as well as maladaptive use that does not meet clinical criteria for a specific diagnosis. The advantage of this definition is that it reflects the fact that substance use lies on a continuum that ranges from abstinence to experimental use, to recreational use, to problem use, to substance abuse (a DSM-IV diagnosis), and finally to substance dependence (also a DSM-IV diagnosis). The majority of youth (generally teenagers) who use drugs or alcohol do not progress to substance abuse or dependence; only a subset of adolescents meet clinical criteria for these disorders. Although substance use is not sufficient for a diagnosis of abuse or dependence, it may be associated with adverse consequences. The present discussion applies to SUDs in general, rather than any to specific substance use diagnosis or specific type of substance.

Commonly misused drugs in the adolescent age range include those commonly misused by adults: alcohol, marijuana, cocaine, heroin, inhalants (e.g., sniffable glue), hallucinogens, prescription drugs, and tobacco. Alcohol and cigarettes are two of the most widely used and misused substances in the teenage years (Weinberg, Rahdert, Colliver, & Glantz, 1998). Anabolic steroid misuse is also growing in this age range.

The clinical features of SUDs vary with the type of substance used, the amount used in a given time, the setting and context of use, the individual's experience with the substance, his or her expectations, and the presence or absence of any comorbid psychopathology. Significant changes in mood, cognition, or behavior are often manifested (AACAP, 1997b). Marked impairment in social and academic functioning may occur. Associated features of adolescent SUDs may include risk-taking behaviors, accidents, violence, school failure, risky sexual behavior with increased risk of pregnancy for females and exposure to sexually transmitted diseases for both sexes, and involvement in delinquent and other antisocial behaviors.

Adolescent SUDs share a significant co-occurrence with other psychiatric disorders and behavioral problems. A high prevalence of comorbidity has been documented in both population-based and clinical samples of adolescents with SUDs. CD, ADHD, MDD, and MDI have been most consistently identified as comorbid with adolescent SUDs (Bukstein, Glancy, & Kaminer, 1992; Lewinsohn, Hops, Roberts, Seeley, & Andrews, 1993; Wilens, Biederman, Abrantes, & Spencer, 1997). Comorbidity in adolescent SUDs may vary by gender, with higher rates of disruptive behavior disorders in males and higher rates of mood disorders in females (see Brook, Whiteman, Finch, & Cohen, 1995). Anxiety disorders are also found to be comorbid with adolescent SUDs (Bukstein, Brent, & Kaminer, 1989). An emerging literature is beginning to describe a relationship between early childhood experiences of physical and/or sexual abuse and victimization and later SUDs, especially in women (Miller, Downs, & Testa, 1993).

Recent surveys have documented a rise in prevalence rates for adolescent SUDs beginning in the early 1990s. In 1996, the annual Monitoring the Future Study (Johnston, 1996) found that almost 33% of high school seniors reported having been drunk in the preceding month, and that 20% of high school seniors and sophomores reported using marijuana in that period. Daily marijuana use was reported by 4.9% of surveyed high school seniors. In other community surveys, lifetime prevalence of alcohol abuse or dependence has ranged from 5.3% in 15-year-olds to 32.4% in 17- to 19-year-olds. For illicit drugs, 23.8% of high school seniors reported use during the 30 days preceding the survey (see AACAP, 1997b).

The prevalence of SUDs in specific populations of adolescents is often higher, especially in those with serious emotional problems. In populations of juveniles who have committed offences or those adolescents with CD, the prevalence of SUDs can be greater than 80% (Bukstein et al., 1992). In a random sample of all youth who were active in at least one of five sectors of care, lifetime rates of SUDs were reported for 82.6% of those in drug and alcohol programs, 62.1% in the juvenile justice system, 40.8% in mental health care, 23.6% of seriously emotionally disturbed youth in school-based services, and 19.2% in child welfare services (Aarons et al., 2001).

The Relationship between SUDs and Aggression

There appears to be a robust relationship between SUDs on the one hand, and aggression and related behaviors on the other (Brady, Myrick, & McElroy, 1998). This association has been documented in population-based studies from many countries such as the United States, France, and India. It has also been documented in experimental studies where a laboratory measure of aggression is used. In both types of research, adolescents with SUDs have been found to be more aggressive than adolescents without SUDs (Allen, Moeller, Rhoades, & Cherek, 1997; Kingery, Pruitt, & Hurley, 1992; Varma, Basu, Malhotra, Sharma, & Mattoo, 1994). Moreover, adolescents with early-onset aggression have been found to have more SUDs than adolescents without a significant aggressive history (Choquet, Menke, & Manfredi, 1991; Valois, McKeown, Garrison, & Vincent, 1995).

However, the nature of the relationship between SUDs and aggression is presently unclear. Several different possibilities exist: (1) A developmental history of early-onset aggression may influence the risk for later SUDs; (2) SUDs may influence the risk for the expression of aggression and related behaviors; (3) aggression and SUDs may be part of a larger syndrome of underlying psychopathology; or (4) comorbidity with other psychiatric disorders may influence the relationship between SUDs and aggression.

There is evidence that early-onset childhood aggression influences the risk for later SUDs in adolescence and adulthood. Several prospective longitudinal studies have documented this relationship. In a study of lower-socioeconomic-status (lower-SES) African American children living in Chicago, Kellam, Brown, Rubin, and Ensminger (1983) found that aggressive first-graders were at increased risk for drug use during adolescence. In a 20-year longitudinal study, aggressive behavior with onset between the ages of 5 and 10 years significantly predicted SUDs during adolescence and young adulthood; this relationship held for both males and females in the sample (Brook et al., 1995; Brook, Whiteman, Finch, & Cohen, 1996). In another study of psychiatrically referred adolescents, the onset of CD by age 10 years and a greater diversity of early-onset CD symptoms were predictive of SUDs during adolescence (Myers, Stewart, & Brown, 1998). Mediating variables between early aggression and later substance use may include depression and anger–impulsivity (Brook et al., 1995, 1996) resulting in impaired information processing, poor social judgment, or possible self-medication of dysphoric affects—all of which may increase risk for later SUDs.

SUDs can also increase the risk for behavioral expressions of aggression. This relationship may be mediated in part through specific physiological and behavioral effects of the drug being misused. An example would be differences in behavior during states of intoxication versus states of withdrawal. Substance withdrawal is an adverse experience that can motivate an addicted individual to seek more of the substance in order to avoid the experience. This may increase the chance of an aggressive or antisocial encounter. The risk of aggression while intoxicated appears to vary by which type of substance is being misused and by whether blood levels of the substance are rising or falling in the body. For example, alcohol appears to have a stronger association with aggression when it acts as a stimulant during absorption and when blood alcohol levels are rising, rather than during periods when blood alcohol levels are falling (Chermack & Giancola, 1997). Cocaine intoxication may also increase risk for aggression (National Institute on Drug Abuse, 1995), whereas cannabis intoxication and opiate intoxication (but not opiate or cocaine withdrawal) may decrease risk for aggressive responding (Chermack & Giancola, 1997). In addition, substance use can influence the risk for aggression and violence through environmental and contextual variables. These include the presence of interpersonal provocation or perception of threat while using a substance, social pressure, or prior experience with and expectations about the substance (Chermack & Giancola, 1997).

Aggression and SUDs may not even be separate disorders, but may be part of a larger syndrome of underlying psychopathology (Brady et al., 1998). Evidence for this is found in research investigating the neurotransmitter 5-HT, SUDs, and antisocial behaviors. For example, adoption studies of individuals with alcoholism have identified a subtype of alcoholism characterized by high heritability, early age of onset (generally in the teenage or young adult years), relative independence from environmental and contextual factors, and a strong association with aggression and criminal behavior (Cloninger, 1987a). Numerous investigations have found reduced brain 5-HT function in this type of alcoholism. Specifically, a low concentration of a CNS metabolite of 5-HT (5-hydroxyindoleacetic acid, or 5-HIAA) has been found in individuals with early-onset antisocial alcoholism (Fils-Aime et al., 1996), persons with impulsive alcoholism and criminal behavior (Linnoila et al., 1983), and individuals with alcoholism who set fires (Linnoila, DeJong, & Virkkunen, 1989). This relationship has recently been found to have a possible genetic basis. Investigating 166 adults with alcoholism and criminal offenses, 261 relatives, and 213 healthy controls, Lappalainen et al. (1998) found a genetic locus predisposing to antisocial alcoholism linked to a specific type of 5-HT receptor: the 5-HT_{1B} gene. For this type of SUD (i.e., alcoholism), these data suggest the possibility that impulsive aggression and alcoholism may be different behavioral expressions of a more fundamental underlying psychopathology—that is, deficits in 5-HT neurotransmission. This type of research has not yet been completed for other types of SUDs, nor has it been studied in children or adolescents. Yet the results are intriguing and may point the way to a deeper understanding of the neurobiological relationships between SUDs and aggression.

More evidence suggesting that SUDs and aggression are part of a more fundamental psychopathology comes from neuropsychological studies documenting executive cognitive function (ECF) deficits both in persons with SUDs and in persons with impulsivity and aggression. ECFs are those brain functions that encompass "higher-order" cognitive abilities. These include attention and vigilance to task, hypothesis generation, abstract reasoning, planning, and self-monitoring. The use of these cognitive abilities results in behavioral inhibition; a decrease in impulsive responses to the environment; and the cognitive generation of multiple, alternative strategies to allow an individual to cope favorably with environmental challenges. Several studies have investigated a relationship among SUDs, compromised ECFs, and aggression. Lau, Pihl, and Peterson (1995) separated normal males into high- and low-functioning groups based on neuropsychological tests of ECFs. These individuals were then given alcoholic or nonalcoholic beverages and tested on a laboratory paradigm of aggression. Results indicated that individuals who received alcohol and those with compromised ECFs displayed higher levels of aggression. In a study of 291 boys aged 10–12 with and without a family history of SUDs, results supported a relationship among ECFs, a family history of SUDs, and aggressive behavior (Giancola, Martin, Tarter, Pelham, & Moss, 1996). Further support for this relationship is found in studies of brain-injured individuals. Individuals with certain types of brain injury may become impulsive and behaviorally disinhibited. These investigations have found high rates of postinjury aggressive behavior and a relatively high incidence of alcoholism resulting in arrest in such patients (Kreutzer, Marwitz, & Witol, 1995). Other studies have found that ECF deficits continue to be related to aggressive behavior even when drug use is controlled for in the experimental design (Giancola, Mezzich, & Tarter, 1998b). These studies suggest the possibility that underlying ECF impairments may increase vulnerability both to SUDs and to aggression and related behaviors.

Finally, high rates of psychiatric comorbidity in adolescents with SUDs may also explain the relationship with aggressive and related behaviors. CD, which is associated with a high frequency of aggressive and antisocial behaviors, has been found to be a prevalent comorbid psychiatric diagnosis in clinical samples of adolescents with SUDs (S. A. Brown, Gleghorn, Schuckit, Myers, & Mott, 1996; Myers et al., 1998). Depression can be associated with increased aggression, possibly as a result of increased irritability and hostility in depressed individuals. Depression is also a frequently occurring comorbid psychiatric diagnosis in individuals with SUDs. High rates of aggression and related behaviors found in youth with SUDs may reflect the interplay of these comorbid psychiatric diagnoses with the physiological and behavioral effects of substance misuse.

In summary, the relationship between SUDs and aggression is a complicated one. Characteristics of the type of drug being misused, physiological states of intoxication or withdrawal, environmental and contextual variables, and characteristics of the individual (including prior history, cognitive experiences and expectancies, and comorbid psychopathology) all may interact to increase risk for aggressive responding in an individual with a SUD.

PERSONALITY DISORDERS

As it does for other mental disorders, DSM-IV (APA, 1994) utilizes a categorical diagnostic approach to personality disorders; that is, it defines them as qualitatively distinct medical syndromes. This stands in contrast to conceptualizations of personality disorders as maladaptive variants of personality traits that exist on a spectrum from normality to pathology and are dimensionally distributed in a population, with no clear boundary marking the onset of a psychopathological syndrome. The categorical approach has been found to have clinical utility for adults, for whom reliable and valid personality disorders can be recognized (Blais, Hilsenroth, & Castlebury, 1997).

It is much less clear, however, that the categorical approach to identifying personality disorders as discrete medical syndromes is useful or valid for children or adolescents (Becker et al., 1999). Studies of the relationship between personality *traits* and disturbances of behavior, cognition, and mood may prove more fruitful in youth, because of their developmental immaturity. An example of this approach is research identifying an undercontrolled (e.g., impulsive, distractible, overactive) temperament at age 3 years as being associated with an increased risk for ASPD in young adulthood (Caspi, Moffit, Newman, & Silva, 1996). Nevertheless, because DSM-IV is widely used in clinical work with referred children and adolescents, this section discusses what is presently known about personality disorders in youth and their linkages to aggression and related behaviors. The discussion focuses on personality disorders in general, rather than on any specific personality disorder in particular.

Description and Prevalence

As defined by DSM-IV, a personality disorder is a durable pattern of behavior and internal experience that differs sharply from the expectations of the individual's culture, is rigid and pervasive, begins in adolescence or early adulthood, is stable over time, and leads to impairment or distress (APA, 1994). DSM-IV notes that the categorical diagnosis of a personality disorder may be applied to a child or adolescent in those fairly unusual circumstances in which the youth's particular maladaptive personality traits appear to be persistent, pervasive, and unlikely to be restricted to a certain developmental stage or an episode of discrete psychiatric illness (APA, 1994). For a personality disorder to be diagnosed in a child or adolescent, the clinical features must be present for at least 1 year. In this categorical diagnostic system individual personality traits (e.g., extroverted, introverted, impulsive, undercontrolled, overcontrolled, obsessive, thrill-seeking, or anxious traits) become personality disorders only when they are inflexible, are maladaptive, and cause significant functional impairment or distress to the individual.

Ten specific personality disorders grouped into three clusters are recognized in DSM-IV. Cluster A personality disorders include paranoid, schizoid, and schizotypal personality disorders. These individuals often appear odd or eccentric. Cluster B includes ASPD, as well as borderline, histrionic, and narcissistic personality disorders. These individuals often appear dramatic, emotional, or erratic. Individuals with Cluster C personality disorders often appear anxious or fearful; this cluster includes avoidant, dependent, and obsessive–compulsive personality disorders. Although this system of grouping the personality disorders can be useful, it presently lacks empirical support and has not been consistently validated, especially with youth (Becker et al., 1999).

Research on the personality disorders has largely focused on adults (Blais et al., 1997). However, the past decade has seen a growing body of studies focusing on children and adolescents. Accumulating evidence suggests that although personality disorders as defined by DSM-IV diagnostic criteria can be reliably diagnosed in children and adolescents, there exists much less evidence to support the *validity* of these disorders in youth (Becker et al., 1999; Brent, Johnson, et al., 1994). Existing investigations of validity in children and adolescents are more strongly supportive of categorically diagnosed personality disorders for adolescents than for younger children (Bernstein et al., 1993). Studies of community samples have found that obsessive–compulsive personality disorder (Cluster C, anxious), and ASPD and borderline and narcissistic personality disorders (Cluster B, impulsive and dramatic), are the most common types of these disorders in nonreferred adolescents and young adults (Bernstein et al., 1993; Lewinsohn, Rohde, Seeley, & Klein, 1997). In psychiatrically referred adolescents, borderline personality disorder is most common, especially in females (Lofgren, Bemporad, King, Lindem, & O'Driscoll, 1991). Of the DSM-IV personality disorders investigated in clinically referred children and adolescents, empirical support is strongest for the validity of avoidant and borderline personality disorders (Guzder, Paris, Zelkowitz, & Feldman, 1999; B. A. Johnson et al., 1995).

The clinical features of the various personality disorders vary with the specific disorder. Regardless of the specific diagnosis, numerous studies document that adolescent personality disorders are associated with a considerable degree of functional impairment. The type of personality disorder most highly associated with aggression and antisocial behavior is ASPD. In the DSM categorical system, this personality disorder is only diagnosed in individuals at least 18 years of age. As such, it is largely a diagnosis of adults rather than youth, but it overlaps to a considerable degree with the diagnostic criteria for

CD (Eppright, Kashani, Robison, & Reid, 1993). Adolescent-onset Cluster A and Cluster B personality disorders appear to increase risk for violent behavior that persists into early adulthood (Johnson et al., 2000).

The prevalence of diagnosable adolescent personality disorders in community samples has been studied and has usually been found to be low. In a study of 299 youth aged 14–18 years, Lewinsohn et al. (1997) found that only 3.3% met diagnostic criteria for a personality disorder. A higher prevalence was found by Bernstein et al. (1993). In a randomly selected community sample of youth aged 9–19 years, 17% qualified for a diagnosis of severe personality disorder when reassessed at a 2-year follow-up. The rates of personality disorder in psychiatrically referred or juvenile justice samples of youth are generally much higher (Brent, Johnson, et al., 1994; Eppright et al., 1993).

The Relationship between Personality Disorders and Aggression

Not all personality disorders in youth have an association with aggression or related behaviors. Cluster C (anxious) personality disorders actually appear to have a decreased association with aggression. In a study of psychiatrically referred adolescents, for example, those meeting criteria for avoidant personality disorder had lower rates of comorbid CD than a psychiatrically referred comparison group (B. A. Johnson et al., 1995). An anxious personality may thus exert a protective effect against aggressive responding.

Cluster A and Cluster B personality disorders have a much stronger association with aggressive behavior (Guzder et al., 1999; Johnson et al., 2000). This appears especially true of youth meeting criteria for borderline personality disorder and of those meeting criteria for ASPD (except for the ASPD age requirement of at least 18 years). This association may be explained in part by several factors. First, impulse control deficits have a relationship to increased risk for aggressive responding (Hart, Hofmann, Edelstein, & Keller, 1997). Adolescents with Cluster B personality disorders, especially borderline personality disorder, have been shown both to be very impulsive (Brodsky, Malone, Ellis, Dulit, & Mann, 1997) and to have high lifetime rates of impulsive violence directed against the self (suicide attempts) and against others (assaults) (Brent, Johnson, et al., 1994). The relationship between aggressive outcome and impulsivity is further underscored by longitudinal studies examining personality *traits* in young children followed over time into adulthood. Children with undercontrolled personality traits (impulsivity, restlessness, and distractibility, as well as deficits in attention, motor control, and perception) have been found to be at significantly higher risk for the development of various personality disorders in adolescence (Hellgren, Gillberg, Bagenholm, & Gillberg, 1994), of aggressive behavior in adolescence (Hart et al., 1997), and specifically of ASPD as young adults (Caspi et al., 1996).

Second, children and adolescents meeting diagnostic criteria for Cluster A and B personality disorders have significant rates of psychiatric comorbidity with depression, PTSD, and CD, as well as high rates of developmental traumas (e.g., physical abuse, sexual abuse, and the experience of pathological parenting) in their lifetime histories. Bernstein, Cohen, Skodol, Bezirganian, and Brook (1996) investigated the childhood antecedents of adolescent personality disorders and found CD to be an independent predictor of personality disorders in all clusters. Garnet, Levy, Mattanah, Edell, and McGlashan (1994) found high rates of comorbidity with CD and MDD in their sample of adolescents with borderline personality disorder. Childhood borderline pathology is also highly comorbid with CD (Guzder et al., 1999). Lewinsohn et al. (1997) found adolescent personality disorders in a community sample to be significantly associated with anxiety disorders, SUDs, depressive disorders, and two of the disruptive behavior disorders (CD and ADHD). Sexual abuse, physical abuse, parental neglect, and parental criminality and SUDs were found to be significant risk factors for the development of borderline pathology in children (Guzder, Paris, Zelkowitz, & Marchessault, 1996). An association with aggression in youth meeting diagnostic criteria for personality disorders may be mediated through these comorbid conditions by increasing the severity and/or intensity of hostility, irritability, rage, sensitivity to fear of threat (fear conditioning), or affective instability; all of these may contribute to lowered impulse control and increased risk of aggressive responding.

In summary, although categorical diagnostic criteria for personality disorders do not have established validity in the child and adolescent age range, they do seem to identify youth at risk for a wide variety of maladaptive outcomes. An association with aggression and related behaviors is strongest for those personality disorders with impulse dyscontrol (Clusters A and B) as a core feature, and for those personality disorders having frequent comorbidity with psychiatric conditions such as depression, the disruptive behavior disorders, and PTSD, which are also known to increase risk for aggression.

PSYCHOPATHY

The concept of a "psychopathic personality" is among the most thoroughly investigated of all personality types. Although psychopathy is not a psychiatric diagnosis, it overlaps to a considerable degree with the diagnosis of ASPD, which is such a diagnosis. Some, although not all, psychopathic individuals may be very aggressive and engage in chronic antisocial behavior. This section first focuses on issues in adult psychopathy, and then discusses research on the emerging concept of child and adolescent psychopathy.

Adult Psychopathy: Description

It has long been recognized in society that some individuals persistently fail to conform to moral and legal expectations of behavior, willfully engage in recidivistic criminality, are self-centered, do not plan for the future, have little empathy for others, lack the emotional capacity for remorse, are capable of

impulsive rage and aggression, do not seem to change their maladaptive behaviors despite punishment, and yet possess no deficits in their intelligence or
reasoning ability. Benjamin Rush used the term "moral insanity" in 1835 to
support his view that these individuals suffer from a constitutional or organic
deficit. The neurologist Philippe Pinel identified *manie sans délire*—a disorder
of aberrant affect, proneness to impulsive rage attacks, and intact reasoning
abilities—in 1801. (For a review of these and other historical concepts of psychopathy, see Sutker, 1994.)

It remains unclear whether the construct of psychopathy is learned or
constitutional, whether it is of a discrete categorical nature or is a dimension
of personality in the population, and whether it measures social deviance or
personality traits (Harris, Rice, & Quinsey, 1994; Lilienfeld, 1994; Sutker,
1994). The personality-based conceptualization of psychopathy was first described by Cleckley (1941). He delineated 16 criteria for a diagnosis of psychopathy. Most of these are personality traits and include such characteristics
as superficial charm, lack of anxiety, lack of guilt, undependability, dishon-
esty, egocentricity, failure to form lasting or close intimate relationships, failure to learn from punishment, poverty of emotions, lack of insight into the impact of one's behavior upon others, and failure to plan ahead. Adherents of
the personality-based conceptualization of psychopathy argue that many individuals meeting personality trait criteria for psychopathy are not antisocial,
violent, or otherwise aggressive, and that many persons who chronically commit violent offenses are not psychopathic (Lilienfeld, 1994).

The behavior-based conceptualization of psychopathy emphasizes chronic
and recidivistic antisocial behaviors as the defining criteria (Cloninger, 1978).
Adherents of this approach argue that personality trait criteria require too
much inference on the part of clinicians and thus possess low interrater reliability. This view became operationalized in DSM-III (APA, 1980) and later
editions of the DSM (APA, 1987, 1994) as ASPD. This categorical personality
disorder requires a chronic history of antisocial behavior as both necessary
and sufficient for diagnosis. As currently described, ASPD (APA, 1994) is a
syndrome characterized by a pattern of disregard for and violation of others'
rights since age 15 years, as shown by three (or more) antisocial behaviors;
present age of at least 18 years; no evidence of schizophrenia or mania; and
evidence of CD beginning prior to age 15 years. Because this syndrome is
operationalized in terms of readily agreed-upon antisocial behaviors, interrater reliability for the diagnosis is much improved over personality-based approaches; moreover, ASPD is more strongly associated with criminal behavior
than are personality-based criteria.

The DSM approach to psychopathy has also been criticized, however
(Hare, Hart, & Harpur, 1991). Since the DSM does not include many of
the classical personality trait indicators of psychopathy (e.g., selfishness,
egocentricity, callousness, poverty of emotions, lack of empathy, manipulativeness), it results in a diagnostic category with good interrater reliability,
but the possibility of diminished content-related validity. As such, the con-

struct of psychopathy as embodied in the diagnosis of ASPD demonstrates a lack of congruence with classical conceptions of psychopathy (Hare et al., 1991).

Because of these concerns, an alternative to the conceptualization of psychopathy as ASPD was developed. The Psychopathy Checklist (PCL; Hare, 1980) and the Psychopathy Checklist—Revised (PCL-R; Hare, 1985; Hare, 1991) are clinical rating scales with items designed to assess the traditional clinical construct of psychopathy, best exemplified in the work of Cleckley (1976). The 22 items of the PCL and the 20 items of the PCL-R measure behaviors and inferred personality traits considered fundamental to the clinical construct of psychopathy. The information needed to score these rating scales is obtained from a semistructured interview with the subject and from institutional files. Despite the subjective nature of most items, the PCL and PCL-R have reasonable interrater reliability and high internal consistency (measures of internal validity) when populations of adults convicted of crimes and forensic psychiatric patients are assessed. Factor analyses of scores from the PCL and PCL-R reveal a two-factor internal structure. Factor 1 reflects a set of interpersonal and affective characteristics (egocentricity, lack of remorse, callousness, etc.) considered fundamental to clinical personality trait conceptions of psychopathy. Factor 2 reflects those behavioral aspects of psychopathy related to an impulsive, antisocial, and unstable lifestyle. The items in the PCL-R are presented in Table 4.1.

Factor 1 positively correlates with clinical ratings of psychopathy, with ratings of narcissistic and histrionic personality disorder, and with self-report measures of narcissism. It is inversely correlated with measures of empathy and anxiety (Hare, 1991; Harpur, Hare, & Hakstian, 1989; Hart & Hare, 1989). Factor 2 is positively correlated with the categorical psychiatric diagnosis of ASPD, with criminal behaviors, and with self-report measures of anti-

TABLE 4.1. Items Loading on the Two Factors of Hare's (1991) Psychopathy Checklist—Revised (PCL-R)

Factor 1: Emotional Detachment	Factor 2: Antisocial Behavior
Glibness/superficial charm	Proneness to boredom
Grandiose sense of self-worth	Parasitic lifestyle
Pathological lying	Poor behavior controls
Conning/manipulative	Early behavior problems
Lack of remorse or guilt	Lack of realistic, long-term goals
Shallow affect goals	Impulsivity
Callous/lack of empathy	Irresponsibility
Failure to accept responsibility	Juvenile delinquency
	Revocation of conditional release (from an institution)

Note. Three items did not load on either factor (promiscuous sexual behavior, numerous short-term marital relationships, and criminal versatility). Data from Hare (1991).

social behavior (Hare et al., 1991). Among adult criminal offenders, Factor 1 correlates with high SES, and Factor 2 correlates with low SES. Factor 1 also correlates with higher, and Factor 2 with lower, Verbal IQ (Patrick, Zempolich, & Levenston, 1997). Individuals scoring high on Factor 1 are less likely to come from single parent homes than those scoring high on Factor 2 (Patrick et al., 1997). Comparison of the criteria for ASPD and the criteria for psychopathy as defined by the PCL and PCL-R reveal that they are not interchangeable and may measure very different constructs.

The two-factor model of psychopathy embodied in the PCL and PCL-R has generated an extensive amount of research. The PCL and PCL-R have generally been found to have better predictive validity than the psychiatric diagnosis of ASPD in assessing recidivism and postrelease criminal behavior in incarcerated adults (Cunningham & Reidy, 1998; Lilienfeld, 1994). High scores on the PCL and PCL-R also significantly predict violent behavior in adult psychiatric patients hospitalized in forensic institutional settings (Pham, Remy, Dailliet, & Lienard, 1998). Age-related differences in the two-factor model have been studied and suggest that mean scores on Factor 2 (antisocial behavior) decline with age, while mean scores on Factor 1 (personality traits) are stable with age, in a male prison population varying between 16 and 69 years old (Harpur & Hare, 1994). The validity of the PCL and PCL-R has been supported in studies of males incarcerated in both America and Europe (Pham, 1998).

Gender differences in adult psychopathy are beginning to be explored with the PCL and PCL-R. In studies of incarcerated adult females, the validity of these checklists in predicting criminal recidivism and convergence with staff ratings of aggression, manipulativeness, lack of remorse, and noncompliance has been demonstrated (Salekin, Rogers, & Sewell, 1997; Salekin, Rogers, Ustad, & Sewell, 1998). A different factor structure may emerge for females with psychopathic offenses as compared to males on this instrument (Salekin et al., 1997). Other gender differences in psychopathy have been revealed. Unlike males, for whom PCL-R Factor 2 scores (antisocial behavior) have a stronger correlation to DSM ASPD diagnosis, for females Factor 1 scores (personality traits) have been found more strongly correlated with diagnosis of ASPD (Rutherford, Alterman, Cacciola, & McKay, 1998). These results support the need for additional research into gender differences in psychopathy.

The two-factor model has also facilitated research on neurocognitive, neurophysiological, and biological variables in psychopathy. On neurocognitive measures, individuals with psychopathy have been found to have diminished emotional responsivity to negative emotional stimuli, low fear reactions to threatening environmental cues, relative insensitivity to the emotional connotations of language, unusual proficiency at selectively focusing attention on events that interest them, reduced breadth of attention, reduced attention to secondary tasks because of excessive attention to immediate goals, and a dominant response set for immediately rewarding activities (Day & Wong, 1996; Kosson, 1996; Louth, Williamson, Alpert, Pouget, & Hare, 1998; Patrick et al., 1997). Relative to individuals who score low on measures assessing psychopathy, high-scoring individuals demonstrate reduced CNS arousal to fearful stimuli, including diminished skin electrodermal reactions, cardiovascular reactivity, and facial muscle responses (Patrick, Cuthbert, & Lang, 1994). Increasing research attention is focusing on neurobiology and psychopathy, including investigations of genetics, neurochemistry, and electrocortical physiology (Dolan, 1994). Behaviorally, adults with psychopathy have been found to commit more instrumental acts and less reactive acts of aggression than aggressive adults without psychopathy (Cornell et al., 1996).

Child and Adolescent Psychopathy: Description

Interest in psychopathic children occurred later than society's attention to psychopathic adults. By the early 20th century, medical professionals (generally pediatricians) began to study and attempt to provide treatment for children who were called "psychopathic" and exhibited chronic behavior problems. For example, a group school–home for psychopathic children was founded in Sweden in 1928. Between 1928 and 1956, 387 boys and 235 girls were admitted to this program (Fried, 1995). During this time, the study of childhood psychopathy was heavily influenced by psychoanalytic thinking. More recent interest in the investigation of child and adolescent psychopathy has been fueled by advances in the study of adult psychopathy, as well as by the recognition that personality traits are predictive of recidivism in juvenile delinquent populations above and beyond the effects of criminological factors such as age and number of prior offenses (Lilienfeld, 1998; Steiner, Cauffman, & Duxbury, 1999).

Longitudinal studies have consistently shown that adult antisocial behavior and psychopathy have important roots in childhood. Indeed, the diagnosis of adult ASPD requires the presence of CD as occurring prior to the age of 15 years. However, the study of childhood precursors to adult antisocial behavior has largely focused on the frequency, severity, and types of antisocial behaviors exhibited by youth, and has largely ignored the psychological dimensions that are more specific to the construct of psychopathy. Since studies of developmental psychopathology have consistently reported findings that the predictive power of aggression seems to be contained in a young age at onset of CD-like behaviors, and not in the type of antisocial behaviors displayed by the child, expanding the study of early-onset childhood conduct problems to include conceptualizations of psychopathy might yield important additional information.

There is some evidence that the interaction between psychopathy and antisocial behavior found for adults may also be relevant for children and adolescents. First, children with CD who are also unable to maintain social relationships (i.e., children with undersocialized aggressive CD) are found to be more aggressive, have a poorer longitudinal prognosis, and have different biological correlates than children with CD who are able to maintain social relationships (i.e., children with socialized delinquent CD) (Rogeness, Javors, & Pliszka, 1992). Second, children with CD who lack anxiety are more aggressive, have more conflict with social systems, respond more poorly to treatment, and have different neurochemical correlates than anxious children with CD (Frick, O'Brien, Wootton, & McBurnett, 1994; Frick, Lilienfeld, Ellis, Loney, & Silverthorn, 1999; McBurnett et al., 1991). These studies suggest that dimensions of personality as contained in the concept of psychopathy may be important for the study of childhood CD.

Child and Adolescent Psychopathy: Types

Presently there are three conceptual approaches to the investigation of psychopathy in juveniles. The co-occurrence of hyperactivity, impulsivity, and attention problems on the one hand, and early-onset conduct problems on the other, has been proposed as creating a subtype of CD with a poor prognosis; such youths may eventually become psychopathic adults (Lynam, 1996). In this model, children who are both hyperactive and antisocial are at risk for persistent antisocial behaviors and have a worse outcome than juveniles with hyperactive-only or antisocial-only behaviors. Lynam hypothesizes that children with both sets of behaviors lack a psychological dimension called "psychopathic constraint." Children lacking in such constraint are impulsive, sensation-seeking, and reward-dominant; may have a CNS 5-HT deficit; and have difficulty in response modulation. These youngsters are hypothesized to be at risk to develop adult psychopathy (Lynam, 1996). The Childhood Psychopathy Scale (CPS) measures this approach to juvenile psychopathy (Lynam, 1997).

A second approach to juvenile psychopathy is to investigate the similarities between psychopathic adults and psychopathic youths. In other words, do youngsters who score high on psychopathic traits resemble adults who score high on measures of psychopathy (Forth, Kosson, & Hare, 1997)? This research has employed a downward extension of the dominant measure of psychopathy for adults, the Hare Psychopathy Checklist—Youth Version (PCL-YV) (Forth et al., 1997).

A third approach utilizes concepts of personality traits derived from conceptualizations of adult psychopathy, but focuses on traits found in juveniles. This approach is not simply a downward extension of models of adult psychopathy as applied to youngsters. In a study of 95 clinic-referred 6- to 13-year-old children, many of whom had severe conduct problems, psychopathic traits were found to be assessed reliably with a child version of the PCL-R (Frick et al., 1994). As for adults, factor analysis of responses to the child PCL-R revealed a two-factor solution. The 10 items of Factor 1 are associated with impulsivity, conduct problems and antisocial behavior; this factor is entitled "poor impulse control–conduct problems." Factor 2 includes 6 traits traditionally associated with the concept of psychopathy and is called "callous–unemotional." Although these factors are significantly correlated with each other, they are also separable. The items in the two-factor model of child psychopathy are presented in Table 4.2.

It should be emphasized that the concept of childhood psychopathy is not synonymous with the categorical psychiatric diagnosis of CD. Psychopathic traits may identify a subgroup of youth with CD who possess characteristics of low anxiety and increased sensation seeking, and who do not have information-processing deficits such as low verbal intelligence (Frick et al., 1994). Similarly, the subgroup of children with CD who demonstrate callous–unemotional traits on the child PCL-R may show a very severe type of CD and may be at risk for the eventual development of adult psychopathy (Christian et al., 1997).

The identification of reliable instruments for assessing psychopathy in children and adolescents has facilitated renewed interest and research in this area of childhood aggression. In a study of 430 boys aged 12 and 13 years, children with psychopathic personalities, like their adult counterparts, were serious and stable in their offending, impulsive, and more prone to externalizing than internalizing disorders (Lynam, 1997). Childhood psychopathy also provided additional statistical power in predicting serious, stable antisocial behavior in adolescence, over and above other known predictors and classification approaches in this same study (Lynam, 1997). Adolescents with psychopathy and CD have been found to be more aggressive and violent, to be more self-centered, to have decreased interpersonal attachments to others, and to demonstrate less anxiety than adolescents with CD but without psychopathic traits (Myers, Burket, & Harris, 1995; Rogers, Johansen, Chang, & Salekin, 1997; Smith, Gacono, & Kaufman, 1997). SUDs also appear signifi-

TABLE 4.2. Items Loading on the Two Factors of Psychopathy in Clinic-Referred Children

Factor 1: Poor impulse control–conduct problems	Factor 2: Callous–unemotional
Brags about accomplishments	Unconcerned about schoolwork
Becomes angry when corrected	Does not feel bad or guilty
Thinks he/she is more important than others	Emotions seem shallow and not genuine
Acts without thinking of the consequences	Does not show feelings or emotions
Blames others for own mistakes	Acts charming in ways that seem insincere
Teases or makes fun of others	Is unconcerned about the feelings of others
Engages in risky or dangerous activities	
Engages in illegal activities	
Does not keep the same friends	
Gets bored easily	

Note. From Frick (1998). Copyright 1998 by Kluwer Academic/Plenum Publishers. Reprinted by permission.

cantly correlated with psychopathic characteristics in incarcerated adolescent males (Mailloux, Forth, & Kroner, 1997).

Juvenile Psychopathy, Antisocial Behavior, and Anxiety

The interaction between antisocial behavior and anxious personality traits has been of interest in the study of antisocial children and adolescents. Antisocial children who also have the capacity for anxiety have been found to be more likely than nonanxious antisocial children to inhibit their behavior in response to environmental cues of nonreward or punishment (Walker et al., 1991). In addition, the behaviors of children with CD but without anxiety appear to be governed by a reward-dominant style. This means that such children are more likely to engage in behaviors that are immediately reinforcing (i.e., that satisfy appetitive drives) and to pay less attention to the consequences (i.e., punishment) of their behavior in choosing how to act.

It has been unclear whether a reward-dominant style is associated with antisocial behavior in general, psychopathy, or both. In investigations of this question, the strongest evidence for a reward-dominant style exists for nonanxious children with CD and psychopathic personality features (Fisher & Blair, 1998; O'Brien & Frick, 1996). This suggests that nonanxious antisocial children with psychopathic personality traits may be particularly unlikely to alter their behavior in response to punishment. Further support for this concept comes from studies of ineffective parenting styles and CD in children (Wootton, Frick, Shelton, & Silverthorn, 1997). Only in children with CD but without psychopathic traits was antisocial behavior related to ineffective parenting. In children assessed as having callous–unemotional (psychopathic) personality traits, antisocial behavior occurred at high rates regardless of the quality of parenting they received. These children appear unable to alter their CD-like behaviors, despite cues of nonreward and punishment from their parents.

The research described above indicates that the concept of psychopathy can reliably and validly be applied to some antisocial children. Although psychopathy is not a psychiatric diagnosis, it does identify a type of antisocial youth with unique characteristics (Frick, 1998). The presence of hyperactivity, impulsivity, and attention problems; adult psychopathic traits and/or callous–unemotional psychopathic personality traits; and significant conduct problems may designate a subgroup of children and adolescents who show a more severe pattern of antisocial behavior and aggression, who are more resistant to treatment, and who correspond closely to adult conceptualizations of psychopathy (Christian et al., 1997). Further research on juvenile psychopathy is needed and should focus on longitudinal studies. Specifically, prospective research is needed to demonstrate that youth with high PCL or PCL-R Factor 1 scores do indeed grow up to become adults with psychopathy. If this continuity can be demonstrated, psychopathy as an important subtype of antisocial youth will be further supported.

PSYCHOTIC DISORDERS

Psychosis implies a serious disturbance in an individual's "reality testing." Impaired reality testing is reflected by a number of specific pathological signs and symptoms, including hallucinations, delusions, and disorganized thought processes (Volkmar, 1996). Disorganized thought processes reflect information-processing deficits in psychotic children, adolescents, and adults. Psychotic symptoms occur in a wide variety of neuropsychiatric conditions in children and adolescents, and are not pathognomonic for any one disorder. For example, disorganized thought processes and illogical thinking are found in children suffering from generalized and complex partial epilepsy (Caplan et al., 1997). A thought disorder needs to be distinguished from expressive and receptive language disorders, which are classified as learning disabilities. Hallucinations can be found in youth suffering from illicit substance intoxication, mood disorders (e.g., psychotic depression and MDI), sexual and physical abuse, posttraumatic stress syndromes, and bereavement following the loss of a loved one (Caplan & Tanguay, 1991). Hallucinations can rarely occur as a side effect of prescribed medications such as stimulants. Indeed, in clinical practice, psychotic symptoms occur much more commonly as part of these disorders than in schizophrenia-spectrum disorders. Most children who have psychotic symptoms are not schizophrenic. The onset of schizophrenia in childhood is relatively rare (McClellan & Werry, 1994).

Developmental issues need to be considered in childhood psychotic disorders. Because psychotic symptoms can generally only be assessed by an evaluation of how a child uses language, little is known about psychotic processes in preschoolers. As a result of cognitive immaturity, preschool children do not yet utilize adult rules of logic and causality. Thus illogical thinking and loose associations of ideas are common in normal preschoolers. After about 7 years of age, these are not so commonly observed in normally developing children (Caplan, Guthrie, Fish, Tanguay, & David-Lando, 1989; Caplan, Perdue, Tanguay, & Fish, 1990). Hallucinations are rare in children younger than 8 years (Caplan & Tanguay, 1991). The presence of pervasively disorganized thinking after age 7 years can clearly be understood as indicating pathology (Caplan, 1994; Caplan, Guthrie, Tang, Komo, & Asarnow, 2000).

Psychotic phenomena are relatively uncommon in the elementary school years. Their presence generally indicates severe psychopathology. Hallucinations are much more prevalent than delusional thinking in psychotic 6- to 12-year-old children, probably because of cognitive immaturity. The content of hallucinations in this age group often reflects developmental concerns, such as monsters, ghosts, pets, or toys. Delusions are rare in this age group; when they do occur, they are more simply organized and less complex, entrenched, and systematic than in psychotic adults (Volkmar, 1996).

During adolescence, the frequency of psychotic illness increases markedly, and symptomatology becomes generally similar to that of adults. The prevalence of delusional thinking increases markedly after age 17 years in psychotic youth, probably reflecting increased cognitive development. Delusions can become organized, systematized, and elaborate in adolescent psychotic disorders, much as they do in adult psychotic disorders. During adolescence, hallucinations and disorganized thinking also begin to take on an adult psychotic form and appearance (Caplan & Tanguay, 1991; McKenna, Gordon, & Rapoport, 1994).

Schizophrenia: Description and Prevalence

Although very rare in childhood and early adolescence, schizophrenia is the prototypic psychotic disorder or group of disorders. It is characterized by one or more of a core group of symptoms, such as bizarre delusions; hallucinations; thought disorder; grossly disorganized behavior; blunted, flat, or grossly inappropriate affect; and significant impairment or deterioration from a previous level of functioning (Asarnow & Asarnow, 1996). These youth are often described as socially withdrawn, shy, isolated, and odd. Schizophrenia rarely occurs before puberty. When onset does occur in childhood, schizophrenia is usually insidious.

The treated prevalence of schizophrenia in children younger that age 15 years is an estimated 0.14 per 1,000 individuals. Between the ages of 15 and 54 years, the treated prevalence of schizophrenia is 50 times higher (McKenna et al., 1994). In the prepubertal years, males are affected more than females, at a ratio of about 2:1; the ratio becomes 1:1 in adolescence (McClellan & Werry, 1994). Although no longitudinal outcome studies of early-onset schizophrenia have been completed, the consensus is that childhood-onset schizophrenia has a uniformly poor prognosis. There exists an increased risk of suicide or accidental death directly attributable to behaviors caused by psychotic thinking in at least 5% of those suffering from this disorder (McClellan & Werry, 1994).

The Relationship between Psychotic Disorders and Aggression

The association between psychotic disorders such as schizophrenia on one hand, and aggression and related behaviors on the other, in prepubertal children appears very weak. First, the prevalence of these disorders in community populations of children and adolescents is very low, in comparison with the prevalence of other childhood psychiatric disorders with a more robust association with aggression, such as the disruptive behavior disorders and mood disorders (e.g., CD, ADHD, MDD, DD). Second, when psychotic syndromes do occur in prepubertal children and they are brought to clinical attention, they are most often described as shy, withdrawn, socially isolated, and odd, rather than aggressive or violent. Third, because of cognitive immaturity, psychotic children do not generally develop systematized and elaborate delusional systems of the type known to be associated with violent behavior in psychotic adults (Link, Andrews, & Cullen, 1992; Volkmar, 1996; Wessely, 1993). Psychotic symptoms in children most often involve age-constrained developmental themes such as monsters, ghosts, or toys, rather than the paranoid ideas of reference commonly seen in violent adults with schizophrenia. Indeed, when studies examine the predictors of violence and assaultiveness in prepubertal children, a difficult temperament, impulsivity, family dysfunction, physical and sexual abuse, cognitive delays, parental psychopathology, parental SUDs, and parental assaultiveness are much more strongly associated with childhood aggression and violence in both psychiatrically referred and nonreferred community samples than are psychotic symptoms. An association of aggression with childhood schizophrenia and psychotic symptoms is generally not found (Kingston & Prior, 1995; Pfeffer, Plutchik, & Mizruchi, 1983b).

The relationship between psychotic disorders and aggression appears to become somewhat stronger in middle to late adolescence and into young adulthood. This association was reinforced by studies largely published before 1989, which consistently reported a relationship between psychotic symptoms and aggressive behavior in adolescents and young adults. For example, in a study of 51 hospitalized psychotic adolescents from low-SES backgrounds, 34 (67%) were found to have histories of violent behavior. The authors of this report concluded that aggression is a common behavioral manifestation of psychosis in adolescence (Inamdar, Lewis, Siomopoulos, Shanok, & Lamela, 1982). In a predominantly young adult psychotic sample admitted to a state mental health institution, Tardiff and Sweillam (1980) reported that 21% had assaultive or suicidal histories prior to admission. These reports have contributed to the common perception that psychotic disorders in general, and schizophrenia in particular, are highly associated with violent behaviors (Link & Stueve, 1998).

More recent investigations have begun to question findings that strong and direct correlations exist between psychotic symptoms and aggression in adolescents and adults (Appelbaum, Robbins, & Monahan, 2000). These newer studies point out that methodological problems in the earlier reports often limit the generalizability of findings. These include studying samples drawn exclusively from the lowest SES levels (which are known to have increased rates of aggression), lack of nonpsychotic comparison groups, lack of community control groups to determine the baseline rates of violence in the communities from which the patients were selected, and methodological difficulties in the measurement of aggression (such that the most extreme examples of aggression were the only behaviors studied).

Recent studies of the relationship between aggression and psychotic illness have utilized better methodological designs. These investigations suggest that although a relationship between psychosis and aggression does exist, it may be mediated by several nonpsychotic variables. In a study of 137 middle- and upper-SES adolescents admitted to an inpatient psychiatry unit (in contrast to previous studies, which investigated only lower-SES psychotic adolescents), no significant differences in aggression were observed between psychotic and nonpsychotic adolescents (Delga, Heinssen, Fritsch, Goodrich, &

Yates, 1989). Studies that have compared rates of aggression in psychotic adolescents by gender have found that psychotic males are significantly more aggressive than psychotic females (Inamdar et al., 1982), similar to the male–female differences in aggression found for adolescents with nonpsychotic disorders (Delga et al., 1989). Proximity to family, friends, and intimate acquaintances may be another risk factor: Psychotic individuals with close interpersonal relationships and increased time spent in close proximity to these relationships have higher rates of interpersonal violence than psychotic individuals who are socially isolated (Steadman et al., 1998). Co-occurring SUDs were found to be prevalent in one study of psychiatrically referred schizophrenic adolescents and adults, and SUDs significantly raised the rate of violence in these patients (Steadman et al., 1998). However, this same study also found increased rates of violence in substance-misusing nonreferred community controls from the same neighborhoods as the psychotic subjects, indicating that psychosis by itself may not a risk factor for violence. The risk may be mediated through comorbid SUDs (Steadman et al., 1998). These studies suggest that SES, gender, proximity to others, and SUDs mediate some of the relationship between aggression and psychotic disorders.

In summary, a relationship between psychotic symptoms and an increased risk of violent aggression probably does exist. This relationship may first begin in adolescence, when cognitive maturity allows the expression of adult psychotic symptoms such as delusions, ideas of reference, and paranoia. However, the magnitude of this risk may be less than what has historically been assumed. Although this relationship is probably strongest for psychotic patients who come to psychiatric attention and often have comorbid conditions such as SUDs, the risk for violence associated with schizophrenia in the community has been calculated at only 3%. That is, if schizophrenia were eliminated, the amount of violent behavior in the community would decrease by only 3% (Swanson, Holzer, Ganju, & Jono, 1990; Wessely, 1993). Psychotic adolescents and adults at the highest risk for violence include those with organized, systematized, paranoid delusions of threat; those who have had a chronic psychotic illness for several years; those who have drifted out of treatment; those who have intimate relationships and frequent contact with family and friends; and/or those with comorbid SUDs (Steadman et al., 1998; Wessely, 1993).

ANXIETY DISORDERS

General Description and Comments

Anxiety symptoms are very common in children and adolescents; they may often occur during normal development. In general, younger children report more symptoms of anxiety than older children, and girls report more anxiety than boys (Bernstein, Borchardt, & Perwien, 1996). Anxiety disorders may be the most common class of psychiatric disorders in psychiatrically referred children and adolescents. Children and adolescents meeting criteria for these disorders are generally described as shy, withdrawn, fearful of situations or objects in the environment, afraid of new activities or meeting new people, and inhibited. With few exceptions, youth with anxiety disorders are not often described as aggressive, violent, or antisocial. Indeed, as noted in the section on psychopathy, aggressive/antisocial behaviors may be decreased in boys who have preexisting CD accompanied by a comorbid anxiety diagnosis (Walker et al., 1991). As such, a vulnerability to anxiety is often considered a protective factor for decreasing the expression of aggression.

Posttraumatic Stress Disorder

Description and Prevalence

PTSD (APA, 1994) is one exception to the general point made above: It is a recognized anxiety disorder in which aggression and related behaviors may be prominent symptoms. This anxiety disorder may increase the risk for aggressive responding, whereas most other anxiety disorders may exert a protective effect. The essential feature of PTSD is the development of particular symptoms after exposure to an extreme traumatic stressor (APA, 1994). The traumatic event may involve direct personal experience of an event involving threatened or actual death, serious injury, or other threats to physical integrity; witnessing an event involving such factors; or learning about such an event experienced by a family member or a close acquaintance. A traumatic event can often evoke intense fear and feelings of being helpless to escape harm. When such feelings are accompanied by persistent reexperiencing of the traumatic event (even when danger has passed and the individual is safe), the avoidance of stimuli that are reminders of the trauma, and ANS overarousal, with symptoms that last for more than 1 month, a DSM-IV diagnosis of PTSD may be made (APA, 1994). The ICD-10 criteria for PTSD (WHO, 1992) are somewhat different. ICD-10 requires only the exposure to a traumatic stressor and symptoms of unwanted reexperiencing of the event. Symptoms of avoidance or ANS overarousal are optional and not required for an ICD-10 PTSD diagnosis.

Examples of traumatic events include violent personal assault, rape, sexual abuse, physical abuse, kidnapping, robbery, mugging, severe accidents, life-threatening illness, natural disasters, human-made disasters (war, combat, torture), domestic violence, gang-related violence, or injury or death to another person. Some traumatic events are single acute occurrences, such as a shooting or a natural disaster. Others are chronic and ongoing, such as physical and sexual abuse that occurs over many years in a child's life. A traumatic event may be reexperienced in various ways. Commonly, recurrent memories or dreams occur in which the traumatic event is replayed. Dissociative states may occur in which the person relives the traumatic event for a brief time period, as if the danger were occurring all over again (flashbacks). Reminders of the trauma are actively avoided. Thoughts, feelings, activities, situations, or people who arouse recollections of the trauma are deliberately forgotten, numbed, or avoided. The traumatized individual may withdraw from life, become emotionally constricted, or feel as if he or she has no future. Persistent symptoms of anxiety, not present before the trauma, may cause irritability, anger outbursts, an exaggerated startle response, and a persistent need to scan the environment for further threats of danger (hypervigilance).

The symptoms of PTSD are generally similar in children, adolescents, and adults; however, some developmental differences have been noted. Adolescents with PTSD exhibit symptoms similar to those of adults and are most likely to develop full DSM-IV criteria. Elementary-school-age children may not develop avoidance symptoms, such as amnesia for the trauma, active avoidance of reminders of it, or a numbing of emotions and feelings associated with it. Instead of dissociative experiences and visual reliving of the trauma (flashbacks), children of this age may reenact the trauma in repetitive play, drawings, or verbalizations. Traumatized children may come to believe that certain omens and "signs" are warnings predicting traumatic events, and that if they are alert enough, they will be able to see these omens. Sleep disturbances are also common in traumatized children. Because of cognitive immaturity, very young children have less of a coping repertoire to help them master a trauma. Preschool-age children who are exposed to severe trauma may not develop DSM-IV PTSD criteria at all. Instead, very distressing events may overwhelm them, leading to a loss of previously acquired skills, such as toilet training or the ability to sleep by themselves at night. Traumatized preschool children may also become aggressive and exhibit severe temper tantrums instead of developing classic PTSD symptoms (AACAP, 1998b; Bernstein & Borchardt, 1991; Fletcher, 1996; Pfefferbaum, 1997; Terr, 1985, 1991).

Behavioral disturbances are common in traumatized children and adolescents. Extreme psychological trauma can be associated with elevated rates of aggression in children and adolescents. This behavioral effect may be mediated by gender, with traumatized boys at greater risk for increased hostility, irritability, and aggression. In contrast, traumatized girls may be at greater risk for elevated rates of internalized hopelessness, helplessness, and mood disorders (Armsworth & Holaday, 1993). Other studies, however, do not report finding a gender effect on aggressive outcomes after exposure to extreme, generally violent traumas (Steiner, Garcia, & Matthews, 1997; Cauffman, Feldman, Waterman, & Steiner, 1998). One particular traumatic stressor that may not show gender differences in subsequent aggressive behavior is physical abuse. Physically abused children have been reported at particularly high risk for continued physical aggression, violence, and antisocial behavior. This has been reported for both boys and girls (Connor, Melloni, & Harrison, 1998; Pelcovitz et al., 1994).

Epidemiological research suggests that it is not rare for children, adolescents, and young adults to be exposed to extreme or life-threatening traumatic events. In a random sample of 1,200 young adults enrolled in a health maintenance organization, 19% reported exposure to traumatic events in a 3-year prospective follow-up (Breslau, Davis, & Andreski, 1995). The definition of traumatic events in this study closely followed the one used in DSM-IV (APA, 1994). In another random sample of nonreferred urban youths exposed to community violence, 34.5% met full criteria for PTSD (Berman, Kurtines, Silverman, & Serafini, 1996). In a study of 384 older working-class adolescents assessed in the community, 43% reported experiencing at least one significant trauma by age 18 years, and 6.3% of the sample developed PTSD (Giaconia et al., 1995). Traumas reported included experiencing physical violence, witnessing physical violence, rape, natural disaster, sudden injury or accident, or hearing news of a friend or relative's sudden death or accident. Of the adolescents reporting traumatic events in this study, 26.8% experienced trauma by age 14 years, and 12.2% experienced trauma before age 10 years (Giaconia et al., 1995). Clearly, a great many children and adolescents are exposed to traumatic events in their developing years.

Subtypes

Acute, Chronic, and Delayed-Onset PTSD. Three subtypes of PTSD, based on symptom duration, are specified in DSM-IV. If the symptoms have lasted less than 3 months since exposure to the traumatic stressor, the acute type is diagnosed. In the chronic type, symptoms have lasted for 3 months or longer. In the delayed-onset type, symptoms begin after a delay of 6 months or longer following the trauma. When characteristic symptoms appear within 1 month of exposure to a traumatic stressor, but do not last longer than 1 month, a distinct diagnosis of acute stress disorder may be given. In other words, in acute stress disorder, the posttraumatic symptoms appear and resolve within 4 weeks of exposure to the traumatic event.

Type I and Type II Trauma. Another PTSD typology has been conceptualized, though it is not formally recognized in DSM-IV; this typology is based on the nature of the trauma experienced (Terr, 1991). In this classification, Type I traumas are distinguished from Type II traumas. The former are defined as acute, one-time traumatic events, such as a motor vehicle accident, a tornado, or a murder. The latter are defined as multiple, ongoing, chronic traumas in which multiple varieties of trauma may be experienced or witnessed over an extended time period. An example would be ongoing physical abuse with intermittent sexual abuse of a child in a family where the children also witness repeated domestic violence between family members. Type I traumas may result in classic DSM-IV PTSD symptoms of reexperiencing, avoidance, and ANS overarousal. Type II traumas may be different, resulting in accommodation to the trauma over time. Symptoms may include denial, dissociation, suppressed rage, hostility, irritability, and numbing of feelings.
    Empirical studies have begun to document support for this framework.

Famularo, Fenton, Kinscherff, and Augustyn (1996) described distinct symptomatology between children experiencing Type I and Type II traumas. This study reported that Type I traumas were associated with more sleep difficulties, physiological hyperarousal, and reexperiencing of events, and that Type II traumas were more prominently linked with dissociation, restricted affect, sadness, and detachment. In a meta-analysis of 2,697 children reported in 34 studies of PTSD, many differences in symptoms and symptom rates were observed, depending on the type of trauma experienced (Fletcher, 1996). More symptoms were observed among child victims of chronic or abusive stressors than among children with Type II stressors. Children exposed to Type II stressors were observed to have more symptoms of avoidance, numbing of feelings, actively trying to forget about the traumatic events, bad dreams, symptoms of overarousal (including irritability and an exaggerated startle response), aggression, and antisocial behaviors than children exposed to Type I traumatic events. These symptom differences may reflect a dependent child's attempts at accommodation in the face of inescapable and chronic abusive events (Fletcher, 1996).

The Relationship between PTSD and Aggression

One way the association between PTSD and aggression may be mediated is through individual neurobiological responses to fears of threat. It is well known that individuals have evolved adaptive responses to threats occurring in the environment. These adaptive responses are controlled by the CNS and increase the organism's probability of survival. In the past decade, much knowledge has been gained about the neurobiological basis of anxiety and fear, and about an individual's adaptation to stress and threat in his or her environment. This research is also beginning to reveal how these adaptational neurobiological systems can become dyscontrolled in the face of sudden, life-threatening, or chronic extreme trauma (Charney, Deutch, Krysta, Southwick, & Davis, 1993; Charney, Grillon, & Bremner, 1998).

Acute, sudden, life-threatening stress activates many alarm systems in the CNS that are designed to perceive and evaluate threat, and to organize an adaptive response that will increase the individual's chances of survival and avoidance of injury. The brain structures that participate in the fear response are both cortical and subcortical. Evaluation of fear of threat can occur without conscious awareness (Charney et al., 1998). If the threat is too intense, too uncontrollable, too inescapable, or too chronic, these neurobiological mechanisms can become disorganized and are no longer adaptive. The higher brain functions that organize adaptive responses to threat and generally exert inhibition over lower brain structures that subserve memory, behavior, and emotion may become impaired. Diminished inhibition may then result in the release of explosive moods and behaviors. Even when the acute trauma has resolved, increased rage, hostility, irritability, and aggression in the face of memories or reminders of the traumatic event may then occur (Kolb, 1987).

This process is called "fear conditioning" (Charney et al., 1993), and it appears to occur similarly in animals and humans. Like the evaluation of fear of threat, fear conditioning can also occur via unconscious emotional processes that operate outside an individual's awareness (Charney et al., 1998).

There is some empirical support for the relationship among psychological trauma, fear of threat, and increased aggression. For example, there is evidence that adolescents suffering from PTSD are more aggressive than adolescents without PTSD. In a study of male adolescents with CD in a juvenile detention setting, those with PTSD were compared to those without it. In the youth with PTSD, traumatic events were usually of a violent nature, including murder, abuse, grave injury, and witnessing violence in the community. The males with CD and comorbid PTSD were significantly more likely to have diminished impulse control and failure to suppress aggressive behavior than males with CD who did not meet criteria for PTSD (Steiner et al., 1997). This finding has been replicated for female adolescents with CD and PTSD in juvenile detention (Cauffman et al., 1998).

Another way in which the association between PTSD and aggressive/antisocial behaviors may be mediated is through the presence of comorbid psychiatric disorders. As noted previously, child and adolescent psychiatric disorders rarely occur in isolation. PTSD has been associated with CD and ADHD at rates that exceed chance levels (Giaconia et al., 1995; McLeer, Callaghan, Henry, & Wallen, 1994; Pelcovitz et al., 1994). Developmentally, these disorders can precede the diagnosis of PTSD. A child or adolescent meeting criteria for these comorbid conditions may be exposed to traumatic events at rates above those of children without preceding externalizing behavior disorders. In other words, a child with CD or ADHD may already be involved in activities in which traumatic stressors have a high likelihood of occurrence. Moreover, CD and ADHD increase the prevalence of aggression and antisocial behaviors in their own right.

PROBLEMS WITH UNDERSTANDING AGGRESSIVE BEHAVIORS WITHIN A CATEGORICAL DIAGNOSTIC CONTEXT

There exist several problems with understanding aggression within the categorical structure of psychiatric diagnoses. Focusing only on aggression as an associated symptom of a categorical psychiatric diagnosis may often ignore the environmental context in which aggression occurs (Jensen & Hoagwood, 1997; Wakefield, 1996). An understanding of environmental cues for aggressive responding is exceedingly important in the study of aggression. For example, the prototypic DSM-IV (APA, 1994) aggressive mental disorder found in children and adolescents is CD. A child who is subjected to physical or sexual abuse or severe neglect in a chaotic and violent home environment may run away, lie, steal, and be truant from school while trying to survive a trauma of this magnitude and severity. Although this child may satisfy the DSM-IV criteria for CD, a better explanation for this behavior is *not* that the child has a mental disorder, but that he or she is adjusting to an overwhelmingly maladaptive and threatening environment with an adaptive survival strategy. Aggression only discussed within the context of a categorically diagnosed psychiatric disorder may obscure the importance of environmental context.

A second problem with the relationship of aggression to categorically diagnosed psychiatric disorders is the heterogeneity inherent in the symptom lists for psychiatric diagnosis (Clark, Watson, & Reynolds, 1995; Sonuga-Barke, 1998). To continue considering CD as an example, the criteria for this mental disorder mix different types of aggressive behaviors. A child or adolescent who engages in purely overt aggression—in which there is a hostile confrontation between the youth and the environment (e.g., physical violence, use of weapons, extortion, or armed robbery)—may satisfy criteria for CD. Conversely, someone who engages in purely covert aggression—acts that are furtive and hidden (e.g., shoplifting, vandalism, or fire setting)—may also satisfy criteria for CD. These two subtypes of aggression are very different. The problem in discussing aggression only as an associated symptom of a categorical psychiatric diagnosis is that meaningful subtypes of aggression may be obscured.

A third problem is the diagnostic comorbidity very commonly found when categorical systems are used to diagnose psychiatric disorders (Caron & Rutter, 1991). For all of the discrete psychiatric diagnoses associated with aggression and related behaviors in youth, other such diagnoses co-occur with them at rates much greater than chance. This comorbidity further obscures understanding of the relationships between discrete psychiatric disorders and aggression, and additionally diminishes the possibility of identifying meaningful subtypes of aggression in youth.

As a result of these problems, alternative approaches to classifying aggressive behavior have been investigated. Many of these alternatives have utilized empirical methods that result in aggressive symptoms' being grouped statistically into factors and clusters in which symptoms are meaningfully related to one another (see Chapter 1). These approaches often result in a dimensional approach to aggressive and antisocial behaviors in which symptoms are continuously distributed in a population, without a clear "cutoff" that identifies them as being present or absent. For example, in a statistical examination of the internal structure of 10 common categorical mental disorders (including ASPD) in an epidemiological study of a U.S. probability sample, factor analysis identified a broad internalizing factor with the elements of "anxious–misery" and "fear," and a broad externalizing factor with the element of "antisocial disruptive behavior." These two factors largely explained the comorbidity between categorical psychiatric diagnoses in the study population (Krueger, 1999). Because these broad internalizing and externalizing factors have been empirically identified, the problems inherent in categorical diagnostic systems, such as symptom heterogeneity and diagnostic comorbidity, are avoided.

CHAPTER SUMMARY

Although most children and adolescents who are referred for clinical services and meet criteria for a categorically diagnosed psychiatric disorder are not violent or otherwise aggressive, these behaviors are among the most common reasons for referral of youth to mental health services. This chapter has reviewed some of the more common and important psychiatric diagnoses that have a relationship with aggression.

Aggression in the context of these categorically diagnosed disorders has multidimensional, diverse, and complex etiologies. These may include biological, developmental, environmental, psychosocial, and neuropsychological causes. The diversity of etiologies points out the inadequacy of any simple, unitary hypothesis of the pathogenesis of aggression in neuropsychiatric illness, and thus the inadvisability of adopting unduly simplified, unifocal, or overgeneralized explanations or psychiatric diagnoses to explain aggressive youngsters. In other words, there is no single aggression diagnosis that exists for all aggressive individuals.

It is clear that the relationship of aggression to psychiatric illness is complex, and that achieving a better understanding of this relationship in youth requires a broad multimodal, multidisciplinary approach. At the same time, clinicians faced with evaluating aggressive juveniles are obligated to assess for the presence of common psychiatric diagnoses associated with aggressive and related behaviors, because they may offer hope of specific treatment.

Risk and Protective Factors in Aggression and Related Behaviors

The importance of identifying risk and protective factors for youthful aggression and related behaviors lies in the hope of (1) improving recognition of at-risk youngsters before the onset of serious maladaptive behavior; (2) clarifying protective buffers against the development of a stable pattern of early-onset maladaptive behavior; and (3) providing an empirical guide for rational individual, family, and community treatment interventions for aggressive youth. "Risk factors" are conditions and influences that predispose children and adolescents to the maladaptive expression of aggressive behavior. "Protective factors" are contingencies that shield youngsters from the influence of risk factors. This chapter reviews and discusses risk factors, protective factors, and their interactions in juvenile aggressive behavior in children and adolescents.

There are several points to keep in mind during any discussion of risk and protective factors. First, in order to devise rational prevention and treatment efforts for aggressive youth, it is important to understand causal mechanisms—the reasons why some youth become aggressive and others do not. However, causality in the development of aggression and related behaviors is very difficult to demonstrate scientifically. The most powerful explanatory tool in the scientist's armamentarium is the experimental method, in which subjects are randomly assigned to at least one experimental and at least one control condition. Ideally, with enough subjects in a sample, the individuals in the groups being compared will be equivalent at the start of the experiment on all variables except the variables to be studied in the experiment. Unfortunately, the experimental method cannot be used to study risk and protective factors in juvenile aggression, because such factors cannot be randomly assigned to children and adolescents. Consequently, the study of risk and protective factors and aggression will *always* be confounded by other characteristics.

Much research in this area has focused on revealing correlates of conduct disorder (CD) or more broadly defined "conduct problems." Correlates are factors that are statistically associated with these problems, or factors that statistically distinguish between groups of youth with and without these problems. Theories are then offered to explain the association of these correlates with the behaviors under investigation. However, correlations do not imply causality. For example, if it is found that Factor A is statistically correlated with aggressive behavior, then one or more of three different explanations may exist: Factor A may cause aggressive behavior; aggressive behavior may cause Factor A; or a third, unrelated factor (Factor B) may mediate the association between Factor A and aggressive behavior. Correlates have many different ways of fitting into causal explanations, and knowing a correlation does not tell us what causal explanation fits best. As such, great care must be taken in interpreting correlative findings.

Next, correlations do not tell us what factors are specific for the development of aggression and related behaviors and what factors are generalized risks for the development of global psychopathology, one aspect of which may be aggression. For example, parental criminality is a risk factor for the development of childhood delinquency (Cadoret, Yates, Troughton, Woodworth, & Stewart, 1995), but it is also a risk factor for the development of general psychopathology in youth, only one aspect of which is delinquency (Rutter, 1979). Similarly, correlations do not tell us what constitutes a direct risk factor for the development of conduct problems, as opposed to a risk factor that is indirect and mediated through other mechanisms. For example, evidence exists that dysfunctional family functioning is correlated with the development and maintenance of childhood antisocial behavior (Dodge, Bates, & Pettit, 1990). However, this is an indirect effect that appears to be mediated by other variables in complex ways. These include poor parental supervision of offspring, low levels of parental involvement in their children's activities, and harsh and inconsistent disciplinary practices (Loeber & Stouthamer-Lober, 1986). The identification of specific and direct risk factors for the development of childhood aggression and related behaviors is a necessary step in uncovering causal processes that can then rationally inform prevention and treatment efforts.

Finally, most correlational research has focused on single variables and sought to determine their significance in the development of aggressive/antisocial behaviors. These are called "univariate," or "main-effects" models. However, causal mechanisms for these behaviors are multifaceted, complex, and transactional (i.e., multiple risk and protective factors that feed forward and backward to influence one another over the course of a youngster's development). The field is rapidly moving away from single-variable, main-effects perspectives and toward viewpoints that attempt to integrate developmental, psychobiological, personological, familial, community, cultural, and socioeconomic factors in more ecologically valid models (Cicchetti & Lynch, 1993).

Readers should keep this discussion in mind during the review of risk and protective factors that follows. For ease of exposition, risk factors among individual, family, and extrafamilial influences are considered first, in that order; protective factors are then more briefly discussed.

INDIVIDUAL RISK FACTORS

Heritable Factors

Neuropsychiatric genetic research is increasingly recognizing the importance of heritable factors in aggression and related behaviors. These heritable influences appear strongest for overt types of aggression, but have also been found for covert and oppositional behaviors (Eaves et al., 1997; Hewitt et al., 1997; Hudziak, Rudiger, Neale, Heath, & Todd, 2000). Although it has been known for a long time that a high degree of familial influence exists in aggressive/antisocial behaviors, it has been unclear to what extent this reflects genetic influences, shared environmental factors, or some interaction between the two. Recent reviews have consistently concluded that there is a substantial genetic component to these behaviors, as well as a substantial interaction between biological vulnerability and adverse environmental factors in the development of these behaviors (Cadoret et al., 1995; Mason & Frick, 1994; Rutter, Silberg, O'Connor, & Simonoff, 1999).

Research into heritable factors in aggressive and antisocial behaviors generally employs several different types of methodological design strategies. These analyses are generally ordered as a series of related steps. The first-step investigations are called "family aggregation studies." These studies seek to determine whether, say, CD runs in families. However, if CD is found to be familial, aggregation studies cannot answer the question of what portion of this is due to genetics and what portion to a shared family environment. In other words, these studies cannot tease out the answer to the "nature versus nurture" question. In this type of research, biological parents and relatives of youth who meet psychiatric diagnostic criteria for CD are themselves evaluated for the presence of psychiatric disorder. Rates of antisocial personality disorder (ASPD) in biological parents and adult relatives, and of CD in child relatives, are ascertained and compared to rates in biological relatives of control children who do not have CD. A variation of this type of study is to examine the offspring of parents with ASPD or antisocial personality traits for the presence of CD in their children. For example, in a study of the latter type, parental ASPD was found to be strongly and specifically associated with child CD, indicating familial aggregation of antisocial behaviors (Faraone, Biederman, Keenan, & Tsuang, 1991). In an example of the former strategy, evidence of familial clustering of CD was found in a general population-based sample (Szatmari, Boyle, & Offord, 1993). These types of investigations have established that antisocial behaviors, such as those defining CD, and early-onset and persistent problems with aggression cluster in families.

If a disorder is found to be familial, the next step is to ascertain "heritability." That is, does the disorder have a genetic component? Studies that utilize adoption and twin designs can begin to answer this question. In adoption methodologies, biological children of antisocial parents who are adopted away at birth to nonantisocial adoptive parents are compared on rates of conduct problems in later childhood or adulthood to rates of antisocial behaviors in adopted-away offspring of nonantisocial parents. These studies are consistent in finding a genetic influence for antisocial behavior, aggression, and adult crime. Studies consistently document statistically significant associations between ASPD and crime in biological parents and similar disorders in adopted-away offspring. Although the absolute rates of adult ASPD in the biological offspring of criminal parents are fairly low in many studies (ranging from 6% to 36%), they are significantly higher than in control adoptees (Cadoret et al., 1995; Rutter et al., 1990, 1999). Since adoption paradigms also produce family members who share the adopted family environment but are not genetically related, these studies can also provide information about shared environmental risks that influence the development of conduct problems. Since not all (less than 100%) adopted-away offspring of antisocial parents develop antisocial problems, environmental factors have also been identified as important in the risk for such problems (Plomin, DeFries, McClearn, & Rutter, 1997).

Another strategy uses twin methodologies. Twins are accidents of nature in which identical or monozygotic (MZ) twins (derived from one fertilized egg or zygote) share 100% of genes, but fraternal or dizygotic (DZ) twins (derived from separately fertilized eggs) share only 50% of genes, as any other sibship does. If aggressive and antisocial behaviors in youth have a genetic basis, concordance rates for such problems should be higher for MZ twins than for DZ twins. This method assumes that the environment is roughly the same for both individual twins reared in the same family. If this equal-environments assumption is correct (and there is evidence to support it), then, because of genetic influences, MZ twins must be more similar than DZ twins on a complex trait such as antisocial behavior. There is now a substantial body of data from twin studies demonstrating a substantial genetic component for both criminality and ASPD in adults. Weighted concordance rates for adult criminality range between 13% and 22% for DZ twins, and between 26% and 51% for MZ twins (Rutter et al., 1990). The data are somewhat different in child studies. In a study pooling all twin data on concordance rates for juvenile delinquency, McGuffin and Gottesman (1985) showed an 87% concordance rate for MZ pairs, compared with 72% in DZ pairs. What stands out in comparison to adult criminal twin studies is the high concordance rate for juvenile DZ twin pairs, indicating that in addition to genetic factors, the family environment shared across siblings is exerting an important influence in juvenile delinquency (Rutter et al., 1990).

These studies support genetic influences in juvenile aggressive and antisocial behaviors. They also support the importance of shared environmental factors in these problems, especially in youth. What is the magnitude of genetic heritability in such behaviors? A quantitative summary of 12 twin studies and three adoption studies published since 1975 was completed to answer this question (Mason & Frick, 1994). The 15 studies reviewed contained 3,795 twin pairs and 338 adoptees. Approximately 50% of the difference between measures of antisocial and nonantisocial behaviors was found to be attributable to genetic effects. Significantly larger estimates of genetic effects were found for more severe than for less severe behaviors, and in clinic-referred as opposed to community samples.

More recent research has begun to focus on investigating the interactional effects between genetic and environmental risks in the development of antisocial behavior. These studies generally report the highest risk for antisocial outcomes when a genetic risk interacts with an adverse environment (Bohman, 1996; Cadoret et al., 1995). For example, in an adoptee study of adult petty criminality, Bohman (1996) found that in the absence of either genetic or environmental risk, the rate of adult criminality was just 3%. When there existed environmental risk but not genetic risk, the rate rose to 6%. With genetic liability but no environmental risk, the rate was 12%. However, with both genetic and environmental risk factors present, the rate of adult criminality was 40%. This interactive effect is illustrated in Figure 5.1.

A similar finding was reported by Cadoret et al. (1995) with an adoption paradigm. In this study, offspring of parents with ASPD and/or substance use

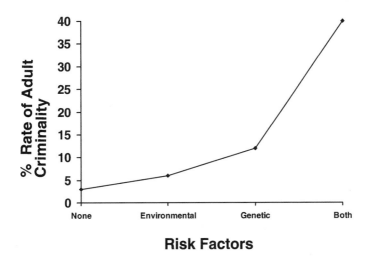

Risk Factors

FIGURE 5.1. Interactional effects on rates of adult criminality for environmental risks, genetic risks, and combined risk factors. Data from Bohman (1996).

disorders (SUDs) who were adopted away at birth were assessed for adolescent and adult aggression and CD. Both a biological background of ASPD and rearing in an adverse adoptive home environment (characterized by marital problems, adoptive parent psychopathology, or legal problems) predicted increased adolescent and adult aggression and CD in adoptees. However, adverse adoptee home environments interacted in such a way as to result in significantly increased aggression and CD in adoptees only in the presence of—not in the absence of—a biological family background of ASPD. These studies shows that environmental effects and genetic–environmental interactions are important and powerful in the genesis of aggression and antisocial behaviors.

Subtypes of aggression and related behaviors may be informative as to genetic influences (Stanger, Achenbach, & Verhulst, 1997). When subtypes of aggression (see Chapter 1) are investigated using rating scales, evidence suggests that the "aggressive" factor as identified in studies by Achenbach, Edelbrock, and colleagues (i.e., overt aggression) is more heritable than the "delinquent" factor (i.e., covert aggression). Edelbrock, Rende, Plomin, and Thompson (1995), for example, studied problem behaviors in twins aged 7–15 years. Results revealed stronger heritability for the aggressive factor and weaker heritability for the delinquent factor. The importance of familial influences on overt aggression is further strengthened by the finding of low cultural influences on the expression of overt aggression in a study reporting child and adolescent problem behaviors across 12 different cultures from around the world (Crijnen, Achenbach, & Verhulst, 1999). Other research has supported stronger genetic influences for early-onset subtypes of aggression that persist into adulthood, as compared to childhood-limited types of aggression that do not persist into the adult years (Lyons et al., 1995). Still other investigations have examined the relationship between aggressive CD and attention-deficit/hyperactivity disorder (ADHD) or its core symptom of hyperactivity–impulsivity. In a twin study of adolescent males, a strong genetic influence was found for symptoms of both ADHD and CD. However, almost no genetic influence was found for "pure CD" without hyperactivity–impulsivity. In the "pure CD" type, strongly shared environmental influences were found (Silberg et al., 1996). This suggests that a subtype of aggression characterized by hyperactivity–impulsivity has a more heritable influence than subtypes of aggression without hyperactive–impulsive components (Rutter et al., 1999). Finally, there is some suggestion that psychopathy is a distinct subtype of aggression that may show heritable tendencies. Aggressive children with psychopathic personality traits show differences in neurochemical and physiological functioning—specifically, autonomic nervous system (ANS) underarousal—compared to nonpsychopathic aggressive children (Lahey, Hart, Pliszka, Applegate, & McBurnett, 1993). These neurochemical and physiological differences in psychopathy may indirectly reflect meaningful genetic differences in this aggressive subtype (Frick, 1998). Genetic findings have been informative, therefore, in suggesting how the heterogeneous, broad category of aggressive and antisocial behaviors can be meaningfully subdivided.

In subtypes of behaviors that reveal a genetic influence, the last step in genetic analysis is to ask what precisely is inherited. Research in neuropsychiatric molecular genetics is only beginning to approach this question, and no definitive answers are yet available. Certainly there is no single gene for aggression. However, future studies in this area offer hope that genetic influences will become more clearly defined in the 21st century and facilitate a broader understanding of gene–environment interactions in the etiology of early-onset, persistent aggressive and antisocial behaviors.

In summary, heritable influences are important for childhood and adolescent aggression and related behaviors. Heritable effects appear strongest for early-onset subtypes of overt aggression that persist into adulthood, are associated with hyperactivity–impulsivity, and possibly include psychopathy. For nonpersistent forms of aggressive behavior that do not continue into adult life, shared environmental influences are stronger for childhood than for adult behaviors. Similarly, shared environmental influences appear stronger for covert forms of aggression. Interactions between genetic influences and adverse environments increase risk for aggressive and related behavior, over and above risk resulting from each factor individually. Molecular genetic investigations into neurotransmitter systems may clarify what is specifically inherited to increase vulnerability in these disorders. (For a more detailed discussion of neurotransmitter research to date, see Chapter 7.)

Temperament

Individual differences in infant and child temperament have long been recognized. "Temperament" is defined as an individual's characteristic style of emotional and behavioral response in a variety of differing situations and to a variety of differing environmental stimuli (Prior, 1992). Temperamental patterns are discernible quite early in life and generally persist over time and across situations. Temperament has been defined as "how" a child behaves. This contrasts with "why" the child does what he or she does (motivation) or "what" he or she does (ability).

Temperament has heritable, biologically based aspects as well as environmentally mediated aspects. Temperamental characteristics are presumably derived from a combination of genetic, intrauterine, central nervous system (CNS), and postnatal environmental factors. Although not rigid and fixed, an individual's temperamental style is likely to be relatively constant over time, especially when the interplay between the individual and his or her environment is relatively stable across development. As the child grows older, temperamental characteristics shade imperceptibly into personality traits. Although temperament is not the same as personality, temperament is one core feature of personality (Rothbart & Ahadi, 1994). An individual's personality is the expression of the interaction between his or her characteristic temperament and life experience.

The structure of temperament has been the focus of extensive research

(Prior, 1992). One important contribution has been the work of Chess and Thomas (1986) in the New York Longitudinal Study of temperament. The authors have defined nine dimensions in modeling the temperament of infants and young children (see Table 5.1).

A cluster of temperamental dimensions described as the "difficult temperament" has been shown to correlate with concurrent and future behavioral adjustment in children of varying ages and different socioeconomic and ethnic

TABLE 5.1. Temperamental Characteristics

Characteristic	Description	Easy	Difficult
Activity level	The motor component present in a given child's functioning	Is able to inhibit motor activity when necessary	Is constantly on the move and cannot inhibit activity when necessary
Rhythmicity (regularity)	The predictability–unpredictability in time of any function, such as sleep–wake, hunger, or elimination patterns	Regular patterns	Irregular patterns
Approach–withdrawal	The nature of the initial response to a new stimulus	Positive approach	Negative approach
Adaptability	Responses to new or changed situations	Quickly accepts new situations	Difficulty adjusting to new situations
Threshold of responsiveness	The intensity level of stimulation necessary to evoke a discernible response	High; enjoys stimulation	Low; easily startled, does not enjoy stimulation
Intensity of reaction	The energy level of response	Mild	Intense
Quality of mood	The amount of pleasant, joyful, and friendly behavior, in contrast to crying, unpleasant, unfriendly behavior	Positive	Negative
Distractibility	The effectiveness of extraneous stimuli in interfering with ongoing behavior	High	Low
Attention span and persistence	The length of time a particular activity is pursued by a child; continuation of an activity in the face of obstacles or distractions	Long	Short

Note. Adapted from Chess and Thomas (1986). Copyright 1986 by The Guilford Press. Adapted by permission.

groups. Although many definitions exist, the "difficult temperament" is generally characterized by qualities of overactivity, undercontrol, high intensity of responses, inattention, predominantly negative mood, and low adaptability to new situations. Chess and Thomas (1986) did not conceptualize the difficult temperament as psychopathology. In their study, they described 10% of their normal, non-clinic-referred sample as exhibiting this cluster of temperamental dimensions. However, research has documented that children with difficult temperaments are at increased risk for the development of psychopathology, especially if other stressors (such as family conflict) are also present (Tschann, Kaiser, Chesney, Alkon, & Boyce, 1996).

Cross-sectional studies document a relationship between difficult temperament and generalized psychopathology, including conduct problems in childhood, adolescence, and adulthood (Giancola, Mezzich, & Tarter, 1998a; Merikangas, Swendsen, Preisig, & Chazan, 1998). Longitudinal studies assessing the relationships between difficult temperament as assessed early in the preschool years and behavior problems later in life are also largely consistent in finding a relationship with increased risk for generalized psychopathology, including aggression, CD, delinquency, and other antisocial behaviors (Caspi, Henry, McGee, Moffitt, & Silva, 1995; Gjone & Stevenson, 1997; Sanson, Smart, Prior, & Oberklaid, 1993). This risk appears for both boys and girls (Caspi et al., 1995), but may be stronger for boys (Gjone & Stevenson, 1997). It should be emphasized that difficult temperament by itself is a relatively weak predictor of the development of conduct problems. When a negative child temperament is combined with family dysfunction, marital conflict, poverty, upbringing in a high-crime neighborhood, and/or parental psychopathology, prediction for aggression and CD is stronger (Maziade et al., 1990).

Other temperamental dimensions have been described. One is "novelty seeking" or "sensation seeking." Children who are high in this trait are described as outgoing, actively pursuing stimulation, impulsive, and lacking in anxiety and fear. Because they are driven to seek stimulation and lack fear, they may have a more difficult time learning from experience and inhibiting their behaviors than children who do not exhibit these temperamental qualities. These children may appear undercontrolled (Caspi et al., 1995). Temperamentally undercontrolled children at age 3 years have been found at age 18 years to have personality traits characterized by impulsivity, danger seeking, and aggression (Caspi & Silva, 1995). In several investigations, children and adolescents with high levels of novelty seeking and fearlessness had higher levels of aggression, conduct problems, criminal involvement, and other antisocial behaviors than youth low on these temperamental dimensions (Raine, Reynolds, Venables, Mednick, & Farrington, 1998; Ruchkin, Eisemann, Hagglof, & Cloninger, 1998; Ruchkin, Eisemann, & Cloninger, 1998). The temperamental dimension of novelty seeking may have a genetic basis. In molecular genetic studies, polymorphisms in dopamine D2 and D4 receptors have been significantly associated with personality traits of novelty seeking in both a European American population (Noble et al., 1998) and a Japanese population (Ono et al., 1997).

In summary, early preschool temperamental dimensions have a relationship with generalized psychopathology in later childhood, adolescence, and adulthood. Some specificity is found for links between the "difficult temperament" cluster and novelty seeking and fearlessness on the one hand, and later aggression and related problems on the other. This relationship may be mediated in part by gender (findings are stronger for boys than girls) and by associated family dysfunction or other environmental stressors. These temperamental dimensions thus appear to have both a genetic and a genetic–environmental interactional basis.

Infant–Caregiver Attachment

It has long been recognized that early environmental influences may make significant contributions to the development of individual personality and risk for psychopathology, including aggression. Among such early environmental influences are the quality and pattern of an infant's attachment to a caregiver (Shaw, Owens, Giovannelli, & Winslow, 2001). During the first year of life, an infant exhibits a repertoire of preadapted behaviors (orienting, crying, clinging, proximity seeking, signaling) that are directed toward the caregiver under conditions of fatigue, illness, threat, or stress; these behaviors serve to promote proximity to the caregiver, with the goal of reducing infant distress. Over time, the repeated interactions of an infant's preadapted behaviors with respect to a caregiver become organized and serve to regulate the infant's emotions and behaviors. This emerging regulation and organization of infant behavior in reciprocal interaction with a caregiver is called "attachment" (Carlson, 1998). Attachment becomes an organized strategy on the part of the infant to obtain attention and care from a particular caregiver—a strategy molded by both participants.

Attachment theory was originally described by John Bowlby (1969), a London psychiatrist, who combined ideas from psychoanalysis and ethology. He argued that the affectional ties between children and caregivers have a biological basis that is best understood in an evolutionary context and serves to promote children's survival. The concept of attachment includes reciprocal social, emotional, cognitive, and behavioral characteristics of both the infant and the caretaker (Goldberg, 1991). Attachment patterns are largely mediated by environmental relational factors, not heredity (Rutter, 1995). First attachments are usually formed by 7 months of age, and are formed to only a few persons in the infant's environment; virtually all infants become attached to their caregivers (Main, 1996). Infants become attached not only to both sensitive and caring parents, but to insensitive and maltreating parents.

Initially, attachment theory focused largely on infants and preschoolers in stable, low-risk families. More recent research has applied attachment theory to individuals across the lifespan and to high-risk infants and families (Main, 1996). Four patterns of attachment have reliably been demonstrated in a separation and reunion paradigm (called the Strange Situation procedure) in laboratory studies of 1-year-old infants, their mothers, and an examiner. These attachment patterns include one secure pattern and three insecure patterns; the four patterns are described in Table 5.2. A recent meta-analysis of attachment studies in infants of low-risk families yielded a distribution of 55% secure, 22% avoidant, 8% ambivalent, and 15% disorganized attachments (van IJzendoorn, 1995).

Characteristics of the caregiver and family environment appear especially important in the genesis of infant attachment patterns. Risk for insecure infant attachment is significantly increased in families with more than four stressors present, such as parental criminality, maternal psychopathology, overcrowding in the home, and diminished or stressful quality of the marital relationship. Risk for infant insecure attachment appears especially increased when family stressors are closely associated with impaired maternal functioning (Shaw & Vondra, 1993). In a meta-analysis of 34 attachment studies, psychopathology in the caregiver led to more deviant infant attachment patterns than did characteristics of the child, such as deafness (van IJzendoorn, Goldberg, Kroonenberg, & Frenkel, 1992). These investigations support the hypothesis that caregiver characteristics appear to play a more important role than child

TABLE 5.2. Attachment Classification

Attachment pattern	Description
Secure	Infant shows signs of missing caregiver upon separation and seeks consolation and physical proximity to caregiver upon reunion. After consolation, returns to active exploration of environment. Caregiver is experienced by infant as available, responsive, and sensitive to infant signals.
Insecure–avoidant	Infant shows no signs of missing caregiver upon separation and actively avoids or ignores caregiver upon reunion. Continues to explore the environment and pays no attention to caregiver. Unemotional. Caregiver is experienced by infant as only intermittently available and responsive.
Insecure–resistant or insecure–ambivalent	Infant overly preoccupied with caregiver throughout the separation–reunion procedure. May seem angry, alternately seeking and resisting caregiver, or overly passive. Fails to be comforted by caregiver upon reunion, continues to focus on caregiver and cry, does not return to exploring the environment. Caregiver is experienced by infant as only intermittently available and responsive.
Insecure–disorganized	Infant shows a blend of contradictory features of several coping strategies to deal with the stress of caregiver separation and reunion. Disorganized behaviors displayed in caregiver's presence, including freezing behaviors, slowed movements, depressed affect, and apprehension and anxiety toward caregiver. Caregiver is experienced by infant as frightening.

Note. Data from Constantino (1995) and Main (1996).

attributes in shaping the quality of the infant–caregiver attachment relationship (Shaw et al., 2001).

Patterns of attachment have been implicated as one of several risk factors in the development of generalized psychopathology, including aggression and antisocial problems, in children and adolescents. This appears particularly true of the avoidant and disorganized patterns of infant attachment (Constantino, 1995; Lyons-Ruth, 1996). Several longitudinal studies are beginning to document relationships between these two patterns of insecure attachment in infancy and increased risk for later psychopathology, including deviant levels of hostility and aggression in later childhood and adolescence. Table 5.3 lists recent longitudinal studies.

The avoidant pattern of insecure attachment appears related to later aggression only in the presence of added caregiver and family risk factors. By itself, the avoidant pattern does not appear related to later aggression (Fagot & Kavanaugh, 1990). These additional risk factors include poverty, adolescent motherhood, intrusive or hostile caregiver parenting style, maternal psychopathology, and family psychosocial problems (see Table 5.3). The disorganized pattern of infant attachment appears more strongly related to later childhood psychopathology and aggressive behavior (Carlson, 1998; Lyons-Ruth, 1996). Disorganized attachment constitutes the collapse of organized, strategic efforts on the part of the infant to obtain security from the caregiver.

TABLE 5.3. Attachment Patterns and the Development of Aggression

Study	Infant attachment type	Mediating variables	Outcome
Renken et al. (1989)	Avoidant	Low SES; maternal hostile, intrusive style	↑ aggression at age 6–8 yr
Fagot and Kavanaugh (1990)	Avoidant	Middle-class, stable families	No relationship with aggression at age 4 yr
Egeland et al. (1993)	Avoidant	Maternal intrusive style	↑ psychopathology at age 42 mo
Hann et al. (1991)	Disorganized	Low SES; adolescent mothers	↑ aggression at age 20 mo
Lyons-Ruth et al. (1993)	Disorganized	Maternal psychopathology; maternal psychosocial problems	↑ risk for aggression and hostility at age 5 yr
Hubbs-Tait et al. (1996)	Disorganized	Maternal depression; adolescent mothers	↑ risk for externalizing behavior problems 10 mo later
Carlson (1998)	Disorganized	Maternal psychosocial problems	↑ risk for psychopathology at age 19 yr

This collapse is thought to be related to caregiving behavior that evokes fear in the infant; possibly the caregiver's own lack of resolution of previous traumatic developmental experiences or ongoing psychopathology leads to a hostile, intrusive style of care that lacks sensitivity to infant needs (Lyons-Ruth, 1996). Disorganized patterns of infant attachment are strongly associated with characteristics of high-risk families (i.e., maternal alcoholism, maternal depression, adolescent parenthood, child abuse, or multiproblem families). In low-risk two-parent families, the prevalence of disorganized attachment patterns is 15% (van IJzendoorn, 1995); this prevalence rises to 82% among high-risk maltreating families (Lyons-Ruth, 1996). In a review of the attachment literature, the relative risk for deviant aggressive outcomes with the avoidant or disorganized infant attachment pattern was found to be elevated, at 1.98 (Constantino, 1995).

Studies in adolescence also demonstrate an association between attachment patterns and antisocial outcomes. In a cross-sectional research design, psychiatrically referred adolescents with an insecure attachment were more likely to develop CD than adolescents demonstrating secure attachment patterns (Rosenstein & Horowitz, 1996). In a longitudinal design, psychiatrically referred adolescents assessed as having an insecure pattern of attachment at age 14 years were more likely to self-report criminal behavior at age 25 years than securely attached adolescents (Allen, Hauser, & Borman-Spurrell, 1996). These studies support the continued association between insecure patterns of attachment and aggressive/antisocial outcomes later in development.

In summary, attachment theory demonstrates that early childhood–caregiver relational variables are important in the etiology of later childhood and adolescent aggression. The caregiver's contribution to infant attachment patterns appears substantial. In addition, this theory reveals that many of the correlates of later childhood aggression are already evident in infancy, as indicated by the quality of infant–caregiver attachment patterns. Risk for insecure attachment increases with increasing numbers of family stressors and decreasing levels of maternal functioning. This upholds the need for increased resources to support highly stressed families with infants, to decrease risk for later aggressive outcomes. Finally, insecure attachment patterns are not a direct cause of psychopathology and aggression, but serve as an initiator of developmental pathways that increase the probability of later psychopathology and aggression (Sroufe, Carlson, Levy, & Egeland, 1999).

Exposure to Neurotoxins

Individual exposure to neurotoxic substances during the course of development is associated with many adverse neurocognitive, neurobehavioral, and structural anatomical abnormalities. The effects of neurotoxins vary across individuals. There are no pathognomonic outcomes that are consistent across all affected individuals. Effects vary depending on cumulative dose; the point in development at which exposure occurs; and associated parental, familial, and environmental risk factors that may interact with the effects of toxins to increase or mitigate risk for individual adverse outcomes. Many of these sequelae may increase risk for aggressive and related behaviors in some, but not all, affected children and adolescents. This section reviews prenatal exposure to alcohol, tobacco, and cocaine, and prenatal and childhood exposure to lead.

Prenatal Alcohol Exposure

Alcohol is a known behavioral and physical teratogen with wide and devastating effects on the developing fetal CNS. Alcohol interferes with all stages of brain development, and the severity of damage depends on the amount of alcohol intake, characteristics of maternal drinking, level of fetal exposure to alcohol, and the developmental timing of exposure. Evidence suggests that the neocortex, hippocampus, cerebellum, and hypothalamic–pituitary–adrenal axis, as well as the developmental patterns of various neurotransmitters, may all be disrupted by fetal exposure to alcohol (Guerri, 1998). Although not every individual exposed prenatally to alcohol shows deficits, grouped animal and human data show that teratogenic alcohol effects occur across the continuum of prenatal exposure according to a dose–response relationship (Olson et al., 1997). Effects of lower levels of alcohol exposure, most often emerge as problems in behavior and adaptive functioning. The heavier the prenatal alcohol exposure or the earlier in pregnancy heavy maternal drinking occurs, the greater the likelihood that physical and anatomical abnormalities will occur along with difficulties in functioning. At its most extreme, prenatal exposure to alcohol results in a medically recognized syndrome called "fetal alcohol syndrome" (FAS). FAS is defined by the triad of pre- and postnatal growth retardation, CNS dysfunction, and a particular pattern of facial characteristics. It has been estimated that only 10% to 40% of the offspring of alcohol-misusing women meet the criteria for a medical diagnosis of FAS (Roebuck, Mattson, & Riley, 1998). Still, the available data suggest that although many children exposed to high amounts of alcohol prenatally are spared physical and anatomical consequences, they remain at risk for cognitive and behavioral problems (Roebuck et al., 1998).

Prenatal alcohol exposure is not rare. In an epidemiological study completed in 1992 that included 29,494 pregnant women from 202 hospitals, a high rate of alcohol use was found (Noble et al., 1997). Specifically, the prevalence of alcohol use detected at childbirth through urine drug screening was 6.72% (1,982 infants exposed to maternal alcohol). Unlike illicit drug and tobacco use, which tended to vary according to social and demographic factors in this sample, alcohol use rates among pregnant women were fairly stable. Incidence rates of children affected by prenatal exposure to alcohol have resulted in figures varying between 0.5 and 3 per 1,000 live births (Weinberg, 1997). The National Institute on Drug Abuse estimates that 7.62 million of all children living in the United States are exposed to alcohol during gestation

(Young, 1997). More severe FAS affects 0.29 to 0.48 per 1,000 live-born children in the United States, with Native American populations reporting FAS incidence rates up to 2.99 per 1,000 live births (Mattson & Riley, 1998).

Prenatal exposure to alcohol may adversely affect cognition; mental retardation and learning disabilities, as well as visuospatial deficits, language delays, and motor coordination delays, are commonly found in affected children. Information-processing deficits may occur even in the absence of mental retardation (Mattson & Riley, 1998; Olson, Feldman, Streissguth, Sampson, & Bookstein, 1998; Weinberg, 1997). Elevated rates of psychopathology are reported in alcohol-affected children, adolescents, and adults relative to control groups. Response inhibition deficits, sustained attention deficits, increased impulsivity, and motor overactivity are commonly found in individuals prenatally exposed to alcohol (Steinhausen, 1995) and are stable over time and development (Steinhausen & Spohr, 1998). These cognitive and behavioral deficits frequently lead to problems in academic and adaptive functioning in affected individuals.

Individuals with FAS or prenatal exposure to alcohol have been found to engage more frequently in impulsive aggression and antisocial behavior than comparison groups do. For example, Streissguth, Randels, and Smith (1991) found that approximately 50% of a sample of adolescents and adults with FAS or known prenatal exposure to alcohol had engaged in bullying and impulsive aggressive behavior. However, in this study the effects of prenatal exposure to alcohol could not be disentangled from the environmental effects of rearing by an alcoholic parent. In a more recent study of the association of prenatal alcohol exposure with behavioral problems in adolescence, many confounding variables were controlled. In a 14-year longitudinal study, 464 children were first assessed at delivery and then again at age 14 years. Adolescents who were prenatally exposed to alcohol had higher rates of antisocial and aggressive problems at age 14 years than prenatally nonexposed comparison children. This finding persisted even after the investigators controlled for 78 confounding variables, including prenatal exposure to drugs other than alcohol, family demographics, postnatal characteristics of the family, and other child characteristics (Olson et al., 1997). A dose–response relationship was also evident: More problems were found in those exposed to higher levels of prenatal alcohol, maternal drinking earlier in pregnancy, and maternal drinking patterns characterized by binge drinking. In another study assessing the association between fetal alcohol exposure and later antisocial behaviors, adolescents with FAS or fetal alcohol effects appeared to be disproportionately represented in the juvenile justice system. For adolescents remanded during a 1-year period to a forensic juvenile justice unit, the prevalence of FAS was 3–10 times and the prevalence of fetal alcohol effects was 10–40 times the accepted worldwide rate (Fast, Conry, & Loock, 1999). These studies suggest that youth affected by FAS or fetal alcohol exposure may be at greater risk for aggressive/antisocial behaviors than youngsters who were not exposed to alcohol *in utero*.

Fetal Nicotine Exposure

In animal models of prenatal nicotine exposure, nicotine is a neuroteratogen (Slotkin, 1998). Evidence is less clear in human populations. However, evidence is emerging that fetal exposure to maternal nicotine may have long-term behavioral consequences (Brennan, Grekin, & Mednick, 1999; Weissman, Warner, Wickramaratne, & Kandel, 1999). Nicotine targets specific neurotransmitter receptors in the fetal brain, eliciting abnormalities of cell proliferation and differentiation; these lead to reduced numbers of cells in the CNS, and eventually cause altered synaptic activity. Adverse effects of nicotine on the developing fetal brain include fetal hypoxia, as well as alterations in cholinergic and catecholaminergic neurotransmitter systems and eventual alterations in synaptic competence. These alterations influence not only immediate developmental events in the fetal brain, but long-term CNS developmental events, which may eventually appear as deficits in cognitive or behavioral competencies in childhood or adolescence after a prolonged period of normality (Slotkin, 1998; Weitzman, Gortmaker, & Sobol, 1992).

The prevalence of maternal smoking during pregnancy remains relatively common. Epidemiological studies of pregnant women admitted to the hospital for obstetrical care continue to find high rates of self-reported smoking. In one such study, 8.82% of 29,494 pregnant women self-reported tobacco use while pregnant (Noble et al., 1997). This translates into 2,601 babies exposed to maternal tobacco products *in utero*. Tobacco use occurs in approximately 25% of all pregnancies in the United States (Slotkin, 1998). This rate overshadows rates of illicit drug use during pregnancy, including cocaine.

Maternal prenatal smoking has been associated with adverse behavioral events in offspring. These include increased rates of delinquency, impulsivity, CD, truancy, and attentional difficulties (Bagley, 1992; Fried, Watkinson, & Gray, 1992; Wakschlag et al., 1997; Weitzman et al., 1992). These associations retain their statistical significance despite controls for such potentially confounding variables as race, age, sex, birth weight, maternal education, maternal use of alcohol during pregnancy, family income, parental divorce, quality of the home environment, parental psychopathology, pregnancy risks, number of schools attended, and parenting practices (see Brennan et al., 1999).

Four longitudinal studies using different birth cohorts have been completed, and all agree in documenting an association between prenatal nicotine exposure and eventual antisocial outcome. Using a Finnish birth cohort of 5,966 subjects, Rantakallio, Laara, Isohanni, and Moilanen (1992) found that individuals whose mothers smoked during pregnancy were twice as likely to have a criminal record at age 22 years as were age-matched controls. Using the same cohort, Rasanen et al. (1999) reported that male offspring of mothers who smoked during pregnancy showed higher risk for violent offenses and recidivism at age 18 years than males whose mothers did not smoke during pregnancy. This relation was specific for violent as opposed to nonviolent crime, and it retained its statistical significance even after the investigators controlled for demographic variables, parental mental illness, pregnancy and birth complications, and various family and parenting factors.

Investigating a cohort of 4,129 Danish males followed from birth until the age of 34 years, Brennan et al. (1999) found a linear relationship between the percentage of violent offenders in their sample and the number of cigarettes the mothers smoked daily during the third trimester of pregnancy. In addition, maternal smoking during the third trimester of pregnancy was statistically associated with higher rates of persistent (as opposed to time-limited) criminal offending. These associations remained significant even after the authors controlled for potential confounds, including socioeconomic status (SES), maternal rejection of an infant, maternal age, pregnancy and delivery complications, maternal use of drugs during pregnancy, paternal criminal and arrest history, and parental history of psychopathology. Compared with males whose mothers did not smoke during the third trimester of pregnancy, males whose mothers smoked more than 20 cigarettes daily during the third trimester were 1.6 times as likely to be arrested for a nonviolent crime, 2.0 times as likely to be arrested for a violent crime, and 1.8 times as likely to commit persistent (as opposed to time-limited) criminal offenses (Brennan et al., 1999). Weissman et al. (1999) found a greater than fourfold increased risk of prepubertal-onset CD in boys whose mothers smoked 10 or more cigarettes daily during pregnancy. These effects persisted despite controls for such variables as maternal misuse of other substances during pregnancy, parental psychopathology, and family risk factors. The effect on boys was relatively specific for CD as opposed to generalized psychopathology. These studies suggest that fetal exposure to nicotine is a risk factor in the later development of aggression and antisocial behaviors in adolescence and young adulthood.

Fetal Cocaine Exposure

Scientific study of prenatal exposure to illicit drugs and child developmental outcome began a period of growth in the 1970s with a focus on exposure to opiates. By the mid-1980s, attention had shifted to the study of cocaine. We now have over 15 years of research on the developmental effects of prenatal exposure to cocaine (Smeriglio & Wilcox, 1999).

Because cocaine use is illegal, and because fear of prosecution may deter women who use cocaine from admitting to this or obtaining medical care, the prevalence of maternal cocaine use during pregnancy is difficult to ascertain. In a study of infants in Georgia, 0.5% were found to have had perinatal exposure to cocaine in 1994 (Centers for Disease Control and Prevention [CDC], 1996a). Early studies documented many deleterious effects of prenatal cocaine exposure on the newborn and developing child. However, these studies largely lacked appropriate methodological controls for the confounding effects of maternal cigarette and polydrug use, poverty, altered maternal nutrition during pregnancy, and a suboptimal maternal–child caregiving environment. As studies began to include longer follow-up periods and more sophisticated control groups necessary to evaluate the unique effects of cocaine, the harmful effects of prenatal cocaine exposure were not as apparent (Landry & Whitney, 1996). Presently, the research picture is decidedly mixed.

Most studies of prenatally cocaine-exposed children have assessed infants, usually within hours or days after delivery. Some of these studies find these infants to have higher risk for intrauterine growth retardation, smaller head circumference, and neurological abnormalities (Chiriboga, Brust, Bateman, & Hauser, 1999; Eyler, Behnke, Conlon, Woods, & Wobie, 1998a). Other studies document neurocognitive deficits in cocaine-exposed infants, such as decrements in state regulation, span of attention, and responsiveness to environmental stimulation (Eyler, Behnke, Conlon, Woods, & Wobie, 1998b). Evidence of a dose–response relationship has been reported: Prenatal exposure to cocaine earlier in pregnancy and at higher concentrations is associated with more risk for physiological and neurocognitive deficits in infants (Delaney-Black et al., 1996; Jacobson, Jacobson, Sokol, Martier, & Chiodo, 1996). However, other studies of infants who are prenatally exposed to cocaine report only minor differences relative to control groups (Bada et al., 1998), or only transient effects of cocaine exposure that disappear within days of birth (Chiriboga, 1998; Richardson, Hamel, Goldschmidt, & Day, 1996). No structural brain abnormalities have been reported in newborns prenatally exposed to cocaine, unlike those prenatally exposed to alcohol (Behnke et al., 1998).

More recent investigations have followed prenatally cocaine-exposed children into the elementary school years. These studies continue to report mixed results. Some of these longitudinal studies report lower IQ and language difficulties in children who were exposed to cocaine *in utero*, despite controls for the potential confounds of an adverse rearing environment (Koren et al., 1998). Other longitudinal studies report a higher incidence of child behavior problems in 3- to 6-year-olds as assessed by classroom teachers, even after potentially confounding environmental, parental, and demographic variables are controlled for (Chasnoff et al., 1998; Delaney-Black et al., 1998; Richardson, 1998). However, just as many studies report no statistically significant differences between prenatally cocaine-exposed children aged 4–9 years and nonexposed controls on measures of cognition, behavior, academic achievement, or physical growth (Hurt et al., 1997; Richardson, Conroy, & Day, 1996; Wasserman, Kline, et al., 1998).

In summary, the developmental impact of prenatal cocaine exposure is at present much less clear than that of prenatal alcohol exposure. Importantly, unlike prenatal exposure to alcohol or tobacco, no direct links to aggressive or related behaviors have yet been found for children prenatally exposed to cocaine.

Prenatal and Childhood Lead Exposure

Concern about the adverse health consequences of childhood lead poisoning was first raised in Australia 100 years ago. Since then, much research has examined the detrimental effects of lead exposure on childhood development. Although high-dose lead poisoning was a focus of early research, subsequent studies have shifted to examining the consequences of low-dose lead exposure. In response to concern that lead is associated with toxic effects even at very low blood levels, the CDC has progressively decreased the threshold blood level used to define lead toxicity in children. In 1991 the CDC recommended that the blood lead level be considered elevated at 10 µg/dl, and that universal childhood screening be implemented (Schaffer & Campbell, 1994).

Lead is ubiquitous in the environment. Sources include lead-based paint, which was sold in the United States until the mid-1970s and may still be present in an estimated 57 million occupied housing units built prior to 1970 (CDC, 1991). In deteriorated housing, contaminated dust and soil as well as flaking paint chips ingested by children are major sources of lead. Other sources include drinking water obtained from lead-containing pipe, and family members whose occupations or hobbies expose them to high levels of lead and who subsequently expose children by wearing work garments or bringing scrap materials home. Elimination of the use of lead in gasoline in the 1970s has helped reduce blood lead concentrations in U.S. residents.

The prevalence of lead toxicity in the population has changed as the threshold level for defining toxicity has been reduced. As this level has been progressively reduced (from 60 µg/dl prior to 1970, to the presently defined threshold of 10 µg/dl), the number of children identified as lead-toxic in epidemiological samples has multiplied. For example, in 1990–1991 the Massachusetts Lead Epidemiology Study assessed the distribution of blood lead levels among 3,599 children from infancy to 4 years of age. A more than fourfold increase in the percentage of children designated as having elevated lead levels (from 5% to 22%) resulted when the threshold level was reduced from 25 µg/dl to 10 µg/dl (see Schaffer & Campbell, 1994).

Since 1943, most studies of the behavioral effects of childhood lead exposure have focused on assessment of psychometric intelligence (IQ). The weight of current evidence supports a significant yet modest association between childhood lead burden (either lifetime or assessed concurrently) and a lower Full Scale IQ at school age (Bellinger, 1995; Bellinger & Dietrich, 1994). When confounding variables such as family sociodemographics and family functioning are controlled for, the association is small. The common effect estimate based on a number of studies is a decline of 2 IQ points for a blood lead increase from 10 to 20 µg/dl (Bellinger & Dietrich, 1994). These studies also note that the effects of prenatal lead exposure appear weaker and more transient than the effects of early postnatal childhood lead exposure. Whereas prenatally exposed children with low blood levels (<10 µg/dl) generally demonstrate less persistent neurocognitive effects, postnatally exposed 1- to 3-year-old children with levels of greater than 15–20 µg/dl demonstrate more enduring neurocognitive deficits into the school-age years. This suggests that exposure early in postnatal life may be more detrimental than prenatal lead exposure, although dose effects need to be considered as well (Bellinger & Dietrich, 1994).

More recent investigations have studied the effects of childhood lead burden on childhood psychopathology and behavioral problems. Unlike earlier studies, this later research has controlled for confounding variables, such as the impact of family dysfunction, parental psychopathology, maternal intelligence, child attributes (e.g., individual temperament), family sociodemographics, and occupational and family residential characteristics. These investigations have generally assessed the consequences of low-dose lead exposure (generally defined as a blood lead level of ≤15 µg/dl) and have largely focused on studying postnatal as opposed to prenatal exposure. In these reports lead burden is ascertained in a variety of ways, including blood lead concentration, bone lead density, and dentine lead levels. A statistically significant but small association between childhood lead burden and increased rates of generalized childhood psychopathology is consistently reported, despite statistical controls for confounds (Bellinger, Leviton, Allred, & Rabinowitz, 1994; Burns, Baghurst, Sawyer, McMichael, & Tong, 1999; Needleman, Riess, Tobin, Biesecker, & Greenhouse, 1996; Sciarillo, Alexander, & Farrell, 1992; Thomson et al., 1989; Wasserman, Staghezza-Jaramillo, Shrout, Popovac, & Graziano, 1998). Increased rates of parent- and teacher-reported internalizing and externalizing behavioral problems are found for lead-exposed children compared to non-lead-exposed controls. Again, however, the effects are small and modest. For example, in the study of Wasserman, Staghezza-Jaramillo, et al. (1998), blood lead effects on generalized child psychopathology ratings (explaining 1% to 4% of the variance) were less than the effects of family sociodemographic factors (explaining 7% to 18% of the variance) and child temperament variables (explaining 2% to 5% of the variance). These results indicate that social factors and individual child characteristics are more powerful than blood lead effects in explaining risks for child psychopathology.

Relevant to our discussion of aggression and related behaviors is the fact that these studies have failed to find a specific effect of lead toxicity on such behaviors. Lead toxicity appears to elevate risk for generalized childhood psychopathology, as opposed to risk for a specific type of psychopathology such as aggression or CD. Small gender effects are found in some studies, suggesting that lead-intoxicated boys are more specifically at risk for externalizing disorders (attention problems, delinquency, and aggression), whereas lead-intoxicated girls are at higher risk for both internalizing (anxiety, depression, social problems) and externalizing problems (Burns et al., 1999).

In summary, childhood lead burden accounts for only a small amount of the variance in children's learning and behavioral performance. Earlier reports suggesting robust associations between childhood lead levels and cognitive decrements and psychopathology largely failed to control for confounding variables that have stronger effects than lead on childhood development. Little specific effect of childhood lead on aggression has been found. Lead intoxication may indirectly elevate risk for childhood aggression by modestly increasing risk for generalized psychopathology and learning problems in children.

Academic Underachievement and Academic Failure

Academic failure is a multidetermined outcome in which a youngster fails to meet the academic requirements of the school setting. This can be reflected in grade retention; placement in a special education classroom; low grades; low scores on standardized achievement tests; school suspension or expulsion; or the presence of significant discrepancies between grades that would be expected, based on the child's intelligence, and his or her actual academic achievement (Brier, 1995).

For almost 70 years, a strong association has been found between academic failure on the one hand, and antisocial behaviors and aggression on the other. For example, in a longitudinal study completed in the 1920s, 54% of youngsters who developed a delinquent pattern were achieving below grade level, compared with only 24% of youngsters who did not develop such a pattern (Wolfgang, Figho, & Sellin, 1927). More recently, a cross-sectional study of 2,000 delinquent urban youth (average age of 14 years) found severe academic deficits. Academic achievement scores in reading, math, and vocabulary ranged from the third- to the fourth-grade level in these eighth-grade students (Zagar, Arbit, Hughes, Busnell, & Busch, 1989). These and similar studies support the view that academic underachievement is associated with antisocial behavior patterns in youth (Davis, Byrd, Arnold, Auinger, & Bocchini, 1999).

The linkage between aggressive/antisocial behaviors and academic problems appears complex and indirect. First, it is controversial whether academic failure and underachievement precede or are consequences of these behaviors (Brier, 1995). Second, developmental shifts in this relationship are important. There exists a large overlap between ADHD symptoms and conduct problems in children (see Chapter 4). The specific association between academic failure and aggressive behavior in early to middle childhood appears to be mediated by associated attention problems, impulsivity, and hyperactivity (Hinshaw, 1992; Frick et al., 1991). Only by the adolescent years are aggression and antisocial behaviors clearly linked to school underachievement and failure in some, but not all, youth. Third, the relationship between academic failure and aggression seems to be mediated by other variables as well. School-age children with aggressive conduct problems often exhibit early reading problems and deficits in verbal skills. Moffitt (1993b), in a review of 47 published studies, concluded that one of the most robust findings in youth with CD is an IQ deficit of about 8 points, compared to peers without CD. This deficit is manifested primarily in Verbal IQ, so that performance IQ consistently exceeds Verbal IQ among children and adolescents with CD. Types of verbal deficits found include deficient word knowledge, meager supply of verbally coded information, and poor verbal reasoning skills (Brier, 1995). A deficit in verbal information processing may contribute to academic underachievement. In addition, a lack of verbally mediated regulation of behavior may create a predisposition toward delinquency and other antisocial behaviors.

Still other variables that mediate the association between academic failure and aggressive/antisocial behaviors include poverty, negative school attitudes, SUDs, association with a deviant peer group, and parents who do not support academic achievement as important for their offspring (Brier, 1995; Hinshaw & Anderson, 1996). In short, the relationship between scholastic underachievement and aggression/conduct problems appears multifactorial and reciprocally deterministic, with multiple risk factors involved that influence one another over time and development, finally resulting in a youngster who is both aggressive/antisocial and failing academically (Hinshaw & Anderson, 1996).

Body Size and Build

Body size and build have an association with aggressive behaviors. Research shows that aggressive juveniles tend to have a body build that is more mesomorphic or endomorphic (muscular, bulky, or fat) and less ectomorphic (slight and thin); however, this relationship is not independent of social factors known to promote aggressive behavior (Farrington, 1989). Other studies have shown that developmental effects such as height measured early in life at ages 8–10 years, but not when measured later at ages 12–14 years, predict violence at ages 16–18 years (Sampson & Lamb, 1997). A longitudinal study found that large body size when measured at age 3 years, but not when measured at age 11 years, predicted aggression in 11-year-old children. This effect occurred for both boys and girls, and continued to be statistically significant even after family SES was controlled for (Raine, Reynolds, Venables, Mednick, & Farrington, 1998). Although the effect of body build on later aggression is modest, these findings suggest that children with increased body size and height early in life may, through instrumental learning processes, discover that aggression may be a successful strategy in dominating social conflicts. This early social learning may eventually increase risk for aggression in the adolescent years (Raine, Reynolds, et al., 1998).

FAMILY RISK FACTORS

One of the best-documented and most consistent findings in the area of child psychopathology is the relation between family risk factors and aggressive/antisocial behavior problems in offspring. This relationship has been reported as early as 2 years of age (Campbell, 1991), and has been emphasized in most social science theories of the etiology of conduct problems in youth (Capaldi & Patterson, 1994). This section reviews the influence of ineffective parenting practices, family functioning, parental psychopathology, child maltreatment, and family structure on the development of aggression in children and adolescents.

Ineffective Parenting Practices

Several ineffective parenting practices have been implicated in the onset and maintenance of aggressive and antisocial behaviors in children and adolescents. These include harsh and inconsistent discipline practices, poor monitoring and supervision of offspring, and low levels of positive involvement with offspring.

A comprehensive model of poor parental disciplinary practices that is very influential in the field is Patterson's "coercive family process" theory (Patterson, 1982; Patterson, Reid, & Dishion, 1992). This model (which is described more fully in Chapter 8) postulates that harsh and inconsistent conflictual interchanges between parents and a child over disciplinary issues in the family eventually train the child in aggression and antisocial behaviors. Parents with poor disciplinary skills inadvertently train their child in an aversive manner through negative reinforcement of the child's behavior. For example, negative reinforcement of the child's coercive behavior occurs when the parent makes a request of the child, the child refuses to comply or ignores the request, and the parent does not follow through. Often the child's refusal to comply is aversive, aggressive, or threatening, in order to intimidate the parent into backing down. When the parental request is successfully avoided, the child learns that aggressive behaviors are a winning social strategy in the home. These behaviors then generalize to environments outside the home (e.g., the school classroom), where arguing, bullying, noncompliance, and fighting may occur. The child's aggression is especially strongly reinforced when stressed or frustrated parents follow a pattern of ineffective discipline with episodic, explosive, harsh behaviors directed toward the child (Capaldi & Patterson, 1994). Parent–child interactions marked by this parental inconsistency (laxness, then harshness), as well as by high conflict and intense negative affect, are particularly likely to train the child in the use of aggression as a social strategy for negotiating interpersonal relationships.

There is much evidence to support the importance of coercive parenting practices in the etiology of aggressive and antisocial behaviors in youngsters. Studies have shown that harsh and inconsistent parenting practices account for 30% to 52% of the variance in the development of antisocial behavior (Capaldi & Patterson, 1994; Patterson et al., 1992), and that coercive parenting practices leading to parent–child conflict in the home form a strong independent predictor of later youth conduct problems (Wasserman, Miller, Pinner, & Jaramillo, 1996).

Poor monitoring and supervision of children constitute another parenting practice linked to aggression and conduct problems in youngsters (Loeber & Stouthamer-Loeber, 1986). Parents of children with these behaviors often do not know where, how, or with whom the children spend time. Lack of, or inconsistent, parental monitoring is a powerful predictor of juvenile delinquent behavior (Wasserman et al., 1996). By supervising their offspring's free time, parents may influence their child's selection of friends and activities and decrease risk for development of conduct problems over time (Patterson et al., 1992).

A low level of positive involvement with children is still another parenting practice associated with elevated risk for eventual conduct problems in children and adolescents. Positive involvement includes such parenting techniques as giving praise for desirable behavior; providing clear guidance, suggestions, and directions for achieving prosocial behaviors; using positive incentives to increase a child's task motivation; giving suggestions and choices, as opposed to controlling commands, to a child; and responding favorably to a child's self-initiated behavior. These broad indicators of parental approval and acceptance of a child are associated with less risk for development of antisocial behaviors. In contrast, parental nonacceptance, intrusive controlling, or rejecting attitudes toward a child are strongly associated with risk for development of such behaviors (Rothbaum & Weisz, 1994).

It should be noted that adolescent parents are at particularly high risk for engaging in the poor parenting practices described above. Although the children of some adolescent parents do very well, generally the younger a mother is (especially if she is below age 15), the greater the risk for poor outcomes in her child (Osofsky, Hann, & Peebles, 1993). A large body of research indicates that adolescent mothers differ in their interactions with their children (generally infants). Teenagers engage less with their offspring, talk less, give more intrusive commands and authoritarian statements, are less affectionate, and provide less stimulation than older, more skilled mothers (see Zeanah, Boris, & Larrieu, 1997). Adolescent mothers are also perceived as less sensitive and responsive to their children, more punitive, and more physically intrusive in their child-rearing practices than older mothers. These are parenting practices that are related to impulsivity and aggression in children (Zeanah et al., 1997).

Research is increasingly recognizing bidirectional influences on family socialization related to child aggressive behavior (Lytton, 1990). Characteristics of the child, such as temperament, impulsive responding, attention span, and oppositionality, can strongly influence parenting behavior. It is conceivable that negative parenting practices may largely be a reaction to the difficult, oppositional, and aggressive behaviors displayed by the child with developing CD (Hinshaw & Anderson, 1996). The child's behaviors can shape parenting techniques, and the parents can shape the child's behaviors. There is no single familial cause of aggressive/antisocial childhood behavior patterns; reciprocal multideterminism over time and development is most likely.

Family Functioning

The broad domain of "family functioning" includes such areas as parental separation or divorce, marital conflict, and domestic violence. A large body of research demonstrates that children from maritally dissolved homes consistently evidence significantly diminished rates of well-being, and higher rates of externalizing and antisocial behaviors, than children from intact and well-functioning two-biological-parent families (Amato & Keith, 1991; Hetherington & Stanley-Hagan, 1999; Najman et al., 1997). This is potentially important, as rates of marital dissolution have been rising over the past four decades. For example, 50% of American marriages currently end in divorce (Glick, 1989). In the early 1960s, almost 90% of children spent the majority of their youth in homes with two biological parents. Presently this is true for only about 40% of children in the United States and about 50% in the United Kingdom (see Hetherington & Stanley-Hagan, 1999). These statistics conceal important ethnic differences. Although 38% of European American children in the United States experience parental divorce prior to age 16, almost 74% of African American children encounter their parents' separation or divorce by the same age (McLanahan & Bumpass, 1988).

The greatest effect of divorce appears to be on children's antisocial and aggressive behaviors (Hetherington & Stanley-Hagan, 1999). Compared to peers from well-functioning nondivorced homes, adolescents in divorced families are two to three times as likely to drop out of school, to engage in delinquent and other antisocial behavior, and to associate with delinquent peers. These relationships retain their statistical significance despite controls for confounds such as maternal age and family income (Najman et al., 1997). The association between divorce and increased risk for antisocial behavior appears to be mediated in part by the child's age and gender. In early and middle childhood following parental divorce, boys appear at greater risk for externalizing behavioral problems than girls (Najman et al., 1997). However, by adolescence female conduct problems become statistically associated with parental divorce (Amato & Keith, 1991).

Recent studies have been consistent in showing that the relative impact of parental separation and divorce on children's risk for conduct problems is largely mediated by dyadic conflict and aggression between parents prior to, coincident with, and following marital breakup (Amato & Keith, 1991). Although falling maternal income after divorce and the absence of a divorced parent in a child's daily life contribute to the drop in children's postdivorce well-being (Amato & Keith, 1991), marital status appears less important than parental interpersonal conflict in determining rates of subsequent conduct problems in children and adolescents from divorced homes (Najman et al., 1997). The importance of marital conflict in increasing risk for offspring's antisocial behavior is strengthened by findings reporting similar rates of externalizing behavior disorders in children from high-conflict intact families and children from divorced families (Hetherington & Stanley-Hagan, 1999).

It appears that risk for childhood aggression and antisocial behaviors in dissolving families is largely mediated by parental conflict and not by actual marital breakup.

Physical aggression and domestic violence between marital partners are particularly severe forms of marital conflict that appear to be strong risk factors for the development of aggression and antisocial behaviors in offspring. Men raised in aggressive families have higher rates of aggression and participation in antisocial behavior as adults, compared to men not brought up in such families (McCord, 1988). Parental aggressiveness and marital conflict have an important impact on risk for later participation in criminal activity and other antisocial behavior, especially for men (McCord, 1979). Nonreferred children from homes characterized by physical conflict between parents have more adjustment problems, including more externalizing behavior problems, than children from families with no conflict or only verbal conflict between parents. This effect holds for both boys and girls (O'Hearn, Margolin, & John, 1997). In children clinically referred for psychiatric hospitalization, parental violence in the home is a strong predictor of homicidal threats or acts, as well as of extreme physical assaultiveness (Lewis, Shanok, Grant, & Ritvo, 1983; Pfeffer, Plutchik, Mizruchi, & Lipkins, 1987). The witnessing of domestic violence between caretakers may sensitize a child to violence as a means of interpersonal problem solving either through social learning mechanisms (i.e., modeling of behavior) or through fear conditioning and hypervigilance to threat.

Family Structure

Some characteristics of family structure have been associated with an increased risk for juvenile delinquency and other antisocial behaviors. These include family size, birth order, and parenting status. Large family size, defined as the presence of four or more children in the family, is associated with a predisposition toward conduct problems and aggression in youth (Raine, 1993; Reiss & Roth, 1993). A review of 32 studies on family size and antisocial behavior found a significant positive relationship in 31 reports (Ellis, 1988). Farrington (1989) found that large family size at age 10 years was predictive of violent criminal offending at age 32 years. These studies indicate that family size is an important variable associated with increased risk for antisocial behaviors in youngsters.

However, not all children from large families grow up to be aggressive or antisocial. Large family size is not by itself deterministic of such outcomes. Other variables may interact with family size to increase risk; these modifying variables appear to include gender, family SES, and birth order. For example, several studies report that large family size is a risk factor for antisocial outcomes only for the number of male children in a large family. Having sisters may actually protect against the development of antisocial problems in brothers (Jones, Offord, & Abrams, 1980). Family size may only be a risk factor for conduct problems in low-SES families (see Raine, 1993); this association does not appear significant in high-SES families. Finally, being the middle male child of a large, low-SES family appears to increase risk for aggression and conduct problems (Tygert, 1991). Being the first- or last-born male child may actually be protective against the development of antisocial behaviors (Reiss & Roth, 1993).

Parenting status is also associated with risk for conduct problems in offspring. Single-mother family structures have been associated with lack of authority acceptance and aggression in children (Pearson, Ialongo, Hunter, & Kellam, 1994). This relation may be mediated by male gender of the offspring, low family SES, and residence in urban environments. With the presence of these additional factors, alternative single-mother family structures such as mother–grandmother or mother–male partner dyads may not protect children from eventual conduct problems (Pearson et al., 1994).

As suggested above, the effects of large family size, birth order, and single-mother parenting status on increased risk for juvenile antisocial behavior and aggression may all be mediated by low family SES. With diminished family economic resources, parents may not be available to supervise and monitor offspring, and thus may be unable to provide sufficient nurturance, guidance, or structure for children to develop self-control. In higher-SES families, resources outside the family may be available to compensate for family structure risk factors.

Parental Psychopathology

Children of parents who demonstrate psychopathology have higher rates of emotional or behavioral difficulties than children of parents who have no psychiatric difficulties (Cantwell & Baker, 1984). Types of parental psychopathology that appear related to increased risk of child psychopathology (including aggression and antisocial behavior) are parental SUDs, maternal depression, maternal somatization, and parental ASPD.

The rate of behavioral problems in children of parents with alcoholism seems increased over that of children whose parents are not alcoholic. Early studies of children of alcoholic parents found an increase in the rates of externalizing behavior problems in offspring, including ADHD (Earls, Reich, Jung, & Cloninger, 1988), CD (Merikangas, Weissman, Prusoff, Pauls, & Leckman, 1985), and oppositional defiant disorder (ODD) (Earls et al., 1988). Later studies either failed to replicate an association between parental alcoholism and child conduct problems (Hill & Hruska, 1992), or found an increased risk for generalized psychopathology in offspring that was not specific for aggression and conduct problems (Hill & Muka, 1996). This is supported by recent studies reporting elevated rates of both externalizing and internalizing problems (such as anxiety) in children of alcoholic parents (Dierker, Merikangas, & Szatmari, 1999). Parental alcoholism is probably not a direct and specific risk factor for childhood aggression and antisocial behaviors, but is indirect and mediated by other variables. For example, the number of alcoholic parents may be important. Rates of childhood conduct problems, anxiety, and generalized psychopathology increase as the number of alcoholic parents increases from zero to two (Dierker et al., 1999; Reich, Earls, Frankel, & Shayka, 1993). The gender of the alcoholic parent may also be important: Children of alcoholic mothers may exhibit more psychological problems than children of alcoholic fathers (Werner, 1986). The gender of the child is important as well: Sons of alcoholic parents appear at risk for conduct problems, whereas daughters may be at risk for anxiety disorders (Kuperman, Schlosser, Lidral, & Reich, 1999).

Children of parents with a history of other SUDs, such as opiate dependence, also have higher rates of internalizing and externalizing psychopathology, attention problems, and impulsivity than children whose parents have no such history (Nunes et al., 1998; Stanger et al., 1999; Wilens, Biederman, Kiely, Bredin, & Spencer, 1995). Similar patterns are found for males and females, despite controls for confounding variables such as informant, family SES, and ethnicity. Effect sizes are generally modest but significant (Stanger et al., 1999). A specific effect on aggression or serious antisocial behavior is not found. However, children of opiate-dependent parents demonstrate increased rates of less severe conduct problems, in addition to increased rates of generalized psychopathology (Wilens et al., 1995). Risk for aggression and antisocial behavior may be mediated by gender of the offspring, gender of the addicted parent, and comorbid parental psychopathology. Sons of opiate-dependent mothers with comorbid major depression appear especially at risk for conduct problems. This relation retains its statistical significance even after offspring age, family living situation, and parental educational level are controlled for (Nunes et al., 1998).

Maternal depression has been linked to an increased risk of aggression in offspring in some studies. In an investigation of depression in multiple familial generations, a threefold elevated risk for conduct problems and disruptive behavior disorders was found for children of depressed parents compared to children of nondepressed parents. An increased risk for early-onset anxiety disorders was also found, indicating that the effect was not specific for conduct problems (Warner, Weissman, Mufson, & Wickramaratne, 1999). The effects of maternal depression on risk for offspring conduct problems may be indirect. An investigation into the relation between maternal depressive symptomatology and the development of externalizing behavior problems in their children found that mother–child interaction quality partially mediated this association, even when the effects of social class were taken into account (Harnish, Dodge, & Valente, 1995). Depression may adversely affect parenting ability in several ways: An increase in negative parent–child interactions may occur because of parental irritability or hostility, or parental monitoring and supervision of offspring may break down.

Other research has linked somatization in mothers and antisocial behavior. A study in mothers of clinically referred children found evidence that maternal somatization and child antisocial behaviors might be related syndromes, and that behavioral disinhibition may be a common predisposition underlying both (Frick, Kuper, Silverthorn, & Cotter, 1995).

Parental ASPD and criminality, especially in fathers, appear to be strong and more specific risk factors for the development of child antisocial behavior and aggression. Children who have both parents criminally involved are at very high risk for the development of such behaviors (Robins, West, & Herjanic, 1975). Loeber and Dishion (1983) found that parental criminality assessed when children were 10 years of age was highly predictive of later delinquency, and that family criminality was a strong predictor of recidivistic offending. Childhood risks may be greater when two or more parental psychopathological risk factors are present. For example, early-onset childhood conduct problems, as opposed to those with later onset, have been found to be associated with both alcoholism and ASPD in parents (Kuperman et al., 1999).

With the exception of familial ASPD, parental psychopathology appears to have an indirect relationship with child antisocial behavior and aggression. This relation may be mediated by contextual variables, such as the number of parents who are impaired, the number of psychopathological conditions present in parents, the quality of parent–child interactions, the availability of parental monitoring and supervision of offspring, family SES, family adversity, and the quality of the neighborhood environment (see Capaldi & Patterson, 1994). Direct effects are strongest for the influence of parental criminality on risks for conduct problems in children. It is also important to remember that the influence of parental psychopathology on offspring may be genetically, as well as environmentally and psychologically, mediated. That is, parental psychopathology may predispose a child to impulsive, aggressive, and antisocial behaviors not solely because of social or experiential factors, but because parents pass along genes to their offspring that may predispose them to such behaviors. This is supported by the adoption studies mentioned earlier. Finally, interactive effects between heritable factors and environmental factors operating across both parents and child may be important.

Child Abuse and Neglect

"Child abuse" is usually defined as sexual and/or physical maltreatment of a dependent child by a generally older caretaker. Documented physical abuse of a child generally entails evidence of physical injury (bruising, bone fracture, burns, welts, etc.). Cases of sexual abuse generally encompass a variety of acts, including assault and battery on a child with intent to gratify sexual desires (Maxfield & Widom, 1996). A wide range of abuse severity is covered by these definitions, including differing frequencies, types of acts, and degrees of injury to a child. "Child neglect" is a separate area of child maltreatment, but may occur in concert with abuse. Child neglect is generally defined as a judgment by protective service agencies that parents' deficiencies in child care are beyond those generally found acceptable by current community and professional standards (Maxfield & Widom, 1996). Child neglect includes parental failure to care for the food, clothing, shelter, and medical needs of a dependent child.

Child abuse appears quite prevalent in the United States. In 1995, a survey of child protective services in all 50 states revealed 3 million cases reported in the community, of which 996,000 were substantiated by child welfare workers as having a high probability of abuse. Physical neglect of the child occurred in 54% of the substantiated cases, physical abuse in 26%, sexual abuse in 11%, and other forms of child maltreatment in 9% (Emery & Laumann-Billings, 1998). This translates into an annual reported community prevalence rate of 15 cases of child maltreatment per 1,000 children. Reported rates are higher in mental health settings, ranging between 23 and 42 cases per 1,000 clinically referred children (Emery & Laumann-Billings, 1998). Prevalence rates vary by child gender and by type of abuse, with higher reported sexual abuse rates for females than for males: Recent studies give prevalence rates of 12% to 17% for females and 5% to 8% for males. Physical abuse prevalence rates are reported at 6% for females and 5% for males (Stevenson, 1999). However, there is some evidence that the prevalence of physical abuse may be higher in the population. An epidemiological study of a community probability sample of 665 youth aged 9–17 years reported finding physical abuse in 25.9% (Flisher et al., 1997).

Substantial empirical evidence supports a correlation between a history of child maltreatment and psychopathology in childhood, adolescence, and adulthood. Childhood physical abuse, sexual abuse, and a history of neglect are all associated with an increased risk for a wide variety of both internalizing and externalizing behavior problems in children and adolescents (Finkelhor & Berliner, 1995; Flisher et al., 1997; Kendall-Tackett, Williams, & Finkelhor, 1993). No specific psychiatric syndrome has been linked to childhood experiences of maltreatment; rather, such experiences seem to be risk factors in the development of many different problems in youth. It is also important to note that many survivors of childhood maltreatment do not later demonstrate many of these sequelae.

Childhood physical abuse and neglect may be particular risk factors for the later development of aggressive behavior. This association is found for both community and clinically referred youth. The methodologically soundest study conducted to date on the effects of different forms of early maltreatment on later development of crime and violence in a nonreferred community sample found that physical abuse and neglect early in childhood were significantly associated with arrest for violent crime in adulthood by age 32, after a 22- to 26-year follow-up (Maxfield & Widom, 1996; Widom, 1989a). This association retained its statistical significance even after the investigators controlled for the confounding effects of age, gender, and race. In this longitudinal study, the risks for violence varied by type of maltreatment. Childhood physical abuse, childhood neglect, and the combination of physical abuse and neglect were associated with differing (though elevated) arrest rates for violent offenses in adolescence and adulthood, as illustrated in Figure 5.2. (By contrast, childhood sexual abuse was not associated in this study with increased rates of arrest for violent offenses, relative to controls.) Both physically abused and/ or neglected males (Widom, 1989a) and females (Maxfield & Widom, 1996) were at risk for elevated rates of violence; however, males and African Americans who were abused and/or neglected as children were subgroups demonstrating especially high risks for violence in this longitudinal study.

A relationship between early physical abuse and chronic aggression is also found in psychiatrically referred samples. In a study of 51 youth referred to a psychiatric residential treatment center, physical abuse was a statistically significant predictor of treatment resistant aggression, despite intensive and long-term multimodal psychoeducational therapies (Figure 5.3) (Connor, Melloni, & Harrison, 1998). There existed a statistical trend for sexual abuse to be associated with ongoing aggression in this sample. The relationship between sexual abuse and aggression in this population of seriously emotionally disturbed youth may have been weak because of the small sample size utilized in this study.

Sexual abuse in childhood may also be associated with the development of aggressive behavior and conduct problems in childhood and adolescence. However, childhood sexual abuse is associated with a wide range of developmental outcomes, including no symptoms of psychopathology at all. There exists no specific sexual abuse syndrome, and aggression is one of many symptom patterns that may occur in sexually maltreated youth (Finkelhor & Berliner,

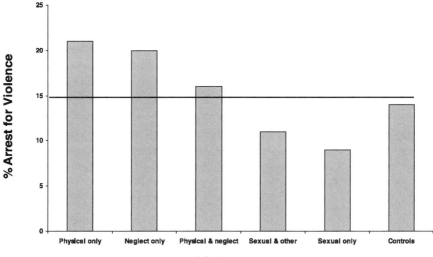

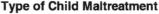

Type of Child Maltreatment

FIGURE 5.2. Increased rates of arrest for violent offenses in adulthood in subjects who were physically abused or neglected as children. Data from Maxfield and Widom (1996).

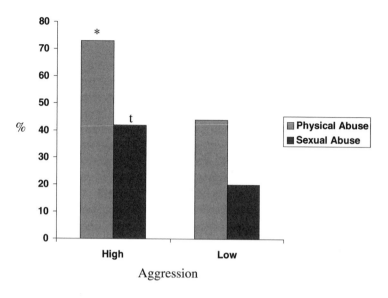

FIGURE 5.3. Relationship between lifetime history of physical abuse or sexual abuse on the one hand, and aggression on the other, in 51 psychiatrically referred children and adolescents. *$p < .05$; t = trend ($p < .10$). Data from Connor, Melloni, and Harrison (1998).

1995). More specific risks for aggression appear to occur in physically abused and/or neglected children.

The relationship between child maltreatment and elevated risk for later psychopathology may be mediated by several factors. Age at onset of maltreatment may be important. In a study examining the relationship between age at onset of sexual abuse in childhood and later functioning, onset of abuse prior to age 7 years resulted in significantly worse outcomes for children than a later onset (McClellan et al., 1996). Other studies have replicated this finding that the earlier the maltreatment occurs in a child's development, the higher the risk for subsequent psychopathology. The highest risk appears to occur in children abused prior to age 5 years (Glod & Teicher, 1996). Gender and ethnicity also appear to be important mediators. As noted above, risk for violence was elevated among males and African Americans who were physically abused and/or neglected in childhood, compared to females and European Americans (Maxfield & Widom, 1996).

Cognitive factors may play a role. Early experiences of childhood physical abuse are associated with impaired social information processing in youth. Specifically, in an investigation of social information-processing patterns, childhood physical abuse was associated with misattribution of neutral social cues as hostile, preferential accessing of aggressive behavioral responses to social stimuli (as opposed to nonaggressive responses), and an endorsement of aggressive responses to social cues as possessing positive outcomes (Dodge,

Pettit, Bates, & Valente, 1995). Comorbid psychopathology may also mediate risk between physical abuse and aggressive outcomes.

Physical abuse, sexual abuse, and neglect may result in a wide variety of emotional and behavioral problems. One such outcome is increased risk for depression in maltreated children (Kaufman, 1991). A study has reported an interactional effect between physical abuse and depression in childhood, such that the risk for heightened aggression was mediated by the presence of both physical abuse and depression and not by either one alone (Scerbo & Kolko, 1995).

Finally, CNS biological factors may be involved in the risk for aggression in abused children. Physical or sexual abuse occurring prior to age 18 years has been found to have a greater impact on two areas of the brain than abuse first occurring later than age 18 years. These are the cortex and the limbic system. These areas are important in the processing of cognitive and emotional information, including inhibitory impulses. Damage to these areas is associated with motor hyperactivity, catecholaminergic dysregulation, electroencephalographic (EEG) abnormalities, and impaired information transfer between the cerebral hemispheres (Glod & Teicher, 1996; Teicher, Ito, Glod, Schiffer, & Gelbard, 1996)—all of which may increase risk for aggressive responding to environmental cues. Clearly, the mechanisms that may mediate the risks for aggression and other psychopathology in abused (and neglected) children are not specific, linear, or causal, but multiple, indirect, correlational, and interacting. A challenge for further research in the area of aggression and childhood maltreatment is to further clarify these complex interactions.

In summary, there is evidence that maltreatment in childhood leads to increased risk for aggression in adolescence and adulthood. This appears especially true for physical abuse; neglect may also be an independent risk factor for later aggression. Sexual abuse appears to have a weaker relationship with subsequent aggression. It is important to note that only 8% to 26% of those maltreated in childhood become violent or otherwise aggressive (Widom, 1989b). The majority of such children do not grow up to be violent. Furthermore, maltreatment is not a specific risk factor for aggression; rather, it increases risk for the development of multiple diverse forms of psychopathology, one of which may be heightened aggression. Finally, it is also important to realize that the effects of maltreatment on later aggression appear indirect, are not causal, and are mediated by a diverse array of other psychosocial and neurobiological factors.

EXTRAFAMILIAL RISK FACTORS

Extrafamilial risk factors for aggression include those that occur in the neighborhood or community, or in association with a deviant peer group. Larger trends in society, such as deprivation, the easy availability of firearms, and mass media violence, are also important. This section examines the relationship between aggression and factors outside the family.

Peer Factors

The association between peer factors and aggression encompasses two distinct yet interrelated phenomena: early rejection of an aggressive child by peers, and later association with a deviant peer group. In the early school years, aggression toward peers is highly associated with social rejection (Coie, Dodge, & Kupersmidt, 1990) and social group victimization (Schwartz, McFadyen-Ketchum, Dodge, Pettit, & Bates, 1998) of the aggressive child. This child is disliked and singled out by the social peer group and then excluded from participation in the peer group's activities. Both rejection and victimization appear to be associated in turn with increased risk for subsequent aggression and antisocial behaviors in the aggressive child. A causal model has been postulated suggesting that aggressive behavior leads to low acceptance by peers, which in turn leads to further development of aggressive behaviors and eventual association with like-minded, similarly rejected, and similarly aggressive peers (Parker & Asher, 1987). Therefore, peer rejection is presumed to set the course toward continued maladaptive aggression and antisociality as development progresses.

However, it is unclear whether early peer rejection of the deviant child causes aggression or whether early-onset aggression in the child causes subsequent peer rejection. Kupersmidt, Coie, and Dodge (1990) argue that peer rejection may be a "marker variable" that suggests the presence of more fundamental risk factors in the child, which may account for the relationship between peer rejection and aggression. Such basic risk factors may involve neurobiological and heritable traits in the child, such as low Verbal IQ, psychopathic traits, high degrees of impulsive and hyperactive responding, low levels of behavioral inhibition, and/or high levels of irritability—all of which may increase risk for aggression, subsequent peer rejection, and eventual poor adult outcome.

In later childhood and adolescence, there is a trend for rejected aggressive youth to associate less and less often with popular, successful, skilled members of the social group, and more and more with other rejected youth who are similar in behavior, goals, and values. In these deviant peer groups, there exists little opportunity for positive peer interactions, which appear to play an important role in the eventual development of cognitive and social skills. The deviant peer group becomes a training ground for aggression, antisocial behaviors (including delinquency and criminality), and drug and alcohol use (Pepler & Slaby, 1994); it thus increases the risk for the individual's continued maladjustment into adulthood.

Several caveats about the relationship between peer factors and subsequent aggression are important to note. First, a child's differential association with deviant peers is only one of a number of correlational factors in the etiology of aggression and conduct problems. Second, peer factors may interact with family factors to increase risk for aggressive/antisocial outcomes. Youth with both poor family relationships and a deviant peer group are at particular risk for such outcomes. Deviant peer influences appear only weakly related to antisocial behavior in those with supportive families (Henggeler, 1989; Raine, 1993). Third, the influence of antisocial peers may explain more minor forms of antisocial behavior, such as truancy, substance misuse, stealing, or rule breaking, but not serious and recidivistic violent crime (Raine, 1993). Finally, deviant peer group associations may be more important in explaining adolescent-onset antisocial behavior (which is more likely to cease when adulthood is attained) than early-onset antisociality (which has a higher risk of persisting into adulthood) (Moffitt, 1993a).

Social Deprivation

General social deprivation includes such factors as individual poverty, low SES, unemployment, poor housing, and overcrowded living conditions. A relationship exists between indices of general social deprivation and increased rates of aggression, crime, and other antisocial behavior in youngsters. Low SES and poverty may be related to serious criminal offenses. In a review of the relationship between SES and violence, Ellis (1988) found that 100% of 46 studies relating low SES to serious crime involving a victim reported a significant relationship, whereas only 68% reporting on less serious crime not involving a victim found this relationship. Similarly, low family income and poor parental work record measured when a child was 8–10 years old predicted violence and recidivistic offending in adulthood at age 32 years (Farrington, 1991). There is more violent crime per capita in urban environments than in rural environments (Ellis, 1988). Children who grow up in deprived inner-city urban environments are at higher risk for delinquency and other antisocial behaviors than children who grow up in more affluent circumstances (Kolvin, Miller, Fleeting, & Kolvin, 1988). This relationship may be specifically mediated by poor housing conditions and overcrowded living conditions, which are more often present in urban than in rural environments (Rutter & Giller, 1983).

However, the relationships between indices of general social deprivation and increased risk for aggression, delinquency, and crime in youth are more complicated than they first appear. Poverty, meaning simply insufficient family income, is not primarily implicated in violence. Most poor individuals are not criminals, nor are they aggressive. Rather, the absence of sufficient income to meet basic family necessities in a given community and in a specific geographical context, compounded by lack of opportunity to access needed resources, is what may be associated with violence (Pepler & Slaby, 1994). A poor parental work record and periods of unemployment are not related to youth violence in high-SES families, as they are in low-SES families (Raine, 1993). This suggests that the impact of parental unemployment on delinquency may vary as a function of family SES. The effects of low family income and family poverty on later adult violent crime also appear to be influenced by the age of the child when family poverty occurs. Unlike family poverty and pa-

rental unemployment occurring early in a child's life, low family income measured later in development (at age 14 years) does not relate to later criminal
offending in adulthood. This suggests that family poverty may have its most
important impact early in a child's development (Farrington, 1991).

On the level of the individual family and child, the effects of general social deprivation on youth conduct problems may be mediated by the individual parenting factors discussed earlier. As the number of stressors grows
in an individual family, and as economic resources become increasingly con-
strained, the ability of parents to supervise and monitor their offspring in a
manner conducive to the promotion of prosocial behavior may be increasingly
limited. In other words, the effects of individual family poverty, unemployment, low family SES, poor housing, and overcrowded living conditions may
ultimately be mediated by the availability and skills of individual parents.
Some evidence supports this concept. In a study of a representative sample of
585 children followed from preschool to third grade, family SES was negatively correlated with eight measures of child socialization: parental discipline
practices (harsh and inconsistent discipline); lack of maternal warmth; exposure to aggressive adult role models; maternal aggressive values; family life
stressors; mother's lack of social support; peer group instability; and lack of
cognitive stimulation of the child. These factors in turn predicted a child's aggressive behavior in school (Dodge, Pettit, & Bates, 1994). Sampson and Laub
(1994) have proposed a two-step hypothesis concerning the effects of social
deprivation on juvenile delinquency. In Step 1, family poverty inhibits family
processes of informal social control; in Step 2, a lack of family social control
increases the likelihood of youth delinquency. Therefore, the effects of poverty
and social deprivation on juvenile delinquency for the individual family appear mediated in part by poor parental discipline techniques, poor monitoring
and supervision of offspring, and weak or conflicted parent–child attachments.

Community Factors

Collective Efficacy

Social scientists have long recognized that violent crime rates vary widely
among the neighborhoods of U.S. cities. These variations cannot be entirely
attributed to the aggregation of individual risk factors for violence. In addition to the individual family indices of general social deprivation discussed
above, certain social and organizational characteristics of neighborhoods help
explain the relationship between sociodemographic factors and violence. One
such characteristic is termed "collective efficacy." Collective efficacy is defined as the differential ability of neighborhoods to realize the common values
of residents and maintain effective social controls. Neighborhood residents are
then regulated according to agreed-upon desired principles, in order to realize
collective goals as opposed to coerced, forced, or individual goals (Sampson,

Raudenbush, & Earls, 1997). Among such collective neighborhood goals are safety and freedom from violence.

Several social factors influence collective efficacy in any given neighborhood. The first is residential mobility. The fostering of community ties to local institutions and neighbors takes time. A high rate of residential mobility in any given community, especially in areas of decreasing population, fosters institutional disruption and weakened social controls over community life. The second is access to resources. Resource availability acts to enhance both an individual and a collective sense of power in controlling and shaping characteristics of the community. Social deprivation weakens collective efficacy.

Studies are beginning to reveal that the construct of collective efficacy can be reliably measured, and that it appears to mediate the association between multiple measures of community violence on the one hand and neighborhood social composition and social disadvantage on the other (Sampson et al., 1997). In other words, it is not poverty or high resident turnover per se that causes violence in a community. On an organizational level, these social stressors decrease collective efficacy in a neighborhood, and this decrease is then associated with increased rates of violence and crime. Higher levels of community collective efficacy are related to lower levels of neighborhood violence (Sampson et al., 1997).

There may also be an interaction between the neighborhood's and an individual's qualities in predicting antisocial behavior. In a cross-sectional study of 13-year-old inner-city boys, and in a longitudinal study of 17-year-old inner-city boys, the relationships among impulsivity, neighborhood context, and juvenile offending were examined (Lynam et al., 2000). Across both studies, results indicated that the effects of impulsivity on juvenile offending were stronger in poorer neighborhoods. Nonimpulsive boys in poor neighborhoods were at no greater risk for delinquency than nonimpulsive boys in better-off neighborhoods.

Neighborhood Violence

Over the past decade, a growing body of evidence has indicated that many youngsters are exposed to considerable amounts of life-threatening violence and other aggression in their neighborhoods, schools, and communities. This is particularly true for youth growing up in urban areas, especially disadvantaged city neighborhoods. Exposure to violence may take many forms, including direct experience (e.g., being shot/shot at, stabbed, or raped/otherwise sexually assaulted) or threats (being chased by an individual or gang intent on harm). Violence exposure also includes witnessing or hearing about violence, viewing dead bodies, or having friends or family members experience violence. For youth in such an environment, exposure to violence is often chronic throughout their developing years, with multiple exposures to many different violent acts (Jenkins & Bell, 1997).

Despite recent trends toward decreasing rates of youth violence in the inner city, the level of violence exposure remains very high among urban youth—and much higher than exposure rates prior to the 1980s, when the surge in youth violence first began to be documented (Group for the Advancement of Psychiatry, 1999). A number of studies report very high rates of both witnessing and direct experience of violence among urban inner-city elementary school children and adolescents. For example, Richters and Martinez (1993) conducted a study of 165 children aged 6–10 years living in a moderately violent neighborhood in Washington, D.C., and attending the same elementary school. These children reported high rates of both witnessing and experiencing violent acts (see Figure 5.4). These acts included shootings, stabbings, sexual assaults, muggings, physical threats, use of illegal weapons, seeing a dead body, and illegal drug transactions. Other studies from 1985 to 1993 have largely replicated these results (see Jenkins & Bell, 1997). Figure 5.5 presents data from several studies describing lifetime self-report rates of witnessing a shooting among urban youth.

Chronic exposure to neighborhood violence has clear consequences for children and adolescents. Increased rates of psychopathology, distress, fear, and academic underachievement are reported in inner-city youth exposed to violence (Jenkins & Bell, 1997; Schwab-Stone et al., 1995). One consequence is an association between violence exposure and a greater willingness to use physical aggression. In a survey of 2,600 urban 6th-, 8th-, and 10th-grade stu-

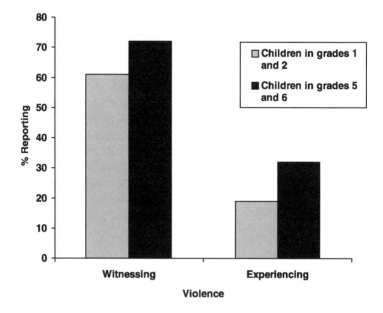

FIGURE 5.4. High levels of violence witnessing and direct violence experience among 6- to 10-year-old elementary school students in Washington, DC. Data from Richters and Martinez (1993).

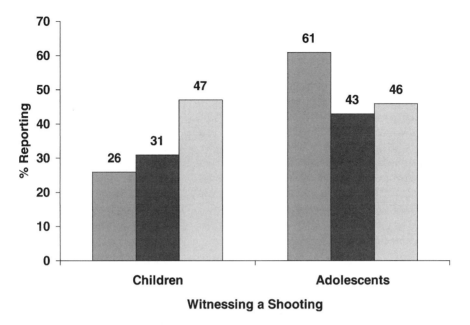

FIGURE 5.5. Witnessing violence: Percentages of urban youth self-reporting lifetime rates of witnessing a shooting. Data from (left to right): Osofsky, Wewers, Hann, and Fick (1993), New Orleans; Richters and Martinez (1993), Washington, DC; Richters and Martinez (1993), Washington, DC; Jenkins and Bell (1994), Chicago; Singer, Anglin, Song, and Lunghofer (1995), Denver; Schwab-Stone et al. (1995), New Haven, CT.

dents, exposure to violence was prevalent (Schwab-Stone et al., 1999). Of the adolescents sampled, 36% reported experiencing at least one type of violent act in their lifetimes, and between 48% and 63% had witnessed violence. In this study, a high correlation (.75) was found between exposure to violence and antisocial behaviors and a willingness to utilize aggression; in other words, those who committed aggressive acts also reported greater violence exposure. The correlation between violence exposure and anxiety, depression, and somatic symptoms was statistically significant but lower (.40) (Schwab-Stone et al., 1999). Violence exposure has been associated in other research with use of physical aggression, diminished perception of risk, lowered personal expectations for the future, heightened antisocial behaviors, use of illegal substances, dysphoric mood, and school underachievement (Schwab-Stone et al., 1995).

Several factors appear to mediate the effects of chronic violence exposure on outcome. Gender is one such mediator: Females generally report lower rates of directly experiencing violence for all categories except sexual assault. Females also report higher rates of internalizing psychopathology after witnessing or experiencing violence, whereas males report higher rates of externalizing behaviors (Schwab-Stone et al., 1999). Age also appears to be a mediator: Younger children who are exposed to violence report more anxiety and fear in their reactions, whereas older children and adolescents report more externalizing behavior symptoms (Schwab-Stone et al., 1999). Family composition is important as well. Urban children in families without mothers appear to be at more risk for violence exposure than urban children living in families with the presence of a maternal figure (Jenkins & Bell, 1997). Children without a maternal figure may be less monitored and supervised in the neighborhood. Finally, geographical location mediates risk of violence exposure. Youth exposure to violence is clearly greater in inner-city urban neighborhoods than in small towns or suburbs (Singer, Anglin, Song, & Lunghofer, 1995).

The Availability of Firearms

Youth living in the United States have an unprecedented access to firearms. These weapons are increasingly easy to use, small, concealable, and lethal. There is evidence that the availability of firearms in the U.S. population is rising: There are an estimated 200 million firearms, including an estimated 60 million handguns, in households in the United States (Christoffel, 1997; Berkowitz, 1994). This easy availability of guns has increased the lethal potential of youth aggression.

The vast majority of firearm deaths (either homicides or suicides) affect 15- to 19-year-old adolescents. In 1990, in fact, deaths due to firearms outnumbered deaths due to natural causes among 15- to 19-year-olds for the first time (Fingerhut, Jones, & Makuc, 1994), Although teenagers and young adult males are the most directly affected by firearm violence, all pediatric age groups are involved. Figure 5.6 shows the number of youth firearm homicide victims by age for the year 1997. No age is spared; even infants are victims of firearms.

The majority of teenage firearm deaths occur among African American male adolescents. Figure 5.7 shows the increase in adolescent male firearm homicides by race for the years 1985 to 1993. Firearm injury deaths are in fact the leading cause of death for young African American males, accounting for almost half of all deaths from any cause among this group (Group for the Advancement of Psychiatry, 1999).

Despite the astounding minority race youth mortality rates from gun-related injuries in the inner cities from the mid-1980s to the 1990s, the issue of children and firearms did not capture widespread media and political attention until the violence appeared in largely white suburbia. This violence took the form of school shootings. Between 1997 and 2001, armed youth in Alaska, Arkansas, Oregon, Pennsylvania, Mississippi, Kentucky, California, and Colorado invaded their schools and opened fire on fellow students and teachers. To date, over 40 parents, students, and teachers have died. These

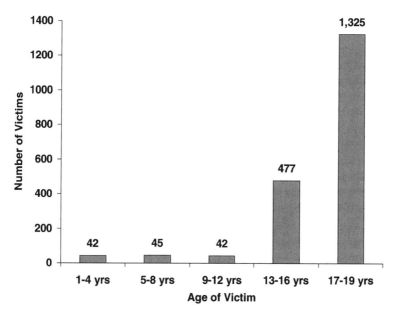

FIGURE 5.6. Firearm homicide victims by age for 1997. Data from Maguire and Pastore (1999, p. 289).

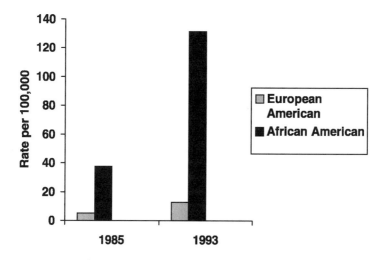

FIGURE 5.7. Rising rate of firearm homicides for the years 1985 through 1993 among adolescent males aged 15–19 years, by race. Data from Fingerhut (1993).

tragedies have refocused debate on the association among youth, lethal violence, and firearms in the United States.

There appears to be a relationship between gun availability and violent death. Of 10 studies investigating the association of firearms and homicide completed between 1973 and 1994, 9 demonstrated a statistically significant correlation between firearms and violent death and injury; in these 9 investigations, handguns were responsible for 73% to 94% of firearm homicides for both youth and adults (see Christoffel, 1997). Another study demonstrated a statistically significant association between the availability of firearms in each of 16 European countries and the United States with homicide rates in those countries (Lester, 1991). Berkowitz (1994) rank-ordered 10 Western industrialized nations in terms of the percentages of their households having firearms and the countries' rates of homicides with guns, and found a statistically significant correlation ($r = .61$). Although such relationships cannot demonstrate causality, they do suggest that the availability of firearms is related to risk for violent death and injury.

Several factors may account in part for the relationship between firearm (predominantly handgun) availability and lethal aggression in youth. First, the great number of available firearms in U.S. society heightens the chance that violence-prone youngsters will be able to obtain a weapon quickly and inexpensively. In contrast, reducing the number of firearms in the population should make it difficult or impossible for youth to purchase scarce (and therefore more expensive) firearms, or to find a gun when violence is their goal. Second, handguns are more lethal now than in the past. Automatic and semiautomatic handguns are readily available, are relatively inexpensive to purchase, and are smaller in size and therefore easier to conceal. All of these characteristics make them easier to use. Finally, there may exist a "weapons effect" (Berkowitz, 1994). That is, in aggressive and underinhibited persons, the presence of stimuli in the environment that symbolize aggression or violence may cause them to respond with more heightened aggression than was otherwise intended. Guns, having a clear aggressive meaning, may give youth holding or seeing them hostile ideas and increase the possibility that they may be impulsively used. In other words, under certain environmental conditions (aggressive experience, aggressive intent, hostile cues, lack of behavioral inhibition), the mere presence of a gun may dictate its use. Although several studies have failed to replicate the existence of a weapons effect, a number of investigations have supported the existence of such an effect (see Berkowitz, 1994).

Media Violence

Movies, broadcast television, and cable television are ubiquitous in American culture. Over 98% of all households in the United States own at least one television set (Huston et al., 1992). Approximately 70% of households own a cable television hookup, which allows access to a far greater variety of programming (Singer, Slovak, Frierson, & York, 1998). In the average U.S. home environment, the television is on about 28 hours per week for children 2–11 years of age and about 23 hours per week for adolescents (Donnerstein, Slaby, & Eron, 1994). Children in the United States view approximately 3–4 hours of television per day (Liebert & Sprafkin, 1988). It is now known that television viewing occupies more time than any other nonschool activity and accounts for more than half of all leisure activity time for children (Donnerstein et al., 1994).

For several decades, increasing concern has been expressed by social scientists about the violent content that is standard fare in American mass media. This content is now available on a daily basis and through multiple venues (broadcast and cable television, video games, home video movies, the cinema, and now the Internet) to the youth of America. Most of the research on violence in the mass media has focused on television. Research indicates a consistently high level of violence in American television programming over the past 25 years (Gerbner & Signorielli, 1990; Lichter & Amundson, 1994). A survey of broadcast and cable television conducted in Washington, D.C., in a 1-day period between 6 A.M. and 12 midnight revealed 1,846 violent scenes in 1992; the figure rose to 2,605 violent scenes when the survey was repeated in 1994, a 41% increase (Lichter & Amundson, 1992, 1994). On prime-time television, five to six violent acts are broadcast per hour (Donnerstein et al., 1994). The American Psychological Association concluded that the average American child has witnessed 8,000 murders and more than 100,000 acts of violence by the time he or she graduates from elementary school (Huston et al., 1992).

The studies cited above provide clear evidence of the prevalence of violence on television, and suggest that youngsters are exposed to wide varieties of violent images while they are watching television. Substantial empirical evidence spanning the past 25 years has consistently linked media violence to violent attitudes, values, and behaviors in children, adolescents, and adults. However, this remains a highly controversial subject: Despite the many studies (reviewed below) linking media violence and juvenile violence, some have argued that this effect occurs only in children already predisposed to violence, and that violent TV does not make nonpredisposed youth more aggressive and violent. Indeed, investigations do suggest that media violence is more popular among violent than among nonviolent viewers (Cantor, 2000). Research is complicated by the fact that we cannot use the experimental method; that is, we cannot randomly assign children to watch heavy doses of media violence during their formative years and compare their later violent criminal acts with those of children in an unexposed control group. Nevertheless, there is ample research evidence that exposure to violence—especially repetitive exposure to violence as it is most frequently presented in the media—is unhealthy for children and adolescents (Cantor, 2000).

In 1972, the U.S. Surgeon General's office reviewed the existing literature on the relationship between violence on television and its impact on children. Strong evidence was found that across several measures of aggressive behavior, there was a significant and consistent correlation between exposure to televised violence and subsequent aggressive behavior on the part of viewers (Surgeon General's Scientific Advisory Committee on Television and Social Behavior, 1972). Ten years later, the National Institute of Mental Health (NIMH) replicated the finding that violence on television leads to aggressive behavior by children and adolescents who watch such programs (NIMH, 1982). These findings were reconfirmed 10 years after the NIMH report by the American Psychological Association, Commission on Violence and Youth, which endorsed the finding that televised violence has a causal effect on aggressive behavior (American Psychological Association, 1993; Huston et al., 1992). These investigations represent diverse perspectives and encompass correlational studies, laboratory research paradigms, field trials, longitudinal research, and meta-analytic reviews. They are consistent in their conclusions that media violence affects aggressive behavior in viewers (see Donnerstein et al., 1994; Murray, 1997). A sampling of these studies is reviewed here.

In one of the largest correlational studies conducted to date, Singer et al. (1998) surveyed 2,245 elementary school students about their television viewing habits and behaviors. Of the children in the sample, two-thirds watched 3 or more hours of TV per day, and one-third watched TV for more than 5 hours per day. Children who reported watching greater amounts of television each day reported more violent behaviors than children who reported watching lesser amounts of TV per day. Moreover, children who reported a preference for TV programs involving action and fighting reported higher levels of violent behaviors than children who watched other types of programming. The number of hours spent watching TV was directly correlated with violent behaviors, such that children who reported watching 6 or more hours of TV per day scored highest on ratings of such behaviors. Since this study was correlational in its methodological design, no inferences about causality can be drawn. It is as possible that more violent children watch more violent TV as that viewing violence on TV results in more violent behaviors.

Early studies used laboratory paradigms to investigate the relation between media violence and aggressive behavior. These studies were largely consistent in demonstrating elementary school children's increased willingness to hurt other children after viewing violent television programming as opposed to neutral programming (Ellis & Sekyra, 1972; Liebert & Baron, 1972). In more recent field experiments, investigators have presented television programs in the normal viewing environment and observed behavior where it naturally occurs. Results indicate that children who are predisposed to aggression become more aggressive when viewing violent programming in their natural environment, and that children who view prosocial TV programming in their natural setting become less aggressive and more cooperative (see Murray, 1997). Longitudinal studies also support the relation between media violence and aggressive behavior. In a 22-year study, Huesmann, Eron, Lefkowitz, and Walder (1984) found a clear and significant relation between early exposure to television violence at age 8 years and adult aggressive behaviors (serious criminal acts) at age 30 years. This suggests that viewing television aggression not only may lead to subsequent aggression, but that such behavior can become part of a lasting behavioral pattern. Finally, a meta-analysis of 217 studies conducted between 1957 and 1990 investigating television violence and aggressive behaviors found that exposure to portrayals of violence on television was consistently associated with subsequent aggressive behavior. Effect sizes were modest yet significant, ranging from 5% to 15% (Comstock & Paik, 1994).

With such evidence, the scientific debate has moved beyond asking whether the viewing of violence in the media has an effect, to asking what the possible mechanisms of this effect are. The viewing of media violence appears to have a direct effect on the young viewer. Although not all children are affected, and not all children are affected in the same way, youth who watch a lot of violence on television may become more aggressive through developing favorable attitudes and positive values about the use of aggression to solve interpersonal problems and social conflicts. In other words, they become more likely to see violence as a valuable tool for the resolution and management of such problems. Next, research has shown that youth who view large amounts of media violence can become desensitized to the effects of violence on others. These youth may become less empathic and more callous and apathetic toward the suffering of those experiencing violence in the real world. In addition, they appear willing to tolerate ever-increasing amounts of violence in their daily lives. Finally, children who watch a lot of television violence may begin to believe that the world is a more violent and threatening place than in fact it actually is. These children may possess heightened fears about being aggressed against and may take extreme steps (such as obtaining a weapon) to defend themselves. All of these mechanisms can increase risk for aggressive behaviors (Donnerstein et al., 1994; Murray, 1997). Indeed, a study of the effects of reducing television, videotape, and video game use on aggressive behavior and perceptions of the world as a violent and scary place in third- and fourth-grade students showed that youth in the intervention group had statistically significant decreases in aggressive behaviors (Robinson, Wilde, Navracruz, Farish Haydel, & Varady, 2001).

Specific subsets of youth may be more susceptible to the risks of viewing media violence. For example, children with various emotional and behavior disorders appear particularly vulnerable to the influence of television violence (Gadow & Sprafkin, 1993). Grimes, Cathers, and Vernberg (1996) found that 8- to 12-year-old children who were diagnosed as having either ADHD, ODD, or CD manifested less emotional concern for sufferers and were more willing to accept violence as justified when viewing media violence than did a matched group of children who did not have these disorders.

In summary, societal violence and media violence are not related in any direct and simple manner; multiple causes for both phenomena exist, and media violence affects different youngsters in different ways. Nevertheless, although controversies remain, the weight of the scientific evidence over the past 25 years indicates that viewing violence in the mass media is a significant contributor to aggressive attitudes and behaviors in children and adolescents, as well as adults (Villani, 2001).

GENERAL DISCUSSION OF RISK FACTORS

Several points about the relation between risk factors and youth aggression need to be emphasized. The beginning of this chapter has emphasized the importance of identifying direct and specific risk factors for childhood aggression, so that we can begin to determine distinct mechanisms of risk. Once these mechanisms are understood, the hope is that they can be subjected to specific and targeted prevention efforts and treatments, in order to interrupt more precisely the development of maladaptive aggression in at-risk youth. However, with the exception of heritable genetic factors (which remain presently poorly clarified and understood), the vast majority of risk factors reviewed in this chapter are nonspecific, increase risk for a wide variety of general childhood psychopathology (only one aspect of which is aggressive behavior), and exert their influence on aggressive outcomes by indirect rather than direct means. Furthermore, risk factors rarely exist in isolation from one another; they are generally multiple and interact in complicated transactions over the course of a child's development. As a result, research is beginning to highlight multiple-risk-factor models and interactions among risk factors in the genesis of aggressive and antisocial behaviors. An example of this type of research is the finding of markedly increased risk for adult criminality when both environmental and heritable risk factors for antisocial behavior are present in an individual's life, as compared to either type of risk factor operating alone (Bohman, 1996). Another example is the impact of maladaptive parenting practices on the development of youth conduct problems. Poor parenting is found to be a risk factor for childhood antisocial behavior only in those children without temperamental characteristics of psychopathy. In children who have callous–unemotional personalities (possibly determined by genetic influences), risk for conduct problems occurs independently of either effective or ineffective parenting practices (Wootton, Frick, Shelton, & Silverthorn, 1997).

   The next point to be made is that psychosocial variables are not independent of genetic and thus of psychobiological and neurobiological influences (which are discussed in greater detail in Chapters 6 and 7, respectively). It is known that genetic influences affect individual differences in psychosocial risk exposure (Plomin & Bergeman, 1991). Consequently, psychosocial influences on the development of aggression and related behaviors in youngsters may actually in part be genetically mediated (O'Connor, Deater-Deckard, Fulker, Rutter, & Plomin, 1998; Rutter, 1999). This relation appears bidirectional. Genetic effects in an individual may bring about increased exposure to environmental risks. This is the effect of people's behavior on the environment. For example, symptoms of ADHD with its attendant risk for impulsivity may be genetically determined. Impulsive individuals can be risk takers and sensation seekers, and generally do not think through the consequences of their actions before they initiate them. This may predispose such individuals to greater exposure to psychosocial risk factors known to be associated with the development of maladaptive aggression, such as association with a deviant peer group. On the other hand, genetic effects may also cause increased vulnerability to environmental risks in an individual. This is the effect of the environment on people's behavior. For example, youth with low verbal intelligence (a genetically mediated effect) appear to be at higher risk for the development of aggression and antisocial behaviors in high-risk, as opposed to low-risk, environments characterized by much psychosocial adversity (Tiet et al., 1998). Findings such as these begin to weaken the dualism between psychosocial risk factors and psychobiological/neurobiological risk factors in the etiology of aggression.

Finally, this review supports the importance of a cumulative risk model for onset and maintenance of maladaptive aggressive behaviors in youth. Risk factors do not occur in isolation from one another and are frequently multiple and chronic in a child's life. Since most psychosocial risk factors are nonspecific and exert their effects on risk for aggressive behaviors indirectly, the specific type of risk factor appears less important for the development of such behaviors than the total number of risk factors present. Cumulative effects of multiple risks (i.e., parental psychopathology; low SES; adverse life events; poor parenting practices; heritable risk factors for psychiatric disorders or psychopathy) have been demonstrated to have a far more serious impact on developmental outcomes in children than any specific type of risk factor (Seifer, Sameroff, Baldwin, & Baldwin, 1992). For antisocial behavior, findings from a Christchurch, New Zealand longitudinal study illustrate the point well: There existed a 100-fold difference in the rate of such behavior between those subjects who experienced the highest cumulative index of risk factors (some reflecting genetic as well as psychosocial influences) and those who experienced the lowest cumulative index (Fergusson & Lynskey, 1996). Another example comes from a study by Rutter (1979). Six family factors that were strongly and significantly associated with child psychopathology (including aggressive/antisocial behaviors) were severe marital discord, low social status, overcrowding or large family size, paternal criminality, maternal psychiatric disorder, and a family history of admission of a child into the care of local child protective services. Children with just one risk factor were no more likely to evidence disorder than children without any risk factor (a 1% increment in risk for psychiatric disorder). However, when two or three risk factors were present together, the level of risk went up fourfold (a 5% to 6% rise in disorder rate). With the presence of four or more risk factors, the risk to a child was several times higher (a 21% rise in the risk for psychiatric disorder) (Rutter, 1979). A similar example from a third study is the finding that youth with cumulative psychosocial stressors (more than five) are at much greater risk for violence than youth exposed to fewer than two risk factors (Herrenkohl et al., 2000). The more stressors present in a child's life, the greater the risk for psychopathology. In the etiology of aggressive/antisocial behaviors in youth, therefore, the total number of risk factors appears more important than the specific types of risk factors.

PROTECTIVE FACTORS

Even in situations of cumulative risk, a proportion of children and adolescents do not develop significant psychopathology, including aggression and related behaviors. In other words, not every youth who experiences a risk condition will have a negative outcome. The study of "protective factors" has the goal of identifying those variables that exert a buffering effect on high-risk youth. Specifically, protective factors modify, ameliorate, or alter a person's response to some environmental hazard that predisposes him or her to a maladaptive outcome (Rutter, 1985). In the discussion that follows, protective factors are not specific for aggression or antisocial behaviors; they relate to child and adolescent psychopathology in general, one aspect of which may be these types of behaviors. The study of protective factors is a younger and less mature field than the study of risk factors. A closely related area of study is research on so-called "resilient" youth. The term "resilience" is used to describe three kinds of phenomena: (1) good outcomes despite high-risk status, (2) sustained competence under conditions of stress, and (3) recovery from trauma (Werner, 1994).

Different types of protective factors exist. There are factors that exert beneficial effects on children's welfare at all times, regardless of a high or low level of risk; these are called "resource factors" (Tiet et al., 1998). Examples are sufficient family income, adequate family functioning, and an absence of parental psychopathology. The variables of most interest for this discussion are those whose effects are most salient when risk is highest, but have less impact when risk to the child is minimal. These are "true protective factors" (Seifer et al., 1992).

Like risk factors, protective factors in three different domains can be considered: child, family, and extrafamilial factors (Rae-Grant, Thomas, Offord, & Boyle, 1989; Wyman et al., 1992). Factors in each of these domains are listed in Table 5.4. These protective factors appear to interact with risk factors to partially buffer youth from maladaptive outcomes, especially in high-risk environments (Jenkins & Smith, 1990; Rae-Grant et al., 1989; Seifer et al., 1992; Tiet et al., 1998; Werner, 1994). Some mediating variables may exist in the interaction of protective factors with risk factors. For example, some stud-

TABLE 5.4. Protective Factors

Child factors	Family factors	Extrafamilial factors
Easy temperament	Good parent–child relations	External supports
Higher IQ		Friendships
Internal locus of control		Availability of opportunities
High self-esteem		
Academic competence		
Social competence		
Competence in activities		

ies have found that girls are more resilient than boys to risk factors that involve marital disharmony and divorce (Block, Block, & Gjerde, 1986). Girls may also be more buffered than boys by the presence of a good mother–child relationship (Wyman et al., 1992) or by the presence of a confiding friendship (Rae-Grant et al., 1989). However, other studies report no gender differences in the operation of protective factors (Siefer et al., 1992). Another mediating factor appears to be developmental age. The impact of protective factors may change in importance at differing periods of development. For example, Rae-Grant et al. (1989) found that the presence of a confiding friendship was protective for adolescent females, but not for younger children living under stressed conditions.

Several authors have proposed ways in which risk and protective factors may interact with one another to determine child behavioral outcomes. Rutter (1985) has outlined three possible models of interaction. "Multiplicative interaction" occurs when the presence of one factor multiplies the effect of another factor. "Potentiating interaction" occurs when the presence of one factor potentates the effect of another. "Catalytic transactional interaction" occurs when factors affect child behavioral outcomes only in the presence of other factors, but do not independently alter behavior. An alternative set of models to explain the interaction between risk and protective factors has been proposed by Garmezy, Masten, and Tellegen (1984). In the "compensatory" model, stressors, risks, and vulnerability factors combine additively. In the "challenge" model, competence and resilience are enhanced as long as stress does not exceed a threshold; once the threshold is exceeded, competence is overwhelmed and breaks down. In the "protective" model, buffering factors modulate the impact of stressors—for example, by improving individual coping skills, adaptation, and the building of competence. Some have suggested that the interaction of risk and protective factors is a balance between the power of the person and the power of his or her social and physical environment, with the adaptational outcome depending on the relative balance at specific periods of development (Werner & Smith, 1982).

CHAPTER SUMMARY

This chapter has reviewed individual, family, and extrafamilial risk and protective factors in the development of aggressive and related behaviors in youth. Some of these factors (e.g., genetics) are biological, while others are psychosocial. These factors do not operate independently of one another; behavioral outcomes are mediated by a complex interplay between risk and protective factors at specific times of development. Most of the associations between these factors and behavioral outcomes are correlational and not causal. A challenge for further investigation is to develop more detailed models of the interactions between multiple risk and protective factors in the determination of outcomes for youth at specific times of development—models that include psychobiological/neurobiological as well as psychosocial variables.

◈ CHAPTER 6

Psychobiology: Neuropsychology, Psychophysiology, Brain Imaging, and Minor Physical Anomalies

Maladaptive aggression and related behaviors in children and adolescents have great social importance. The individual, familial, and extrafamilial psychosocial risk factors discussed in Chapter 5, provide an important, yet incomplete, understanding of the etiologies of these behaviors. In recent years it has been realized that the investigation of psychobiological variables may also help shed light on the development and maintenance of aggressive behaviors in youngsters. Psychobiology is a field of study that investigates complex behavioral, cognitive, physiological, and anatomical manifestations that result from the output of more fundamental and elemental CNS neurobiological systems. This avenue of study has been pursued for several reasons (see Lahey, Hart, Pliszka, Applegate, & McBurnett, 1993). First, a better understanding of the psychobiological correlates of these behaviors may lead to a better understanding of their psychosocial etiologies. For example, psychosocial factors may cause aggression, but the effects of these factors on the development and chronicity of aggressive behaviors may be mediated by neuropsychological and/or psychophysiological events in the central nervous system (CNS). Second, the high familial loading of conduct problems and antisocial behaviors found in studies of high-risk families suggests the possibility that genetic variables may be operative in the genesis of these behaviors. Since genetic factors may express themselves phenotypically through neuropsychological and psychophysiological mechanisms, these variables are important to investigate. Third, since aggression and related behaviors in youth are heterogeneous in nature, a better understanding of neuropsychological and psychophysiological variables may help us classify these behaviors into more conceptually and physiologically relevant subtypes. Finally, an enhanced understanding of psychobiological variables may promote the development of improved psychosocial and psychopharmacological treatments for aggressive behaviors in children and adolescents.

It should be emphasized that the study of neuropsychological and psychophysiological variables in these behaviors is not independent of the study of psychosocial factors, but is a complementary avenue of investigation. Biological determinism in the etiology of aggressive/antisocial problems is rejected. The challenge for investigators is to understand how psychosocial risk and protective factors interact with neuropsychological and psychophysiological risk and protective factors over the course of development to result in behavioral outcomes.

Relationships between neuropsychological variables and aggressive behavior problems in youngsters have been the focus of much research over the past two decades. Much less methodologically sound research is available on the psychophysiological correlates of these behaviors; in this area of research, most findings remain correlational and are not causal. Moreover, most of the available studies in both areas investigate male subjects. Little research is available on gender differences in neuropsychological and psychophysiological correlates of conduct problems. Finally, although most studies present their findings as univariate main effects, the true challenge is to understand the interactions between psychosocial and psychobiological variables in the etiology of these behaviors over the course of an individual's development. This chapter focuses primarily on the neuropsychological and psychophysiological correlates of aggressive behaviors in youngsters. Briefer discussions of brain imaging findings and so-called "minor physical" anomalies (MPAs, which are included here because they may be markers for problems in CNS development) are also provided.

NEUROPSYCHOLOGY

Children and adolescents who exhibit persistent, early-onset aggression, delinquency, and other antisocial behaviors, have been studied via neuropsychological procedures, in order to investigate evidence for any neurological or cognitive dysfunction that may account for their behaviors. "Neuropsychology" is a subspecialty of neuroscience that uses indirect, specialized testing procedures to explain the way in which activity of the brain is expressed in observable behavior. In this way, neuropsychology attempts to clarify relationships between the brain and behavior (Beaumont, 1983).

One of the basic principles underlying neuropsychology is the idea that certain brain functions are to some degree localized within certain areas of both cerebral hemispheres, whereas others (such as language) are lateralized to one cerebral hemisphere or the other. Neuropsychology has commonly studied patients with damage to specific parts of the brain who then perform poorly on selected neuropsychological tests. In this manner, performance on neuropsychological tests can indirectly reveal information about regional brain functioning. Some common neuropsychological tests and the approximate brain areas they assess are outlined in Table 6.1. This list is not meant to be exhaustive or complete, but simply to give the reader several examples of neuropsychological tests commonly used with youth and the ages for which the tests are validated.

TABLE 6.1. Some Common Neuropsychological Tests for Children and Adolescents

Test	Domain measured	Approximate cortical location	Age range (yr or grade)
Kaufman Assessment Battery for Children	Global intelligence	Nonspecific	2½–12½
Wechsler Intelligence Scale for Children—III	Global intelligence	Nonspecific	6–16
Verbal subtests	Verbal information	Left hemisphere	
Performance subtests	Visuospatial–motor information	Right hemisphere	
Stanford–Binet Intelligence Scale, 4th edition	Global intelligence	Nonspecific	2–23
Wechsler Individual Achievement Tests	Academic achievement	Nonspecific	5–19
Woodcock–Johnson Achievement Tests	Academic achievement	Nonspecific	2–90
Peabody Individual Achievement Tests	Academic achievement	Nonspecific	K–grade 12
Rey–Osterrieth Complex Figure	Perceptual organization/visual memory	Frontal/parietal	4–adult
Facial and Vocal Affect Recognition Test	Social-emotional cognition	Limbic/orbital frontal/right hemisphere	6–17
Clinical Evaluation of Language Fundamentals	Linguistic skills/ rules	Left frontal/ temporal	K–grade 12
Test of Language Development	Receptive/ expressive language	Left frontal/ temporal	2–12
Continuous-performance tests	Vigilance	Frontal (R > L)	4–adult
Stroop Color–Word Interference Test	Executive functions	Orbital frontal	7–adult
Wisconsin Card Sorting Test	Executive functions	Dorsolateral frontal	6½–adult

Note. Data from Boll, Williams, Kashden, and Putzke (1998) and Harris (1995).

Before a discussion of neuropsychological findings in juvenile aggression and antisocial behaviors can proceed, several limitations of neuropsychological testing need to be clarified. First, as should be evident from Table 6.1, such testing is not a direct method for obtaining precise locations of neuronal activity as they relate to behavior. Rather, this method is indirect and can only give general neuroanatomical guidelines. This is because localization of brain function is relative, not absolute. For any one specific form of CNS information processing, several different brain areas may be involved sequentially or simultaneously. As such, neuropsychological testing can only give a general idea of brain regions involved in complex behaviors. Next, the various tests differ in the degree to which they are sensitive and specific to brain dysfunction. Some tests appear more sensitive to brain dysfunction in specific locations (e.g., the Wisconsin Card Sorting Test and dorsolateral frontal lobe dysfunction); others are more global and appear sensitive to dysfunction in almost any cerebral region (e.g., the Digit Symbol test, one of the Verbal subtests in the Wechsler Intelligence Scale for Children—III). Finally, it should be emphasized that findings on neuropsychological tests in aggressive and antisocial youngsters does not imply that these juveniles are "brain-damaged." Rather, findings from these tests identify individual differences in the quality of functioning of different parts of the brain, and these differences may correlate with a vulnerability for aggressive acts. As such, neuropsychological tests of youth with aggressive and related behaviors do not identify a subset with "brain damage." Instead, they document that this population may show more dysfunction in certain brain areas than youth without aggression. A better understanding of the various brain dysfunctions in this population may facilitate future prevention and treatment efforts.

A Brief Review of Neuroanatomy

To give readers a better understanding of the brain areas that are tested by neuropsychological techniques, a brief review of neuroanatomy is provided here. The brain can be roughly divided into cortex and subcortex. The cortex is the phylogenetically newest part of the brain and covers the outer surface of the brain. Its surface is extremely convoluted. The subcortex lies beneath the cortex and is made up of evolutionarily older structures. Beginning at the level of the midbrain (diencephalon) and up through the cortex, the brain is divided into two hemispheres, which are connected by a series of commissures. Apart from these commissure links, the two cerebral hemispheres are quite independent at the cortical level and have their own specialized functions. The left cerebral hemisphere is specialized for verbal and symbolic information processing, and in most individuals language function is lateralized to the left hemisphere. The right hemisphere is specialized for visuospatial information processing. The cortex in each hemisphere is divided into four different regions or lobes: frontal, temporal, parietal, and occipital. These lobes are illustrated in Figure 6.1 (top).

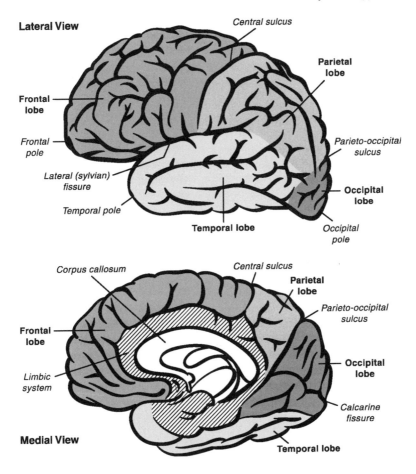

FIGURE 6.1. Diagram of the lateral regions (top) and medial regions (bottom) of the brain, illustrating the frontal, parietal, temporal, and occipital lobes and the limbic system.

Most of the neuropsychological findings in aggression and antisocial behaviors have generally focused on anterior regions of the cortex (which include the frontal and temporal lobes), and have generally emphasized findings relating to the left as opposed to the right cerebral hemisphere. Subcortical systems (especially the limbic system; see below) are also important in regulating emotion and aggression, but these are largely inaccessible to neuropsychological techniques.

The frontal lobes of the cerebral cortex are generally considered to have evolved most recently, and traditionally they have been viewed as the site of "higher" mental functions. Neuroanatomical sites for the production of expressive language are located in the inferior posterior frontal cortex in Broca's area (left hemisphere). The importance of the frontal lobes in human evolution is revealed by the fact that they constitute about one-third of the cortex (Walsh, 1987).

The bottom illustration in Figure 6.1 is a medial view of the brain (cut along the midline that includes a schematic outline of another important region—the limbic system, which lies deep in the brain, bilaterally on either side of the midline. The limbic system is a series of interconnected subcortical structures connected to higher cortical structures by neuronal axons ("white matter"). This phylogenetically old system consists of the hippocampus, amygdala, fornix, septal region, cingulate gyrus, and mammillary bodies, together with connections to the thalamus and hypothalamus. The limbic system is involved in learning and memory processes, and in emotional and aggressive behavior.

Recent research has documented several types of associations between neuropsychological test findings and aggressive/antisocial behaviors in children and adolescents. These findings involve deficits in global intelligence (IQ) and verbal intelligence (Verbal IQ); the possibility of reduced cerebral hemisphere lateralization for language skills; and dysfunction in the frontal lobes (hypofrontality), characterized by deficits in several higher cognitive functions. These are discussed in turn below.

Global and Verbal Intelligence

One of the most robust findings in the neuropsychological study of antisocial youth is a global IQ deficit of about half a standard deviation (about 8 IQ points), relative to nonantisocial youngsters (Moffitt & Lynam, 1994). When high-risk children characterized by early onset and developmental persistence of aggressive/antisocial behaviors are studied, the IQ deficit can be even more striking—about one standard deviation, or 17 IQ points (Moffitt, 1990b). This finding has been replicated in many subsequent investigations, including epidemiological samples (Goodman, Simonoff, & Stevenson, 1995), cross-sectional studies of clinically referred youth (Goodman, 1995), and longitudinal studies of high-risk samples (Lynam, Moffitt, & Stouthamer-Loeber, 1993; Moffitt & Silva, 1987, 1988a; Pine, Wasserman, & Workman, 1999). The correlation between global IQ deficits and antisocial behavior continues to hold despite controls for the potentially confounding effects of social disadvantage (Moffitt & Silva, 1988a); socioeconomic status (SES) (Goodman, 1995); race (Moffitt & Silva, 1988b); legal detection of delinquent acts (antisocial children with lower global intelligence may get caught by the authorities for illegal acts more frequently than antisocial children with higher IQs, and may therefore be recognized more frequently in research studies)(Moffitt & Silva, 1988b); parental IQ (Goodman et al., 1995); and scholastic attainment (Goodman, 1995).

Conversely, studies have found a protective effect of high global IQ in nonpsychopathic subjects at high risk for juvenile delinquency. In a longitudinal investigation of 1,037 children, whose risk status for delinquency was first assessed at age 5 years, outcome was determined at ages 13 and 15 years. Delinquent male and female adolescents were found to have significantly lower IQ scores than nondelinquent adolescents. A very high IQ was found to help boys at high risk stay free of delinquency altogether (White, Moffitt, & Silva, 1989). Although youth with psychopathy (who often are very intelligent) must be excluded, these findings suggest that high IQ may protect children in high-risk environments from developing adolescent CD (Kandel et al., 1988).

There also exists evidence for a more specific Verbal IQ deficit in antisocial youngsters. For over 60 years, neuropsychologists have consistently noted that Performance IQ test scores (roughly measuring right-hemisphere functioning) are greater than Verbal IQ test scores (roughly measuring left-hemisphere functioning) in delinquent youth (Moffitt & Lynam, 1994). Since language functions are primarily subserved by the left hemisphere in almost all individuals, this Performance > Verbal score finding has been taken as evidence of language-based deficits in antisocial youngsters. The existence of such deficits is further supported by findings of increased rates of reading and spelling learning disabilities in children with conduct problems, even after controls for global intelligence and SES (Prior, Smart, Sanson, & Oberklaid, 1999).

Reduced Cerebral Laterality for Language Functions

The consistent finding of reduced Verbal IQ scores relative to Performance IQ scores across multiple neuropsychological studies has given rise to a theory of relative left-hemisphere dysfunction in youth with early-onset, persistent developmental histories of aggressive conduct problems. This theory states that such youngsters may have less lateralized linguistic functions and have relatively inefficient left-hemisphere information processing, compared to individuals who are not at risk for early-onset aggressive conduct problems (Raine, 1993). Support for this theory comes from several sources.

Psychopathic individuals often show an unusual use of language. Their language can be loquacious and deceitful, and there is often a dissociation between what they say about themselves and how they actually behave. These individuals can be of high intelligence and have superficial charm; yet they are often untruthful, insincere, self-centered, and lacking in remorse and shame for their antisocial acts. They have little insight into their behavior and do not appear to learn from the consequences of their actions. The dissociation between what they say about themselves and how they truly act, as well as their lack of insight, may represent a form of aphasia (so-called "semantic dementia") that may reflect less specialized left-hemisphere verbal information processing (Cleckley, 1976). Experimental evidence indicates that persons with psychopathy process and express language differently from nonpsychopathic individuals (Day & Wong, 1996; Louth, Williamson, Alpert, Pouget, & Hare, 1998).

Other evidence comes from verbal dichotic listening studies in children and adolescents with aggression and conduct disorder (CD). Dichotic listening tests measure lateralization of brain functioning by assessing ability to perceive competing auditory stimuli presented simultaneously to both cerebral hemispheres. A subject listens through a headset while a series of randomly paired stop consonants and vowels ("ba," "da," "ga," "ka," "pa," "ta") is presented simultaneously to both ears. At the end of the series, the subject must report the stimuli heard. The ear associated with more correct responses is described as showing an ear advantage. The neural systems for processing language are predominantly contralateral (although an ipsilateral pathway also exists). That is, auditory stimuli presented to the right ear are largely processed in the left cerebral hemisphere, and auditory stimuli presented to the left ear are largely processed in the right hemisphere. Beginning in early childhood, subjects typically show higher scores on right-ear as opposed to left-ear measures, reflecting the left cerebral hemisphere's dominance for language (Pine, Bruder, et al., 1997).

Several studies have now documented a reduced right-ear advantage on verbal dichotic listening tests for children and adolescents with psychopathy and disruptive behavior disorders. In a study of 40 adolescents aged 13–18 years who met multiple overlapping behavioral and personality criteria for psychopathy, reduced ear asymmetries on a verbal dichotic listening task were found in comparison with nonpsychopathic subjects (Raine, O'Brien, Smiley, Scerbo, & Chan, 1990). Specifically, the psychopathic adolescents expressed less right-ear advantage, indicating reduced lateralization for verbal information processing to the left hemisphere. This finding remained statistically significant despite controls for age, ethnicity, IQ, left-handedness, and selective attention to one ear during testing. Reduced right-ear advantage was also documented in 6- to 10-year-old children meeting diagnostic criteria for attention-deficit/hyperactivity disorder (ADHD), oppositional defiant disorder (ODD), or CD—clinical diagnoses with high risk for aggression and conduct problems in youth (Pine, Bruder, et al., 1997). Deficits in reading and language ability on academic achievement tests were also correlated with reduced right-ear accuracy for dichotic syllables in this same study, further supporting language-based deficits in this sample.

The hand dominant for writing ability has also been used to assess hemisphere laterality. This is because contralateral neural pathways also tend to predominate between hand and brain, with the left hemisphere controlling the right hand (and vice versa). About 90% of people are right-handed, because the left hemisphere is dominant in most people. The vast majority of people who are right-hand-dominant for writing are left-hemisphere-dominant for language. Left-handed subjects are less clearly lateralized for linguistic processes, with approximately 70% having these processes lateralized to the left hemisphere, 15% having them lateralized to the right hemisphere, and 15% having some bilateral representation for language (Raine, 1993). As such, handedness may be taken as a crude indication of cerebral hemisphere lateralization for language.

If youth with aggressive and antisocial behaviors demonstrate reduced hemisphere lateralization for language, one would expect a higher incidence of left-handedness in such youngsters. To date, the evidence is mixed. In a prospective study of 265 Danish children, a left-side preference measure at age 11 years predicted delinquency at age 17 years (Gabrielli & Mednick, 1980). This finding was not accounted for by low Verbal IQ, suggesting that gross left-hemisphere dysfunction did not account for the effect. However, there have been failures to replicate this finding. In a study of the lateral preferences of 881 children aged 7 years, left-hand or left-foot dominance was found to be unrelated to delinquency measures at ages 13–15 years (Feehan, Stanton, McGee, Silva, & Moffitt, 1990).

In summary, findings from global and verbal measures of intelligence (see above) and from dichotic listening studies provide the most support for a theory of reduced language processing and reduced cerebral hemisphere lateralization in early-onset, persistent aggression and antisocial behavior. However, some failures to replicate these findings do exist, and further research is necessary to clarify these brain–behavior relationships (Sanford et al., 1999). Youth with the psychopathic subtype of aggression may demonstrate effects on reduced hemisphere lateralization (but not IQ) most clearly. The results from studies of hand and foot dominance are inconclusive.

Deficits in Verbal IQ and hemispheric lateralization for linguistic processing may result in higher risk for aggressive and related behaviors through several mechanisms (see Moffitt & Lynam, 1994). First, diminished linguistic processing may contribute to inefficient use of internal language to modulate behavior. Children with language inefficiencies may have difficulty thinking through the consequences of their actions before acting. As such, they may be more impulsive, and demonstrate reduced self-control of aggressive/antisocial behaviors. Second, inefficient verbal information processing may result in a present-oriented cognitive style, which in turn may foster more irresponsible and exploitative behavior. Third, reduced verbal skills may interfere with children's ability to label their perceptions of the emotions expressed by others, and thus may contribute to diminished empathy or perspective taking. This in turn could limit behavioral response options in ambiguous social situations and contribute to risk for aggressive responding. Finally, less verbally proficient children may be at increased risk for academic and school failure, which is correlated with CD and other aggressive/antisocial outcomes.

The Frontal Lobes and Executive Cognitive Functioning

The frontal lobes are important in the self-regulation of goal-directed behavior. An important subdivision of the frontal lobes is the prefrontal cortex (PFC). This is the very anterior part (frontal pole; see Figure 6.1) of the mammalian brain, and is generally defined neurophysiologically as the part of the cortex that receives neuronal projections from the mediodorsal nucleus of the thalamus (a subcortical structure) (Fuster, 1997). The PFC is extremely important for abstract cognitive functions and higher intelligence; the temporal organization of goal-directed behavior; attention; sequential planning; behavioral inhibition; short-term (working) memory; and the regulation of emotions and affect, including aggression. These have been called "executive cognitive functions" (ECFs) by neuropsychologists (Giancola, 1995).

The frontal cortex is further subdivided into three regions, called the dorsolateral, medial/cingulate, and orbital frontal cortex. These regions, which may have importance for the study of maladaptive aggression, are illustrated in Figure 6.2 (where they are referred to simply as the lateral, medial, and orbital regions, respectively). Damage to these regions of the frontal cortex in humans results in different clusters of neuropsychological symptoms, which reveal some clues as to their respective functions (Fuster, 1997). Injury to the dorsolateral frontal cortex can result in a disturbance of attentional regulation that leaves the patient with deficits in goal-directed planning. This region has been implicated in the regulation of physical aggression (Giancola, 1995). The medial/cingulate frontal cortex helps in regulating autonomic nervous system (ANS) and endocrine functions. It is also involved in conditioned

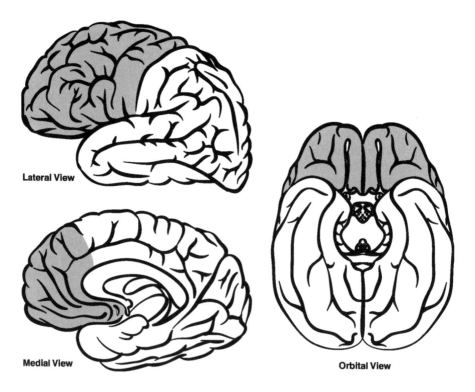

FIGURE 6.2. The frontal lobe: Lateral (top left), medial (bottom left), and orbital (right) regions.

emotional learning, vocalizations associated with expressing internal states, assessments of motivational content, and the assignment of emotional valence to internal and external stimuli. Dysfunction of the medial/cingulate frontal cortex, such as in anterior cingulate epilepsy, often results in psychopathic, antisocial, or other aberrant social behaviors (Devinsky, Morrell, & Vogt, 1995). Damage to the orbital frontal cortex may result in increased disinhibition, increased impulsivity, increased irritability, hypermotility, euphoria, and attentional disruption with increased distractibility. Dysfunction in this region is implicated in the psychopathic subtype of aggression (Fuster, 1997; Raine, 1993). These symptoms are all highly relevant to the neuropsychological study of aggressive/antisocial behaviors (Giancola, Martin, Tarter, Pelham, & Moss, 1996; Niedermeyer, 1998).

The importance of the frontal lobes in social behavior is illustrated most famously by the historical case of Phineas P. Gage. As described by Damasio (1994), Gage was a 25-year-old, hard-working, reliable construction foreman working for the Rutland and Burlington Railroad. In 1848 he was in charge of a crew clearing rock that lay in the path of the railroad's expansion into Vermont. Because of the terrain, much blasting with gunpowder was required to remove rock and make the railroad bed straight and level. As a result of an accident during the blasting procedure late one afternoon, an explosion occurred, and a heavy iron rod was blown into Gage's left cheek. It pierced the base of his skull, traversed the front of his brain, and exited through the top of his head.

Most amazingly, Gage did not die from this event. He lived until 1861, almost 13 years after the accident. He regained strength, and his physical recovery appeared complete. He had no physical paralysis and could speak, touch, hear, and use his limbs with dexterity. His only physical disability was complete loss of vision in his left eye. His wound was pronounced cured 2 months after the accident, and he left medical care. However, he still had massive damage to his medial/cingulate frontal lobe, and his personality was irrevocably altered. This former hard-working, reliable family man now drank to excess and got into brawls. Accounts described him as impulsive, with a quick temper, without patience or restraint, cursing, obstinate, and incapable of planning efficiently or following through on his plans to completion. This famous historical case in the annals of neuropsychiatry illustrates the importance of the frontal lobes in the control of aggression and the self-regulation of goal-directed behaviors.

The neuropsychological investigation of frontal lobe functioning in juvenile CD and aggression has been of interest for several decades. Several studies report evidence of frontal lobe dysfunction and ECF deficits in youth with early-onset aggressive conduct problems (although not all studies agree). In a 7-year longitudinal study of 6- to 12-year-old nonreferred boys living in the community, neuropsychological tests distinguished those boys with stable physical aggression (fighting) from nonaggressive boys. Scores on neuropsychological tests measuring ECFs were significantly lower in the aggressive boys than in the nonaggressive boys. These findings could not be explained by differences in global IQ, concomitant ADHD, or SES (Seguin, Pihl, Harden, Tremblay, & Boulerice, 1995; Seguin, Boulerice, Harden, Tremblay, & Pihl, 1999). In another neuropsychological study of ECFs using a measure of response inhibition (called the "stop task"), two groups of children were investigated. One group met diagnostic criteria for ADHD, and the other for CD without ADHD. On testing, response inhibition deficits were found for both groups; this finding indicated that ECF deficits were not specific to the group with ADHD, but were present in children meeting diagnostic criteria for CD without ADHD as well (Oosterlaan, Logan, & Sergeant, 1998). Neuropsychological testing evidence of dysfunction in ECFs (and, by implication, frontal lobe and PFC dysfunction) has been found in aggressive boys at high risk for substance misuse (Giancola, Moss, Martin, Kirisci, & Tarter, 1996), girls with CD (Giancola, Mezzich, & Tarter, 1998a), aggressive girls at high risk for substance misuse (Giancola, Mezzich, & Tarter, 1998b), juveniles with psychopathy (Fisher & Blair, 1998), and aggressive boys with comorbid ADHD and CD (Moffitt, 1990b). These studies provide partial support for a frontal lobe dysfunction hypothesis in youth with CD (with and without comorbid psychopathology).

However, failures to replicate the importance of frontal lobe neuropsychological findings in aggressive youngsters with CD also exist. A study of 59 adolescents sought to determine whether an association existed between neuropsychological deficits and CD with and without concurrent ADHD. Results indicated that ECF deficits were not found in subjects with CD but without comorbid ADHD, relative to controls; such deficits were limited to the CD-ADHD youngsters only (Dery, Toupin, Pauze, Mercier, & Fortin, 1999). A finding of verbal skill deficits in adolescents with CD relative to controls was replicated, indicating that CD in juveniles is associated with lower verbal skills, independently of comorbid ADHD and of ECF/frontal lobe dysfunction (Dery et al., 1999). Other studies have also failed to find neuropsychological evidence of ECF deficits and frontal lobe impairment in youth with CD but without ADHD (Frost, Moffitt, & McGee, 1989; Linz, Hooper, Hynd, Issac, & Gibson, 1990; Pennington & Ozonoff, 1996; Speltz, DeKlyen, Calderon, Greenberg, & Fisher, 1999).

Mixed findings (some positive and some negative) for an association between ECF deficits and frontal lobe dysfunction on the one hand, and CD on the other, may have been obtained for several reasons. First, in both clinical and nonreferred community samples of aggressive juveniles who meet criteria for CD, a large association with comorbid ADHD is found. It is known that a large overlap exists between attention deficits/hyperactivity and conduct problems/aggression (Hinshaw, 1987). For CD and conduct problems in general, overlap with ADHD is reported in 85% of clinically referred children and adolescents (Biederman, Faraone, & Lapey, 1992); in nonreferred youth, the overlap ranges between 35% and 47% (Biederman et al., 1992). Studies that report large ECF deficits on tests of neuropsychological functioning in youngsters with CD often do not control for comorbid ADHD. Indeed, when

ADHD is controlled for, neuropsychological findings of ECF deficits in CD become much weaker (Dery et al., 1999; Pennington & Ozonoff, 1996).

Next, more attention to subtyping aggression needs to be considered in further neuropsychological research on ECF dysfunction in early-onset aggressive/antisocial behaviors. Attention should be focused on two possible subtypes in particular: (1) the co-occurrence of ADHD and CD, and (2) psychopathy. There is evidence from longitudinal studies that a subset of aggressive boys meeting clinical criteria for both ADHD and CD may exhibit a distinct subtype of aggression (Moffitt, 1990a). They demonstrate an early age at onset of aggressive behavior, more varied types of aggression, persistence of aggression across the lifespan, social information-processing deficits, and a poorer prognosis (Hinshaw, 1987). Boys with this subtype also evidence more neuropsychological deficits on measures of verbal skills and ECF than boys with only ADHD or only CD (Moffitt, 1990b; Moffitt & Silva, 1988c). This suggests that the specific comorbidity of ADHD and CD merits further neuropsychological study (Moffitt & Silva, 1988).

Psychopathy is emerging as a distinct personality type with high risk for aggression and related behaviors in youngsters (Frick, O'Brien, Wootton, & McBurnett, 1994). Psychopathic individuals may demonstrate more specific frontal deficits on neuropsychological tests than other individuals with aggression. To date, more work has been completed in adult than on juvenile psychopathy. In comparisons of adult psychopathic and nonpsychopathic criminals, specific deficits on neuropsychological tests assessing orbital frontal and ventromedial frontal lobe functioning emerged in the psychopathic subjects (Lapierre, Braun, & Hodgins, 1995). This suggests that frontal lobe dysfunction as measured by neuropsychological testing may be more specific to the psychopathic subtype of aggression and antisocial behaviors than to other subtypes.

Finally, few neuropsychological studies of ECF deficits in aggression and related behaviors have controlled for environmental stress. An emerging body of research is suggesting that stress can impair PFC functioning in rodent models, primate models, and human beings (Arnsten, 1999; Arnsten & Goldman-Rakic, 1998). For example, in rodent models mild stress such as noise, restraint, or forced swimming stress can impair PFC and take the PFC "off-line." In primates, noise stress reduces PFC functioning. Diminished PFC inhibition of lower subcortical structures (such as the hypothalamus, amygdala, or hippocampus) allows the release of more instinctual behaviors that facilitate organismic survival in stressful environments (Arnsten & Goldman-Rakic, 1998). A consequence of PFC stress-induced inhibition is the emergence of more disinhibited behaviors, including attention deficits, impulsive aggressive behavior, and impairments in working memory. The importance of environmental stress in PFC functioning has also been noted for human beings (Arnsten, 1999). Children and adolescents in stressful environments often demonstrate clinical symptoms suggestive of ECF deficits, including impulsive aggressive behavior and sustained attention deficits. In clinically referred samples of aggressive youngsters meeting criteria for CD, many have experienced chronic trauma and stress, including neglect, abuse, and multiple changes of caregivers (Connor, Melloni, & Harrison, 1998). The possibility of frontal lobe dysfunction in clinically referred traumatized youth is suggested by high comorbidity rates between posttraumatic stress disorder (PTSD) and ADHD. In a study of psychiatric disorders in sexually abused children, ADHD was the most common psychiatric disorder in 46% of the sample; 23% had both PTSD and ADHD; and 15.4% had both PTSD and CD (McLeer, Callaghan, Henry, & Wallen, 1994). These data suggest the possibility that ECF deficits in aggressive/antisocial children could be secondary to the neuropsychological effects of environmental stress on PFC functioning, and not solely due to ADHD, CD, or psychopathy. As such, future research should control for severe environmental stress in investigations of neuropsychological functioning and aggressive CD in youth.

Summary of Neuropsychological Findings

Although not all studies agree, there exists evidence to support correlations between neuropsychological test findings and aggressive/antisocial behaviors in children and adolescents. Global IQ and Verbal IQ deficits in such youngsters have strong scientific support. Reduced efficiency in processing language, reduced cerebral laterality for language, and inefficient frontal lobe functioning in youths with psychopathy, ADHD and CD, and early-onset, persistent aggression are deserving of further neuropsychological study.

PSYCHOPHYSIOLOGY

"Psychophysiology" is the study of the relationships between physiological measures and psychological states or processes, usually relating to such domains as learning, emotion, arousal, and cognition (Dawson, 1990). The psychophysiological measures most commonly recorded from aggressive/antisocial youngsters are electrodermal activity (EDA), heart rate, cortical measures of event-related potentials (ERPs), and cortical measures of the electroencephalogram (EEG). In addition, sensitivity to pain may index some aspects of ANS functioning. These measures are discussed in turn below.

Electrodermal Activity

EDA is a general term encompassing the various indicators of electrical conductance and potential difference measured across the skin of a subject. Skin conductance (SC), one form of EDA, is generally measured by placing electrodes on two sites of the hand (generally the fingers or palm) and passing a very small electrical current between the two electrodes. The current is generally imperceptible to the subject. The amount of current passing across the skin varies as a function of sweat activity, with increased sweating leading to an increase in EDA. Since the sweat glands are innervated by the sympathetic branch of the ANS, various EDA indices are often used as peripheral measures of ANS arousal (McBurnett & Lahey, 1994).

The general concept of EDA can be subdivided into more specific measurements. SC level (SCL) reflects the tonic level of electrical activity measured across skin at rest (without a stimulus presented to the subject). Superimposed upon the SCL are brief spontaneous phasic changes in SC known as "spontaneous fluctuations" (SFs). Phasic changes in SC occurring in response to a stimulus (generally a sound or a mental task) are referred to as SC responses (SCRs). These usually occur from 1 to 3 seconds after the presentation of a stimulus and provide a very sensitive index of what is termed the "orienting reflex" (the "what is it" response). Information-processing models of orienting suggest that individual differences in the size of SCRs reflect the degree to which an individual allocates attentional processing resources to the stimulus, and thus that SCRs vary with the significance to the individual of the eliciting stimulus (Filion, Dawson, Schell, & Hazlett, 1991). SCRs are used as peripheral measures of ANS arousal and reactivity to a stimulus; SCL and SFs are used as measures of basal ANS arousal. There is evidence that the PFC, the pons, and the temporal lobe/amygdala are CNS structures mediating SC orienting in human beings (Raine, Reynolds, & Sheard, 1991).

EDA has been studied in youth with aggression and related behaviors. Results from studies conducted since 1980 are presented in Table 6.2. The findings of eight reviewed cross-sectional studies were mixed, with five studies reporting significantly lower EDA in groups of children and adolescents with aggression and conduct problems, compared to controls or children with other psychiatric disorders. Two studies reported negative results (Garralda, Connell, & Taylor, 1990, 1991). One study reported differences in the opposite direction of the hypothesized lower EDA in youth with CD (Dwivedi, Beaumont, & Brandon, 1984). The differences in outcomes may have resulted from methodological differences across studies, with two investigations using a mental task as the stimulus reporting no significant results across groups, whereas studies using a tone or bell stimulus have generally reported significant findings. The two cross-sectional studies evaluating hyperactivity (Delamater & Lahey, 1983) or ADHD (McBurnett et al., 1993) found no interaction with EDA in their samples. These studies suggest that EDA underactivity in conduct problems is independent of ADHD. All four longitudinal studies are consistent in finding evidence for EDA underarousal in groups of children with CD (see Table 6.2). Taken together, these longitudinal studies support the hypothesis that ANS underarousal as measured by EDA is associated with physical aggression, conduct problems, and delinquency in both clinically referred and community samples of juveniles.

Heart Rate

Both resting heart rate level (HRL) and heart rate reactivity (HRR) to a stimulus have been extensively studied in juveniles with aggressive antisocial prob-

TABLE 6.2. EDA and Aggressive/Antisocial Behaviors in Children and Adolescents

Study	Subjects	Sample	Findings
Cross-sectional studies			
Delamater and Lahey (1983)	36 children/age 10 yr	Children with learning disability/some with hyperactivity	Smaller SCR amplitudes in children with conduct problems. No interaction with hyperactivity.
Dwivedi et al. (1984)	12 boys/age 14–16 yr	High-risk clinical sample	Greater SCR amplitudes in high-aggression boys (opposite finding from what was expected).
Raine and Venables (1984a)	101 boys/age 14–16 yr	Community sample	Reduced frequency of SC orienting to neutral stimuli in antisocial subjects.
Schmidt et al. (1985)	22 children/mean age 9.7 yr	Children with CD/controls	Low SCR to aversive stimuli in subjects with CD.
Garralda et al. (1990)	15 children/age not given	Children with CD and emotional disorders	NSD[a] on mental task as stimulus.
Garralda et al. (1991)	75 children/age 7–13 yr	Children with CD and emotional disorders/controls	NSD on mental task as stimulus.
McBurnett et al. (1993)	57 children/age 5–12 yr	Children with CD/ADHD/controls	Lower EDA in children rated high on aggression. No interactive effects with ADHD.
van Goozen, Matthys, et al. (2000)	64 children/age 8–12 yr	Children with CD/controls	Low SCL in children with CD vs. controls.
Longitudinal studies			
Venables (1989)	1,800 children/assessed at age 3 yr	Community sample	Low SC at age 3 yr predicted fighting behavior at age 9 yr.
Raine et al. (1990a)	101 boys/age 15 yr	Community sample	Adult criminals at age 24 yr had sig. lower resting SCRs when measured at age 15 yr.
Kruesi et al. (1992)	29 children/age 6–17 yr	Children with disruptive behavior disorders	At 2-yr follow-up, lower SCL predicted greater severity of aggression.
Raine, Venables, and Mednick (1997)	1,795 children/assessed at age 3 yr	Community sample	Aggressive children at age 11 yr gave fewer SC orienting responses at age 3 yr than nonaggressive children. Interaction with SES.

[a]NSD, no significant difference (in this and subsequent tables).

178

lems. Many studies have reported that these children and adolescents have lower resting HRL than control groups (Raine, 1993). Heart rate is under the dual control of the sympathetic and parasympathetic branches of the ANS. Lower resting HRL and diminished HRR to a stimulus or mental task can be due either to lower sympathetic ANS activity or to increased parasympathetic ANS activity. Findings of lower resting HRL or diminished HRR in aggressive/antisocial juveniles versus controls can be interpreted as reflecting either characteristically slower basal activity, or lesser cardiac reactivity to novel stressful experimental situations (McBurnett & Lahey, 1994). As such, youngsters with lower resting HRL or less HRR to a stimulus may have either sympathetic or parasympathetic ANS differences (or both) from controls.

Heart rate is one of the simplest psychophysiological measures to collect; anyone can take a pulse. However, it is difficult to interpret. Numerous variables—metabolic demands, age, physical activity, physical fitness level, environmental temperature, oxygen availability, and disease exposure—affect HRL and HRR. Activation of motor activity reliably increases heart rate and can alter measures of HRR unless the subject remains motionless during testing. These potential confounds must be controlled for in experimental investigations, in order to hear a "signal" potentially linking aggressive/antisocial behaviors with ANS changes as measured by these cardiac parameters.

Investigations since 1980 examining the relationships of HRL and HRR to juvenile aggression and conduct problems are presented in Table 6.3. These studies have investigated clinically referred as well as community samples of youth. The majority of studies examined boys, but several included girls as well. Of the 12 cross-sectional studies of resting HRL, 8 were consistent in finding lower resting HRL in aggressive or antisocial youth (Kindlon et al., 1995; Maliphant, Hume, & Furnham, 1990; Maliphant, Watson, & Daniels, 1990; Pitts, 1997; Raine & Venables, 1984b; Raine & Jones, 1987; Rogeness, Cepeda, Macedo, Fischer, & Harris, 1990; van Goozen, Matthys, Cohen-Kettenis, Buitelaar, & van Engeland, 2000). Four studies reported no statistically significant differences in resting HRL across groups (Delamater & Lahey, 1983; Dwivedi et al., 1984; Garralda et al., 1991; Losel & Bender, 1997).

Of the eight reviewed cross-sectional studies investigating HRR to a stimulus, four reported diminished HRR in aggressive juveniles (el-Sheikh, 1994; Garralda et al., 1990; Mezzacappa et al., 1996; Pitts, 1997). Three studies found no significant differences across groups (Dwivedi et al., 1984; Liang et al., 1995; Pine et al., 1998). One study investigating high-risk sons in families with multigenerational alcohol problems obtained results opposing the hypothesis that lower HRR is associated with conduct problems; that is, sons with CD who had alcoholic parents exhibited higher HRR to a stimulus (Harden & Pihl, 1995).

Results from five longitudinal studies of resting HRL and aggressive/antisocial behaviors are also presented in Table 6.3. These longitudinal studies were fairly consistent: Four of five found a significant relationship between

TABLE 6.3. Heart Rate and Aggressive/Antisocial Behaviors in Children and Adolescents

Study	Subjects	Sample	Findings
Cross-sectional studies of resting HRL			
Delamater and Lahey (1983)	36 children/age 10 yr	Learning disability/some with hyperactivity	NSD in resting HRL in children with conduct problems.
Dwivedi et al. (1984)	12 boys/age 14–16 yr	High-risk clinical sample	NSD in resting HRL in children with CD.
Raine and Venables (1984b)	101 boys/age 14–16 yr	Community sample	Lower resting HRL in antisocial boys.
Raine and Jones (1987)	40 boys/age 7–15 yr	Boys with CD	Lower resting HRL in boys with CD.
Maliphant, Hume, and Furnham (1990)	44 girls/age 12–13 yr	Community sample	Lower resting HRL in disruptive girls.
Maliphant, Watson, and Daniels (1990)	50 boys/age 7–9 yr	Community sample	Lower resting HRL in disruptive boys.
Rogeness, Cepeda, et al. (1990)	589 children/age 12–13 yr	Children with CD/depression/anxiety disorders	Lower resting HRL in boys and girls with CD compared to controls.
Garralda et al. (1991)	50 children/age 7–13 yr	Children with CD/emotional disorders	NSD in resting HRL in children with CD.
Kindlon et al. (1995)	138 boys/age 9–12 yr	Community sample	Lower resting HRL associated with physical fighting at age 11 yr.
Pitts (1997)	95 boys/age 9–12 yr	Community sample	Lower resting HRL in aggressive boys.
Losel and Bender (1997)	37 boys/mean age 17.4 yr	High-risk/clinically referred sample	NSD in resting HRL in antisocial adolescents.
van Goozen, Matthys, et al. (2000)	62 boys and girls/age 8–12 yr	Children with CD/clinically referred sample	Lower resting HRL in children with CD.

180

Cross-sectional studies of HRR

Dwivedi et al. (1984)	12 boys/age 14–16 yr	High-risk clinical sample	NSD in HRR in children with CD.
Garralda et al. (1990)	15 children/age not given	Children with CD/emotional disorders	Lower HRR to a mental task in children with CD.
el-Sheikh (1994)	Preschoolers	Community sample	HRR in preschoolers negatively correlated with physical violence in the home.
Harden and Pihl (1995)	28 boys/age 12 yr	Community sample	High-risk boys with conduct problems from families with alcohol problems had greater HRR on a mental task than controls (opposite finding from what was expected).
Liang et al. (1995)	24 boys/age 14–16 yr	Community sample	HRR not independently related to risk behaviors, including physical fighting.
Mezzacappa et al. (1996)	15 children/age 15 yr	Community sample	Lower HRR in aggressive subjects.
Pitts (1997)	95 boys/age 9–12 yr	Community sample	Lower HRR in aggressive boys.
Pine et al. (1998)	69 boys/age 11 yr	High-risk community sample	NSD in HRR between boys with disruptive behavior disorders and others.

Longitudinal studies

Kruesi et al. (1992)	29 children/age 6–17 yr	Children with disruptive behavior disorders	At 2-yr follow-up, severity of aggression predicted by lower resting HRL measured at baseline.
Raine et al. (1990b)	101 boys/age 15 yr	Community sample	Lower resting HRL at age 15 yr in those who were criminal at age 24 yr.
Farrington (1997)	411 boys/age 18 yr	Community sample	Lower resting HRL at age 18 yr predicted violence before age 25 yr.
Raine, Venables, and Mednick (1997)	1,795 children/assessed at age 3 yr	Community sample	Lower resting HRL at age 3 yr predicted high aggression at age 11 yr.
Van Hulle et al. (2000)	601 children/assessed at age 7 yr	Community sample	NSD.

lower resting HRL and later aggressive/antisocial behaviors in children and adolescents. One study did not find a relationship between lower resting HRL at age 14 months and externalizing behavior problems at age 7 years (Van Hulle, Corely, Zahn-Waxler, Kagan, & Hewitt, 2000).

The differing results may be due to study design and methodological differences. For example, heart rate varies inversely with age (Liang et al., 1995). Some studies mixed children with adolescents in their samples, and this may have confounded heart rate findings. In addition, differences in study samples may account for some of the discrepancies. In the study of boys with conduct problems from alcoholic families, higher HRR was found than in controls (Harden & Pihl, 1995). This suggests that aggressive/antisocial youth with alcoholic parents may constitute a subtype with ANS findings distinct from those of youth without such a family history. Some studies report an interaction among resting HRL and HRR, aggression/conduct problems, and SES. Stronger and more consistent psychophysiological findings may be obtained from aggressive juveniles residing in more stable home environments characterized by higher SES (Raine, Reynolds, Venables, & Mednick, 1997). Finally, personality dimensions such as hostility can affect cardiovascular functioning. In adult men who were verbally provoked in a laboratory setting, sustained, enhanced heart rate was seen on a mental task only in subjects with higher hostility levels (Suarez, Kuhn, Schanberg, Williams, & Zimmermann, 1998). Since aggressive/antisocial juveniles are also generally more hostile than nonaggressive youth, hostility may explain some of the differences in cross-sectional studies of HRL and HRR reviewed above.

These results suggest that further investigations of resting HRL and HRR might be fruitful, especially studies controlling for age, SES, aggressive subtypes, and personality dimensions such as hostility. Recent advances in the field include spectral analysis of heart rate variability. This technique decomposes real-time heart rate beat-to-beat variability into its various components. What emerge are contributions of variations in blood pressure (under sympathetic ANS control) and respiration (under parasympathetic ANS control) to the total heart rate variability. These components in turn can be linked to mediation by the two branches of the ANS under certain experimental conditions, and can begin to provide a more detailed analysis of ANS contributions to heart rate variability (Mezzacappa, Kindlon, Saul, & Earls, 1998). Recent studies have documented reduced heart period variability and associations with externalizing behavior disorders (Pine et al., 1998) and stable, predatory aggression (Mezzacappa et al., 1997), suggesting deficient parasympathetic ANS modulation of heart rate variability in boys with stable aggression.

Event-Related Potentials

ERPs provide a way to study information processing in the electrical activity of the brain. Studies of the EEG demonstrate that sensory stimuli provoke a measurable electrophysiological response. This response, the ERP, can be measured from surface electrodes applied to the scalp (according to the stan-

dard International 10-20 System of electrode placement) and the EEG. However, the ERP is much smaller in magnitude than the amplitude of the background EEG. As a result, the ERP signal is drowned out by the background
"noise" of the EEG. This problem is overcome with the use of signal-averaging
techniques. Potentials elicited from multiple repeated ERP trials are superimposed on one another and averaged by computer analysis. Since the background activity from the EEG is random, in repeated trials it averages to zero,
and a specific ERP signal emerges.

ERPs can be reliably elicited with visual, auditory, or somatosensory
stimuli. These potentials have well-defined positive and negative peaks and
represent the electrical activity of the primary neural pathway from sensory
receptors to the cortex. Both the amplitude of the peaks and the latency, or
time from the stimulus until the waveform appears, are measured. An example
of a brainstem auditory evoked potential (AEP) is given in Figure 6.3. Each of
the seven AEP peaks corresponds to neural activity in particular brain structures mediating information processing in the auditory neural pathway from
sensory receptors to cortex. Some of the AEP neuroanatomical correlates are
better known than others.

An ERP occurs within the first 100 milliseconds (msec) after stimulus onset. Early components of the ERP are related to the parameters of the stimulus
(e.g., intensity, duration, complexity) and are termed "exogenous activity."
They occur with a latency of about 1–50 msec after stimulus onset. The mid-

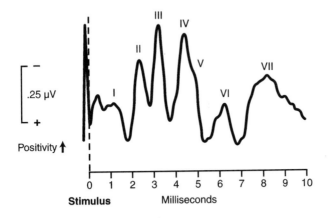

FIGURE 6.3. A brainstem auditory evoked potential (AEP).
Waveform and anatomical relationships after an acoustic
stimulus excites the auditory nerve. I, auditory nerve; II, co-
chlear nuclei (brainstem); III, superior olivary nucleus (brainstem); IV, lateral leminiscus (brainstem); V, inferior colliculus
(midbrain); VI, (?) medial geniculate nucleus (midbrain); VII,
(?) auditory radiations. From Adams and Victor (1981).
Copyright 1981 by The McGraw-Hill Companies. Reprinted
by permission.

dle (50–250 msec) and late (250–500 msec) components are of particular interest because they are thought to reflect increasing psychological processing of the stimulus, independently of the physical properties of the stimulus (e.g., attention and arousal). This "endogenous activity" can be analyzed to study a range of information-processing phenomena.

In experimental paradigms in the laboratory, a standardized procedure for presenting stimuli to a subject is often followed. A target stimulus is presented, and the subject is told to respond, such as by pressing a key or counting the number of times the stimulus is presented. In a variation, a warning stimulus precedes an imperative stimulus to which the subject must react, such as by pressing a lever. In the "oddball" paradigm, rare events (such as a differing tone) are embedded in more frequent common events (the usual tone). The subject gives a motor response, such as pressing a button, to the rare event. When these electrical events are averaged over multiple trials, an ERP waveform that looks like Figure 6.4 is generated.

As a rule, positive-going deflections in the ERP waveform are labeled P, for positive, whereas negative-going deflections are labeled N, for negative. Following the polarity label, a number is affixed to indicate the latency of the component in milliseconds after stimulus onset. It is thought that the amplitude of a given deflection is related to the magnitudes of the intracerebral volume currents that generate it, which in turn are related to the electrical activity of the stimulated neurons generating the current. The latency of a given com-

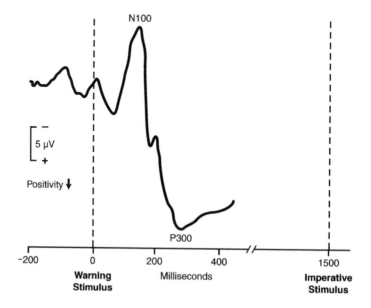

FIGURE 6.4. An event-related potential (ERP) waveform after averaging over multiple trials. In this diagram, positivity is down. Shown are N100 and P300.

ponent reflects transmission time along the neural pathway since stimulus on-set (Nelson & Luciana, 1998). Another convention is to label the first nega-tive deflection N1, the second N2, the first positive wave P1, and so on, and to state the latency in milliseconds.

There are a number of ERP components (or waves), which reflect differ-ent aspects of stimulus information processing. As a rule, these components generally occur more than 100 msec after stimulus onset in the adult. In chil-dren, the latency is somewhat more variable. One of the best studied in neuropsychiatry is the P300 component. The P300 response is generally in-voked by target- or task-relevant events. It occurs anywhere from 300 to 600 msec or more after such an event has been presented to the subject, and is maximal at midline/posterior scalp electrodes. Although there is debate over the precise meaning of P300, there is general agreement that it reflects some aspects of cognitive information processing relating to working memory (Nel-son & Luciana, 1998); to the efficiency of cognitive processing (Gerstle, Mathias, & Stanford, 1998); to task relevance, decision making, orienting, and stimulus salience (Raine & Venables, 1987; Raine, 1989); and to atten-tion (Overtoom et al., 1998). The P300 component may be generated from subcortical sources, including the hippocampus, the hippocampal gyrus, and the amygdala (Raine, 1989). The latency of P300 may reflect stimulus evalua-tion time (Gerstle et al., 1998). Other late components receiving study in neuropsychiatry include N100 (N1), the first negative component, reflecting stimulus intensity as well as some aspects of endogenous information process-ing (McBurnett & Lahey, 1994); N200 (N2), a measure of response inhibition (the opposite of impulsivity) (Overtoom et al., 1998); and N400, which is re-lated to linguistic processing when semantic judgments are required (Nelson & Luciana, 1998). The contingent negative variation (CNV) is a long-latency (several seconds), slow negative shift in the ERP waveform that occurs when a subject is presented with a warning stimulus signaling the arrival of a second imperative stimulus on which the subject must act. The CNV is thought to re-flect higher cognitive behavior—specifically, neural activity preparatory to a goal-directed act (Nelson & Luciana, 1998).

ERPs have been studied in juveniles with aggressive behavior; conduct problems, delinquency, and other antisocial behavior; ADHD; and severe gen-eral psychopathology. Over the years, however, less research has been con-ducted with children and adolescents than with incarcerated antisocial and psychopathic adults. Research since 1980 on ERPs and aggressive and related behaviors in juveniles is presented in Table 6.4. This literature is difficult to interpret precisely. Although information-processing abnormalities as assessed via ERPs are found in many of these reports, no unique ERP signature is pres-ent across all of these studies. This may be due to the fact that various investi-gations have studied differently defined subgroups of "delinquent," "antiso-cial," "hyperactive," and "criminal" juveniles, some with and some without substance use disorders (SUDs), and some with internalizing as well as externalizing comorbid psychopathology. In addition, the ages of subjects in these studies have varied from early elementary school to the college years.

TABLE 6.4. ERPs and Aggressive/Antisocial Behaviors in Children and Adolescents

Study	Subjects	Sample	Findings
Cross-sectional studies			
Dwivedi et al. (1984)	12 boys/age 14–16 yr	High-risk clinical sample	Longer N2 latencies in aggressive boys.
Satterfield and Schell (1984)	141 children/age 6–12 yr	Children with hyperactivity/delinquency/controls	Smaller N2 amplitudes in hyperactive children who were not delinquent.
Raine and Venables (1987)	101 boys/age 14–16 yr	Community sample	P300 amplitude significantly larger in antisocial group.
Herning et al. (1989)	25 children/age 15–16 yr	High- and low-delinquency community sample ± drug use	Longer latency of wave V and faster latency of N100 in high-delinquency subjects (with mild to moderate drug use).
Pickworth et al. (1990)	35 adolescents/age = 16.4 yr	High- and low-delinquency community sample ± drug use	Longer P300 latency in high-delinquency subjects with drug use. Smaller N100 amplitude in high-delinquency subjects without drug use.
Gerstle et al. (1998)	44 young adults/age 18–24 yr	College students ± impulsive aggression	Lower P300 amplitudes in subjects with impulsive aggression.
Overtoom et al. (1998)	32 children/age 6–14 yr	Children with ADHD/controls	Lower P300 amplitudes in children with ADHD compared to controls. Subgroup with ADHD + ODD (verbal aggression and oppositional) had smaller N2 amplitudes compared to controls.
Lincoln et al. (1998)	40 children/age 9–13 yr	Children with borderline pers. disorder/ADHD/controls	Smaller P300 amplitudes in borderline children with greater internalizing and externalizing psychopathology, compared to children with ADHD or controls.
Bauer and Hesselbrock (1999)	257 adolescents/age 15–20 yr	Adolescents with high/low conduct problems	Smaller P300 amplitudes in subjects with greater conduct problems.
Longitudinal studies			
Satterfield et al. (1987)	141 children/age 6–12 yr at initial assessment	Children with hyperactivity/delinquency/controls	At 8-yr follow-up, hyperactive children without delinquency had abnormal maturational changes on auditory ERP, compared to hyperactive children with delinquency and controls.
Raine et al. (1990c)	101 boys/age 15 yr	Community sample	Higher N1 amplitude and faster P300 latencies at age 15 yr in those who became criminal by 9-yr follow-up.

One observation is that ERP measures are sensitive to many different subject characteristics, including various types of aggressive and related behaviors, the presence of hyperactivity or ADHD, the presence of comorbid internalizing psychopathology, and drug use. In addition, the possibility of interactions between age and subject characteristics needs to be considered (McBurnett & Lahey, 1994).

What is clear from Table 6.4 is that unimodal, simplistic models of deficient information processing in aggressive/antisocial juveniles as indexed by ERP components must be rejected. Whereas some studies report lower P300 amplitudes in college students with impulsive aggression (Gerstle et al., 1998), other studies report higher P300 amplitudes in delinquent 15-year-olds (Raine & Venables, 1987). At least some differences may be due to the salience of the stimulus. It is possible that antisocial individuals, especially those with psychopathic qualities, demonstrate enhanced information processing to stimuli that are of much interest to them, at least in the short run (Raine, 1989). For example, these youth may have acutely enhanced information-processing abilities when it comes to eluding detection for their illegal activities. The idea that aggressive/antisocial individuals always demonstrate deficient information processing in all settings must be rethought. This is further supported by the longitudinal study of Satterfield, Schell, and Backs (1987), who found normal maturational ERP changes in delinquent children as compared to controls, but abnormal maturational ERP changes in hyperactive children without delinquency.

Raine (1989), reviewing primarily ERP studies of adults, has argued for a model of psychopathy that involves cortical underarousal (based on the long latency of early ERP components); sensation seeking (based on abnormal middle ERP components); and enhanced attentional processes to stimuli of interest, such as, escape from punishment (based on enhanced late ERP components). This has led to a hypothesis that persons with psychopathy exist in a relative state of cognitive underarousal and stimulus deprivation, and seek out stimulating events in order to optimize their level of cognitive arousal (Raine, 1989). Seeking stimulating events may lead to a higher possibility of engaging in exciting but antisocial behaviors. In antisocial juveniles, there is some support for this theory. Longer latencies of ERP components have been observed in several studies of youth (Dwivedi et al., 1984; Herning, Hickey, Pickworth, & Jaffee, 1989; Pickworth, Brown, Hickey, & Muntaner, 1990), supporting a cognitive underarousal model. Higher P300 amplitudes in delinquents reported by Raine and Venables (1987) support enhanced information processing to stimuli of interest in delinquent adolescents.

The data are also partially supportive of an alternative theory, the two-factor motivational hypothesis of Gray (1982) (see Chapter 7). According to this theory, antisocial and psychopathic individuals would be expected to have an overactive behavioral activation system (BAS) and an underactive behavioral inhibition system (BIS). An overactive BAS would be consistent with enhanced P300 amplitudes to stimuli of interest and reward. An underactive BIS would be consistent with ERP findings of cortical under-arousal (McBurnett & Lahey, 1994).

However, the ERP data in children, adolescents, and young adults are not entirely consistent with the two theories presented above. Instead of higher P300 amplitudes, other studies have reported lower P300 amplitudes in youth with borderline personality disorder and comorbid externalizing and internal-izing psychopathology (Lincoln, Bloom, Katz, & Boksenbaum, 1998), college students with impulsive aggression (Gerstle et al., 1998), adolescents with conduct problems (Bauer & Hesselbrock, 1999), and children with both ADHD and ODD (verbal aggression) (Overtoom et al., 1998). These data sug-gest the importance of subtyping aggression and related behaviors in future ERP studies.

The Electroencephalogram

The EEG is a recording of electrical potentials from the scalp. Voltage is re-corded as the potential difference between what is considered an electrically active site and what is assumed to be an electrically inactive site. Electrodes are placed on the scalp according to the standardized International 10-20 sys-tem. The EEG reflects the electrical activity of the cortex, although subcortical structures such as the thalamus and hippocampus are probably involved in neuronal control of this cortical activity.

EEG activity is classified into four frequency bands: delta (below 4 Hz), theta (4–8 Hz), alpha (8–12 Hz), and beta (above 13 Hz). The alpha and beta frequencies are often further subdivided into slow and fast subcategories. Fre-quency bands are associated with varying degrees of cortical alertness and arousal. Delta is associated with sleep, theta with low levels of alertness such as drowsiness, alpha with relaxed wakefulness, and beta with alertness and vigilance. Although all frequencies are present in an awake individual, the rel-ative power of these frequency bands differs across different people. Quantita-tive methods of analysis can decompose the EEG into fundamental frequen-cies and compute the power spectrum within each of the EEG frequency bands. For example, cortical arousal may be inferred by the frequency that predominates within the alpha bandwidth. A preponderance of slower, lower frequency in the alpha band is termed "alpha slowing" and is taken as evi-dence of relative cortical underarousal (McBurnett & Lahey, 1994; Raine, 1993). Quantitative EEG analysis has revealed maturational changes in these frequencies across development. Very young children exhibit slower frequen-cies; as maturation proceeds, higher-frequency rhythms become more preva-lent (Schmidt & Fox, 1998).

In the past six decades, literally hundreds of studies have assessed the EEG in individuals with criminal activity, delinquency, psychopathy, and recidivistic violent offenses (Raine, 1993). Many of these studies have found evidence of EEG abnormalities in such individuals. These investigations suggest that the prevalence of nonspecific EEG abnormalities in habitually vi-olent adults and adolescents ranges from 25% to 50% (Mednick, Volavka,

Gabrielli, & Itil, 1982). This is greater than the background prevalence of EEG abnormalities found in the general population, which is about 12% (Ounsted, 1969). Many of these studies, however, were done long ago and were technologically primitive (i.e., relying on visual inspection of the EEG instead of quantitative analysis of band frequency). They reported a high amount of slow EEG activity in boys with conduct problems (Coble et al., 1984), and paroxysmal spike and wave abnormalities in repeatedly violent delinquent boys (Lewis, Pincus, Shanok, & Glaser, 1982). However, other studies reported no significant differences in EEG abnormalities between delinquent juveniles and psychiatric controls (Hsu, Wisner, Richey, & Goldstein, 1985). Other investigations found a low prevalence of EEG abnormalities in consecutive case series of children with CD and/or ADHD (9%, as compared to the population background rate of 12% of EEG abnormalities) (Phillips, Drake, Hietter, Andrews, & Bogner, 1993).

Studies reporting a high rate of EEG abnormalities in this population have been criticized on several grounds. First, as noted earlier, the EEG changes with development and CNS maturation (Schmidt & Fox, 1998). EEG abnormalities in children may be unstable, and may also change with time and development; thus their relationship to aggressive and antisocial behaviors is uncertain (Milstein, 1988). Second, most EEG studies have used institutionalized or clinically referred populations, as well as older delinquent individuals. Finally, studies have not controlled for the accumulating effects on the EEG over time of SUDs and head injuries, both of which are highly prevalent in aggressive/antisocial individuals (McBurnett & Lahey, 1994).

These difficulties may be overcome in part by research that examines EEG changes in nonreferred, younger children, before a delinquent lifestyle begins to affect the EEG. A second strategy is the use of prospective longitudinal studies. Post-1980 investigations using these strategies are presented in Table 6.5. These more recent EEG studies suggest two hypotheses: (1) that children who are at risk for externalizing behavior disorders may have EEG evidence for cortical asymmetry, which may be associated with diminished verbal regulation of disruptive behavior; and (2) children who later become delinquent have EEG evidence of cortical underarousal (i.e., alpha frequency slowing).

In a cross-sectional study, 48 children aged 4 were observed in a play quartet session to assess behavior. An EEG was obtained on each child about 2 weeks later. Children who displayed a pattern of right frontal EEG activation and were socially intrusive were more likely to exhibit externalizing behavior problems than were socially intrusive children who exhibited left frontal EEG activation (Schmidt & Fox, 1998). Socially intrusive normal children with relatively greater right frontal EEG activation may not have the characteristics (such as verbal skills, which are thought to be subserved by the left frontal region) necessary for competent regulation of affective and behavioral arousal. As such, they may be more at risk for the development of aggression and related behaviors.

Three of four longitudinal studies and all prospective investigations using community samples have provided congruent EEG evidence of cortical under-

TABLE 6.5. EEG Activity and Aggressive/Antisocial Behavior in Children and Adolescents

Study	Subjects	Sample	Findings
Cross-sectional studies			
Schmidt and Fox (1998)	48 children/age 4 yr	Community sample	Highly sociable children with greater right frontal EEG activation were more likely to exhibit externalizing behavior problems than highly sociable children with left frontal EEG activation.
Longitudinal studies			
Mednick et al. (1982)	129 children/age 10–13 yr at baseline	Community sample	In those who became multiple-delinquency offenders at 6-yr follow-up, the baseline EEG showed significantly greater slow alpha activity (8–10 Hz).
Petersen et al. (1982)	571 children/age 1–15 yr at baseline	Community sample	In those who were convicted of theft at 12- to 13-yr follow-up, the baseline EEG showed significantly greater alpha slowing than in those never convicted of theft.
Satterfield and Schell (1984)	141 boys/age 6–12 yr at baseline	Boys with hyperactivity/ controls	NSD in EEG power spectra when delinquent hyperactive boys were compared to controls at 8-yr follow-up. Most deviant EEG measures found in nondelinquent hyperactive boys (50% abnormal in this group).
Raine et al. (1990b)	101 boys/age 15 yr at baseline	Community sample	At 9-yr follow-up, those who acquired a criminal record had evidence of EEG slowing at age 15 yr (increased delta and slow alpha EEG power spectra).

arousal in youth who went on to become delinquent (Mednick et al., 1982; Peterson, Matousek, Mednick, Volavka, & Pollock, 1982; Raine, Venables, & Williams, 1990b). The one longitudinal study that did not find such evidence assessed a clinically referred sample of hyperactive youth with and without delinquency, as well as controls (Satterfield & Schell, 1984). The hyperactive children without delinquency evidenced the most abnormal EEG findings (in this group, 50% of the EEGs were abnormal), whereas the delinquent hyperactive children were indistinguishable from controls at an 8-year follow-up. This suggests that children from a normal sample who become antisocial and delinquent may differ in some respects from those among a hyperactive group who eventually become delinquent (McBurnett & Lahey, 1994).

Pain Sensitivity

Sensitivity to pain is mediated in part by the ANS. If the ANS is underaroused in individuals who are aggressive/antisocial, they might be expected to have less sensitivity to pain than nonaggressive groups. There is some evidence to support this theory. In a study of 177 adolescent boys who had been initially assessed in kindergarten, those who were persistently aggressive over time into their teenage years were found to have less pain sensitivity in a laboratory paradigm than either nonaggressive boys or boys who were only intermittently aggressive (Seguin, Pihl, Boulerice, Tremblay, & Harden, 1996). The intermittently aggressive boys were found to exhibit the highest pain sensitivity, and also to be most anxious; this suggests that pain sensitivity may be directly related to anxiety.

Cardiovascular reactivity may contribute to increased pain sensitivity. In another laboratory investigation, undergraduate college students with greater cardiovascular reactivity to a psychological stressor (a mental arithmetic task) were found to have a diminished pain threshold (higher sensitivity to pain) to a subsequent cold pressor task. Those with less cardiovascular reactivity demonstrated a higher pain threshold (Caceres & Burns, 1997). This suggests the possibility that youth with lower HRLs and diminished ANS arousal when confronted with environmental stressors may also have higher pain thresholds, which might further contribute to risk for an aggressive lifestyle.

Summary of Psychophysiological Findings

Studies of EDA, heart rate, ERPs, the EEG, and pain sensitivity in juveniles all to some degree support the concept of psychophysiological underarousal as important in the expression of persistently aggressive and antisocial behaviors in youth. Findings from longitudinal prospective studies are generally more consistent than findings from cross-sectional investigations. These results have been interpreted as supporting three theories relating low arousal to the expression of aggression and related behaviors. First, fearlessness theory posits that low levels of psychophysiological arousal are markers of low levels of fear. Lack of fear in stressful or anxiety-provoking situations could predispose youngsters to antisocial and violent behavior, because such behavior requires a degree of fearlessness to execute (Raine, 1993). Second, lack of fear and anxiety, especially in childhood, may lead to poor socialization. Low arousal and anxiety in the face of parental or community punishment or sanction for antisocial deeds committed as a youngster may reduce the effectiveness of behavioral conditioning and the learning of prosocial behavior. Reduced prosocial conditioning in childhood increases the risk for continuing antisocial behaviors in adolescence and adulthood (Raine, 1996). Third, stimulation-seeking theory argues that chronic low arousal represents an aversive physiological state, and that aggressive/antisocial individuals constantly seek out stimulation in order to restore arousal levels to an optimal level (Eysenck, 1964). In this theory, aggressive and related behaviors are seen as forms of stimulation seeking that optimize individual psychobiological arousal levels.

Underarousal, however, cannot account for the full spectrum of antisocial and aggressive behaviors in juveniles. These theories may be more specific to covert forms of such behaviors (e.g., instrumental aggression, theft, burglary, and milder forms of violent behavior or psychopathy) than to overt aggression (Scarpa & Raine, 1997). These theories ignore the role that negative emotion plays in the expression of aggressive behavior. Anger-induced, fear-motivated, irritable, or emotionally driven aggression may be characterized by ANS/CNS overarousal, not underarousal (Zillmann, 1983). Emotionally driven aggression is subsumed under the category of defensive or reactive aggression. Whether or not the actual outcome of ANS arousal will be an aggressive act depends on environmental cues, individual cognitive attributions, prior learning and social conditioning, and the evaluation of the outcome of such an act. Future studies in the psychophysiology of aggression will benefit from further subtyping aggression into psychopathic, instrumental, and reactive (defensive) categories.

BRAIN IMAGING

Neuroimaging technology is a rapidly progressing area and offers the potential to greatly enhance our understanding of neuropsychiatric disorders. Since computed tomography (CT) was developed in the 1970s, structural and functional brain imaging techniques have greatly advanced. Structural brain imaging techniques include CT and magnetic resonance imaging (MRI). These reveal an anatomical picture of the brain in living subjects. Functional neuroimaging techniques reveal a picture of neuronal metabolism and activity of various brain regions; they include such technologies as regional cerebral blood flow (rCBF), single-photon emission tomography (SPECT), positron emission computed tomography (PET), magnetoencephalography (MEG), magnetic resonance spectroscopy (MRS), and functional MRI (fMRI). Of these neuroimaging techniques, MRI, fMRI, MRS, and MEG are uniquely suited to the study of structural, physiological, and developmental brain ab-normalities in children, and to the performance of repeated measures over time and child maturation: They involve no exposure to ionizing radiation or radioactive isotopes, and they have been shown to have an absence of biologi-cal hazards at currently used field strengths (Hendren, De Backer, & Pandina, 2000; Lyon & Rumsey, 1996).

Despite significant advances in the state of the art, the potential clinical applications of neuroimaging technologies to the psychiatric care of children and adolescents have yet to be realized. Neuroimaging remains a research tool, and little research in youth with psychiatric disorders has accumulated to date. Specifically, no neuroimaging studies investigating possible structural or functional brain abnormalities in aggressive youth have been presently com-pleted (Hendren et al., 2000). A small research literature has begun to exam-ine structural and functional neuroimaging and aggression in adults with antisocial personality disorder (ASPD) and psychopathic behavior (Raine, Buchsbaum, & LaCasse, 1997; Raine, Lencz, Bihrle, LaCasse, & Colletti, 2000) and in childhood disruptive behavior disorders, especially ADHD (Semrud-Clikeman et al., 2000).

In a study of men with ASPD and psychopathic behavior who were not clinically referred and who resided in the community, structural MRI was per-formed. Results were compared to neuroimaging data from three control groups: a control group with SUDs, a psychiatric control group, and a healthy control group. Results revealed a subtle yet statistically significant reduction in the prefrontal brain volumes of men with ASPD and histories of violence, compared to the control groups. Findings were correlated with reduced ANS activity (reduced heart rate and reduced skin conductance to a social stressor) in the antisocial men (Raine et al., 2000). Since the PFC is important in the neural regulation of cognition, emotion, and behavior in social contexts, this study supports a neurological basis for ASPD and psychopathic behavior.

Another imaging study explored rCBF as measured by PET and psycho-physiological measures or emotional responsivity in 15 young adult men. The volunteers had no history of abnormal behavior or psychiatric illness. They were imaged while imagining either neutral or aggressive scenarios. Results showed that the aggressive imagined scenarios were associated with signifi-cant emotional reactivity, as well as with rCBF reductions in the ventromedial PFC (Pietrini, Guazzelli, Basso, Jaffe, & Grafman, 2000). This study provides an *in vivo* functional demonstration of the involvement of the orbital frontal cortex in the expression of aggressive behavior (see Figure 6.2, right).

As noted throughout this book, ADHD is highly associated with behav-ioral disinhibition and conduct problems in children. Several functional and structural neuroimaging studies have begun to reveal subtle abnormalities of the basal ganglia (a subcortical brain structure) and of the frontal lobes (a cor-tical brain area) in children with ADHD accompanied by behavioral inhibi-tion deficits and impulsivity (Castellanos et al., 2001; Hendren et al., 2000; Semrud-Clikeman et al., 2000).

Although it is premature to draw any firm conclusions from such early neuroimaging research, these results do suggest that subtle structural and functional CNS deficits can be found in children, adolescents, and adults with psychiatric disorders that predispose them to vulnerabilities for aggressive behaviors. These findings lend support to the hypothesis that subtle CNS neurobiological abnormalities, and their interactions with stressful or maladaptive psychosocial environments, may be important in the etiology of aggression for some (but not all) violent individuals.

MINOR PHYSICAL ANOMALIES

Mpas are various congenital malformations of the head and/or extremities that are considered indicators of disruption in fetal development. The CNS may also be affected by factors responsible for MPAs, because the development of the CNS is concurrent with the development of the organs that show MPAs (Arseneault, Tremblay, Boulerice, Seguin, & Saucier, 2000), and because MPAs have been found to predict behavioral problems and psychiatric disorders. Typical MPAs include hypertelorism (abnormal width between the eyes), large epicanthal folds (folds of skin extending from the root of the nose to the median end of each eyebrow), malformed ears, a curved fifth finger, a high-arched palate, furrowed tongue, and/or a single transverse palmar crease. Because the integument and the CNS share common embryological origins, MPAs are considered possible markers for CNS maldevelopment (Pine, Shaffer, Schonfeld, & Davies, 1997). They are attributed to both genetic and environmental factors affecting the developing fetal CNS. However, their exact origins remain poorly understood.

Studies suggest that MPAs may be biological vulnerability factors in the development of childhood conduct problems and disruptive behavior disorders that persist into adulthood. In a 10-year longitudinal study, MPAs were assessed in youth 11–13 years of age, and police records of criminal behavior were ascertained at 20–22 years of age. Individuals with recidivistic offenses, particularly aggressive and violent crimes, evidenced more MPAs than subjects with only one violent offense or subjects with no violent offenses (Kandel, Brennan, Mednick, & Michelson, 1989). This finding has been replicated in a longitudinal study of 170 adolescent boys. In this study, both the total number of MPAs and the total count of MPAs specifically affecting the mouth were significantly associated with an increased risk of violent delinquency in adolescence, even when childhood aggression and family adversity were controlled for (Arseneault et al., 2000).

A third study suggests that MPAs are not direct risk factors for the expression of conduct problems and aggression in youth, but rather that they modify an individual's vulnerability to environmental risk factors for antisocial behavior and other psychopathology. In a 10-year longitudinal study of 118 adolescents assessed first at age 7 years from a community sample, and reassessed at age 17, there was a significant interaction between MPAs and environmental risk in predicting CD (Pine, Shaffer, et al., 1997). In this study, the association between psychosocial risk factors and CD occurred only among boys with a greater number of MPAs. In boys with MPAs, as the number of psychosocial risk factors increased, so did the risk for CD; this association was not found for boys without MPAs. This study suggests a biosocial interaction in the risk for development of conduct problems, such that subtle biological abnormalities affect the development of antisocial behaviors via interactions with adverse rearing environments.

CHAPTER SUMMARY

This chapter has reviewed psychobiological variables and their relationship to aggression, and related behaviors in youth. The review has been selective for studies since 1980 and has focused on the juvenile rather than the adult literature. A number of correlates with aggression and conduct problems have been identified. These studies suggest that subgroups of aggressive/antisocial children and adolescents can be distinguished from control subjects on a number of neuropsychological, psychophysiological, brain imaging, and MPA variables.

Consistent evidence supports a neurocognitive vulnerability in some youth with early-onset, chronic aggression. Lower scores on neuropsychological tests measuring global intelligence and, more importantly, verbal intelligence have been reported in many such youngsters. There is also evidence for reduced laterality for language functioning, especially in those with psychopathic personality traits. Neuropsychological tests measuring ECFs find evidence of reduced PFC functioning in individuals who are impulsive/aggressive and may misuse substances. Neurocognitive deficits may render youth more vulnerable to the expression of aggressive behaviors because of a reduced capacity to inhibit impulsive behaviors and/or utilize language in the service of solving interpersonal conflicts.

Psychophysiological investigations of EDA, heart rate, ERPs, EEG findings, and pain sensitivity are largely consistent in supporting a relationship between ANS underarousal and aggressive behavior. Lack of fear and anxiety, especially in childhood, may lead to poor socialization. Low arousal and diminished anxiety in the face of parental or community punishment or sanction for antisocial deeds committed as a youngster may reduce the effectiveness of behavioral conditioning and the learning of prosocial behavior. Reduced prosocial conditioning in childhood may increase the risk for continuing aggressive/antisocial behaviors in adolescence and adulthood. ANS underarousal may be especially important in covert types of these behaviors (i.e., deeds done without direct confrontation with the environment). These activities include stealing, shoplifting, lying, cheating, vandalism, and fire setting. ANS overarousal may be important in fear-induced, reactive, or defensive aggression in which aggression can be more overt and involve direct confrontations with others (such as physical fighting and assault).

Weaknesses are also present in the psychobiological literature. Clearly, no single biological signature exists that identifies risk for aggression across all groups of antisocial children and adolescents. Few females have been studied, and so there is no available evidence addressing possible gender differences in the biological correlates of aggressive and related behaviors. Issues in the classification of these behaviors are also pertinent. Distinctions between overt and covert aggression, and between defensive/reactive aggression and instrumental/proactive aggression, may have important implications for the correlation of behaviors with psychobiological variables, beyond the psychiatric diagnosis of CD. This also appears true for psychopathy and, to a lesser extent, sensation seeking as personality dimensions. Further classification issues include the relationship between early-onset (as opposed to adolescent-onset) CD and psychobiological correlates.

C H A P T E R   7

Neurobiology: Biobehavioral Models and Neurological Disorders

Neurobiology is the study of discrete and fundamental CNS neural systems and their function, regulation, and control, and is an emerging field of research in the study of human aggression. As noted in Chapter 6, there is no such thing as biological determinism in the etiology of individual violence; nevertheless, the neurobiological systems in the central nervous system (CNS) that subserve aggressive behavior are important to understand. After all, it is in the brain that experience is processed; that learning occurs; that emotional, cognitive, and motor responses are generated; and that neuropsychiatric medications exert their effects.

Compared to research studying psychosocial correlates of aggression and related behaviors in youth (see Chapter 5), much less information is presently available about neurobiology and aggression. Although the study of human neurobiology and aggression is in its infancy, in the 21st century much more detailed information will become available. As of this writing, the human genome has been mapped, and laboratory techniques are becoming ever more detailed and sophisticated. The study of how neurobiological systems function in aggressive versus nonaggressive individuals will be facilitated by these new technologies. As we achieve a clearer understanding of the complex interactions between environmental stress on the one hand and heredity on the other, the underlying neurobiology of aggression will become more understandable.

This chapter first discusses the relationships between hormones and aggression, and between CNS neurotransmitters and aggression, in children and adolescents. Two neurobiological–behavioral models important to the study of aggression—the biobehavioral model of Gray (1982, 1987), and the emerging area of fear conditioning—are next presented. Finally, the complicated

and historically misinterpreted relationship between certain neurological disorders and aggressive behavior is considered.

STEROID HORMONES

Cortisol

The hypothalamic–pituitary–adrenal (HPA) axis is an intricate control and
feedback system for the neurohormonal regulation of organismic arousal. The
HPA axis is not under direct autonomic nervous system (ANS) control and is
an arousal-regulating system that is distinct from the ANS, but the two systems reciprocally influence one another in physiologically regulating individual response to stress (Nemeroff, 1991). Since arousal mechanisms appear important in the psychobiology of aggression and related behaviors, the HPA
axis has been studied in such behaviors in children and adolescents.

Cortisol is a stress hormone synthesized by the adrenal cortex and is an
index of HPA axis arousal. Cortisol secretion by the adrenal cortex is under
hierarchical control by adrenocorticotropic hormone (ACTH) from the pituitary, which is regulated in turn by corticotropin-releasing hormone (CRH)
from the hypothalamus. The region of the hypothalamus that secretes CRH is
distinct from those hypothalamic regions that govern ANS activity (sympathetic outflow), but the serotonergic, noradrenergic, and other tracts from the
limbic system that affect hypothalamic sympathetic outflow also influence the
centers that modulate HPA activity (Nemeroff, 1991). So these two systems
interact and influence one another in organismic response to environmental
stress and individual physiological regulation of arousal.

In response to stress, the adrenal cortex secretes cortisol into the general
circulation, where it is bound by several plasma-borne proteins. When the circulating levels of cortisol exceed the binding capacity of these proteins, the unbound cortisol fraction is excreted into the urine and saliva. Unbound cortisol
reflects the free, or biologically active, portion of the hormone. Peripherally
circulating cortisol may be measured in plasma, urine, or saliva. These measurements reflect slightly different aspects of HPA function. Urinary cortisol
reflects the integrated function of the HPA over a period of time, whereas salivary and plasma cortisol levels reflect the state of the HPA axis at a specific
point in time. Plasma cortisol measurements reflect both free and protein-
bound cortisol, whereas urine and saliva measurements reflect free, biologically active cortisol (Schulz, Halperin, Newcorn, Sharma, & Gabriel, 1997).

Many factors influence cortisol level. The peripherally circulating level of
cortisol rises and falls in a diurnal rhythm, necessitating cortisol sample collection at the same time of day or over an extended (e.g., 24-hour) collection
time. Novel, stressful, or cognitively demanding psychological tasks elevate
cortisol. Anxiety-arousing events also elevate cortisol. Mood disorders such as
depression may dysregulate cortisol secretion and HPA axis functioning
(Lahey, McBurnett, Loeber, & Hart, 1995; McBurnett & Lahey, 1994).

Numerous studies have investigated the relationship of cortisol to aggressive/antisocial behaviors in adults, adolescents, and children. Post-1980 studies of juveniles are presented in Table 7.1. Most of these studies have utilized cross-sectional methodological designs and have studied males: Of the 24 studies reviewed, 20 were cross-sectional and 4 were longitudinal in design, and 12 of the 20 cross-sectional studies investigated predominantly male study samples. The ages of subjects ranged from 4 to 19 years. Three of the four longitudinal studies were all from the same laboratory, and two of these three longitudinal studies examined cortisol and conduct problems in pregnant adolescent females—a physiologically unique group (see Table 7.1).

This review has provided mixed evidence to support the hypothesis of HPA axis underarousal in youth with aggression or conduct problems. Nine cross-sectional studies found a statistically significant inverse correlation between cortisol concentrations and aggressive behavior as measured in urine (Tennes & Kreye, 1985; Tennes, Kreye, Avitable, & Wells, 1986), saliva (King, Barkley, & Barrett, 1998; McBurnett, Lahey, Capasso, & Loeber, 1996; Moss, Vanyukov, & Martin, 1995; van Goozen, Matthys, Cohen-Kettenis, Gispen-de Wied, et al., 1998; van Goozen, Matthys, et al., 2000; Vanyukov et al., 1993), and plasma (Pajer, Gardner, Rubin, Perel, & Neal, 2001). Ten cross-sectional studies found no significant differences between aggressive or delinquent subjects and controls, or between community samples with "high normal" aggression and controls, on cortisol measures in urine (Kruesi, Schmidt, Donnelly, Hibbs, & Hamburger, 1989), saliva (Banks & Dabbs, 1996; Dabbs, Jurkovic, & Frady, 1991; Granger, Weisz, & Kauneckis, 1994; Jansen et al., 1999; McBurnett et al., 1991; Scerbo & Kolko, 1994), and plasma (Gerra et al., 1998; Schulz et al., 1997; Stoff et al., 1992). One study using plasma concentrations reported an unexpected finding of higher cortisol concentrations in subjects with higher aggression (Gerra et al., 1997).

Stronger support for an inverse correlation between cortisol and aggressive/antisocial problems has been provided by the longitudinal studies. One longitudinal study found inverse relationships between plasma cortisol and conduct disorder (CD) symptoms in a community sample (Susman, Dorn, Inoff-Germain, Nottleman, & Chrousos, 1997). A longitudinal study of pregnant teenagers, while finding no significant effects for plasma cortisol on CD, did find a significant inverse relationship between CRH hormone and CD symptoms (Susman et al., 1999). Another longitudinal study of pregnant teenagers reported opposite findings—that is, higher salivary cortisol and more CD symptoms in pregnant female adolescents (Susman & Ponirakis, 1997). A separate research group reported significant inverse correlations between salivary cortisol and persistent aggression in elementary-school-age boys with disruptive behavior disorders over a 4-year study (McBurnett et al., 2000). Taken together, these longitudinal studies support a relationship between cortisol hyposecretion and HPA axis underarousal on the one hand, and aggression and related behaviors on the other, in youth.

TABLE 7.1. Cortisol Reactivity and Aggressive/Antisocial Behaviors in Children and Adolescents

Study	Subjects	Sample	Source of cortisol	Findings
Cross-sectional studies				
Tennes and Kreye (1985)	70 children/age 6–12 yr	Community sample	Urine	Hostility to teachers negatively associated with urine free cortisol.
Tennes et al. (1986)	30 children/age 7–9 yr	Community sample	Urine	Aggression toward peers negatively associated with urine free cortisol.
Kruesi et al. (1989)	38 boys/age 7–16 yr	Clinic-referred boys with DBDs/controls	Urine	NSD.[b]
McBurnett et al. (1991)	67 boys/age 8–13 yr	Clinic-referred boys with DBDs/controls	Saliva	NSD.
Dabbs et al. (1991)	113 males/age 17–18 yr	Incarcerated males with high/low aggression	Saliva	NSD in cortisol concentration, but cortisol may mediate testosterone–aggression relationship.
Stoff et al. (1992)	31 boys/mean ages 10 and 14 yr	Clinic-referred boys with DBDs/controls	Plasma	NSD.
Vanyukov et al. (1993)	150 boys/age 10–12 yr	Community sample: Sons of substance-misusing fathers/controls	Saliva	CD in sons of substance-misusing fathers negatively associated with salivary cortisol.
Granger et al. (1994)	107 children/age 7–18 yr	Community sample	Saliva	NSD.
Scerbo and Kolko (1994)	40 children/age 7–14 yr	Clinic-referred sample	Saliva	NSD.
Moss et al. (1995)	184 boys/age 10–12 yr	Clinic-referred sons of substance-misusing fathers/controls	Saliva	Aggression in sons of substance-misusing fathers negatively associated with salivary cortisol, compared to controls.
Banks and Dabbs (1996)	65 young adults/mean age 25 yr	Community sample: Delinquent individuals/controls	Saliva	NSD.
McBurnett et al. (1996)	67 boys/age 7–12 yr	Clinic-referred sample	Saliva	Overt (not covert) aggression negatively associated with salivary cortisol.
Gerra et al. (1997)	30 males/age 18–19 yr	Community sample: Males with high/low aggression	Plasma	High aggression positively associated with plasma cortisol.

Study	Sample	N/age	Measure	Findings
Schulz et al. (1997)	Clinic-referred boys with ADHD ± aggression	50 boys/age 7–11 yr	Plasma	NSD.
Gerra et al. (1998)	Community sample with high/low aggression	30 boys/age 12 yr	Plasma	NSD.
van Goozen, Matthys, Cohen-Kettenis, Gispen-de Wied, et al. (1998)	Clinic-referred boys with DBDs/controls	52 boys/age 8–11 yr	Saliva	Boys with DBD had lower cortisol concentrations.
King et al. (1998)	Community sample with ADHD	20 children/age 4–6 yr	Saliva	Aggressive children with ADHD who retained their diagnosis over 1 yr had blunted cortisol responses to a stressor, compared to children with ADHD who did not retain their diagnosis.
Jansen et al. (1999)	Clinic-referred children with DBDs/controls	67 children/age 6–12 yr	Saliva	NSD.
van Goozen, Matthys, et al. (2000)	Clinic-referred children with DBDs/controls	64 children/age 8–12 yr	Saliva	Cortisol lower in children with DBDs under stress, but not at baseline, compared to controls.
Pajer et al. (2001)	Community sample	84 adolescents/age 15–17 yr	Plasma	Cortisol lower in girls with conduct problems.
Longitudinal studies				
Susman and Ponirakis (1997)	Community sample: Pregnant females/controls	128 pregnant adolescents/age 13–19 yr	Saliva	Over 8 mos, increased CD symptoms predicted by higher salivary cortisol.
Susman et al. (1997)	Community sample	36 children/age 9–14 yr	Plasma	Over 12 mos, increased CD symptoms predicted by low plasma cortisol in a novel situation.
Susman et al. (1999)	Community sample	59 pregnant adolescents/age 13–19 yr	Plasma	NSD for plasma cortisol and CD symptoms. CRH negatively associated with CD symptoms over 8 mos.
McBurnett et al. (2000)	Clinic-referred aggressive boys	38 boys/age 7–12 yr	Saliva	Low cortisol levels associated with persistence and early onset of aggression over 4 yr.

[a]DBDs, disruptive behavior disorders (in this and subsequent tables).
[b]NSD, no significant difference (in this and subsequent tables).

Several reasons may account for these inconsistent findings. First, study samples have been heterogeneous with respect to age of subjects (prepubertal vs. postpubertal), referral source (community samples with "high normal" aggression but without diagnosable psychopathology vs. clinically referred youth with aggression or diagnosed disruptive behavior disorders), and type of cortisol measurement (urine, saliva, plasma). Second, studies have been heterogeneous for anxiety as a potential confound of the cortisol–underarousal–CD association. Studies may have mixed a high-anxiety/low-aggression CD subtype with a low-anxiety/high-aggression CD subtype (McBurnett et al., 1991). When anxiety is controlled for, a clearer picture of cortisol, underarousal, and aggressive/antisocial behavior may emerge. Finally, the subtyping of aggression beyond a psychiatric diagnosis of CD may be necessary. An additional analysis of the data from McBurnett et al. (1991) found that the distinction between overt and covert symptoms of aggression was important. Salivary cortisol was significantly inversely correlated with overt aggressive symptoms (e.g., fighting, threats of violence), but not with covert aggressive symptoms (e.g., cheating, lying) (McBurnett et al., 1996). Therefore, some of the failures to find a relationship between cortisol and CD may have been obtained in study samples that mixed less overtly aggressive, more covertly aggressive, high-anxiety, high-cortisol subjects with more overtly aggressive, less covertly aggressive, low-anxiety, low-cortisol subjects. In addition, because youth with early-onset CD tend to have a more severe and stable pattern of aggression over their lifespan than do youth with adolescent-onset CD (Moffitt, 1993a), it may be important to study cortisol associations in the early-onset CD subtype.

Androgens

Androgens are steroid hormones that are derivatives of cholesterol. Commonly studied androgens in youth with conduct problems and aggression are testosterone and its precursors, including dehydroepiandrosterone sulfate (DHEAS). Androgens have two different general physiological effects. "Androgenic" effects include sexual differentiation of brain structure and function, as well as differentiation, growth, and development of the male reproductive tract, external genitalia, and accessory sexual organs. "Anabolic" effects include the stimulation of linear body growth and somatic growth (Rubinow & Schmidt, 1996). These processes represent organizational effects of androgens on physiology and are permanent. Androgens may also exert temporary activational effects on an individual, including changes in sexual and aggressive behavior (Rubinow & Schmidt, 1996).

The most commonly studied androgen is testosterone. Testosterone may be measured in blood serum or in saliva. Serum testosterone reflects both the protein-bound fraction and the free, biologically active fraction. Salivary testosterone is highly correlated with the unbound fraction of circulating testosterone, and is assumed to be a more precise indicator of the behaviorally active fraction of testosterone (Schaal, Tremblay, Soussignan, & Susman, 1996).

Testosterone and its biochemical precursors have been studied for over 30 years in attempts to demonstrate a correlation between levels of these androgens and aggression in humans. Previous reviews have largely focused on aggressive adults. At least one of these has found support for a correlation between testosterone and human aggression (Archer, 1991), but others have questioned the strength of this association (Albert, Walsh, & Jonik, 1993; Pope, Kouri, & Hudson, 2000).

Investigations since 1980 of testosterone and its precursors, focusing on children and adolescents demonstrating aggressive/antisocial behaviors, are reviewed in Table 7.2. Of the 17 studies reviewed, 14 were cross-sectional and 3 were longitudinal in methodological design. Nine of the cross-sectional investigations found a significant positive correlation between higher testosterone levels, measured either in serum or saliva, and aggression or delinquency (Banks & Dabbs, 1996; Brooks & Reddon, 1996; Cohen, Nisbett, Bowdle, & Schwarz, 1996; Dabbs et al., 1991; Gerra et al., 1997, 1998; Mattsson, Schalling, Olweus, Low, & Svensson, 1980; Olweus, Mattsson, Schalling, & Low, 1988; Scerbo & Kolko, 1994). Two studies found a significant positive correlation between DHEAS and CD or oppositional defiant disorder (ODD) (van Goozen, Matthys, Cohen-Kettenis, Thijssen, & van Engeland, 1998; van Goozen, van den Ban, et al., 2000). Four cross-sectional studies found no correlation between testosterone and aggression (Berenbaum & Resnick, 1997; Constantino et al., 1993; Susman et al., 1997; van Goozen, Matthys, Cohen-Kettenis, Thijssen, et al., 1998). The study by van Goozen and colleagues, as noted above, did find a relationship between the testosterone precursor DHEAS and aggression in boys with CD (van Goozen, et al., 1998); however, another study reported no relationship between DHEAS and aggression in young boys (Constantino et al., 1993). Cortisol was found to mediate the testosterone–aggression relationship in one study (Dabbs et al., 1991), but not in another (Scerbo & Kolko, 1994). In general, more studies finding support for a correlation between testosterone and aggression have included pubertal and/or postpubertal adolescents and young adults in their samples. In the negative studies, sample populations have tended to be prepubertal. This is illustrated by the Berenbaum and Resnick (1997) study, which investigated aggression in 2- to 13-year-old children, as well as separate samples of adolescents and adults, all with congenital adrenal hyperplasia (CAH). These subjects were all exposed to high levels of circulating androgens *in utero*. The prepubertal children with CAH were not found to have higher levels of aggression in childhood than controls; however, the adolescents and adults with CAH had significantly higher aggression scores than comparison adolescents and adults. This suggests a possible developmental effect for the relationship between testosterone and aggression, such that it may become stronger after puberty. However, other studies have found no effects of pubertal status on this relationship (Susman et al., 1987).

TABLE 7.2. Testosterone and Aggressive/Antisocial Behaviors in Children and Adolescents

Study	Subjects	Sample	Source of testosterone	Findings
Cross-sectional studies				
Mattsson et al. (1980)	98 males/age 14–19 yr	Incarcerated offenders/controls	Serum	Testosterone positively correlated with aggression in incarcerated adolescents compared with controls.
Susman et al. (1987)	108 children/9–14 yr	Community sample	Serum	NSD.
Olweus et al. (1988)	58 boys/age 15–17 yr	Community sample	Serum	Testosterone positively correlated with provoked aggression.
Dabbs et al. (1991)	113 males/age 17–18 yr	Incarcerated offenders	Saliva	Testosterone positively correlated with aggression. Cortisol modulated testosterone–aggression interaction.
Constantino et al. (1993)	29 boys/age 4–10 yr	Boys with CD/controls	Serum	NSD for testosterone or DHEAS.
Scerbo and Kolko (1994)	40 children/age 7–14 yr	Children with DBDs/controls	Saliva	Testosterone positively correlated with aggression. No interaction with cortisol.
Brooks and Reddon (1996)	194 males/age 15–17 yr	Incarcerated offenders	Serum	Testosterone positively correlated with violence.
Banks and Dabbs (1996)	65 young adults	Community sample	Saliva	Testosterone positively correlated with delinquency.
Cohen et al. (1996)	173 males/college students	Subjects from Northern vs. Southern cultures in United States	Saliva	Testosterone positively correlated with provoked aggression.

Study	N/age	Sample	Measure	Findings
Gerra et al. (1997)	30 males/age 18–19 yr	Community sample with high/low aggression	Serum	Testosterone positively correlated with aggression.
Berenbaum and Resnick (1997)	65 children/age 2–13 yr	Children with congenital adrenal hyperplasia	—	NSD in aggression for prepubertal children exposed to high androgen concentrations *in utero*.
Gerra et al. (1998)	30 boys/age 12 yr	Community sample with high/low aggression	Serum	Testosterone positively correlated with aggression.
van Goozen, Matthys, Cohen-Kettenis, Thijssen, et al. (1998)	40 boys/age 8–12 yr	Boys with CD/controls	Serum	NSD for testosterone. DHEAS positively correlated with aggression.
van Goozen, van den Ban, et al. (2000)	92 children/age 6–12 yrs	Children with ODD/controls	Serum	DHEAS positively correlated with ODD.
Longitudinal studies				
Halpern et al. (1993)	100 boys/age 12–13 yr	Community sample	Serum	NSD for testosterone (measured 1–3 yr before) and aggression at follow-up.
Schaal et al. (1996)	178 boys/age 6–13 yr	Community sample	Saliva	Boys rated high in aggression at ages 6–12 yr, found to have *lower* testosterone at age 13 yr than low-aggression boys. Testosterone positively correlated with social dominance/success.
Finkelstein et al. (1997)	49 children/age 10–19 yr	Children with pubertal delay, on randomized, controlled trial of hormone replacement	Serum	Testosterone (males) and estrogen (females) replacement therapy positively correlated with self-reported aggression.

The environmental context may be important for any interpretation of testosterone and its relationship to aggression. It is well known that testosterone levels rise in male primates and humans in the context of social dominance and success, whereas they decline in the context of social defeat or subjugation (Albert et al., 1993). In the Schaal et al. (1996) study, high testosterone levels were not correlated with aggression, but were significantly correlated with social dominance, success, and assertiveness in boys. This suggests that the relationship between testosterone and aggression may be mediated by environmental context, at least for prepubertal boys.

Type of aggression may also mediate the relationship between testosterone and aggression. Two studies of adolescent and young adult males found that testosterone levels were correlated with provoked aggression, such as readiness to respond aggressively to an insult, but not with unprovoked aggression (Cohen et al., 1996; Olweus et al., 1988).

Findings from the three longitudinal studies investigating relationships between serum and salivary testosterone and aggression have been mixed. One prospective study reported no correlation between aggression and serum testosterone in pubertal boys (Halpern, Udry, Campbell, & Suchindran, 1993). Schaal et al. (1996) reported the opposite finding of *lower* salivary testosterone correlating with high aggression, but a positive relationship between salivary testosterone and social dominance and success in prepubertal and pubertal boys (discussed above). An interesting prospective study of hormone replacement therapy in children and adolescents with pubertal delay utilized a randomized, double-blind, placebo-controlled, crossover methodology that compared self-reported aggression on and off hormone treatment (Finkelstein et al., 1997). Depot testosterone was administered to boys, and conjugated estrogens were given to girls. Results supported a correlation between steroid hormone replacement and increased self-reported aggression in both boys and girls. Type of aggression was important in this study, with hormone replacement therapy correlating with increases in physical aggression and aggressive impulses, but not in verbal aggressive behaviors.

Although much evidence supports a strong relationship between testosterone and aggression in preclinical models of male animals (Albert et al., 1993; Rubinow & Schmidt, 1996), the evidence is somewhat more mixed for a relationship between testosterone and human aggression. In juveniles, this review has found a stronger correlation between testosterone and aggression for pubertal and postpubertal males than for prepubertal males. Type of aggression, including provoked versus unprovoked and physical versus verbal aggression, may be important in clarifying relationships between testosterone and aggression. Finally, environmental factors such as social dominance may also modulate the relationship between testosterone and aggression. In summary, although testosterone may lack a direct relation to aggression, it may have an indirect relationship to aggression mediated by development, gender, environmental context, and individual experience.

MONOAMINES

The monoamines, including serotonin (5-HT), norepinephrine (NE), and dopamine (DA), are important neurotransmitters in the CNS and are involved in the regulation of several behavioral systems that play an important role in the interaction of the organism with its external environment. DA appears to be involved in the CNS regulation of active behavioral patterns, including aggressive and sexual drives. NE and 5-HT appear to regulate CNS behavioral inhibition systems that mediate increased control of organismic response to environmental stimuli (Rogeness, Javors, & Pliszka, 1992). According to Spoont (1992), 5-HT activity stabilizes CNS information flow and thus facilitates controlled behavioral, affective, and cognitive responses to the environment, whereas deviations in 5-HT activity result in altered neural information processing and an increased probability of impulsive or poorly modulated responses.

Serotonin

5-HT is a neurotransmitter that is found in several brain structures and is also found in the periphery, predominantly in the gut (Cooper, Bloom, & Roth, 1986). In the CNS, the major 5-HT tract arises in the dorsal raphe nucleus and projects through the limbic system, including the hippocampus, hypothalamus, and frontal cortex. 5-HT primarily serves as an inhibitory neurotransmitter that appears to modulate emotional behavior and sympathetic ANS outflow (Miczek & Donat, 1989). An important hypothesis guiding psychobiological research in aggression is that abnormalities in CNS 5-HT functioning (particularly underfunctioning of the 5-HT system) are relevant for chronic aggressive/antisocial behavior, particularly overt or physical aggression (Lahey, Hart, Pliszka, Applegate, & McBurnett, 1993).

Extensive preclinical research supports this hypothesis. These studies report that 5-HT plays a role in the modulation of aggressive behavior in every mammalian species in which the relationship has been investigated (Albert & Walsh, 1984). This relationship has also been reported in adults with impulsive aggressive behaviors (Brown et al., 1982; Coccaro, Kavoussi, Sheline, Berman, & Csernansky, 1997; Tuinier, Verhoeven, & van Praag, 1995). For these reasons, 5-HT has become an important focus of psychobiological research on aggression and related behaviors in youth.

5-HT cannot yet be measured directly, economically, or easily in the living human brain with existing technology. As a result, researchers use a variety of indirect assessment methods. These include measurement of the principal 5-HT metabolite, 5-hydroxyindoleacetic acid (5-HIAA) in the cerebrospinal fluid (CSF) or plasma; pharmacological challenge studies; measurement of 5-HT in whole blood; and measurement of 5-HT receptor activity in platelets from peripheral blood samples. Each of these methods is discussed in turn.

5-Hydroxyindoleacetic Acid

Concentrations of CSF 5-HIAA are thought to reflect brain 5-HT activity, based on studies that demonstrate a strong correlation between concentrations of CSF 5-HIAA and 5-HT concentrations in the human frontal cortex at postmortem (Stanley, Traskman-Bendz, & Dorovini-Zis, 1985). Blood 5-HIAA concentrations have been found to be significantly correlated with CSF 5-HT measures in subhuman primates (see van Goozen, Matthys, Cohen-Kettenis, Westenberg, & van Engeland, 1999, for a discussion). However, it should be kept in mind that the 5-HT system is complex, and that some of its complexitites may limit the extent to which measurements of CSF 5-HIAA concentration reflect actual brain 5-HT activity. For example, the sensitivity of 5-HT receptors to concentrations of 5-HT in the synaptic cleft may be an important regulator of 5-HT neurotransmission, but is not reflected in the amount of 5-HT metabolized into 5-HIAA. Measurements of 5-HIAA from peripheral blood are further complicated by the fact that most 5-HT in blood originates in the gastrointestinal system and does not reflect CNS 5-HT activity (Coccaro, Kavoussi, Sheline, et al., 1997).

With these caveats in mind, let us look at studies investigating the hypothesis of an inverse relationship between 5-HIAA concentration in CSF or blood and aggressive behavior. Table 7.3 reviews post-1980 studies in juveniles. Of three recent cross-sectional studies examining CSF 5-HIAA levels and aggression in juveniles, two have found the hypothesized inverse association. Levels of CSF 5-HIAA were lower in newborns with family histories of antisocial personality disorder (ASPD) than in newborns without such histories (Constantino, Morris, & Murphy, 1997). In this study, newborns presented to the hospital with a febrile illness; CSF was obtained from newborns in the course of an infectious disease evaluation, and leftover portions of CSF were used to assay for 5-HT metabolites. Another study involved clinic-referred children and adolescents with disruptive behavior disorders; CSF 5-HIAA was inversely correlated with measures of aggression and positively correlated with measures of social competence (Kruesi et al., 1990). It is to be noted that in both of these studies, rated aggression was moderate to severe in character (ASPD in family members or severe physical aggression in children with disruptive behavior disorders). In the third study, Castellanos et al. (1994) reported the opposite finding—that is, a positive correlation of aggression with CSF 5-HIAA levels. This may have been because this sample was of children with attention-deficit/hyperactivity disorder (ADHD) who exhibited high levels of hyperactivity, but only mild amounts of aggression. Two independent samples of children with CD or ODD (reported together) found an inverse correlation of plasma 5-HIAA concentration and aggression in these children as compared to controls (van Goozen et al., 1999). Plasma 5-HIAA levels accounted for 81% of the variance in aggression in these two samples. However, given the fact that most plasma 5-HT is derived from the gut, these findings remain somewhat difficult to interpret.

TABLE 7.3. 5-HIAA and Aggressive/Antisocial Behaviors in Children and Adolescents

Study	Subjects	Sample	Source of 5-HIAA	Findings
Cross-sectional studies				
Kruesi et al. (1990)	29 children/age 6–17 yr	Children with DBDs/controls with OCD	CSF	CSF 5-HIAA negatively correlated with aggression, positively correlated with social competence.
Castellanos et al. (1994)	29 boys/age 6–12 yr	Boys with ADHD and mild aggression	CSF	CSF 5-HIAA positively correlated with aggression.
Constantino et al. (1997)	193 infants/age 0–3 months	Normal newborns with a febrile illness	CSF	CSF 5-HIAA in infants negatively correlated with family history of ASPD.
van Goozen et al. (1999)	40 boys/age 8–11 yr	Boys with CD/controls	Plasma	Plasma 5-HIAA negatively correlated with aggression.
van Goozen et al. (1999)	48 children/age 8–12 yr	Children with CD/controls	Plasma	Plasma 5-HIAA negatively correlated with aggression.
Longitudinal studies				
Kruesi et al. (1992)	29 children/age 6–17 yr	Children with DBDs	CSF	At 2-yr outcome, lower CSF 5-HIAA predicted increased aggression, independently of age, gender, or race.
Clarke et al. (1999)	73 infants/0–3 mos	Normal newborns with a febrile illness	CSF	Low CSF 5-HIAA levels negatively correlated with increased externalizing behavior at 30-mo outcome, independently of gender, race, or Medicaid status.

Two longitudinal studies reported findings in the hypothesized direction—namely, lower CSF 5-HIAA levels and higher aggression. In a 2-year prospective study, lower CSF 5-HIAA levels predicted increased aggression independently of age, gender, and ethnicity (Kruesi et al., 1992); in this sample, CSF 5-HIAA concentration accounted for 52% of the variance in physical aggression. In a 30-month follow-up of the newborn sample discussed above, Clarke, Murphy, and Constantino (1999) found that low levels of CSF 5-HIAA at baseline predicted higher levels of externalizing behavioral problems in toddlers. However, variations in CSF 5-HIAA levels explained less than 5% of the variance in externalizing behavior in this sample. These authors concluded that 5-HT as measured by CSF 5-HIAA concentration may mediate one component of a vulnerability to aggression, but that the magnitude of the component may be less than suggested by previous reports.

Pharmacological Challenge Studies

Another indirect method for assessing CNS 5-HT functioning in individuals with maladaptive aggression is the pharmacological challenge paradigm. In this paradigm, a drug or a dietary manipulation that is known to affect CNS 5-HT functioning is given to an individual. A physiological variable known to be influenced by CNS 5-HT mechanisms is then measured at outcome. Changes in the outcome variable are then compared across highly aggressive and comparison groups, to ascertain between-group differences in CNS 5-HT functioning.

Prolactin is a hormone produced by the pituitary gland and is secreted into the bloodstream under CNS 5-HT control. In challenge studies, a change in prolactin level in response to a challenge agent is often used as an indirect measure of CNS 5-HT functioning. One commonly used challenge agent has been *dl*-fenfluramine. In 1997 fenfluramine was voluntarily taken off the market by the manufacturer following reports that its use resulted in heart valve complications in some patients. Administered as a single dose, *dl*-fenfluramine enhances 5-HT transmission by augmenting the release of presynaptic 5-HT, inhibiting reuptake of synaptic 5-HT, and both directly and indirectly stimulating postsynaptic 5-HT receptors (Halperin et al., 1994). The net result is enhanced CNS 5-HT activity, which promotes release of prolactin into the bloodstream where it may be obtained and assayed. Another challenge agent is low dietary tryptophan. Tryptophan is an amino acid obtained from the diet, which is a precursor of 5-HT. Dietary depletion of tryptophan results in a decrease in available 5-HT and a decrease in CNS 5-HT (LeMarquand et al., 1998). Change in body temperature has also been explored as an indirect and peripherally measured index of CNS 5-HT function, because 5-HT appears to increase body temperature (Donovan, Halperin, Newcorn, & Sharma, 1999), and pharmacological challenges such as the administration of *dl*-fenfluramine will increase body temperature.

An inverse relationship between aggression and the prolactin response to challenge agents that stimulate CNS 5-HT function, indicating diminished or blunted CNS 5-HT functioning, has been found for adults (Coccaro et al., 1989, Moss, Yao, & Panzak, 1990). This relationship appears more complex in juveniles, however. Table 7.4 presents 5-HT challenge studies since 1980 in aggressive children and adolescents; the hypothesis that diminished CNS 5-HT functioning is correlated with increased aggression, as found for adults, receives little support from the juvenile studies included in this table. Only one study found a significant inverse correlation between an indirect measure of CNS 5-HT function and aggression (Donovan et al., 1999). This study used a change in body temperature to fenfluramine challenge to index CNS 5-HT function, and this methodology is in need of replication before it can be generally accepted. Other studies have reported either no significant differences in CNS 5-HT function between aggressive and nonaggressive youngsters as assessed by prolactin response to fenfluramine challenge (Stoff et al., 1992), or no differences in impulse control between aggressive adolescents and controls when dietary sources of tryptophan are restricted (LeMarquand et al., 1998).

Several challenge studies have reported findings that are the opposite of what would be expected from the hypothesis that aggression is related to diminished CNS 5-HT functioning. Three studies of prepubertal boys reported positive correlations between prolactin response to fenfluramine challenge and aggression (Halperin et al., 1994; Halperin, Newcorn, Schwartz, et al., 1997; Pine, Coplan, et al., 1997). These results indicated enhanced CNS 5-HT functioning in younger, as compared to older, aggressive boys. These studies have facilitated a developmental hypothesis of CNS 5-HT functioning and aggression (Halperin et al., 1994; Pine, Coplan, et al., 1997)—specifically, that the relationship of such functioning to the presence or absence of aggressive behavior in boys (especially those with ADHD) may vary as a function of age. Younger children who are aggressive may demonstrate enhanced CNS 5-HT functioning relative to younger nonaggressive youngsters; as they develop, they may not undergo normal developmental changes in CNS 5-HT function and subsequently have a blunted 5-HT response when assessed as aggressive adults (Halperin, Newcorn, Schwartz, et al., 1997). This is an intriguing hypothesis that remains to be rigorously tested in future studies.

5-HT challenge studies in aggressive youngsters have also found a possible association between CNS 5-HT functioning and familial aggressive behavior. One study of aggressive boys with ADHD and a parental history of aggressive behavior found a significantly lower prolactin response to *dl*-fenfluramine challenge than in aggressive boys without a parental history of aggression (Halperin, Newcorn, Kopstein, et al., 1997). A second study found that adverse rearing environments, including parental aggressive behaviors, were positively correlated with prolactin response to *dl*-fenfluramine challenge in younger brothers of adolescents convicted of delinquency (Pine, Coplan, et al., 1997). Although these two studies found indices of CNS 5-HT functioning to be correlated with familial histories of aggressive behaviors, the direction of the association remains unclear. Differences in study samples

TABLE 7.4. 5-HT Challenge Studies and Aggressive/Antisocial Behaviors in Children and Adolescents

Study	Subjects	Sample	5-HT challenge outcome measure	Findings
Cross-sectional studies				
Stoff et al. (1992)	31 boys/mean ages 10 and 15 yr (two samples)	Boys with DBDs/controls	dl-Fen[a]/prolactin	NSD in dl-Fen-induced prolactin release and aggression in either prepubertal boys or adolescents with DBDs.
Halperin et al. (1994)	25 boys/age 7–11 yr	Boys with ADHD and high/low aggression	dl-Fen/prolactin	Boys with ADHD and high aggression had greater prolactin response to dl-Fen than the low-aggression boys with ADHD.
Halperin, Newcorn, Schwartz, et al. (1997)	25 boys/age 7–11 yr	Boys with ADHD and high/low aggression	dl-Fen/prolactin	Developmental effect: Young boys (< 9.1 yr) with ADHD and high aggression had greater prolactin response to dl-Fen challenge than young boys with ADHD and low aggression. NSD for older (>9.1 yr) boys.
Halperin, Newcorn, Kopstein, et al. (1997)	41 boys/age 7–11 yr	Boys with ADHD	dl-Fen/prolactin	Aggressive boys with ADHD and a parental history of aggression had lower prolactin response to dl-Fen challenge than aggressive boys with ADHD but without a history of parental aggressive behavior.
Pine, Coplan, et al. (1997)	34 boys/mean age 8 yr	Younger brothers of convicted delinquent adolescents	dl-Fen/prolactin	Increasing degrees of aggressive behavior positively correlated with prolactin response to dl-Fen challenge.
LeMarquand et al. (1998)	Adolescents 13–18 yr	Community sample with high/low aggression	Dietary tryptophan depletion/impulsivity	NSD in effects of tryptophan depletion on increasing impulsivity in highly aggressive adolescents.
Donovan et al. (1999)	27 boys/age 7–11 yr	Boys with ADHD	dl-Fen/body temp. change	Inverse correlation between temperature change to dl-Fen challenge and teacher ratings of aggression.

[a] dl = Fen, dl = fenfluramine.

212

(boys with ADHD vs. brothers of delinquent adolescents) may account for some of the discrepancy, and further research is required.

Whole Blood 5-HT

Studies have also assessed the relationship between whole-blood 5-HT and aggression in juveniles. Whole-blood samples (obtained from the peripheral circulation through venipuncture, a standard medical procedure) are much easier to obtain than CSF samples (obtained through lumbar puncture, a more invasive procedure). In addition, whole-blood 5-HT studies do not require a pharmacological agent to be administered, as do the challenge studies discussed above.

The results from studies investigating whole-blood 5-HT and its relationships to aggression and related behaviors in youth are decidedly mixed. Post-1980 studies are presented in Table 7.5. Two studies reported no significant difference in whole-blood 5-HT levels between youth with CD and controls (Rogeness, Hernandez, Macedo, & Mitchell, 1982) or between youngsters with ADHD and with or without comorbid CD (Cook, Stein, Ellison, Unis, & Leventhal, 1995). Two studies reported significant inverse correlations between whole-blood 5-HT levels and aggression (i.e., lower 5-HT levels were found in more aggressive children). In a study of youths with obsessive–compulsive disorder (OCD), some met criteria for a comorbid disruptive behavior disorder and some did not; whole-blood 5-HT was significantly lower in the children with both OCD and a disruptive behavior disorder, than in those without comorbidity (Hanna, Yuwiler, & Coates, 1995). In a study of children of alcoholic fathers, whole-blood 5-HT levels were lower in the children with more behavior problems than in those with low levels of behavior problems (Twitchell et al., 1998). Three studies of clinically referred or incarcerated youth reported positive correlations between whole-blood 5-HT and aggression (i.e., higher 5-HT levels were found in more aggressive juveniles and young adults). In a study of adolescent boys with CD and with or without comorbid mood and anxiety disorders, higher whole-blood 5-HT levels were associated with clinician ratings of conduct symptoms (Pliszka, Rogeness, Renner, Sherman, & Broussard, 1988). Unis et al. (1997) not only replicated the finding of higher whole-blood 5-HT levels in incarcerated juveniles with CD, but found that early-onset as opposed to adolescent-onset CD was positively correlated with higher 5-HT levels. In an investigation of psychiatrically referred children and adolescents, whole-blood 5-HT levels were higher in youth with disruptive behavior disorders than in those with mood disorders or in normal subjects (Hughes, Petty, Sheikha, & Kramer, 1996).

These findings are contradictory. Studies of the relationship between whole-blood 5-HT and aggression have reported no difference, an inverse relationship, or a positive and direct relationship. Discrepancies may be due to methodological differences across studies. Most studies have had very small sample sizes, have been cross-sectional in design, and have investigated differ-

TABLE 7.5. Whole-Blood 5-HT and Aggressive/Antisocial Behaviors in Children and Adolescents

Study	Subjects	Sample	Findings
Cross-sectional studies			
Rogeness et al. (1982)	45 boys/mean age 11 yr	Boys with CD/controls	NSD in whole-blood 5-HT between boys with CD and controls.
Pliszka, Rogeness, Renner, et al. (1988)	44 boys/mean age 15 yr	Incarcerated boys with CD ± mood/anxiety disorders	Whole-blood 5-HT positively correlated with CD. Trend for those with violent offenses to have higher whole-blood 5-HT.
Hanna et al. (1995)	18 children/mean age 13 yr	Children with OCD ± DBDs	Whole-blood 5-HT negatively correlated with DBDs and aggression.
Cook et al. (1995)	52 children/age 4–14 yr	Children with ADHD ± CD	NSD in whole-blood 5-HT between ADHD groups.
Hughes et al. (1996)	118 children/age 8–17 yr	Children with mood disorders or DBDs/controls	Whole-blood 5-HT positively correlated with DBDs.
Unis et al. (1997)	42 males/age 13–17 yr	Incarcerated males with CD (childhood vs. adolescent onset)	Whole-blood 5-HT positively correlated with childhood-onset CD and higher aggression.
Twitchell et al. (1998)	44 children/mean age 10 yr	Children of alcoholic fathers with high/low disruptive behavior	Whole-blood 5-HT negatively correlated with disruptive behaviors.
Moffitt et al. (1998)	781 young adults/age 21 yr	Representative epidemiological sample	Whole-blood 5-HT positively correlated with violence in young men, not young women.

ent populations (either clinically referred youth or youth incarcerated in the juvenile justice system). Different studies have compared children and adolescents with different psychiatric disorders, such as ADHD, CD, or OCD. The ages of subjects have ranged from prepubertal to adolescent. In addition, the overall meaning of results from whole-blood 5-HT studies is difficult to determine. 5-HT in blood is largely produced in the gut, is wholly contained within platelets, and does not cross the blood–brain barrier. Thus its relation to 5-HT function in the CNS remains unclear and speculative (Sarrias, Cabre, Martinez, & Artigas, 1990).

Many of these methodological difficulties can be overcome by the use of a non-clinic referred, representative community sample in an epidemiological study. Moffitt et al. (1998) measured whole-blood 5-HT in a representative birth cohort of 781 women and men aged 21 years . Aggression was assessed by self-report and by official court conviction records. Women constituted 47% and men constituted 53% of the sample. Whole-blood 5-HT was related to violence among men, but not women; the findings for women were not significant. Violent men's mean blood 5-HT level was 0.48 standard deviations above the male population norm and 0.56 standard deviations above the mean of nonviolent men. The finding was specific to violence as opposed to general antisocial behavior or crime. The finding remained significant despite controls for age, diurnal variation in blood sampling, diet, psychiatric medication history, psychiatric diagnosis, illicit drug history, seasonal effects on blood 5-HT concentration, alcohol and tobacco use, body mass, history of suicide attempts, socioeconomic status, IQ, and overall criminal offending (Moffitt et al., 1998). Although it remains unclear just how peripherally obtained whole-blood 5-HT is related to CNS 5-HT functioning, this epidemiological study demonstrates that whole-blood 5-HT is related to violent behavior in men and warrants further investigation.

Platelet 5-HT Models

The human blood platelet has been utilized as a peripheral model of CNS neuronal functioning. Platelet membranes show similarities to CNS 5-HT pre- and postsynaptic membranes (Lesch, Wolozin, Murphy, & Riederer, 1993). Platelet membrane functioning is thought to be similar to CNS 5-HT neuronal membrane functioning in a number of important aspects, such as 5-HT transport from outside to inside the cell (Moss & Yao, 1996). Thus there is evidence that 5-HT-related platelet membrane physiology can serve as a peripheral model of CNS 5-HT neuronal physiology.

Platelet 5-HT functioning is measured in a number of ways. Both the density of 5-HT receptors on the platelet and the speed of serotonin transport into the cell (uptake) can be measured. Radioactively labeled chemicals, called "ligands," bind to 5-HT receptors on platelets, can be measured, and provide understanding of the number (concentration) of these receptors on platelets. Various ligands, such as [^{3}H]imipramine and [^{3}H]paroxetine, are used.

Changes in 5-HT concentration over time in platelet-enriched whole blood serve to measure 5-HT transport (uptake) into platelets. Changes in platelet function, such as platelet activation in response to biochemical signals with subsequent secretion of adenosine triphosphate, may also be used as a peripheral measure to reflect CNS 5-HT function (Moss & Yao, 1996).

Post-1980 studies assessing platelet models of CNS 5-HT functioning and aggression in children and adolescents are presented in Table 7.6. The findings from this research are inconsistent. Six of the reviewed studies six found evidence for the hypothesized inverse correlation between 5-HT underfunctioning and higher aggression (Birmaher et al., 1990; Blumensohn et al., 1995; Modai et al., 1989; Moss & Yao, 1996; Pine et al., 1996; Stoff, Pollock, Vitiello, Behar, & Bridger, 1987). These studies have used a variety of methodologies, including binding with different titrated ligands, measuring platelet 5-HT uptake, and assessing platelet secretory responses (see Table 7.6). These investigations suggest low receptor density, low receptor affinity, and/or underfunctioning of platelet 5-HT receptors in aggressive youth, and support the hypothesis that CNS 5-HT hypofunction is related to aggressive behavior. It should be noted that these studies *consistently* report an inverse correlation between platelet markers of 5-HT function and aggression; there are no findings in the opposite direction. However, four studies have found no significant differences between platelet 5-HT receptor function and aggression (Halperin et al., 1994; Pornnoppadol, Friesen, Haussler, Glaser, & Todd, 1999; Unis et al., 1997; Stoff et al., 1991). These investigations with negative findings weaken the argument that platelet measures of 5-HT functioning are inversely correlated with aggression in children and adolescents. Differences in methodology may account for the discrepancies, and further research is required.

Summary of 5-HT Research

An important hypothesis in psychobiological aggression research is that alterations in CNS 5-HT functioning—most importantly, 5-HT underfunctioning—are related to increased vulnerability to aggressive behavior. Support for this hypothesis is found most consistently in aggression research with adults (Coccaro et al., 1989; Coccaro, Kavoussi, Shaline, et al., 1997). Although the present review of studies in aggressive youth supports an association between aggressive behavior and CNS 5-HT functioning, such abnormalities are found less consistently than in adults. Moreover, the relationship is not a simple inverse correlation.

The strongest support for the involvement of CNS 5-HT function in the etiology of aggressive behavior in youth comes from two longitudinal studies of CSF 5-HIAA (Clarke et al., 1999; Kruesi et al., 1992). Both studies support the hypothesized inverse correlation between lower indices of CNS 5-HT and increased aggressive behavior. However, the magnitude of the effect varies from 5% in infants (Clarke et al., 1999) to 52% in older children and adolescents (Kruesi et al., 1992). Differences may be due in part to the known in-

TABLE 7.6. Platelet 5-HT and Aggressive/Antisocial Behaviors in Children and Adolescents

Study	Subjects	Sample	Methods	Findings
Cross-sectional studies				
Stoff et al. (1987)	20 children/ age 12–17 yr	Children with CD/controls	Platelet IB[a]	IB negatively correlated with aggression and hostility after controls for depression and suicidality.
Modai et al. (1989)	34 adolescents/ age not given	Psychiatric inpatients	SPU[b]	SPU negatively correlated with diagnosis of CD.
Birmaher et al. (1990)	23 children/age 10–16 yr	Children with DBDs	IB	IB negatively correlated with aggression and hostility.
Stoff et al. (1991)	68 boys/mean age 10 yr	Boys with DBDs/controls	IB	NSD in platelet 5-HT receptor density between boys with DBDs and controls.
Halperin et al. (1994)	25 boys/age 7–11 yr	Boys with ADHD and high/ low aggression	Platelet 5-HT levels	NSD in platelet 5-HT levels between high- and low-aggression boys with ADHD.
Blumensohn et al. (1995)	104 adolescents/ age 12–18 yr	Incarcerated youth with CD/ controls	Platelet 5-HT$_2$ receptor binding	Platelet 5-HT$_2$ receptor binding negatively correlated with aggression in youths with CD compared to controls.
Pine et al. (1996)	34 boys/ age 6–10 yr	Younger brothers of convicted delinquent adolescents	Platelet 5-HT$_{2A}$ receptor density	5-HT$_{2A}$ receptor density negatively correlated with parental aggressive and antisocial behaviors.
Moss and Yao (1996)	106 males/mean age 16 yr	Males with CD + SUDs[c]/ controls	Platelet secretory responses	Diminished platelet secretory responses in boys with CD and SUDs compared with controls.
Unis et al. (1997)	42 males/age 13–17 yr	Incarcerated males with CD (childhood vs. adolescent onset)	Platelet 5-HT receptor binding	NSD in receptor binding for childhood-onset versus adolescent-onset CD.
Pornnoppadol et al. (1999)	33 children/ age 7–17 yr	Children with ADHD ± CD	Platelet 5-HT$_{2A}$ receptor binding	NSD in platelet 5-HT$_{2A}$ receptor binding between youth with ADHD with vs. without CD.

[a]IB, [^{3}H] imipramine binding.
[b]SPU, serotonin (5-HT) platelet uptake.
[c]SUDs, substance use disorders.

217

verse correlation of 5-HT with age (Kruesi et al., 1992). Elevated indices of CNS 5-HT functioning in younger children may dilute the postulated effect, which may become more robust in older aggressive youth. The epidemiological study of Moffitt et al. (1998) supports cross-sectional findings that higher whole-blood 5-HT is related to violence. This result obtained in a representative, nonreferred population is important for reporting a gender effect (i.e., higher whole-blood 5-HT relates to aggression in young adult men, not women). As noted previously, however, the meaning of whole-blood 5-HT (largely derived from the gut) for the understanding of CNS 5-HT functioning is difficult to determine.

Although low CNS 5-HT functioning may lead to an increased vulnerability to the expression of aggressive behavior in youngsters, alternative explanations exist and have yet to be rigorously tested. First, aggression may lead to decreased levels of CNS 5-HT activity. This has previously been shown for the relationship between testosterone and aggression: Aggression can raise levels of testosterone, but the converse is not true (Constantino, 1998). Second, environmental factors such as an aggressive rearing environment may produce correlated effects on both aggression and 5-HT. Studies of family functioning and 5-HT functioning in individual children have found modest inverse correlations ($r = -.43$) between a measure of family cohesion and aggression (Clarke et al., 1999). In addition, challenge studies have found a relationship between family and parental histories of aggression and 5-HT functioning in aggressive juveniles (Halperin, Newcorn, Kopstein, et al., 1997; Pine, Coplan, et al., 1997). These studies suggest that the characteristics of the individual aggressive child are not what mediate the relationship with CNS 5-HT functioning; rather, the adverse rearing environment and its subsequent effects on the developing child may be associated with this relationship. Finally, a developmental relationship may exist between CNS 5-HT functioning and aggression in juveniles (Halperin et al., 1994). This relationship may be confounded in studies that assess a wide age range of subjects. The Halperin et al. (1994) study suggests that younger aggressive children may demonstrate enhanced 5-HT functioning, and older aggressive youth may reveal blunted functioning. Possible developmental changes in the relationship between CNS 5-HT functioning and aggression remain to be further researched.

Norepinephrine

NE is a catecholamine that serves as a neurotransmitter in the hypothalamus, the limbic system, and the sympathetic division of the ANS (Cooper, Bloom, & Roth, 1991). In the peripheral circulation, NE is principally derived by release from sympathetic nerve synapses. The sympathetic ANS is regulated by activity in CNS NE neurons originating in the locus coeruleus. An important hypothesis in the psychobiological study of aggression is that externalizing behavior disorders are associated with a decrease in CNS NE functioning (Quay, 1988). Low CNS NE functioning should cause individuals to be less likely to experience anxiety and fear, less sensitive to signals of punishment for aggressive/antisocial behaviors, and therefore less likely to internalize societal rules and inhibit such behaviors.

Biological Markers of NE

Since there currently exists no direct measure of CNS NE activity, measures taken from CSF, urine, or plasma are used as indirect indices of such activity. For example, one metabolic product of NE is 3-methoxy-4-hydroxy-phenylglycol (MHPG), which can be measured in the urine, CSF, or plasma and is thought to reflect a measure of central NE activity. Other metabolic products of NE include normetanephrine and vanillylmandelic acid, which may be measured in urine. Although there exist moderate correlations between central NE and its metabolites in urine and blood (Cooper et al., 1991), the largest proportion of catecholamines in urine and blood have their origin in the peripheral activity of the sympathetic ANS and not in the brain. As such, peripheral measures of NE or its metabolites are at best only approximations of CNS NE functioning. This functioning may be assessed more directly by measuring NE metabolites in CSF.

Dopamine-beta-hydroxylase (DßH) is an enzyme that converts DA (another catecholamine serving as a CNS neurotransmitter; see below) into NE. DßH is under genetic control, and its levels in the peripheral circulation appear stable beginning at about 6 years of age in humans (Weinshilboum, 1983). The major proportion of DßH in the body is located in sympathetic nerve terminals, and DßH is released into the circulation when NE is released. Plasma DßH has also been measured as a peripheral marker of CNS NE activity in research on aggression and related behaviors in youth. Since plasma DßH is genetically determined, it is likely that low peripheral DßH will indicate low CNS DßH as well. Positive correlations between peripheral and CSF DßH have been reported (Rogeness, Javors, Maas, & Macedo, 1990).

Most studies of NE and aggression in children and adolescents are less than definitive, because they assess NE and its metabolites outside of the CNS in blood and urine. Since peripheral sources of NE and its metabolites may confound associations between CNS NE activity and aggression, these studies are not further reviewed here (see Lahey, McBurnett, et al., 1995, for a review). Studies that investigate CSF MHPG and aggression are thought to reflect CNS NE activity more directly; these studies provide support for a correlation between CNS NE dysregulation and aggression. Two such investigations are presented in Table 7.7. In a sample of mildly aggressive boys with ADHD, Castellanos et al. (1994) found a positive association between CSF MHPG and aggression. Kruesi et al. (1990) studied more severely aggressive children with disruptive behavior disorders and found that low CSF MHPG was significantly associated with higher aggression. Although the direction of the correlation is unclear from these two studies, they do support a relationship between CNS NE dysregulation and aggressive behavior in youth.

TABLE 7.7. Markers of CNS NE Activity and Aggressive/Antisocial Behaviors in Children and Adolescents

Study	Subjects	Sample	Findings
Cross-sectional studies: CSF MHPG			
Castellanos et al. (1994)	29 boys/age 6–12 yr	Boys with ADHD/controls	CSF MHPG positively correlated with aggression in boys with ADHD.
Kruesi et al. (1990)	29 children/age 6–17 yr	Children with DBDs/controls with OCD	CSF MHPG negatively correlated with aggression in children with DBDs.
Cross-sectional studies: Plasma			
Pliszka, Rogeness, and Medrana (1988)	42 boys/age 7–14 yr	Clinic-referred boys with CD/other diagnoses	NSD in DßH activity between boys with and without CD.
Pliszka, Rogeness, Renner, et al. (1988)	44 boys/mean age 15 yr	Boys in juvenile detention/clinic-referred comparison group	NSD in DßH between juvenile detention and comparison groups.
Bowden et al. (1988)	72 boys/age 6–14 yr	Boys with ADHD/controls	Low plasma DßH correlated with ADHD and more CD/aggression.
Rogeness, Javors, et al. (1990)	103 boys/age 6–16 yr	Clinic-referred boys with low/high DßH	Low plasma DßH correlated with CD diagnosis.
Galvin et al. (1991)	21 boys/age 9–17 yr	Clinic-referred boys with CD/other diagnoses	Low plasma DßH correlated with CD.
Gabel et al. (1993b)	31 boys/age 7–15 yr	Clinic-referred sample	Low plasma DßH correlated with aggression and antisocial behavior.

As noted above, plasma DßH is important as another possible biological marker reflecting aggressive/antisocial behaviors, because its concentration is genetically regulated and it appears stable from relatively early in childhood. Several studies of DßH are also presented in Table 7.7. In a series of studies on a large sample of psychiatrically hospitalized children and adolescents derived from a single source, results have consistently supported a correlation between low plasma concentrations of DßH in boys classified as having undersocialized aggressive CD, compared to less aggressive CD and other psychiatric diagnoses (Rogeness, Hernandez, Macedo, & Mitchell, 1982; Rogeness et al., 1984; Rogeness, Javors, et al., 1990; Rogeness, Javors, & Pliszka, 1992). Three additional reports from independent investigators have replicated this finding (Bowden, Deutsch, & Swanson, 1988; Gabel, Stadler, Bjorn, Shindledecker, & Bowden, 1993b; Galvin et al., 1991). Two studies have not replicated this finding (Pliszka, Rogeness, & Medrano, 1988; Pliszka, Rogeness, Renner, Sherman, & Broussard, 1988).

Summary of NE Research

Taken together, these studies support a role for CNS NE dysregulation in juvenile aggression. Some support is found for Quay's (1988) hypothesis of CNS NE underfunctioning and externalizing behavior disorders in youth. Statistically significant inverse correlations have been reported between CSF MHPG and aggression, and between plasma DßH and aggressive CD.

However, not all studies have found evidence for the hypothesized relationship between NE underfunctioning and aggression in youth. As a result, other hypotheses have been offered to explain this association. One alternative hypothesis states that there is an association between adverse childhood developmental attachment experiences, including physical and sexual abuse, and CNS NE functioning. In this hypothesis, the adverse rearing environment mediates the relationship between CNS NE functioning and aggression. For example, distress in infants increases CNS NE function and promotes attachment behavior to the caregiver, which optimizes the probability of survival for infant organisms (Kraemer, 1985). Developmental CNS adaptation to chronic experiences of adverse caregiver rearing (e.g., chronic abuse, long-standing neglect, chaotic families, multiple out-of-home placements, multiple disruptions of infant attachment to a caregiver) may result in eventual adaptive downregulation of CNS NE activity, with resultant NE underfunctioning. Since child maltreatment is related to aggression (Connor, Melloni, & Harrison, 1998), the relationship between CNS NE underfunctioning and aggression may be mediated by adverse developmental attachment experiences. Evidence for this comes from studies that find significantly more cases of neglect or abuse in subjects who are psychiatrically diagnosed with aggressive CD and also have low levels of plasma DßH, compared to subjects with higher levels of DßH (Galvin et al., 1991; Rogeness et al., 1984). These results suggest that it is not the characteristics of the individual, but the individual's adaptive response to a chronically adverse developmental rearing environment, that mediates the relationship between CNS NE dysregulation and aggression.

Another alternative hypothesis states that CNS NE function is related to personality traits of sensation seeking. Since sensation seeking has been found to be associated with CD in youth (Russo et al., 1993), the relationship between diminished CNS NE functioning and aggression may be mediated by personality traits involving impulsivity and disinhibited behavior. Support for this hypothesis comes from a study of plasma MHPG and sensation seeking in psychiatrically hospitalized adolescents admitted because of maladaptive aggressive and antisocial behaviors. High sensation seeking, as assessed by personality rating scales, was inversely correlated with plasma MHPG in these adolescents (Gabel, Stadler, Bjorn, Shindledecker, & Bowden, 1994). These findings support the hypothesized link among NE dysregulation, personality traits of sensation seeking, and aggressive/antisocial behaviors.

Dopamine

DA is another catecholamine that acts as a CNS neurotransmitter, with high concentrations in the basal ganglia (caudate and putamen), limbic system, and prefrontal cortex (Cooper et al., 1991). DA is involved in the control of motor movement, in the regulation of attention and vigilance, and in the regulation of reward systems in the brain. It is thought to be important as a neurotransmitter in a generalized behavioral system that functions to mobilize behavior so that active engagement with the environment occurs. Examples of such behaviors include extroversion, sexual behavior, and aggressive behavior (Rogeness, Javors, & Pliszka, 1992). Quay (1988) has hypothesized that individuals who are motivated by immediate gratification of needs and wants, and have little ability to delay rewards—traits found in aggressive/antisocial youth and adults—have higher CNS DA functioning than individuals lacking these traits.

Studies of aggression and CD in youngsters have generally measured a metabolite of DA called homovanillic acid (HVA) in CSF and in the peripheral circulation. The relationship of plasma HVA to CNS DA functioning is presently unclear (Gabel, Stadler, Bjorn, Shindledecker, & Bowden, 1995). Measuring HVA in the CSF may give a clearer picture of DA activity in the brain.

To date, little support has been found for an association between increased CNS DA functioning and conduct problems and aggression in youth. Cross-sectional studies of plasma HVA (Rogeness, Javors, Maas, Macedo, & Fischer, 1987) and of CSF HVA (Kruesi et al., 1990) report no correlation of HVA with aggression or the diagnosis of CD. A longitudinal study found no association between CSF HVA and aggression at 2-year outcome (Kruesi et al., 1992). Two studies have reported an inverse association between plasma HVA and conduct problems in younger children (Gabel, Stadler, Bjorn, Shindledecker, & Bowden, 1993a; van Goozen et al., 1999). However, the correlation of peripheral concentrations of HVA and CNS DA function is unclear.

Monoamine Oxidase

Monoamine oxidase (MAO) is a major enzyme in the metabolic degradation of catecholamines. MAO is localized largely in the outer membrane of mitochondria, which are intracellular organelles. It is largely considered to be an intraneuronal enzyme, but also occurs in abundance extraneuronally. MAO is present in two forms: MAO-A and MAO-B. These forms are defined based on substrate specificity. MAO-A is specific for NE, 5-HT, and DA; MAO-B is specific for DA, beta-phenylethylamine, and benzylamine (Cooper et al., 1991). MAO activity is commonly measured in platelets obtained by venipuncture from the peripheral circulation. Platelet MAO activity is remarkably stable in the individual over time, is under genetic control, and demonstrates a heritability of about .75 as revealed by twin studies (Pedersen, Oreland, Reynolds, & McClearn, 1993).

Since platelet MAO is involved in the regulation of catecholamines, it has been studied as a marker in psychobiological studies of aggression and related behaviors in children, adolescents, and adults (Alm et al., 1994). There is evidence to indicate that platelet MAO activity may reflect some properties of CNS 5-HT functioning. There exists a positive correlation between the 5-HT metabolite 5-HIAA in the CSF and platelet MAO activity in the peripheral circulation (Oreland et al., 1981). MAO may also reflect some aspects of CNS DA functioning, although the data are somewhat weaker (Davidson et al., 1987). The importance of MAO in the study of aggression in humans has been highlighted by a case report of a family in which a point mutation in the gene encoding MAO-A abolished MAO-A enzymatic activity. The males of the family demonstrated chronic, excessive, inappropriate aggressive behaviors (Brunner, Nelen, Breakefield, Ropers, & van Oost, 1993).

Cross-sectional studies of platelet MAO activity in youth with aggressive/antisocial behaviors have largely been contradictory. Evidence for positive correlations between platelet MAO activity and such behaviors has been found for CD-diagnosed sons of substance-misusing fathers versus non-CD-diagnosed sons of similar fathers (Gabel et al., 1995), and for boys with disruptive behavior disorders and high impulsivity versus controls (Stoff et al., 1989). On the other hand, evidence for inverse correlations between platelet MAO activity and CD in boys with ADHD has also been reported (Bowden et al., 1988). Other studies have reported no significant differences in platelet MAO activity among boys with CD, boys with other psychiatric diagnoses, and controls (Pliszka, Rogeness, & Medrano, 1988; Rogeness et al., 1982). These discrepant findings may be due to differences in methodology and sample ascertainment.

The strongest evidence for an association between platelet MAO activity and antisocial behaviors comes from two longitudinal studies conducted in Sweden. In a 25-year longitudinal study, Alm et al. (1996) first evaluated a community sample of boys between the ages of 11 and 14 years. Indices of criminal activity, biological measures, and rating scales assessing psychopathic personality traits were first assessed in adolescence, and then again when subjects were between 38 and 46 years of age. Results indicated a fourfold increased risk of persistent criminality into adulthood in adolescents with low platelet MAO activity. The combination of psychopathic personality traits and low platelet MAO activity increased risk over either factor alone. This study supports the finding that psychopathic traits and low platelet MAO are independent risk factors for early-onset adolescent antisocial behavior and persistent criminality (Alm et al., 1994, 1996). In a 14-year longitudinal study, af Klinteberg (1996) found that adolescent norm breaking and externalizing behavior first assessed at ages 13–15 years was significantly associated with low platelet MAO activity at age 27 years. This finding held for both males and females.

Low platelet MAO activity could be related to early-onset and persistent aggressive/antisocial behavior in several ways. First, low platelet MAO activity has been found to be related to certain personality traits—such as sensation seeking, impulsivity, aversion to boredom, and monotony avoidance—in both males and females (Schalling, Aberg, Edman, & Levander, 1984), and in both psychiatric patients and normals (Zuckerman, 1991). These impulsivity-related personality traits are also found in individuals at risk for early-onset and persistent psychopathy and other antisocial behaviors (Zuckerman, 1991). Second, since platelet MAO activity is positively correlated with the 5-HT metabolite 5-HIAA in CSF (Oreland et al., 1981), low platelet MAO activity could reflect CNS 5-HT underfunctioning, which is also related to aggressive behavior (Kruesi et al., 1992).

General Summary of Monoamine Research

The studies reviewed in this section of the chapter suggest that measures of CNS 5-HT and NE are associated with aggressive/antisocial behaviors in children and adolescents. The evidence for an association between CNS DA functioning and such behaviors in youth appears much weaker. Evidence is strongest for longitudinal studies relating measures of CNS 5-HT metabolism to aggressive behaviors; cross-sectional studies linking CSF MHPG and plasma DßH to aggressive behaviors; and longitudinal studies reporting low platelet MAO activity to be associated with risk for early-onset and persistent antisocial behavior across development.

However, this evidence cannot be accepted without several caveats. The studies reviewed here are marked by lack of standardization in relation to subject recruitment; definitions of aggression (e.g., a categorical psychiatric diagnosis of CD vs. the dimensional measurement of externalizing behavior problems); differing psychiatric diagnoses in subjects studied; frequent lack of controls for the effects of diurnal variation, season of the year, concomitant drug intake, and nutritional intake on biochemical dependent variables; and low statistical power in study samples. In addition, the studies reviewed here are based on samples in which the vast majority of subjects are male. As a result, no information on possible gender differences in the relationship of monoamines to aggression is available.

Finally, this review emphasizes that different subtypes of aggression may have different biochemical correlates. Overt physical aggression may be more strongly linked to neurotransmitter variables than nonphysical, hidden, or covert subtypes of aggression may be. As such, youth meeting criteria for highly aggressive forms of CD may show stronger correlations on these variables than do youngsters who demonstrate less aggressive forms of CD. Next, personality traits may be correlated with monoamine neurotransmitter variables and mediate the relationship between biochemical indices and aggressive behavior. As such, further research exploring relationships between personality traits of psychopathy, impulsivity, sensation seeking, and monotony avoidance on the one hand, and aggressive/antisocial behaviors and biochemical variables on the other, are needed. Finally, characteristics of the rearing environment and the quality of a youth's attachment to a caregiver may also mediate the relationship between monoamines and aggressive behavior. Developmental adaptation to a chronically fear-producing and/or aggressive rearing environment may produce adaptive CNS changes that are reflected in the relationship between monoamines and aggressive behavior in youth.

NEUROBIOLOGICAL–BEHAVIORAL MODELS

The Biobehavioral Systems Model of Gray

Jeffrey A. Gray (1982, 1987) has proposed a comprehensive biobehavioral theory of brain functioning. Gray posits that diverse forms of normal and abnormal personality variants, emotions, and behaviors have their etiology in the relative balance between identifiable and separate neurological systems that serve to mediate organismic activation and inhibition to environmental stimuli. This theory has relevance for a classification of aggressive behaviors. Gray has proposed three primary brain systems: a behavioral inhibition system (BIS), a behavioral activation system (BAS) (Fowles, 1994), and a flight–fight system. These brain systems appear to be phylogenetically conserved in evolution, since they are hypothesized to mediate approach behavior and inhibition to environmental stimuli in a wide number of species, as well as in human beings. In humans, the integrated functioning of these systems is postulated to determine many aspects of learning, personality, emotional behavior, and psychopathology, including aggressive/antisocial behaviors.

The BAS is an action system controlling behavioral approach when signals of reward (conditioned stimuli) are received by an individual (see Table 7.8). The BAS is also important in facilitating active escape from a threatened punishment or other aversive situation. This behavioral system governs predatory or instrumental aggression in Gray's model. Human emotions associated with this system include hope (of reward) or relief (escape from punishment). Empirical data from nonhuman animals suggest that the neuroanatomical lo-

TABLE 7.8. Gray's Model of Systems for the Control of Emotional Behavior

	BAS	BIS	Flight–fight
Reinforcing stimuli	Conditioned stimuli for reward and nonpunishment (reward learning and escape from punishment)	Conditioned stimuli for punishment and nonreward	Innate threat stimuli (unconditioned)
Emotion	Hope (of reward); relief (escape from punishment)	Anxiety, apprehension, worry	Fear
Behavior	Active approach (to reward); predatory aggression; active avoidance (escape punishment)	Inhibition	Instinctive (unconditioned) escape; defensive aggression
Neuroanatomy	Ventral tegmental area (A10 nucleus); medial forebrain bundle (DA); nucleus accumbens; ventral striatum	Septo-hippocampal system; Papez circuit; medial forebrain bundle (NE and 5-HT); neocortical structures (entorhinal, prefrontal, cingulate cortex)	Amygdala; medial forebrain bundle (NE); ventromedial nucleus of hypothalamus; central grey of mesencephalon

Note. Data from Gray (1982, 1987).

cus of the BAS includes DA pathways that mediate reward responding, arising from the ventral tegmental area of the brainstem and terminating in the nucleus accumbens and ventral striatum (Gray, 1987) (see Figure 7.1).

The BIS inhibits or decelerates behavioral responding under signals (conditioned stimuli) of impending punishment, nonreward, frustration, or novelty. Essentially, the BIS is thought to function by continuously comparing actual environmental circumstances with learned concepts of expected outcomes of behavior. In theory, when mismatches occur, the BIS inhibits the BAS from active response (Gray, 1982; Rogeness et al., 1992). Human emotions associated with the BIS include anxiety and apprehension (see Table 7.8). Gray's conceptualization of the BIS is based on extensive empirical evidence from nonhuman animals suggesting that the locus of this system resides in the septo-hippocampal complex and its neuroanatomical connections to deeper brainstem structures and to higher neocortical structures. The neurotransmitters important to the BIS appear to include NE and 5-HT.

The empirical evidence for the BIS rests on neuroanatomical lesion studies and pharmacological investigations. First, anatomical lesions of the septohippocampal and related areas in animals produce behavioral effects that Gray interprets as indicative of decreased anxiety and lessened behavioral inhibition. These include impaired suppression of rewarded behavior by punishment in passive avoidance conditioning, impaired acquisition of conditioned

Behavioral Activation System (BAS)

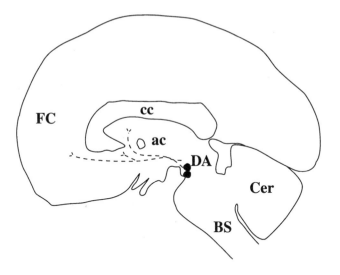

FIGURE 7.1. Schematic drawing of a sagittal view of the human brain illustrating the behavioral activation system (BAS). Ascending dopamine (DA) fibers originating from the substantia nigra and ventral tegmental area project to the caudate–putamen, nucleus accumbens, and frontal cortex (FC). ac, anterior commissure; BS, brainstem; cc, corpus callosum; Cer, cerebellum.

emotional responses, increased aggression in response to provocation, increased exploration of novel environments, and increased sociability (Gray, 1982, 1987). Next, substances (benzodiazepines, barbiturates, alcohol) that decrease anxiety in humans also produce much the same changes in animals' behavior as septo-hippocampal lesions do (Gray, 1982, 1987). Thus the BIS in Gray's model is viewed as responsible for both the expression of anxiety and the inhibition of behavior in the presence of cues signaling impending punishment or lack of reward (see Figure 7.2).

Gray has conceived of a third system, called the flight–fight system, which responds to unconditioned (not learned, innate) stimuli such as pain, punishment, and frustration (see Table 7.8). The human emotion mediated by this system is fear. Unconditioned escape and defensive aggression are the main behaviors produced by this system. The principal brain structures involved are the amygdala, the ventromedial hypothalamus, and the central grey of the mesencephalon, with associated ascending NE tracts (see Table 7.8). Fear conditioning is discussed in more detail below.

The relative balance in functioning between the BAS and the BIS has been

Behavioral Inhibition System (BIS)

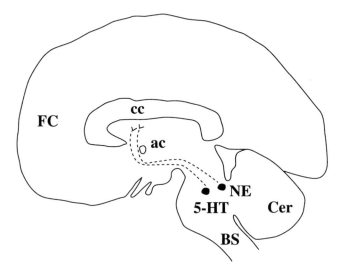

FIGURE 7.2. Schematic drawing of a sagittal view of the human brain illustrating the behavioral inhibition system (BIS). Ascending norepinephrine (NE) and serotonin (5-HT) fibers originate from the locus coeruleus and the raphe nuclei, respectively. Other abbreviations as in Figure 7.1.

postulated to be important in psychopathology (Fowles, 1994). Gray (1982) has hypothesized that an individual with a stronger BIS should be prone to anxiety. An individual with a more responsive BAS should be impulsive and prone to disinhibited behavior (Quay, 1993). The relative strengths of these two biobehavioral systems may have important implications in mood disorders, schizophrenia, and addictions (Fowles, 1994). This two-factor model (BAS and BIS) also has implications for aggression and related behaviors. In Gray's (1987) model, such behaviors should be most severe and persistent in individuals with both excessive BAS activity and deficient BIS activity. These individuals should be reward-driven despite cues of punishment, be relatively resistant to anxiety conditioning, demonstrate impulsivity, and have difficulty withholding behavioral responses that are inappropriate and likely to elicit punishment.

Direct tests of the relationships between the BAS/BIS and aggressive behavior are more difficult in humans than in animal models. However, some evidence does exist to support Gray's model in children with conduct problems, though this evidence is more indirect than the lesion studies and pharmacological challenge studies in nonhuman animal paradigms. Tests of Gray's hypothesis involve three approaches: (1) differential aspects of learning and behavior; (2) pharmacological evidence; and (3) psychophysiological indices of sympathetic ANS system functioning, such as heart rate and electrodermal activity (EDA).

Because the BAS and BIS control different aspects of instrumental learning and behavior, an individual's performance in different aspects of learning and behavior may reflect differences in the operation of the two systems. For example, the BAS is felt to be activated when conditioned signals of reward are received by an individual. A youth with a more responsive BAS will be more sensitive to rewards, even in the face of punishment or nonreward experiences, than a youth with a less responsive BAS. Gray's theory postulates that an individual with a strong BAS and a weak BIS will be prone to aggressive/antisocial behavior (i.e., will lack anxiety, will not learn from punishment, will persist in reward-driven activities despite cues of punishment, will seek sensation, and will be skilled at escaping punishment). Remember also that the BAS controls predatory and instrumental aggression. An individual with an active BAS should be more skilled at instrumental aggression than a child with an underactive BAS or a strong BIS, and may engage in this form of aggression more frequently. There is evidence in support of these predictions. Children and adolescents meeting psychiatric diagnostic criteria for CD demonstrate many more features of instrumental aggression than children who do not meet these criteria (Quay, 1993). Children with CD and psychopathic traits are also more skilled at instrumental and predatory forms of aggression than are children with CD who are not psychopathic (Christian, Frick, Hill, Tyler, & Frazier, 1997).

In laboratory paradigms investigating perseverative responding for reward in the face of cues of nonreward, children with CD demonstrate behavior that is reward-dominant. For example, in one laboratory paradigm, subjects play a computerized card game in which the probability of correct responses (which are reinforced with money) declines over subsequent trials, and the probability of losing money because of incorrect responses increases over trials. Compared to control children, youth with CD continue to play on more trials and lose more money, despite being free to play or pass on each trial (Daugherty & Quay, 1991; Shapiro, Quay, Hogan, & Schwartz, 1988). Within the context of Gray's theory, these results suggest that a child with CD (expecially one with psychopathy) will have a strongly responding BAS and demonstrate reward-dominant behavior.

In contrast, according to Gray's theory, a youth with an active BIS is more prone to anxiety. If the BIS inhibits the BAS, and a youngster with a strong BAS is more prone to CD, then a youth with anxiety should demonstrate less antisocial behavior. Several investigations have found evidence to support this. In a study of 177 clinic-referred boys, Walker et al. (1991) found that boys with CD and comorbid anxiety disorders were significantly less deviant on several measures of antisocial behavior than boys with CD but without anxiety. The anxious boys with CD had fewer police contacts and were nominated by their peers as less aggressive than the nonanxious boys with CD.

In a follow-up study, the anxious boys with CD were found to have higher salivary cortisol levels than the nonanxious boys with CD, suggesting that cortisol may be important in further attempts to elucidate physiological processes involving anxiety, behavioral inhibition, and CD (McBurnett et al., 1991). Other support comes from longitudinal studies. In a 3-year follow-up of early adolescent boys from an economically depressed urban area, indices of behavioral inhibition (defined as a tendency to be anxious, fearful, or afraid in new situations) protected against the development of delinquency and other antisocial behavior at outcome (Kerr, Tremblay, Pagani, & Vitaro, 1997). Within the context of Gray's theory, a strong BIS, as reflected in increased vulnerability to anxiety, constrains the BAS and results in less antisocial behavior.

Neurochemical studies have also provided some support for Gray's theory in children and adolescents. Remember that the neurotransmitters hypothesized to be most important for the BIS are NE and 5-HT. DA appears to be the most important neurotransmitter for the operation of the BAS. Biochemical evidence of inefficient NE and 5-HT activity in youth with conduct problems would support the hypothesis of an inefficient BIS in these youth. Evidence of more efficient DA functioning than expected in these same youth would support enhanced activity of the BAS. To date, evidence is stronger for inefficient NE and 5-HT functioning in youth with CD than for enhanced DA functioning.

As noted earlier in the chapter, DßH is an enzyme important in the biochemical conversion of DA to NE. Its activity in plasma (blood) is relatively constant in an individual over time. Lower levels of DßH (and thus less conversion of DA to NE) in children and adolescents with CD suggest inefficient NE functioning in these same youth. Several investigations of plasma DßH have reported significantly lower levels in youth who meet criteria for CD. However, not all studies have been able to replicate this finding (for a review, see Rogeness et al., 1992). Similarly, many studies using a variety of methodologies, have reported evidence of diminished 5-HT functioning in youth with disruptive behavior disorders and measures of increased aggressiveness (for a review, again, see Rogeness et al., 1992). These data are consistent with an association between decreased NE and 5-HT functioning on the one hand and aggressive/antisocial behaviors on the other, as predicted by Gray's theory. Current neurochemical data do not show the predicted association between increased DA function and CD.

Psychophysiological indices have also been used to test Gray's hypothesis. These include heart rate under a variety of environmental conditions and the EDA. In this model, cardiac acceleration as measured by increased heart rate is thought to reflect appetitive motivational states and to index activity in the BAS (Fowles, 1988). If this is the case, then increased heart rate in the face of reward in children with CD versus controls should reflect increased activity in the BAS. Heart rate acceleration to reward has largely been studied in laboratory paradigms with adult subjects, where this hypothesis has been supported

(Fowles, 1994). At present, there are few data on the reward paradigm and accelerated heart rate in children and adolescents with CD. Most psychophysiological data on heart rate measurement in such youth index resting heart rate. These studies find that noninstitutionalized, nonclinic-referred youth with milder forms of antisocial behavior demonstrate lower tonic heart rates than nonantisocial controls. Lower resting heart rates in these youth correlate with cross-sectional and longitudinal risk for increased conduct problem behaviors and aggression (Raine, 1993). These findings have been interpreted as supporting theories of fearlessness or ANS underarousal and associated sensation seeking in the etiology of antisocial behavior in youth, as opposed to supporting Gray's theory of a strongly responding BAS (Raine, 1993).

EDA is usually measured by placing electrodes on two sites of the hand and passing a small electrical current across the two electrodes (see Chapter 6). Increased sweating leads to an increase in EDA that can be measured with a polygraph. The eccrine sweat glands are innervated by cholinergic fibers from the CNS. Novel stimuli, emotional stimuli, threatening stimuli (i.e., cues of impending punishment or nonreward), and attention-getting stimuli can elicit measurable EDA. EDA is a peripheral measure of sympathetic ANS activity and CNS information processing; within Gray's model, it is thought to index activity in the BIS (Fowles, 1988). If this is the case, diminished BIS functioning in children with CD should be reflected in lower EDA than that of control children. In seven studies of EDA in children and adolescents (which used widely varying criteria for subject selection), youth with aggression, antisocial behavior, or conduct problems manifested diminished EDA responsiveness to external stimuli when compared to control groups (see Quay, 1993, for a review). The consistency of results in these seven studies is striking; to interpret the results within Gray's theory, they suggest evidence of BIS underactivity in children and adolescents with aggressive and related behaviors.

Interestingly, two recent studies support the hypothesis that antisocial adolescents who desist from crime demonstrate *greater* physiological ANS arousal and reactivity (reflecting an underactive BAS and a strong BIS, in Gray's model) than antisocial adolescents who persist in criminal behaviors as adults. In a cross-sectional study of males, subjects with criminal fathers who did not themselves become criminal as adults were found to have significantly greater EDA and heart rate orienting reactivity than criminal subjects with criminal fathers (Brennan et al., 1997). In a 14-year longitudinal study, antisocial adolescents who ceased a criminal lifestyle by age 29 years demonstrated significantly higher EDA orienting than a persistently criminal comparison group (Raine, Venables, & Williams, 1995). The findings suggest that individuals predisposed to adult crime and other antisocial behavior, by virtue of showing antisocial problems in adolescence, may be protected from persistent antisociality in adulthood by high levels of ANS arousal and reactivity. These factors may reflect not only increased BIS and decreased BAS activity, but also more efficient information processing and attentional resources, which can protect high-risk adolescents from persistent antisocial lifestyles (see Chapter 6).

Gray's biobehavioral systems model of anxiety and psychopathology is potentially very useful to the study of aggression for several reasons. It provides a neurobiological–behavioral hypothesis that potentially underlies neuropsychological, psychiatric, and personality trait descriptions of impulsive aggression and concepts of psychopathy. Unlike studies of aggression and antisocial behaviors that utilize observer-completed or self-report behavioral rating scale methodologies, Gray's concepts of the BAS and BIS are grounded in CNS neuroanatomy and neurobiology; as such, it has the potential to be tested. Newer laboratory techniques, including noninvasive radiological functional imaging technologies that have a minimal radiation cost to the subject (see Chapter 6), may be very informative in the study of the septo-hippocampal and ventral tegmental systems in aggressive/antisocial youth compared to controls. In addition, Gray's model predicts that pharmacological interventions that block DA neurotransmission (decrease BAS overactivity) and enhance NE and/or 5-HT functioning (enhance a deficient BIS) may be helpful in the treatment of youth with CD. This can be directly tested. For example, antipsychotic medication blocks DA neurotransmission and has been found effective in youth with explosive aggression and CD (Campbell, Gonzalez, Ernst, Silva, & Werry, 1993). Lithium enhances 5-HT functioning (among its other pharmacological actions) and has also been found effective in treating hospitalized aggressive children with CD (Campbell, Adams, et al., 1995). These studies provide indirect evidence suggesting that the hypothesized BAS and BIS may be pharmacologically manipulated for therapeutic benefit in youth with CD. As such, the testing of Gray's theory deserves more research attention in the study of aggressive children and adolescents.

Traumatic Stress and Fear Conditioning

As discussed, previous research on the psychobiology of aggression has emphasized the importance of sympathetic ANS underarousal in contributing to aggressive/antisocial behavior (Raine, 1993). Such underarousal has been documented in lower EDA and lower heart rates in undersocialized aggressive children with conduct problems, and in aggressive youth with psychopathic traits, as compared to control children (see Chapter 6). These children also appear to have less anxiety when faced with cues of nonreward or punishment. In contrast, some children and adolescents behave aggressively because they are chronically fearful. These youth exhibit sympathetic ANS overarousal as a result of traumatic experiences in their lives that have resulted in behavioral sensitization to cues of fear and threat. Such youth are hypervigilant, scan the environment for threats, easily misinterpret threat where none actually exists, and have a low threshold for defensive behaviors (including defensive aggression). Occasionally, their traumatic symptoms can be severe enough to qualify for a psychiatric diagnosis of posttraumatic stress disorder (PTSD) (see Chapter 4). Aggression occurring in the face of perceived threat and sympathetic ANS overarousal may be very different from aggression occurring because of underarousal in neurobiological systems controlling inhibition.

Emerging evidence on the neurobiological basis of human fear is beginning to delineate the neuroanatomy and neurobiology of CNS pathways that mediate fear responses to threat. When these systems are active, increased sympathetic ANS arousal occurs, with an increased possibility of defensive behaviors such as active escape or defensive aggression. Since it is known that children and adolescents who experience traumatic, threatening stressors such as physical abuse in their developing years may be more aggressive than children who have not experienced such trauma (Connor, Melloni, & Harrison, 1998; Fletcher, 1996), any discussion of a classification of aggressive behavior in children and adolescents needs to include a discussion of fear and fear conditioning.

Children and adolescents who have directly experienced or witnessed traumatic events in their developing years—events that are outside the range of normal human experience, terrifying, and threatening to life or body integrity—may develop pervasive symptoms of chronic sympathetic ANS overarousal. These symptoms may include easy startle reactions, irritability, hostility, a low threshold for aggressive responding, and impulsive reactions to sensory environmental or cognitive stimuli that others would not perceive as threatening. These symptoms may persist for long periods of time even when the threat is past. Although fears may eventually be attenuated and partially masked by the passage of time, reminders of the fearful events may easily reactivate an intense and long-lasting fear reaction in traumatized individuals, often many years after the actual trauma.

Classical fear conditioning, easily demonstrated with animals in the laboratory, may explain some of these observations. Animals exposed to a visual or auditory conditioned stimulus (i.e., the stimulus to be fear-conditioned, such as a light or a sound) in conjunction with an aversive unconditioned stimulus (i.e., a foot shock) will subsequently exhibit a conditioned emotional (fear) reaction to the conditioned stimulus in the absence of an unconditioned stimulus. These behavioral changes can last for years in laboratory animals (Charney, Deutch, Krystal, Southwick, & Davis, 1993). In humans, investigations have demonstrated that fear conditioning may be mediated by subcortical CNS mechanisms and can occur without conscious awareness or conscious learning (Charney, Grillon, & Bremner, 1998; LeDoux, 1996).

Three interconnected brain regions regulate fearfulness (Kalin, 1997). The prefrontal cortex interprets sensory information and assess potential for danger. In the absence of threat, the prefrontal cortex inhibits activation of the fear pathways. The amygdala, a part of the limbic system, generates emotions including fear. It becomes active when danger is signaled. In the presence of threat, the hypothalamus secretes CRH, which acts on the anterior pituitary to secrete ACTH, which acts on the adrenal cortex to secrete cortisol, which then activates the body for defense in the face of perceived danger (see the "Cortisol" section earlier in this chapter). This system is commonly referred to as the HPA axis. The neuroanatomy of the threat defensive system is well understood both in laboratory animals and in humans (Lang, Bradley, & Cuthbert, 1998; LeDoux, 1998). A flow chart of this pathway is presented in Figure 7.3, and placed in context in a sketch of the human brain in Figure 7.4.

Traumatic stress produces profound alterations in multiple neurotransmitter systems. The NE, 5-HT, DA, opiate, and neurohormonal systems are all involved in the modulation of acute and chronic responses to overwhelming threat. There is evidence that in the face of chronic life-threatening stress, these systems can become dysregulated. Stress, particularly uncontrolled stress, is known to produce fear and anxiety and to increase NE turnover in

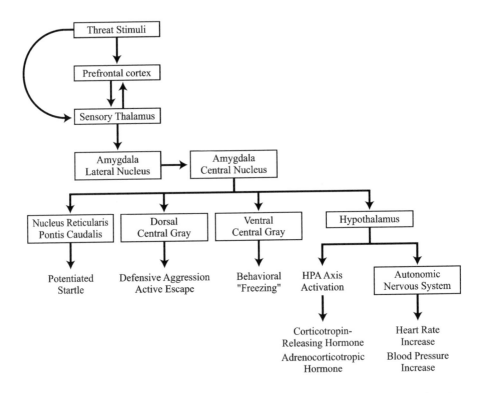

FIGURE 7.3. Brain pathways involved in fear conditioning. The basic neural pathways underlying fear conditioning involve transmission of sensory stimuli about a threat (conditioned stimulus) to the amygdala from the thalamus and cortex. Signals first reach the lateral nucleus of the amygdala and then project to the central nucleus of the amygdala. Output from the central nucleus controls the expression of defensive responses. These include a potentiated startle reflex; defensive aggression; active escape from threat; behavioral immobility ("freezing"—a form of camouflage from predators); activation of the stress response via the hypothalamic–pituitary–adrenal (HPA) axis; and activation of the sympathetic branch of the autonomic nervous system. Data from Lang, Bradley, and Cuthbert (1998) and LeDoux (1998).

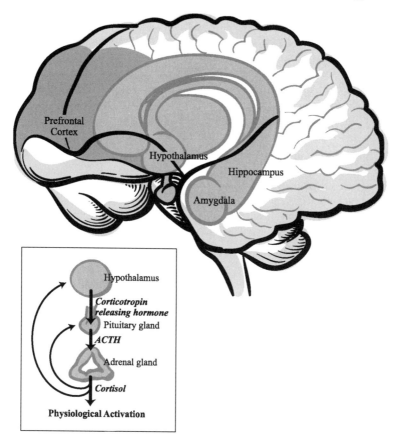

FIGURE 7.4. Brain regions that are critically important in regulating fear-induced behaviors. The prefrontal cortex participates in assessing signals of danger and threat. The amygdala produces the emotion of fear. The prefrontal cortex, amygdala, and hippocampus signal the hypothalamus to activate the HPA axis to secrete hormones that help activate and support individual responses to danger. Data from Kalin (1997).

specific brain regions (the locus coeruleus, hypothalamus, hippocampus, amygdala, and cerebral cortex) and to increase the responsiveness of the NE system to excitatory stimulation in animal models (Simson & Weiss, 1988). In human research, there is emerging evidence of dysregulation in the NE system in adults meeting criteria for PTSD (Southwick et al., 1997) and in sexually abused girls (DeBellis, Lefter, Trickett, & Putnam, 1994). There is also evidence of dysregulation in 5-HT system following severe stress in both animal and human research, although this has been less well studied (Arora, Fitchner, & O'Connor, 1993; Southwick et al., 1997). Increased NE functioning, elevated sympathetic ANS arousal, and diminished 5-HT functioning can elevate risk for impulsive aggression in traumatized individuals (Southwick et al., 1997). Stress-induced hyperactivity of CNS DA systems may be linked to hypervigilance, paranoid thinking, and exaggerated startle reactions in traumatized individuals (Charney et al., 1993). Children and adolescents experiencing chronic trauma and uncontrollable stress may exhibit analgesia and a diminished responsiveness to painful stimuli, a consequence of stress-induced release of endogenous opiates (Charney et al., 1993). Chronic high levels of stress-induced circulating neurohormones such as corticotropin and corticosterone may cause injury to hippocampal neurons, which are important in cognitive functions such as memory, and thus may result in the memory disturbances seen in traumatized individuals (Lombroso & Sapolsky, 1998).

Once established, fear conditioning can be resistant to change. Ordinary anxiety tends to become less intense upon repeated exposure to an anxious stimuli if negative reinforcement such as escape from the anxious stimulus is prevented; this process is known as "habituation" or "extinction." Fear conditioning, however, may be relatively permanent and not easily extinguished, in humans as well as laboratory animals (Charney et al., 1993). For example, in a study of adult women, those with childhood histories of sexual or physical abuse were found to exhibit increased pituitary–adrenal and ANS activation responses to a mild stress, compared to never-abused control women (Heim et al., 2000). This suggests that early stress may sensitize the HPA and ANS systems, and cause them to overreact to mild stimuli in a persistent and chronic manner years after the acute trauma is over. In addition, a process known as "behavioral sensitization" may occur. Individuals who have been traumatized demonstrate an increased vulnerability to stress in general. Eventually, environmental stimuli that bear only a distant relationship to the original traumatic event may trigger fear-conditioned behaviors (Charney et al., 1993; Heim et al., 2000).

All of the neurobiological changes occurring as a result of chronic, uncontrollable stress such as childhood trauma can have an enduring and profound impact on the emotional, behavioral, cognitive, social, and physical functioning of children. For example, noninvasive neuroimaging studies are beginning to document changes in specific CNS structures as a result of childhood trauma. Magnetic resonance imaging has revealed hippocampal atrophy in adult patients with PTSD who experienced childhood physical and sexual abuse (Bremner, et al., 1997). Perry and Pollard (1998) point out that a child or adolescent, with an immature and still developing CNS, is more vulnerable to traumatic stress than an adult, who possesses a fully developed CNS. A child's brain develops capacities that best suit adaptation to the environmental milieu in which he or she is raised and must live day to day. If the child is exposed to chronic neglect, physical abuse, sexual abuse, or other trauma during the developing years, fear-inducing stimuli may constitute the original organizing experience for the child's CNS. Since the human CNS is profoundly efficient at learning from and adapting to environmental stimuli, the longer the developing child is exposed to ongoing trauma, the more these fear-conditioned neural systems may become "hard-wired" in a use-dependent fashion (Perry, Pollard, Blakley, Baker, & Vigilante, 1995). With time, these neurobiological systems may become increasingly resistant to change. The traumatized child thus becomes fear-conditioned, with increased vulnerability to hypervigilant, fearful, overaroused, impulsive, aggressive, hostile, and irritable responding to the environment.

NEUROLOGICAL DISORDERS THOUGHT TO BE RELATED TO AGGRESSION

Most reviews of the neurobiology of aggression do not include a discussion of neurological disorders and aggression. This is unfortunate, since some such disorders directly alter brain biology and can result in altered behavioral functioning. An extensive clinical case report literature describes the relationship between neurological diseases affecting the CNS and disorders of impulsive aggression in adults (Silver & Yudofsky, 1994; Silver, Hales, & Yudofsky, 1992). This literature largely focuses on adults with brain tumors, epilepsy, traumatic brain injury (TBI), and episodic behavioral dyscontrol (Elliott, 1987). These reports often lead clinicians evaluating aggressive/antisocial youth with a history of TBI or epilepsy to wonder whether the neurological disorder may be causing the youth's problem behaviors.

Methodologically rigorous investigations of the relationship between neurological disorders and aggressive behavior are few in number, especially in children and adolescents. What follows is a review of the association between two disorders common in youth—TBI and epilepsy—and aggression and related behaviors.

Traumatic Brain Injury

TBI is an insult to the brain caused by an external force that results in impairment of cognitive, behavioral, emotional, or physical functioning. Postinjury impairment may be transient or permanent. TBI is divided into two categories: "open" and "closed" head injuries. Open head injury is defined by penetration of the brain, such as might occur by a gunshot wound; it usually results in more localized damage than closed head injury. The severity of damage is related to the kinetic energy of the penetrating object. Closed head injury does not involve penetration of the brain, but is related to translational and rotational forces on the brain within the closed volume of the cranium. With translational forces, the brain moves within the skull. As the moving brain strikes the hard, rough edges of the cranial vault, contusions may occur. Brain contusions most commonly involve the inferior frontal and temporal lobe surfaces (Guthrie, Mast, Richards, McQuaid, & Pavlakis, 1999) (see Chapter 6, Figures 6.1 and 6.2). The moving brain may collide with a skull surface and rebound, striking the opposite skull surface; this is known as a "coup–

contrecoup" injury. In addition to contusions, translational forces in the brain can result in hemorrhages in various brain tissues and locales. Rotational forces can cause the brain to twist on its axis, and this may lead to diffuse damage to axons via shearing forces. Areas commonly affected by shearing injury include subcortical white matter, the upper brainstem, the basal ganglia, the hippocampus, the grey–white matter junction (the interface between neuronal cell bodies and their myelinated axons), and the interface between the brain and its covering membrane (the dura) (Guthrie et al., 1999). Closed head injuries in the pediatric age range are most commonly caused by falls, motor vehicle accidents, bicycle accidents, sports injuries, and physical abuse (Guthrie et al., 1999; Silver et al., 1992). TBI is a major cause of morbidity and mortality among children, with a prevalence estimated to be between 180 and 295 per 100,000 children and adolescents in the United States (Guthrie et al., 1999).

A broad range of severity is present in TBI. The vast majority of TBI in youngsters is classified as mild. Severe TBI accounts for approximately 10% of toddler head trauma (usually a result of child abuse), decreases during the school-age years, and rises to an incidence of approximately 20% among adolescents with TBI (usually as a result of motor vehicle accidents and violence) (Guthrie et al., 1999). Severity is measured in a variety of ways. The length of posttraumatic amnesia appears important. Disturbances of memory lasting less than 7 days after head injury characterize mild to moderate TBI, whereas memory loss lasting more than 1 week after head injury identifies severe TBI (Brown, Chadwick, Shaffer, Rutter, & Traub, 1981). Loss of consciousness after injury is another important variable. Mild TBI is defined as unconsciousness for less than 5 minutes, moderate TBI by unconsciousness lasting between 5 minutes and 24 hours, and severe TBI by coma lasting more than 24 hours (Guthrie et al., 1999; Silver et al., 1992). The Glasgow Coma Scale (GCS; Jennett, 1976) measures responsiveness following TBI as expressed by eye opening, motor response, and verbal response. Each domain is rated on a scale of 1–5, and an aggregate score is summed for all three domains. The higher the total score, the more responsive the patient, and the better the prognosis. A GCS score of 13 or more identifies mild TBI, a score between 9 and 12 identifies moderate TBI, and a score less than 9 identifies severe TBI (Guthrie et al., 1999). Often all three measures—length of posttraumatic amnesia, duration of loss of consciousness, and GCS score—are combined to estimate TBI severity. The severity of TBI appears important in prognosis.

Longitudinal studies of TBI have identified risk factors for new-onset psychiatric illness after head injury in children who did not have a psychiatric illness before injury. These factors include severity of TBI. Youth with mild TBI are indistinguishable from controls without head injury in the development of new psychiatric disorder following TBI (Max & Dunisch, 1997), whereas juveniles with severe TBI have a clearly elevated risk for developing such a psychiatric disorder (Brown et al., 1981: Max et al., 1997). Family functioning and the degree of family psychosocial adversity are also powerful predictors of new-onset psychiatric illness after TBI. Youth with TBI from families with greater adversity and poorer functioning are at increased risk for the development of a novel psychiatric disorder in the 2 years following TBI (Max et al., 1997). Finally, lifetime history of psychiatric disorder in the individual prior to TBI is also an important predictor of the development of new-onset psychiatric illness following TBI (Max et al., 1997). In a study of children 6–14 years of age with TBI, severity of injury, family functioning, and history of previous psychiatric illness accounted for 76% to 81% of the variance in the development of a novel psychiatric disturbance following TBI (Max et al., 1997).

Important for our discussion of any relationship between TBI and aggression and related behaviors in juveniles are repeated findings that when new-onset psychopathology occurs following TBI, it is generalized and is not specific to aggression (Brown et al., 1981; Deb, Lyons, Koutzoukis, Ali, & McCarthy, 1999; Max et al., 1997; Max & Dunisch, 1997). The most common psychiatric finding after TBI is socially disinhibited behavior—namely, behavior that violates social norms but is not frankly aggressive (Brown et al., 1981). Examples include making lewd comments to strangers or disrobing in public. Other psychiatric disorders that frequently develop after TBI include depression and anxiety (Deb et al., 1999). New-onset aggression, CD, or delinquent behaviors are not frequently found (Max & Dunisch, 1997). Although psychiatric case reports from the adult TBI literature identify injury to the inferior orbital surface of the frontal lobe and anterior temporal lobes as being specifically associated with outbursts of rage and violence (Silver et al., 1992), this is not frequently reported in children following TBI. Rather, youth who are antisocial, hyperactive, or aggressive after TBI generally have a psychiatric history of such behaviors prior to injury and live in families with high rates of psychosocial adversity (Brown et al., 1981; Max et al., 1997). In summary, there is little evidence to support the idea that TBI is causative of aggressive behavior in youth. However, the inverse statement has support from research: Aggressive, hyperactive, and antisocial youth may be at much higher risk for TBI than youth without these behavioral problems (Gerring et al., 1998; Guthrie et al., 1999).

Epilepsy

A "seizure" can be defined as a sudden, involuntary, transient alteration in cerebral function due to the abnormal, hypersynchronous electrical discharge of neurons (Holmes, 1987). A seizure may be caused by an acute neurological disturbance (e.g., a head injury) or a systemic illness (e.g., hypoglycemia), or it may occur idiopathically in an individual who is prone to spontaneous seizures. Epilepsy is a chronic condition characterized by recurrent, unprovoked seizures, with a tendency toward spontaneous seizure recurrence. Epilepsy may result from CNS trauma, infection, or tumor. Certain types of epilepsy appear to have a strong familial tendency, and some of these types have been linked to chromosomal defects (Thiele, Gonzalez-Heydrich, & Riviello, 1999).

The clinical manifestations of a seizure are determined by the location and characteristics of the abnormal discharge, including where it originates in the brain; whether it spreads and, if so, where; or whether it involves both brain hemispheres at onset. The Commission on Classification and Terminology of the International League Against Epilepsy (1981) has proposed a classification of seizures into a broad typology of "generalized" and "partial" seizures, based on clinical and electroencephalographic (EEG) manifestations. Generalized seizures at onset involve both cerebral hemispheres, and consciousness is impaired. Partial or focal seizures initially involve only a part of one hemisphere, but may secondarily generalize to involve both hemispheres. Simple partial seizures may involve no impairment of consciousness, whereas complex ones may cause impairment of consciousness. The clinical symptoms of a partial seizure depend on the area of the cortex in which the abnormal electrical discharges first begin, and on the function this cortical area serves. If a focal seizure originates in the motor cortex, the clinical manifestations will involve motor movement of the face, arms, or legs. If the seizure focus is in the temporal lobe, clinical manifestations may include psychic sensations such as a sensation of fear or *déjà vu* (Thiele et al., 1999).

Seizures and epilepsy are common neurological disorders in children and adolescents, probably secondary in prevalence only to headache. The incidence of seizures is higher in children than in adults, with the greatest incidence occurring within the first year of life (Thiele et al., 1999). It is estimated that 75% of epilepsies have their onset before 20 years of age (Lennox & Lennox, 1960). By the age of 20 years, up to 5% of children in the United States and western Europe will have experienced a seizure, but only 25% of these will go on to develop epilepsy (Hauser, 1995). There is a high remission rate in many children, with 80% of children expected to be seizure-free within 5 years of seizure onset. Even among children with seizures as a result of a congenital disorder, up to 40% may eventually become seizure-free (Thiele et al., 1999).

The association of epilepsy and generalized psychiatric disorder is complex. Although not all children with epilepsy suffer from psychiatric disorders, the empirical evidence indicates that they may be at greater risk for a variety of psychiatric problems than children without epilepsy. The Isle of Wight Study, an epidemiological study of the rates of childhood psychiatric disorder from a single geographical area, found a 29% prevalence of psychiatric disorder in children with idiopathic epilepsy. This rate was much higher than that for a control group of children with physical disorders not involving the brain (12%), or for children free of epilepsy or other physical disease (7%), but less than the rate of psychiatric disorder in children with structural brain disease such as cerebral palsy (44%) (Rutter, Graham, & Yule, 1970). This finding was replicated in a survey study of 308 school children with epilepsy compared to nonepileptic controls: Behavioral disorders were found in 27% of the epileptics, but only in 15% of the controls (Mellor, Lowit, & Hall, 1974). Although children with epilepsy have higher rates of psychiatric disorder than controls, the nature of their psychiatric problems is not specific. In the Isle of Wight Study, over 90% of the epileptic children who had a psychiatric problem had either a conduct problem or an emotional disorder, or a mixture of the two (Rutter et al., 1970).

The relationship between aggressive behavior and epilepsy remains controversial. In the late 19th century and on into the 20th there existed a widespread although scientifically unproved assumption that violence is directly associated with epilepsy. Well over 100 years ago, Gowers (1881) described "epileptic mania" as sudden paroxysmal outbursts of violence to others. In the late 20th century, epilepsy was still being used as a legal defense, similar to the insanity defense, in individuals on trial for homicide (Treiman, 1986). There existed—and to some extent still exists—a common belief that epilepsy is inextricably associated with unpredictable, irrational violent behavior, and that epileptic individuals are to be feared because they are at risk for sudden outbursts of violent and aggressive behavior. A scientific understanding of the relationship between epilepsy and aggression is more complex.

Any scientific approach to the relationship between aggression and epilepsy must recognize the concept of hierarchical control of brain functions (see Benjamin, 1999). According to this model, basic homeostatic functions are subserved by diencephalic brain structures such as the hypothalamus and brainstem. These functions include the regulation of temperature, thirst, satiety, biological rhythms, sexual drives, and aggressive drives. The limbic system, consisting of the anteromedial temporal lobe (including the amygdala), is the next level and serves as an important link between incoming sensory and sensory association signals and outflow to the hypothalamus. The limbic system serves to regulate the hypothalamus and lower brainstem centers by providing a sort of "bridge" between externally perceived reality and basic physiological organismic drive states. In this hierarchy, the highest level is the frontal neocortex, consisting of dorsolateral, orbital, and medial/cingulate frontal cortex (see Chapter 6, Figure 6.2). The orbital frontal cortex, connected with the amygdala and hypothalamus and (via the frontal dorsolateral convexity) with the rest of the brain, exerts control over the limbic system and amygdala. Theoretically, seizure activity involving any of these areas could result in the release of aggressive behavior, because of either overstimulation of the hypothalamus or loss of control over aggressive drive states from higher regulatory centers (Benjamin, 1999).

Studies investigating the occurrence of aggression during an actual seizure episode (so-called "ictal" aggression) have found little evidence to support a relationship between directed or organized violence and seizures. When aggression does occur during a seizure, it has characteristics that would be expected of any behavior during seizure activity. There is impairment of consciousness, and the aggressive activity is usually carried out in a disordered, uncoordinated, nonpremeditated, and nondirected manner (Fenwick, 1993).

In the most comprehensive study to date of this topic, 5,400 videotaped seizures from different epilepsy hospital wards around the world were viewed by a panel of epilepsy experts and rated for their degree of ictal aggression. Only 13 cases of aggressive behavior during a seizure were found, and only 3 of these involved attacks on people. The experts concluded that ictal aggression is a rare phenomenon (Delgado-Escueta et al., 1981). "Postictal" aggression is more common. In the confusional state following a seizure, individuals may be irritable, misinterpret others' attempts to help them as threatening, and actively resist attempts at restraint. The characteristics of postictal aggression reveal it also to be unplanned, undirected, and unsustained (Benjamin, 1999).

"Interictal" aggression refers to aggression that occurs at a time when the individual is not having a seizure. Interictal aggression is controversial. However, there does exist some support for an tendency toward increased interictal aggression in individuals having complex partial seizures (CPSs), especially those involving the temporal regions of the brain (Benjamin, 1999).

Up to 45% of seizures in youth are CPSs (Rothner, 1992). Temporal lobe epilepsy (TLE) is a common type of epilepsy that occurs in childhood and involves CPSs (Kim, 1991). CPSs may result in a wide range of psychiatric and behavioral problems, including mood, anxiety, psychotic, cognitive, personality, and disruptive behavior symptoms (Kim, 1991). There is support for an association between CPSs involving the temporal regions of the CNS and interictal aggressive behavior in children and adolescents. Evidence for an association comes from two sources. First, children with CPSs (especially TLE) have been found to have a high prevalence of aggression and higher rates of aggression than children with other types of seizures or epilepsy. Nuffield (1961) developed an aggression score for 322 children with TLE, petit mal epilepsy, or grand mal epilepsy. The children with TLE had aggression scores four times higher than those of children with petit mal epilepsy. Over a 30-year period, Ounsted and Lindsay (1981) longitudinally studied 1,000 children with every type of seizure disorder and found 100 with TLE. Rage attacks were found in 36 of the 100 children with TLE, and these predicted a poor adult outcome in general, as well as specific associations with adult antisocial behaviors and psychiatric disorders. In this childhood TLE sample, no gender difference was found for aggressive behavior; girls and boys with TLE were equally aggressive. A high rate of aggression was reported in youth referred for inpatient psychiatric hospitalization who also were found to have CPSs (Szabo & Magnus, 1999). Second, youth with early-onset, chronic, and severe aggression and conduct problems have been found to have a high rate of CPSs. In a study of 97 incarcerated delinquent boys, 18 were found to have CPSs. This was a much higher rate of CPSs (about 5%) than was thought to exist in the background population (Lewis, Pincus, Shanok, & Glaser, 1982). In this study, the number of epileptic psychomotor symptoms was correlated with the degree of violence in the study sample.

Although there is evidence that CPSs and especially TLE have an association with aggression, the strength of the correlation weakens when controls for psychosocial variables and brain damage are utilized. In the Ounsted and Lindsay (1981) study, most of the children with aggressive outbursts suffered their first seizure early in life, exhibited hyperactive–impulsive behavior, and had cognitive delays. Children with TLE alone, without other evidence of neurological dysfunction, did not exhibit rage attacks. A study of patients with TLE and aggressive behavior found that the factors correlating most strongly with aggression were nonspecific and not related to the severity of the epilepsy; they were more closely related to social factors and the extent of brain damage (Herzberg & Fenwick, 1988). Psychotic symptoms and illogical thinking have been reported to be more common in epileptic children and adolescents, especially those with CPSs (Caplan et al., 1997). These neurocognitive symptoms could also account for the statistical association between CPSs and aggression. Indeed, Lewis et al. (1982) found that epileptic psychomotor symptoms also correlated independently with the presence of psychotic symptoms, including hallucinations, thought disorder, and paranoid ideation. These symptoms may have contributed to the risk of aggression in this sample, independently of any association with epilepsy. Studies have examined the relative role of parent–child relationships, family stress, and seizure factors in predicting behavior problems in children with epilepsy. These investigations have found evidence that the quality of child–parent relationships predicts the development of externalizing behavior problems in boys with epilepsy, over and above the influence of seizure-related factors (Pianta & Lothman, 1994). Finally, some controlled studies have not reported an increase in aggressive behaviors in children suffering from CPSs compared to children with idiopathic generalized epilepsies (Whitman, Hermann, Black, & Chhabria, 1982).

In summary, aggression is a complex behavior with multiple determinants; it is typically not caused by a single factor, such as a seizure disorder. A relationship between aggressive behavior and epilepsy, especially CPSs or TLE, probably does exist. However, the nature of the association is not clear. The relationship is most likely due to nonspecific risk factors that are common to patients with both aggressive behavior and epilepsy. The extent and location of brain damage, and antecedent and ongoing psychosocial variables (such as family stress, family psychopathology, and the quality of the child–parent interaction), may be most important in predicting externalizing behavior problems in youth with epilepsy.

CHAPTER SUMMARY

This chapter has reviewed hormones, neurotransmitters, neurobiological–behavioral models, and neurological disorders that are important in understanding human aggression. Findings from studies assessing possible associations of cortisol, testosterone, and the monoamines with aggression and related behaviors are presented. The findings regarding cortisol and androgens are mixed. Some evidence has been found to support the hypothesis that low

CNS 5-HT functioning is linked with diminished inhibition, and thus with aggressive and related problems. Other evidence supports the hypothesis that low CNS NE functioning contributes to low levels of anxiety and thus to increased risk for aggressive/antisocial behaviors. Little evidence presently indicates that enhanced CNS DA functioning contributes to reward-driven behaviors, and thus to aggressive/antisocial behaviors.

Larger neurobiological–behavioral models and their relationship to aggression and related behaviors are increasingly receiving research attention. These include the biobehavioral systems model of Gray and the neurobiological understanding of fear conditioning. The relationship between neurological disorders (specifically, TBI and epilepsy) and aggression remains complicated and unclear.

⊠ CHAPTER 8

Integrated Models of Aggression and Related Behaviors

The previous chapters demonstrate that many psychosocial, psycho-biological, and neurobiological variables are correlated with aggression and related behaviors in youth. Indeed, much is presently known about factors that have a relationship with early-onset, maladaptive aggressive behavior in the young. These include intrinsic child factors, parenting factors, and environmental factors. Clearly, aggression research does not lack data.

However, much less is known about how to integrate disparate, correlational data into working models that explain how a particular child with a specific set of risk and protective factors, living with a certain set of parents in a specific environment, does or does not develop maladaptive aggression at a particular time in his or her development. In other words, aggression research lacks models for integrating data that are able to account for multiple factors over the course of development to determine risk. Such models would indeed be useful in identifying high-risk children before maladaptive aggressive behavior becomes entrenched, and in developing targeted prevention efforts for these children.

Such integrated models with high predictive accuracy do not yet exist in the field to guide prevention and clinical efforts. However, recent developments in two areas have helped move aggression research from an emphasis on univariate, main-effects models toward more multivariable, integrated models. These recent developments include the emerging field of developmental psychopathology and the study of biosocial interactions in the genesis of aggression.

DEVELOPMENTAL PSYCHOPATHOLOGY

The study of childhood psychopathology, including aggression and related be-haviors, is complicated by the fact that it does not come in neat little packages that are separate and distinct from one another. Most types of childhood psychopathology are known to overlap and to coexist with other problems. This remains evident whether childhood psychopathology is considered as a group of categorical psychiatric diagnoses or as continuous dimensions of problem behavior in the population.

It has also become increasingly clear that aggression and antisocial behaviors cannot be attributed to a single unitary cause. These behaviors are likely to result from multiple, frequently co-occurring, reciprocal, and inter-acting risk factors, causal events, and processes, all of which may differ depending on a child's gender and developmental age (Mash & Dozois, 1996).

In response to the challenges that arise in attempting to study complicated, reciprocal, transactional developmental processes in youth, there have been calls for integration of findings from diverse fields. A new holistic field of inquiry has emerged in the last 20 years, called "developmental science" (Magnusson, 1999). Developmental science constitutes a scientific discipline whose focus is on individual functioning as a total, integrated, complex, and adaptive system—a system that is contextually dependent on environmental factors, and that develops and changes across the individual's lifespan. Developmental science seeks to understand all of the mental, psychological, biological, behavioral, and environmental factors that interact at particular points in an individual's development to form the potentialities and set the restrictions for a nested developmental process of maturation and experiences (Magnusson, 1999). These factors function simultaneously in the individual, and developmental science seeks to place them in a coherent theoretical frame-work, in which the individual in his or her environment forms the organizing principle. Developmental science is conceptualized as drawing on cross-disci-plinary collaboration among the fields of developmental biology, physiology, molecular biology, neuroscience, developmental psychology, sociology, and anthropology. As such, it takes its place at the interface among the behavioral, biological, medical, and social sciences (Magnusson, 1999).

"Developmental psychopathology" is a subset of developmental science that seeks to provide a broad template and general principles for understanding the development of psychopathology in children. The purview of the field of developmental psychopathology includes the range of processes and mechanisms underlying why and how psychopathology emerges in children and adolescents, how psychopathology changes in an individual over time, and how it is influenced by the child's developmental capacities and by the contexts in which development occurs (Cicchetti, 1984; Kazdin, 1989; Mash & Dozois, 1996). Sroufe and Rutter (1984) define the field as the study of the origins and course of individual patterns of behavioral maladaptation, whatever the age of onset, causes, transformations in behavioral manifestation, and other complexities may be. Developmental psychopathology seeks to provide a general framework within which to understand both normal and maladaptive development. As such, the field does not focus exclusively on the study of childhood disorders, categorical psychiatric diagnoses, or problematic dimensions of maladaptive behavior; instead, it serves to inform the understanding and treatment of these problems in youth through the study of a full range of developmental processes and outcomes. The field emphasizes multiperspective and interacting influences on maladaptive childhood behavior, and stresses the importance of individual biological and psychological factors, parental and family factors, and environmental factors in predicting and understanding adaptive and maladaptive individual developmental changes. Therefore, individual psychological processes cannot be studied in isolation from individual biological factors or from the parental, familial, and environmental contexts to which the individual must adapt and with which he or she must cope.

Four principles that define the field of developmental psychopathology have been articulated (Sroufe & Rutter, 1984): (1) an interest in childhood problem behaviors, but also in the relationships between psychopathology and normal development and socialization across time and development; (2) the examination of disordered behaviors in terms of their deviation from the usual patterns of adaptation within a given developmental period; (3) an interest in nonpathological childhood behavior patterns that may predict risk for later disorder; and (4) an interest in patterns of childhood behavior that generally predict later disorder but do not do so in a particular subset of children (i.e., prediction of resilience).

A developmental psychopathology perspective is guided by a number of assumptions that characterize organizational theories of development more generally (Rutter et al., 1997). These include the following:

1. Individuals differ in their reactivity to features of the environment. For example, extroverted individuals may react differently from introverted individuals to a particular stimulus.

2. A two-way interaction exists between individuals and their environments. For example, in males high levels of testosterone are associated with aggression (an example of hormones influencing behavior). But dominance in social situations also raises testosterone levels in males (an example of behavior influencing hormones) (see Rutter et al., 1997).

3. The interplay between the person and the environment needs to be considered within a broader social context. For example, the association between antisocial behavior and low socioeconomic status (SES) may lie in family interaction patterns, such that families in poverty may promote beliefs supporting aggression in children (Guerra, Huesmann, Tolan, Van Acker, & Eron, 1995).

4. Children and adolescents process their experiences rather than serve as passive recipients of environmental forces. For example, Dodge and Frame (1982) have shown that aggressive boys develop biases toward misattributing hostile intent to others in ambiguous social situations where in fact no hostile intent actually exists.

5. Children and adolescents act on their environments so as to shape and select their experiences. For example, children with difficult temperaments may elicit more harsh parental discipline than children with easy temperaments (Lahey, Waldman, & McBurnett, 1999).

6. Surface behavioral patterns for an individual may change over the course of development, whereas underlying vulnerabilities to disorder persist over time. This phenomenon is termed "heterotypic continuity." For example, antisocial traits may show moderate to strong stability over the course of development, yet the surface manifestations of the underlying propensity will change with growth and development. In a toddler, this propensity may express itself as irritable, oppositional behavior; in a school-age child, as fighting and stealing; and in an adolescent, as substance misuse, irresponsible sexual behavior, or crime (Hinshaw & Anderson, 1996).

7. All forms of childhood psychopathology are best conceptualized in terms of longitudinal, developmental trajectories, rather than as static entities at particular points in development. The expression and outcome for any problem for a particular child will depend on the configuration and timing of a host of surrounding circumstances, which include events both within and outside of the individual child.

A developmental psychopathology approach is well suited to the study of aggression and related behaviors in youngsters. Univariate, main-effects models of aggression have failed to explain the complicated person–environment transactions that predispose some individuals to persistent aggression across development. Main-effects models have also proven inadequate to explain why some high-risk youth do not develop chronic aggressive/antisocial behaviors. The framework of a developmental psychopathology approach to such problems in youth allows for consideration of a broad range of interacting individual child, parental, family, and environmental variables, including biological as well as psychological processes, in the development, maintenance, and/or desistance of maladaptive aggression across development.

However, the field of developmental psychopathology is relatively new, and a robust scientific literature utilizing its principles is just now accruing. As a result, less is known about the developmental psychopathology of aggression than is needed to allow for accurate predictions of risk and to precisely inform treatment for specific children and adolescents. In the following sections, several models of juvenile aggression and related behaviors, that utilize principles of developmental psychopathology are described. All of these models emphasize the importance of studying disordered behaviors by following at-risk children over time, using developmental trajectories to help predict which individuals will persist in such behaviors and which individuals will eventually desist from such behaviors (i.e., continuities and discontinuities in development). In addition, all of the models emphasize the importance of investigating multiple person–environment factors that interact in reciprocal ways over development to influence final outcomes.

Coercive Family Process

In their very influential research on the development of antisocial and aggressive behavior in children, Gerald Patterson and his colleagues studied children with conduct problems and their families. Over 200 families and their children referred for treatment at the Oregon Social Learning Center were compared with hundreds of normal control families. Patterson's group studied family structure and processes on multiple levels to determine what individual child, parent, and family/contextual variables result in the formation and persistence of aggressive/antisocial behaviors in children (Patterson, 1982). Patterson's "coercive family process" theory posits that parents and children in families with aggressive/antisocial children interact in such a way that the children's negative behaviors are behaviorally reinforced. This integrated theory (which has been mentioned briefly in Chapter 5) has the support of much empirical evidence (Patterson, 1982; Patterson, Reid, & Dishion, 1992). An illustration of the theory is presented in Figure 8.1.

Patterson's theory focuses on negative reinforcement of aggressive/antisocial behaviors. A behavior is negatively reinforced when it allows an individual to escape from a noxious, aversive, anxious, or unpleasant situation or task. In coercive family process theory, the negative behavior of one member of a parent–child dyad serves to terminate the ongoing negative behavior of the other, thereby negatively reinforcing the first member's original negative behavior. For example, if a parent attempts to impose a command that the child finds aversive, the child may resist the command by engaging in oppositional, aggressive, or noncompliant behavior. In the face of such behavior, the

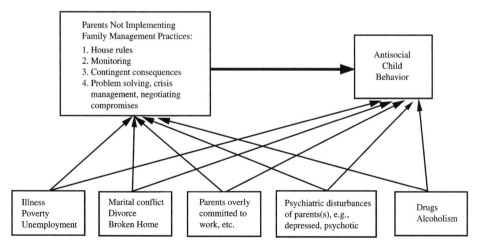

FIGURE 8.1. The relationships among family management practices, contextual variables, and antisocial child behavior. From Patterson (1982, p. 217). Copyright 1982 by Gerald R. Patterson. Reprinted by permission.

parent may abandon his or her original command, and the child escapes from the aversive task. The child's success at escaping the command, no matter how temporary it may be, increases the likelihood that the child will resist again. The more a parent persists in repeating an aversive request, the more intense the child's resistance may become. The child's resistance may habitually become so intense that the parent habitually backs down. The child thus learns that negative behavior is successful. A parent may acquire aggressive or coercive behavior toward a child in much the same manner. The parent may be temporarily successful at getting a noncompliant child to obey by yelling, threatening, or using physical aggression against the child. If the parent is successful and the child obeys, the adult is negatively reinforced for his or her behavior by escaping the aversive situation of the child's disobedience. In this manner, a coercive cycle is born. Over time the coercive cycle escalates and may generalize out of the home into school or the community. The child has learned that aggressive/antisocial behaviors "work" to solve social problems.

Patterson depicts a breakdown in positive parenting practices at the core of coercive family process theory. In families of aggressive/antisocial children, parents stop implementing house rules, monitoring their children's whereabouts, using appropriate negotiating techniques, and uniformly and consistently applying consequences that fit the children's negative behaviors. Family/contextual variables also play a role in diminishing positive parenting practices (see the lower boxes in Figure 8.1). Thus coercive family process theory is an integrated understanding of child, parent, and family/environmental variables in the formation of juvenile aggression and antisocial behaviors.

The Developmental Progression from Early Oppositional Behavior to Later Conduct Disorder

Another line of inquiry concerns the developmental progression from oppositional and difficult behaviors in infancy to oppositional defiant disorder (ODD) in early childhood, and finally to conduct disorder (CD) in late childhood and adolescence. This research utilizes categorical psychiatric diagnoses and asks which children meeting diagnostic criteria for ODD in the preschool years will go on to develop the more serious diagnosis of CD in later childhood. A general model for this progression is presented in Figure 8.2.

As Figure 8.2 shows, normative infant and early childhood oppositional behaviors may actually follow one of two developmental pathways, depending on the influence of various interacting individual, parental, and peer factors (Loeber, Green, Lahey, Christ, & Frick, 1992; Loeber, Keenan, Lahey, Green, & Thomas, 1993; Loeber, Wung, et al., 1993; Loeber & Hay, 1994). In the normative pathway, infant oppositional behaviors undergo a slow process of progressive socialization under the influence of normative and appropriate parenting and school pressures, which results in a general lessening of oppositional and defiant behaviors. This lessening first begins to be noticeable at about age 6 years and continues to diminish throughout the elementary

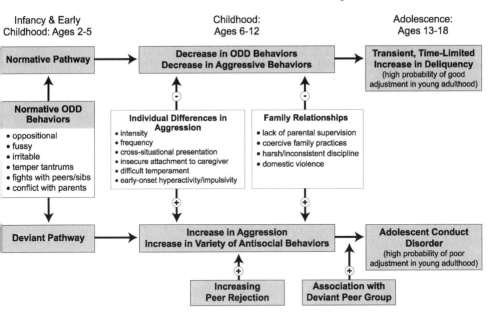

FIGURE 8.2. The developmental pathway leading to CD in later childhood and adolescence, beginning with difficult infant temperament and early ODD-like behavior. Data from Loeber, Keenan, Lahey, Green, and Thomas (1993).

school years. Under the influence of adolescent development and teenage peer influences, premature experimentation with adult activities such as drinking alcohol, smoking, and staying out late at night may occur, and transient and time-limited increases in delinquency are frequently observed. In the normative pathway, however, the prognosis for eventual good adjustment in the early adult years is high.

In contrast, a second, more deviant pathway is highlighted. In this pathway, normative early childhood oppositional behaviors become influenced by a variety of individual difference factors, parenting and family factors, and peer factors to result in the development of CD by elementary school age or early adolescence. These risk factors have been more fully discussed in Chapters 4–7 of this book. As various maladaptive behaviors emerge in elementary school, the aggressive child is increasingly rejected by more successful and prosocial classmates and begins to associate with a deviant peer group. This sets the stage for serious aggressive/antisocial behavior in adolescence. The prognosis for eventual good adjustment in the early adult years becomes progressively weaker.

Evidence to support an orderly sequence in the emergence of CD from early ODD has come from the Pittsburgh Youth Study, a longitudinal investigation of the emergence of these disorders, in a sample of 177 clinic-referred boys who were aged 7–12 years at the time of initial assessment (Loeber,

Keenan, et al., 1993). They were reevaluated at approximately yearly intervals, with a nearly universal retention rate across follow-up assessments. The
research design allowed the emergence of disruptive behavior disorders to be
observed prospectively. Results showed that oppositional behaviors generally
emerged before more serious antisocial behaviors in boys who progressed
from ODD to CD (Loeber, Wung, et al., 1993; Loeber & Hay, 1994). Figure
8.3 depicts this progression.

Although there was a wide range in the age of onset and a large overlap
of symptoms in boys, stubborn behaviors tended to emerge first, followed by
defiant behaviors including disobedience. Minor covertly aggressive acts, such
as lying and shoplifting, occurred next. Mild aggression such as bullying was
followed by acts of property damage, including vandalism and fire setting. In
the early adolescent years, more serious maladaptive behaviors emerged; these
included physical fighting and violence, as well as avoidance of authority (e.g.,
truancy from school, runaway behavior, and staying out late at night). Data
are much more sparse on the development of CD in girls (see Chapter 9), but
the Pittsburgh results indicate a recognizable developmental pathway in the
progression of ODD to CD for at least some boys.

The next question concerns the predictive utility of ODD in early childhood. In other words, which boys who manifest early-onset ODD will progress to more serious CD by middle childhood or early adolescence? Data
indicate that the majority of boys with early-onset ODD behaviors do not
progress to CD. In the Pittsburgh Youth Study (Loeber, Keenan, et al., 1993),
about 33% of boys initially diagnosed with ODD went on to develop CD at

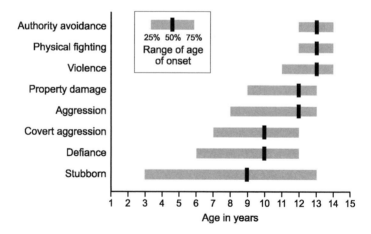

FIGURE 8.3. The orderly emergence of CD behaviors from early
ODD symptoms. From Loeber, Wung, et al. (1993). Copyright
1993 by Cambridge University Press. Reprinted by permission.

the 3-year follow-up. However, 66% did not. Of the youth who did progress to later CD, all met criteria for earlier ODD. As CD developed, these boys generally retained the symptoms of earlier ODD as well (Loeber, Keenan, et al., 1993). In other words, ODD symptoms were not replaced by CD symptoms; symptoms of CD were added to the already existing ODD symptoms. Although many boys meeting psychiatric diagnostic criteria for earlier ODD did not progress to CD, in this study a prior diagnosis of ODD led to a three-fold increase in risk for the development of CD by the 2-year follow-up (Loeber, Keenan, et al., 1993).

Thus the prediction of CD from a prior diagnosis of ODD appears to be highly sensitive. Hinshaw and Anderson (1996) note that over 90% of boys with CD have previously met (and retain) diagnostic criteria for ODD. However, the positive predictive power of the association (i.e., the ability to determine *which* boys with ODD will progress to CD) is far lower than the sensitivity; only about one-third of boys with ODD progress to CD. Hinshaw and Anderson (1996) found that approximately one-half of boys diagnosed with ODD maintained this diagnosis over the follow-up study period without progressing to CD, and that a lesser percentage of boys diagnosed with initial ODD desisted over time and did not meet diagnostic criteria for ODD or CD at follow-up. Therefore, although a clear developmental pathway from early-onset ODD to later CD appears to exist, it does so for only a minority of boys.

Different opinions about the importance of these findings exist. On the one hand, the ability to identify young boys with ODD who are at increased risk of developing more serious antisocial behavior in later childhood is very important. Later CD is very resistant to change, and early identification of at-risk boys might allow early intervention strategies to be delivered at a younger developmental period, where symptoms may prove to be more amenable to change. It is known that the stability coefficients of antisocial behaviors and CD increase with age, and that treatments for CD are less effective than treatments for ODD (Loeber, Lahey, & Thomas, 1991). Therefore, the early identification of boys meeting diagnostic criteria for ODD is very important. On the other hand, with such a low positive predictive power, most boys with ODD will not progress to CD. Early intervention efforts that target all boys with ODD will be expensive for society and may be misguided. The data suggest that infants and preschool children who exhibit early-onset hyperactivity, have frequent and intense attacks of temper, and live in families characterized by nonoptimal parenting practices and domestic violence are at high risk for progression to more serious and stable antisocial behaviors. These children should qualify for early intervention services to prevent the formation of later stable patterns of aggression. Highly needed is more precise research investigating the specific risk and protective factors that propel some boys with ODD toward a more stable antisocial developmental trajectory and cause other boys to follow a nonantisocial life course.

Antisocial Propensity and the Risk for Antisocial Behavior

The next model identifies a construct labeled "antisocial propensity" and integrates it with developmental trends to help explain the growth of antisocial behavior in certain individuals (Lahey, Waldman, et al., 1999). Antisocial propensity is defined as a quality of the individual and is inferred from individual differences and individual variations in aggressive, criminal, and other antisocial behaviors (Gottfredson & Hirschi, 1990). Youngsters with greater antisocial propensity are thought to be more likely to engage in physically aggressive/antisocial behaviors, to begin these behaviors at an earlier age of onset, and to persist in them through the teenage and young adult years.

In order to prevent circularity of reasoning, constituents of an individual's antisocial propensity have been hypothesized. These include male gender, impulsive responding, daring, low intelligence, a high motor activity level, and physical strength (Farrington, 1995; Gottfredson & Hirschi, 1990). These person-specific differences in antisocial propensity interact with environmental and situational influences across development to result in individual differences in the expression of antisocial behavior. Thus this model attempts to integrate person and environmental variables in a model of causation of the development of antisocial behavior (Lahey, Waldman, et al., 1999).

Many factors contribute to antisocial propensity through multiple overlapping and mutually influencing causal sequences. The model proposes that the same causal sequences apply to youth whose antisocial behavior emerges at all ages (from early childhood through late adolescence), and in girls as well as boys, but that the relative strength of the influences changes with age and gender. For youngsters with earlier-onset antisocial behavior, antisocial propensity is the net result of multiple aspects of genetically influenced temperament and neurocognitive vulnerabilities that are transformed into aggressive/antisocial behaviors through successive transactions with the social environment. The causal role of genetic factors is indirect and is mediated through heritable effects on individual temperament and neurocognitive abilities. As youngsters become older, the role of genetic influences in antisocial behavior declines, and the importance of purely environmental factors increases. Thus peer influences are more important in the genesis of antisocial behaviors at older ages of onset. For girls, earlier development of verbal communication skills (Keenan & Shaw, 1997), higher levels of empathy and guilt (Kochanska, De Vet, Goldman, Murray, & Putnam, 1994), and different parental disciplinary responses to difficult child behavior and temperament (Keenan & Shaw, 1997) may contribute to differences in the levels and effects of causal variables in antisocial propensity. However, the model proposes that these variables remain the same in girls and boys (Lahey, Waldman, et al., 1999).

The key variables that influence individual antisocial propensity, which then determines individual differences in antisocial outcome across time and development, are depicted schematically in Figure 8.4. These variables include temperamental, neurocognitive, parental, and environmental variables, all of

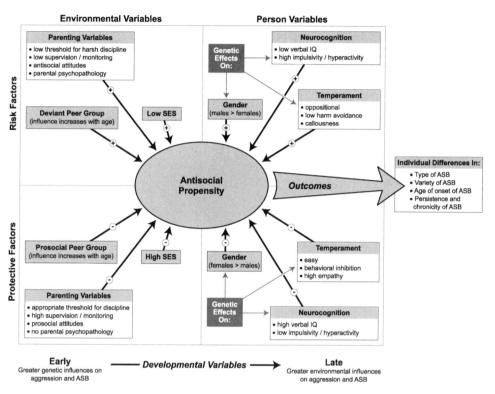

FIGURE 8.4. Antisocial propensity, developmental trends, and individual differences in antisocial behavior (ASB) outcomes. Data from Lahey, Waldman, and McBurnett (1999).

which are discussed more fully in Chapters 4–7. Temperamental contributions to antisocial propensity include oppositional (or difficult) temperament, low levels of the dimension of "harm avoidance," and high levels of the personality dimension of "callous–unemotional behavior" (see Chapters 4 and 5). In childhood, maladaptive interactions with parents and others in the child's life transform difficult infant temperament into arguing, defiance, vindictiveness, and intentionally annoying others—the symptoms of ODD. The dimension of harm avoidance was first described by Cloninger (1987b) and has also been called "behavioral inhibition" (Kagan, 1994). Infants and children high in harm avoidance are anxious, shy, inhibited, and apprehensive. Such children are less likely to engage in antisocial behaviors than children low in harm avoidance (Tremblay, Pihl, Vitaro, & Dobkin, 1994). A dimension of personality in children similar to psychopathy in adults has been described as callous–unemotional behavior (Frick, O'Brien, Wootton, & McBurnett, 1994; see Chapter 4). Children high in such behavior display more conduct problems (Frick et al., 1994).

Neurocognitive contributions to antisocial propensity include high levels of impulsivity–hyperactivity and low verbal intelligence (see Chapters 4 and 6 for discussion). Better-developed verbal communication skills protect against the development of antisocial behavior (Lynam, Moffitt, & Stouthamer-Loeber, 1993). More verbally proficient toddlers and preschoolers may be easier to parent and to socialize, and may prove less frustrating to parents; lower verbal ability in offspring may interfere with parents' early efforts to socialize their children. At older ages, children with better-developed verbal skills may be more adept at anticipating the consequences of their antisocial behaviors and at adopting more prosocial alternative strategies. Early-onset impulsivity and hyperactivity are robust predictors of future conduct problems (Loeber, Green, Keenan, & Lahey, 1995).

Parenting factors that contribute to risk for antisocial outcomes in youth include harsh and inconsistent discipline, low levels of supervising and monitoring offspring in the home and neighborhood, and parental attitudes that do not define antisocial behavior as something that should be discouraged in offspring (see Chapter 5 for discussion). Parenting practices may interact with demographic variables to explain the well-known inverse relationship between SES and antisocial behavior. Across gender and ethnicity, much of the relationship between low family income and delinquency, crime, and aggression in children can be accounted for by less parental monitoring and supervising of offspring behavior at lower levels of family SES (Lahey, Waldman, et al., 1999). Daily life stressors, more common in families of lower SES, may also contribute to a lower threshold for inappropriate parental responses to child misbehavior—responses that serve to foster, rather than discourage, the development of children's antisocial behavior.

Peer influences on the development of antisocial behavior appear to vary with age. The association of antisocial children with similar peers during elementary school does not seem to influence risk for displaying antisocial behavior in the future among children who already display such behavior (Bartusch, Lynam, Moffitt, & Silva, 1997). However, the influence of delinquent peers on adolescent-onset antisocial behavior appears much stronger. Association with antisocial peers is related to the later emergence of new antisocial behavior during adolescence among youths who did not exhibit behavior problems as children (Bartusch et al., 1997).

In summary, the model depicted in Figure 8.4 describes an integrative causal approach to the development of antisocial behavior in youth that integrates person and environmental variables, and risk, and protective factors, to help explain variations in individual vulnerability to the expression of antisocial behavior over the course of development. Stable individual differences in antisocial propensity reflect variations in several different temperamental and neurocognitive abilities, each with their own genetic and environmental influences. Individual antisocial propensity in turn interacts with a number of social influences over the course of development. The net result is an individual's risk for the expression of antisocial behavior.

Multiple Pathways to the Development
of Aggressive/Antisocial Behaviors

A final model based on developmental psychopathology illustrates developmental sequences in the crystallization of serious aggressive/antisocial behaviors over time, and demonstrates that multiple pathways within different forms of these behaviors may exist. This model shows that less serious forms of aggression and antisocial behaviors generally precede more serious forms, as noted earlier in discussing the progression of ODD to CD. It also demonstrates that whereas many youngsters may engage in the milder forms of these behaviors, many fewer youth progress over time to the more serious forms. Finally, the model illustrates different developmental pathways for different types of aggressive and antisocial behaviors, including (1) an authority conflict pathway, (2) a covert pathway, and (3) an overt pathway (Loeber, Wung, et al., 1993; Loeber & Hay, 1994; Loeber & Stouthamer-Loeber, 1998).

In a series of studies, developmental sequences in disruptive behavior in three community samples of boys from the first, fourth, and seventh grades were traced both retrospectively and prospectively over a period of 3 years (Loeber, Wung, et al., 1993; Loeber & Hay, 1997). Each group, oversampled to contain high percentages of boys with disruptive behaviors, contained approximately 500 boys. The three developmental pathways in antisocial behavior that were distinguished are illustrated in Figure 8.5.

In this model, the authority conflict pathway is the earliest to emerge and begins in childhood. This pathway begins with stubborn behavior and gradually escalates to defiance (e.g., doing things one's own way, refusing to do things, disobedience). The final stage of this pathway is authority avoidance (e.g., truancy, running away, staying out late at night). This final stage is reached in early adolescence. Of the boys who entered this pathway in Loeber and colleagues' research, about half started with the first step in the sequence, about a quarter entered at the second step and skipped the first step entirely, and slightly more than 16% entered at the third step (Loeber, Wung, et al., 1993). Of the boys entering the authority conflict pathway at the first step, 11% proceeded over time through the full sequence to authority avoidance, 13% showed the first two steps in the sequence, and 16% exhibited stubborn behavior (the first step) only and did not proceed further in the sequence (Loeber, Wung, et al., 1993). In these research studies, the majority of boys fit the proposed developmental sequence, and only 13% of the sample did not fit the succession of stages (e.g., experiencing authority avoidance prior to the onset of stubborn behavior). Of the three developmental pathways, the authority conflict pathway had the earliest age of onset. The outcomes for boys in this pathway was relatively benign. Boys who advanced in the authority conflict pathway experienced some antisocial behaviors at outcome, but had generally low rates of delinquency and low rates of meeting criteria for later CD (Loeber, Wung, et al., 1993).

The next pathway in the model involves escalation in covert problem be-

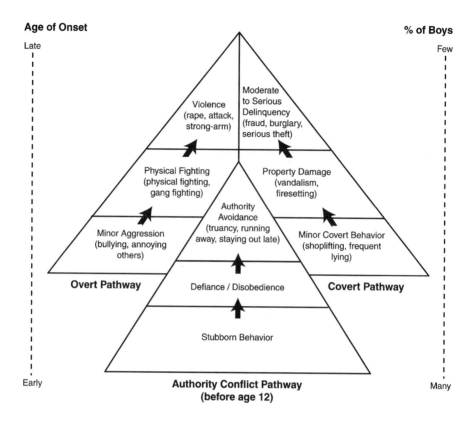

FIGURE 8.5. Multiple pathways to the development of aggression and antisocial behavior. From Loeber and Hay (1994). Copyright 1994 by Blackwell Science Ltd. Reprinted by permission.

haviors. These are defined as hidden, furtive acts that generally do not involve direct physical confrontation with other individuals. The covert pathway starts with minor covert behaviors such as lying and shoplifting. Progression to property damage, such as vandalism and fire setting, defines the next stage in the sequence. Finally, moderate to serious forms of delinquency occur (e.g., car theft, breaking into others' property, drug dealing, and pickpocketing). More than half of the boys studied by Loeber's group entered this sequence at the first step of minor covert behavior. Far fewer boys entered at the second step, and very few boys entered the covert pathway by skipping directly to the third step. Of younger children at study entry, about 10% progressed through all three steps; of older children at study entry, about 20% progressed through all three steps of the covert pathway. The majority of boys fit the developmental sequence of the covert pathway. However, between 22% and 33% of boys experienced the steps out of order (i.e., did not fit the sequence). Prognosis in this pathway was less benign: At outcome, slightly more youth in the covert pathway met criteria for CD and self-reported more delinquency than boys in the authority conflict pathway (Loeber, Wung, et al., 1993).

The third pathway in this model consists of escalation in overtly aggressive behaviors, defined as direct physical confrontation with other individuals. This sequence begins with minor acts of overt aggression, such as bullying and annoying others. The next stage is escalation to physical fighting, either as an individual or as part of a gang. Finally, escalation to serious violence (e.g., attacking others and forcing sexual activity onto others) occurs. In this research, boys who entered the overt pathway, more than half began at the first step of the sequence. Fewer boys entered at the second step, and it was rare for boys to enter the overt pathway at the third step (Loeber, Wung, et al., 1993). Of the youngest boys (first-graders at study entry), almost 74% of those who entered the overt pathway progressed through all the stages to violence. About 56% of the fourth-grade boys and about 37% of the boys who entered the study at seventh grade progressed to the final stage (Loeber & Stouthamer-Loeber, 1998). Thus many more boys who entered the overt pathway completed all steps in the sequence than boys who entered the authority conflict or covert pathways. There may have been less desistance from aggressive behaviors for boys in this pathway than for those in the other two pathways. The data also suggest that the prognosis for youngsters entering the overt pathway varied inversely with age of entry: boys with early-onset overt aggression appeared to have a worse prognosis than boys with overt aggression first displayed later in childhood. At outcome, youth in the overt pathway were slightly more court-involved than youth in the other pathways, but, surprisingly, none met criteria for CD (Loeber, Wung, et al., 1993).

The majority of boys displaying behaviors characteristic of one pathway also displayed behaviors characteristic of other pathways. In other words, most boys advanced on more than one pathway simultaneously over the course of development. For these boys, the prognosis was far worse than for boys who advanced on only one pathway. Boys on all three pathways (authority conflict, covert, and overt) had the highest rates of court involvement at outcome, delinquent acts, and violence. Poor outcomes were also found for boys in the dual covert–overt and authority conflict–covert pathways. These youths achieved rates of CD ranging between 9% and 29% at outcome. In contrast, boys advancing on the overt pathway alone or in the authority conflict pathway alone had the best outcomes, with rates of eventual CD ranging only between 2% and 5% (Loeber, Wung, et al., 1993).

In summary, this model distinguishes among three pathways to the development of aggressive/antisocial behaviors. A multiple-pathways model discriminates better among different degrees and types of deviance than is possible with the formulation of only a single developmental pathway. This model shows that in general less serious behaviors precede more serious ones, and that for the majority of boys aggressive/antisocial behaviors proceed in an orderly and knowable fashion across development. Although many boys may engage in such behaviors early in childhood, far fewer progress to serious forms of violence and delinquency in adolescence, and many desist from further aggression and antisocial behavior. The model also reveals that certain combinations of pathways are more powerful indicators of serious negative outcome than other pathways. This appears particularly true for boys following the triple pathway and for boys in the dual covert–overt and authority conflict–covert pathways. Identification of an individual's position on a pathway not only specifies present problems, but suggests what problems may occur next. Thus such knowledge can promote prevention of future steps in the sequence, in addition to clinical intervention with the current problems (Loeber & Stouthamer-Loeber, 1998).

Summary of Developmental Psychopathology Models

Developmental psychopathology is an emerging field of study that may offer a way to integrate multiple, diverse correlates of aggression and related behaviors into developmentally sensitive models that emphasize interactions between person and environmental variables, as well as between risk and protective factors. Models integrating developmental psychopathology perspectives may prove more facile in predicting risk for antisocial outcomes for individuals than single-variable, main-effects models.

This section has described four models of the development of aggressive/antisocial behaviors in children and adolescents. A model depicting coercive parent–child practices, the importance of negative reinforcement, and the abandonment of positive parenting practices in families with aggressive/antisocial children is presented first. A developmental pathway from difficult temperament in early childhood to later ODD and eventual CD in some, but not all, boys is then discussed. A third model introduces the concept of "antisocial propensity" as a key construct to explain individual differences in the risk for and type of antisocial behaviors at outcome. The multiple-pathways model demonstrates distinctions and differences in the development of aggressive/antisocial behaviors in youth. Eventual antisocial outcome may best be understood by differences in three developmental pathways encompassing sequential steps in conflicts with authority, covertly aggressive acts, and overtly aggressive acts.

Developmental psychopathology as it applies to juvenile aggression is a new and emerging field of study. A major task for the future is to begin to integrate research findings such as autonomic nervous system (ANS) underarousal (discussed in Chapters 6 and 7), indices of reduced central nervous system (CNS) serotonin (5-HT) functioning (discussed in Chapter 7), and perinatal risk factors such as *in utero* nicotine and alcohol exposure (discussed in Chapter 5) into existing developmental psychopathology models of the emergence of these behaviors.

BIOSOCIAL INTERACTIONS

An emerging area of investigation is the study of "biosocial interactions"—that is, interactions between biological variables and social/environmental variables in the etiology of juvenile CD and other forms of aggressive/antisocial behaviors (Brennan & Raine, 1997; Raine, Brennan, & Farrington, 1997). Since human behavior is determined by complex interactions between biological and contextual factors, it is hoped that research into biosocial interactions will prove more powerful in explaining the onset and maintenance of these behaviors than study of each factor individually. Despite the commonsense appeal of this idea, surprisingly little research on such biosocial interactions has been completed to date.

For the purposes of clarification, some definitions are required. A "biological" variable is defined as a biological measure of a biological construct. An example is measuring heart rate as an indicator of ANS arousal. Another example is measuring 5-HT receptors on blood platelets to estimate the integrity of CNS 5-HT neurotransmission. "Social" variables reflect measures of social and environmental constructs. An example is the SES of the family in which a child develops. From the perspective of the growing child, other social variables may include measures of parenting functioning or parental psychopathology, which shape the family environment and the parent–child interactions in which a child learns and matures.

However, some variables defy easy categorization. For example, where do neuropsychological variables such as IQ, infant temperament, or impulsivity fit? Intelligence as measured by IQ results from the interaction between the cognitive capabilities of the child and his or her experience in life over the course of development. Because cognition has substantial biological underpinnings (Afifi & Uc, 1998), for the purposes of the present discussion it is considered a biological variable. Similarly, temperament in infancy, which includes a broad array of behavioral traits, is considered to have a large hereditary component and, as a general construct, appears to be biologically determined (Bates, Pettit, Dodge, & Ridge, 1998). Impulsive responding, or an inability to inhibit behavioral responses to internal or external stimuli, also has a biological substrate in executive cognitive functioning mediated by the prefrontal cortex (Fuster, 1997). Because these neuropsychological variables have a substantial genetic component (and thus biological basis), for ease of exposition they are included in this discussion as biological variables.

Biological and social variables may interact in various ways in the etiology of aggression and related behaviors. Social variables may influence aggression through biological mechanisms. For example, physical abuse in early development (from the perspective of the child, a social variable) may result in head trauma (a biological variable), with a resultant increase in poor impulse control, leading to increased aggressive behavior in the abused child. Conversely, biological variables may influence aggression through social mechanisms. Children with low autonomic nervous system arousal (a biological variable) may be more likely to engage in dangerous behavior such as physical fighting than children with higher ANS arousal when a social conflict situation (an environmental variable) arises.

In research, social and biological variables relate to aggression in various ways. If a researcher demonstrates that biological variables are related to aggression independently of social variables (i.e., if he or she statistically controls for social variables) and vice versa, and both variables sets of make independent contributions to overall aggression, the total contribution of the variables may reflect several interactions. The outcome on aggressive behavior may reflect an additive interaction of biological and social variables (i.e., the sum of the parts). Or the interaction of independent biological and social variables may be nonadditive. This may occur when the final outcome on aggression reflects multiplicative or nonlinear effects of the interaction between biological and social variables on outcomes.

The aim of this section is to provide some examples of biosocial interaction research in the domain of juvenile aggressive/antisocial behaviors. The discussion is not meant to be exhaustive (although to date few biosocial studies of these behaviors have been completed). It is meant to illustrate how research investigating biosocial interactions in the development of early-onset aggressive/antisocial behaviors may offer more detailed explanations than single-variable main-effects models investigating only biological or only social variables in the origin of these behaviors. Some examples of genetic–environmental interactions are first considered, followed by examples of ANS–social interactions, neurological (broadly defined)–social interactions, and finally temperament–socialization interactions.

Genetic–Environment Interactions

Genetic–environmental interaction in the genesis of aggression and antisociality was examined in an adoption study mentioned in Chapter 5 (Cadoret, Yates, Troughton, Woodworth, & Stewart, 1995). In this research, adopted male and adopted female offspring of biological parents with documented antisocial personality disorder (ASPD) or substance use disorders (SUDs) were studied when they were between 18 and 47 years of age. Characteristics of the adoptees and the adoptive home environment (especially adoptive parents' marital problems, divorce, legal problems, SUDs, depression, and/or anxiety) were assessed at outcome. These adoptees were compared with adoptee control subjects whose biological background did not include any family members with ASPD or SUDs. Several interesting results were obtained. First, an adoptee biological background of ASPD predicted increased adolescent aggression and CD, and, when adoptees had grown into adulthood, increased rates of adult ASPD relative to controls. This finding was specific for an adoptee genetic background of ASPD and not for a genetic background of SUDs. Next, adverse adoptive home environments independently predicted increased adult ASPD in grown-up adoptees, but had no effect for early-onset aggression or CD in childhood or adolescence. Most importantly, an adverse adoptive home environment was found to result in significantly increased childhood aggression, childhood CD, adolescent aggression, and adult ASPD in adoptees *only* in the presence of—not in the absence of—a biological (genetic) background of ASPD (Cadoret et al., 1995).

Using similar adoption paradigms, four independent studies have now reported the finding of a nonlinear interactive effect of genetic factors and environmental factors in the genesis of early-onset conduct problems (Cadoret, Cain, & Crowe, 1983; Cadoret et al., 1995; Cloninger & Gottesman, 1987; Crowe, 1974). These studies demonstrates the interaction of genetic factors and adverse social factors in the genesis of aggression, CD, and other antisocial behaviors in children, adolescents, and adults. The interaction effects appear nonlinear and nonadditive (i.e., greater than the simple sum of their parts). Several points need to be emphasized. First, genetic–environmental interactions are frequently found only for early-onset aggression and conduct problems in children and adolescents. Generally, only environmental factors are found significant in the etiology of adult-onset antisocial behaviors. This suggests that genetic–environmental interaction effects may be of particular importance in the origins of early-onset aggression, which has the most chronicity and the worst prognosis (see Chapter 4). Thus further research on biosocial interactions in the vulnerability to early childhood-onset conduct problems is important, because it offers the possibility of yielding knowledge that might facilitate the early identification of children at risk for the worst outcomes, as well as the development of effective prevention strategies for these same children. Next, the Cadoret et al. (1995) study found no gender effects on the interaction of genetic vulnerability and adverse environmental factors in predicting aggressive/antisocial outcomes; the interaction pertained to girls as well as boys. Finally, this same study found that the specific genetic effect was for biological parental ASPD and not for biological parental SUDs. Although there exists little evidence for a direct genetic inheritance of aggression/antisociality, this research thus supports the importance of a biosocial interaction in specific vulnerability to early-onset antisocial behaviors.

ANS–Social Interactions

ANS underarousal has been linked to increased risk for aggression, delinquency, crime, and other antisocial behavior in youngsters. Resting heart rate and electrodermal activity (EDA) are laboratory measures that assess ANS functioning. ANS arousal is associated with laboratory measures of conditionability, which reflects aspects of learning (see Chapter 6). Several studies have examined the interaction between measures of ANS arousal and social characteristics of the families in which subjects were raised, to ascertain effects on aggressive and antisocial outcomes.

Wadsworth (1976) assessed resting heart rate in 1,813 British male children at age 11 years. A low resting heart rate was found to be associated with criminal convictions when subjects were between the ages of 8 and 21 years. The sample was then divided into children from intact family homes and children from homes broken by divorce or separation of parents in the first 4 years of life; low resting heart rate was found to be statistically associated with increased risk for criminal conviction only in the children raised in intact homes. This study suggests a biosocial interaction, such that biological characteristics of the individual (such as low ANS arousal) may have greater explanatory power in predicting antisocial behavior (such as crime) in environments where the social risk factors for antisocial behavior are less (Raine, Brennan, & Farrington, 1997).

Raine and Venables (1981, 1984b) largely replicated this biosocial finding. These two studies investigated 101 males aged 15 years in England. The researchers studied the interaction between psychophysiological functioning and SES in predicting antisocial outcome. Antisocial conduct was measured by self-report and teacher ratings. In the first study (Raine & Venables, 1981), the biological measure used was conditionability as measured by EDA (a measure of ANS arousal) in a laboratory-based classical conditioning paradigm. The social variable was parental SES as measured by parental occupation. A biosocial interaction was found. When subjects from high-SES families were studied, antisocial individuals were found to evidence poorer conditionability. The opposite effect was noted in subjects from low-SES families: Antisocial individuals from these backgrounds were found to demonstrate good conditionability. Since conditionability reflects aspects of learning, these results are consistent with theories that antisocial behavior can result from good learning in an antisocial environmental context, or from poor learning in a prosocial context (where biological factors may posses greater explanatory power).

In a second study using the same subject sample, Raine and Venables (1984b) investigated the interaction between resting heart rate and SES in predicting antisocial outcome. Low resting heart rate characterized antisocial behavior. The sample was then divided into subjects from high-SES and low-SES families. The relationship between low heart rate and antisocial behavior was found in those from high-SES, not low-SES, backgrounds. This biosocial interaction thus supports the conception that individual biological variables may have greater explanatory power in predicting antisocial behavior in more benign (higher-SES) home environments. Thus youths with low ANS arousal as evidenced by poorer conditionability and lower resting heart rates may be protected from learning antisocial behavior in antisocial environments, and thus evidence less antisocial behaviors. Youths in antisocial homes who demonstrate good learning and adequate ANS arousal may well learn antisocial behaviors. Conversely, youth in benign, nonantisocial homes may become antisocial when a stronger biological vulnerability (low ANS arousal) is present.

Neurological–Social Interactions

For the purposes of our discussion, "neurological" variables are here broadly defined as including IQ, early infant birth complications, neuromotor delays, psychiatric vulnerabilities such as psychotic symptoms, and neurological findings such as EEG abnormalities with or without the presence of clinical seizures. All of these factors have strong biological underpinnings. This section discusses research investigating the interaction of neurological factors with social/environmental variables in the genesis of aggressive and antisocial behaviors.

Two studies have examined the interaction of verbal IQ and family functioning in predicting antisocial outcomes. The Dunedin (New Zealand) Multidisciplinary Health and Development Study was a longitudinal investigation of the relationship between neuropsychological functioning and self-reported aggressive acts during adolescence (Moffitt, 1990b). The sample consisted of 1,037 children assessed every 2 years from birth to age 13 years. Neuropsychological status and self-reported antisocial behavior were gathered at age 13 years. Measures of family functioning were gathered at all stages of assessment. Results showed a statistically significant interaction between measures of family adversity and child verbal IQ deficits for self-reported delinquent acts in adolescence involving aggressive confrontation. The group who evidenced both family adversity and neuropsychological deficits was found to have a mean aggression score four times higher than those of the other groups in the sample.

Another longitudinal study that investigated the relationship between verbal IQ and measures of family functioning in predicting antisocial behaviors was the Pittsburgh Youth Study, described earlier in this chapter (Lahey, Loeber, et al., 1995). Family functioning variables included SES and parental ASPD. The 177 male subjects, aged 7–12 years at the time of initial assessment; were oversampled to represent disruptive behavioral disorders. Results showed that only about half of the 65 boys who met criteria for CD at Year 1 continued to meet criteria for CD at Year 2. However, 88% of the boys who initially met criteria for conduct disorder at Year 1 met these criteria at least once again over the subsequent 3 years of the study. The researchers examined factors that led to continued CD symptoms or improvement over the 4 years of the study. The interaction of parental ASPD (from a child's perspective, a social factor) with lower verbal IQ predicted persistence of CD over time. Only boys without a parent with ASPD and with above-average verbal intelligence showed clear improvement in their CD over time. This study is important in demonstrating that age at onset of CD is not related to prognosis and chronicity of symptoms. Rather, the specific interaction of an individual neurologically based deficit with an adverse parenting factor predicts persistence of childhood antisocial behaviors over time.

Another series of studies investigated a different set of neurological vulnerabilities and their interactions with parenting factors in the prediction of adult violent criminal outcomes (Raine, Brennan, & Mednick, 1994; Raine, Brennan, & Mednick, 1997; Raine, Brennan, Mednick, & Mednick, 1996). The first set of studies tested the biosocial interaction hypothesis that birth complications (a biological variable) when combined with early maternal rejection of an infant (a social variable) would predispose the infant to violent crime in adulthood (Raine et al., 1994; Raine, Brennan, & Mednick, 1997). The hypothesis was tested in a cohort of 4,269 consecutive live male births on whom measures of birth complications at age 0 years, maternal rejection at age 1 year, and violent crime at ages 18 and 34 years were collected. Birth complications included forceps extraction, breech delivery, umbilical cord prolapse, preeclampsia, and long birth duration. Variables relevant to maternal rejection at 1 year of age included whether or not the pregnancy was wanted, the mother's attempts to abort the fetus, and placement of the infant for care in a full-time public institution for more than 4 months of the child's first year of life. Results showed a statistically significant interaction between birth complications and early maternal rejection, indicating that subjects who experienced both were most likely to commit violent criminal offenses by age 18 years (Raine et al., 1994; Raine, Brennan, & Mednick, 1997). When subjects were studied at age 34 years, the biosocial interaction was specific for violent but not nonviolent crimes; was specific to more serious forms of violence, such as rape, homicide, and domestic violence; was not specific to threats of violence; and was specific for the development of violent crime at less than 18 years of age, but not for the development of violence first occurring in adulthood (Raine, Brennan, & Mednick, 1997). The biosocial interaction results did not generalize to nonviolent crimes or criminal recidivism. Finally, the interaction between birth complications and early maternal rejection in predisposing to violence was not influenced by psychiatric illness in the mother (Raine, Brennan, & Mednick, 1997).

In another prospective biosocial interaction study, obstetrical risk factors were assessed at birth, and early neuromotor deficits were assessed when subjects were 1 year of age (Raine et al., 1996). Neuromotor measures included the developmental timing of motor milestones, such as an infant's holding his or her head up, crawling, and standing. Social variables included early maternal rejection, paternal criminality, marital stability, family SES, and marital conflict. Family, social, demographic, and behavioral variables were assessed when subjects were 17–19 years of age. Violence and other criminal outcomes were assessed at 20–22 years of age. Cluster analysis of risk factors indicated a group with obstetrical risk factors only, a group with poverty risk factors only, and a biosocial risk factor group with both unstable family environments and early neuromotor delays. Results showed that the biosocial risk factor group had more than double the rates of crime at adult outcome. This group accounted for 70% of all crimes committed in the entire sample. Specifically, the biosocial group had 2.3 times more violent crime than the groups with either risk factor alone (Raine et al., 1996).

The importance of biosocial risk factor interactions during the developing years in predicting risk for adult violent crime was again demonstrated in the study of Lewis, Lovely, Yeager, and Femina (1989). They followed 95 juveniles who were incarcerated for crimes between the ages of 12 and 17 years; subjects were reassessed between the ages of 20 to 25 years. Intrinsic individual biological risk factors included episodic psychotic symptoms, neurological dysfunction, and cognitive impairment. Social risk factors included a family history of violence in general and a specific history of physical or sexual abuse of the child. Evidence for a biosocial interaction was observed, in that delinquents with two or more biological vulnerabilities and at least one social risk factor were more likely to commit violent crimes in adulthood. However, those with only one biological vulnerability coupled with one social risk factor were no more likely to commit violent crimes in adulthood than those with social risks only or those with biological risks only. This study illustrates that biosocial interactions in the origins of violent behavior may be more complex than the interaction of a single biological vulnerability with a single social risk factor.

Temperament–Socialization Interactions

A final example of biosocial interactions in the development of juvenile aggressive/antisocial behaviors is the investigation of child temperament factors and their interactions with qualities of the socializing environment (Bates et al., 1998). These interactive processes have been summarized in terms of the "goodness of fit" between a child's temperament and the expectations and resources of the child's home and school environment (Thomas & Chess, 1977). In theory, temperament does not lead to behavior problems in and of itself; it only does so in conjunction with certain environments.

Bates et al. (1998) studied one child temperament–socialization interaction in the genesis of later aggression and disruptive behavior disorders (i.e., ODD and CD). The child temperamental trait was "impulsivity–unmanageability." The core behavior in this trait is a child's failure to comply with parental attempts to stop or to redirect the child's action. Although temperament reflects more than a pure biological construct (it also includes elements of learning and environmental conditioned experience), as a broad array of behavior traits temperament is generally considered to be biologically rooted (Rothbart & Bates, 1998). "Parental restrictive control" was the socialization variable. This term refers to a parent's behaviors intended to stop, inhibit, or punish the child, such as giving negative commands, removing objects from the child, scolding, and spanking. These behaviors are part of normative parenting and do not encompass abuse, violence, or harsh discipline. In this community sample, temperament and environmental interactions with parents were observed between the ages of 1 and 5 years, and externalizing behavior was assessed between the ages of 7 and 11 years.

A central question of this study concerned the process by which parental restrictive control moderates the link between child temperamental unmanageability and later externalizing behaviors. Results revealed a biosocial interaction. Children's impulsive–unmanageable temperament predicted later externalizing behavioral problems more accurately when parents were low in control actions. When parents were high in restrictive control, children's temperament was less likely to be associated with later behavior problems. This interaction persisted even when statistical controls for child gender and family SES were used (Bates et al., 1998). This study shows that a socialization variable (restrictive parental control) can interact with a child biological variable (a temperamental trait) to produce later externalizing behavior problems in a non-clinic-referred sample.

Summary of Biosocial Interaction Research

The studies described in this section demonstrate that biosocial interaction research may prove more explanatory than single-variable, main-effects models in increasing our understanding of juvenile aggression and related behaviors. This section has reviewed examples of research on genetic–environmental, ANS–social, neurological–social, and child temperament–socialization interactions. This research illustrates the importance of biosocial interactions in the genesis not only of disruptive behavior problems in non-clinic-referred children who are pursuing a largely normative developmental trajectory, but of severe aggression and violence in clinically referred or juvenile-justice-identified youths who are not pursuing normative developmental pathways into adulthood.

The studies reviewed above suggest that interactions between a child's intrinsic biological vulnerabilities and psychosocial risk factors in the child's family and environment may help to explain the development of an early-onset subtype of childhood aggressive/antisocial problems. These types of interactions may also indicate why early-onset CD has such a poor developmental outcome; may help explain some of the mechanisms underlying early-onset violent behaviors as distinguished from adult-onset, nonviolent criminal activity; and highlight the importance of integrating psychosocial with biological factors in efforts to prevent negative outcomes for at-risk youth.

CHAPTER SUMMARY

This chapter has discussed research that attempts to identify and test multi-variable models of the development of early-onset aggression and related behaviors in children and adolescents. These studies begin to integrate biological vulnerabilities with social/environmental risk factors in the genesis of these behaviors over the course of development. Four models from the developmental psychopathology literature are presented: a model of family coercion; a model of early oppositional behavior leading to later childhood CD; a model of antisocial propensity; and a multiple-pathways model of juvenile aggression and antisociality. A complementary approach to studies of developmental psychopathology is research examining the interactions between specific biological and social risk factors. A selective review of biosocial research studying the interactions between genetic–environmental, ANS–social, neurological–social, and temperament–parenting variables has been presented. It is important to highlight the idea that this research does not find biological processes to be deterministic for antisocial outcomes (McCord, 1996); rather, the degree to which biological factors determine outcomes varies in relation to environmental conditions, as well as the variability in biological risk factors. Therefore, both types of variables must be studied in relationship to one another and in relationship to the developmental age of the child in further risk factor research.

⊞ CHAPTER 9

Issues in Female Aggression and Related Behaviors

Gender differences in the quality and quantity of aggression and related behaviors are well documented in the behavioral science and criminal justice literatures. These differences are often cited and, until the past two decades, were largely accepted. Males have been found to be more aggressive than females across various types of scientific studies (Maccoby & Jacklin, 1974, 1980). In animal research, the only exception to the general finding of greater male aggression has been maternal aggression, in which a mother defends her offspring from attack by a predator (Moyer, 1976). In humans, a male preponderance in aggressive behaviors has been found across categorical and dimensional definitions of such behaviors (Achenbach, Howell, McConaughy, & Stanger, 1995a; Zoccolillo, 1993) and categories of aggressive behavior, such as physical and verbal aggression (Hinshaw & Anderson, 1996). Gender differences in aggression and antisocial behavior are supported by cross-cultural studies (Parke & Slaby, 1983) and by studies of violent crime (Hood, 1996). As a result of the generally accepted notion that males are more aggressive than females, the study of female aggression and related behaviors has lagged far behind studies of males.

More recent studies of aggression, however, have begun to challenge the generally accepted idea that males are always more aggressive than females. Beginning in the 1970s, descriptive reviews of the adult aggression literature have not found support for the hypothesis that men are almost always more physically aggressive than women (Frodi, Macaulay, & Thome, 1977). Women have been found to act just as aggressively as men in situations where aggression is perceived as justified, and where protections against retaliation are present. In a meta-analytic review of 63 studies investigating gender differences in adult aggressive behavior, Eagly and Steffen (1986) found that such differences were present, but small. For example, sex differences in aggression were smaller than gender differences in many other common social behaviors, such as helping behaviors and nonverbal communication behaviors. Although adult males were found to express more aggression and to receive more aggression from others than adult females, the magnitude of the differences appeared slight. Men's expression of aggression was less than a third of a standard deviation greater than women's, and men's receipt of aggression differed from women's by only an eighth of a standard deviation. Eagly and Steffen (1986) concluded that gender differences in adult aggression are relatively small when averaged and are quite inconsistent across scientific studies. Similar conclusions were drawn from a quantitative review of 143 studies of gender differences in child and adolescent aggression published between 1962 and 1981: Only 5% of the variance in aggression in the sample population was accounted for by gender (Hyde, 1984). In this review, gender differences in aggression appeared larger than gender differences in adult aggression, but remained slight; boys' aggression exceeded girls' in aggression by only half of a standard deviation (Hyde, 1984). These meta-analytic studies suggest that sex differences in aggression are less than those previously accepted, for both youths and adults.

There may be several reasons why the earlier research emphasized a preponderance of male aggression. First, gender differences in aggression may vary by type of aggression studied. Since behavioral scientists have historically defined "aggression" as behavior intended to inflict harm or injury to others (Eagly & Steffen, 1986), aggression research has generally emphasized the study of overt forms of aggression such as physical fighting, and deemphasized other types such as covert aggression, relational aggression, or indirect aggression. Physical aggression is easy to observe in laboratory and field studies, and therefore lends itself well to measurement and investigation. Covert aggression, relational aggression, and indirect aggression may be more prevalent in females (see Chapter 1) and are much harder to observe and quantify in observational studies. Since males tend to be more physically aggressive than females, a gender bias in aggression research may have been introduced.

Second, gender differences in aggressive behavior may vary by type of study methodology. Commonly used measurement techniques in aggression research include direct observation of behaviors; parent, teacher, or other reports on rating scales assessing aggressive behaviors; peer nomination techniques, in which a child's peers are asked to nominate the most and least aggressive child in the classroom; and self-report of aggressive behaviors. Gender differences in aggression are larger when measured by direct observation or peer nomination (which favor the observation of overt forms of aggression), and smaller when self-report methodologies are used (Hyde, 1984).

Third, gender differences in aggression may vary by the type of setting in which aggression is studied. Sex differences in aggressive behavior are larger in correlational studies completed in naturalistic environments, and smaller in experimental studies of aggression using laboratory paradigms (Hyde, 1984). Finally, the magnitude of gender differences in aggression is inversely correlated with developmental age. Studies assessing children generally report greater male–female differences in aggression than studies evaluating adults (Eagly & Steffen, 1986; Hyde, 1984). Thus gender differences in aggression may have been exaggerated by these potential confounds in the research.

With growing recognition that previous aggression research has neglected aspects of female aggression, studies are now investigating female aggression as a phenomenon in itself. Research has moved beyond simply asking whether men are more aggressive than women, to investigating the development, phenomenology, correlates, and outcome variables of female aggression as an area of investigation in its own right. A more sensitive perception of what constitutes female aggression and how it differs from aggression in males is starting to emerge. This chapter therefore reviews issues in female aggression and related behaviors.

THE FORMS OF FEMALE AGGRESSION

Indirect and Relational Aggression

As noted above, one reason why males may have been identified in previous research as more aggressive than females is that the forms (types or modes) that female aggression takes may have been underrecognized and underappreciated in earlier scientific studies. More recent investigations into female aggression identify two forms of aggression that are more prevalent in females than in males. One type of aggression is called "indirect" aggression (Bjorkqvist, Osterman, & Kaukiainen, 1992), and the other type is called "relational" aggression (Crick & Grotpeter, 1995; Crick & Bigbee, 1998). Indirect aggression is conceptualized as a kind of social manipulation. The aggressor induces others to attack the victim, using the existing social structure in order to harm the target individual. Indirect aggression protects the aggressor from being personally involved in the attack; it thus gives her (or him) a greater chance of going unnoticed and avoiding retaliation (Lagerspetz, Bjorkqvist, & Peltonen, 1988). Relational aggression consists of behaviors that are intended to significantly harm another child's friendships or feelings of inclusion by the peer group. Examples include expressing anger and aggression toward another child by excluding that individual from one's social group; purposefully withdrawing friendship in order to ostracize another child; or socially manipulating other children to reject the target individual, such as by spreading rumors about the child (Crick, Bigbee, & Howes, 1996). It can be seen that in some respects, indirect aggression and relational aggression overlap.

Crick and Grotpeter (1995) propose that when children aggress against other children, they do so in ways that best thwart or damage the goals valued by their respective gender peer groups. Boys tend to harm others through physical and verbal aggression—behaviors that interfere with the types of goals important to boys within the peer group. Such male goals include themes of independent agency, mastery, instrumentality (getting things from another), and establishing social dominance hierarchies within the social group. These types of social goals appear less salient for girls. Girls tend to display a strong affiliative style in their social relationships—a tendency that is often attributed to their biologically driven and/or socially prescribed role of preparing to become primary child caregivers when they reach maturity (Cryanowski, Frank, Young, & Shear, 2000). Relative to boys, girls display a preference for close emotional communication, intimacy, and responsiveness within interpersonal relationships (Feingold, 1994). Thus, when girls aggress against another girl, they do so in ways that will harm affiliative interactions.

When indirect forms of aggression are investigated in non-clinic-referred samples of children, girls are found to be more aggressive in this mode than boys. In a study of Finnish school children aged 8–18 years, boys were consistently more physically aggressive; the two genders were found not to differ significantly from each other with respect to verbal aggression; and girls were estimated by their peers to use indirect means of aggression significantly more than boys in all age groups except for the youngest age range (8-year-olds) (Bjorkqvist et al., 1992). Studies also document that relational aggression is more common in girls than in boys. In a study using a peer nomination instrument, a community sample of 491 third- through sixth-grade children was assessed (Crick & Grotpeter, 1995). Relational forms of aggression were found to be valid modes of aggression, distinct from overt physical forms of aggression. Girls were also found to be significantly more relationally aggressive than boys. Further studies have established that children do indeed view relational aggression as angry, harmful behaviors (Crick et al., 1996), and that relational aggression predicts concurrent psychosocial adjustment problems in girls (Crick & Bigbee, 1998).

These studies support the hypothesis that gender differences with respect to choice of aggressive strategies exist for non-clinic-referred children and adolescents residing in the community. When gender differences in aggression strategies are recognized, the often-cited male preponderance in aggressive behavior begins to weaken. Developmental trends may also be identified. Physical aggression appears at the earliest stages of life; then direct verbal threats appear; and finally indirect strategies that utilize the existing social milieu appear. This sequence may be related to the developmental order of skill acquisition in children (i.e., first physical/motor, then verbal, and finally social) and may reflect the earlier developmental mastery of language in females and their predisposition toward affiliative behaviors.

Conduct Disorder

Another form that aggressive/antisocial behavior may take in females is behavior that meets psychiatric diagnostic criteria for conduct disorder (CD) (see Chapter 4). CD is not well studied in girls. This is unfortunate, because CD is the second most prevalent psychiatric diagnosis in girls, with prevalence rates ranging between 4% and 9.2% in epidemiological studies of non-clinic-referred youth (Zoccolillo, Tremblay, & Vitaro, 1996). In a review of 10 epidemiological studies of the prevalence of CD from five different countries, no gender differences in prevalence during adolescence were found in 40% of the studies (Zoccolillo, 1993). In addition, CD may be the most common persistent psychiatric disorder in girls (Zoccolillo, 1993). Furthermore, girls meeting diagnostic criteria for CD in childhood and adolescence are known to experience poor outcomes across multiple psychosocial domains in young adulthood (Zoccolillo & Rogers, 1991; Zoccolillo, 1993). All of this suggests that female CD is a topic in need of much further investigation.

Symptoms of CD appear to differ between females and males. Girls meeting diagnostic criteria for CD have a preponderance of nonaggressive or covertly aggressive symptoms, whereas boys appear to have a preponderance of overtly aggressive symptoms (McGee, Feehan, Williams, & Anderson, 1992). Common symptoms of adolescent female CD include the following (Zoccolillo, 1993; Zoccolillo & Rogers, 1991):

Chronic violations of rules at school
Chronic lying
School grades below expectations
Substance abuse
Nonconfrontational stealing
Running away from home overnight
Somatization (medically unexplained somatic complaints)
Increased rates of arrest for nonviolent crimes

In a study of 55 girls aged 13–16 years who had been admitted to an inpatient psychiatric unit for CD, nonaggressive or covertly aggressive symptoms predominated over overtly aggressive symptoms. Only 49% of the female adolescent sample self-reported engaging in two or more fights. In contrast, chronic rule violations in school, lying, and academic underachievement were identified in 60% to 73% of these girls (Zoccolillo & Rogers, 1991). Somatization is also commonly found in females with CD; unexplained medical complaints have been much more highly associated with adult female antisocial personality disorder (ASPD) and female childhood CD than in males with these disorders (Zoccolillo, 1993). Thus a preponderance of nonaggressive or covertly aggressive symptoms and somatic complaints may lead to an underrecognition of CD in females.

Another factor that may contribute to the underrecognition of CD in girls is a different developmental trajectory from that of boys. It appears that CD has a later age of onset in girls than in boys. In the review of 10 epidemiological studies of CD from five countries mentioned above, all 10 studies reported an increased prevalence rate of CD favoring boys over girls in the preadolescent years. However, by adolescence this male gender difference was not found in 4 of the 10 studies (Zoccolillo, 1993). In a longitudinal study of CD, clear gender differences at age 11 years were replaced by similar prevalence rates between males and females by age 15 years. The male–female ratio of severe conduct problems decreased from 2.6:1 at age 11 years to 0.7:1 at age 15 years (McGee et al., 1992).

The research described above thus indicates that the increase in rates of female CD in adolescence is accounted for primarily by a rise in nonaggressive or covertly aggressive activity, occurring at a later developmental age than occurs for CD in boys. As a result, psychiatric diagnostic criteria emphasizing overt aggression may lead to higher rates of diagnosed CD in males than in females. Less openly aggressive forms of CD appear to display a nearly equal prevalence during the teenage years. The admixture of overtly, physically aggressive symptoms and covertly aggressive or nonaggressive symptoms in the current official diagnostic criteria for CD (see Chapter 4) tends to obfuscate the nature of this gender-related developmental shift (Hinshaw & Anderson, 1996).

Although a psychiatric diagnosis of CD may be useful in identifying a subset of persistently antisocial teenage girls with poor outcomes across multiple domains of functioning who are in need of broad-based psychoeducational and community treatment interventions, it remains highly unclear that this diagnosis is useful for identifying preadolescent girls with early-onset and persistent antisocial behaviors. Indeed, studies investigating the question of whether the official psychiatric diagnostic criteria for CD can identify girls in the general population with these types of behaviors beginning in elementary school—who thus are in need of early intervention to prevent a poor outcome—have largely been negative. In a longitudinal study of 2,251 girls, first assessed for CD at age 7 years and followed up at age 10 years, Zoccolillo et al. (1996) found that the diagnosis of CD did not identify most preadolescent girls with early-onset, pervasive, and chronic antisocial behaviors. Since one purpose of psychiatric diagnosis is to identify those in need of treatment interventions, this study raises questions about the utility of CD as a diagnosis for elementary-school-age girls who exhibit such behaviors.

The evidence that early signs of CD are more effectively detected in boys, presumably because of the more overtly aggressive form of the syndrome in males, has raised questions about modifying the diagnostic criteria for CD in girls (Zoccolillo & Rogers, 1991; Zoccolillo, 1993). Because CD may be qualitatively different in girls, separate diagnostic criteria may be needed for the two genders. Candidates for different symptoms in girls might be somatization and extensive rule violations (Zoccolillo, 1993). Lower diagnostic criteria thresholds for girls might also help identify more females at risk and allow interventions to occur before problems become intractable. This proposal has sparked a lively debate that presently is not resolved. Concern has been raised that lowering the diagnostic threshold for CD in females could be seen as stigmatizing for girls, by indicating that relatively low levels of rule violations, aggression, or conduct problems would receive pejorative psychiatric diagnostic labeling (Zahn-Waxler, 1993). Further research on the symptoms, outcomes, and biological, familial, and social correlates of CD in females remains much needed.

Psychopathy

Historically, the term "psychopathy" was used to describe those persons who did not appear to have a mental disorder proper, yet were considered deviant and not entirely sane because their emotions and behaviors constantly placed them in conflict with societal laws, rules, and mores. "Psychopathy" currently refers to a large constellation of deviant personality traits and antisocial behaviors (see Chapter 4). These include lying, insincerity, manipulation of others, superficial charm, shallow emotions, unreliability, lack of remorse, poor insight into one's behavior, antisocial acts, and a failure to learn from experience (Myers, Burket, & Harris, 1995). In work with psychopathic adults, two important factors have emerged on rating scales assessing the characterological and behavioral dimensions of psychopathy (Hare, 1991). The first factor includes such personality traits as selfishness, callousness, and remorseless use of others. The second factor includes behaviors that constitute a chronically unstable, antisocial, and socially deviant lifestyle (Rogers, Johansen, Chang, & Salekin, 1997). Psychopathy overlaps with, yet is separable from, categorical psychiatric diagnoses such as ASPD and CD. These disorders consist largely of antisocial behaviors in which the basic rights of others or societal rules are violated. In contrast, psychopathy includes deviant personality traits as well as antisocial behaviors.

Psychopathy is beginning to be investigated in female adults (Rutherford, Cacciola, & Alterman, 1999), adolescents (Myers et al., 1995; Rogers et al., 1997), and children (Frick, O'Brien, Wootton, & McBurnett, 1994; Frick, Lilienfeld, Ellis, Loney, & Silverthorn, 1999). Adult studies of female psychopathy have largely focused on inmate populations (Grann, Langstrom, Tengstrom, & Kullgren, 1999; Salekin, Rogers, Ustad, & Sewell, 1998) and clinically referred populations with substance use disorders (SUDs) (Rutherford, Alterman, Cacciola, & McKay, 1998; Rutherford et al., 1999). These are populations with a high prevalence of psychopathy. Although adult females meeting criteria for psychopathy are consistently identified in these studies, the prevalence rates for women are much lower than for men. For example, 1.5% of 137 clinically referred females with SUDs met robust criteria for psychopathy, as determined by a Psychopathy Checklist—Revised (PCL-R) score greater than 30 (the generally accepted cutoff score on the PCL-R for psychopathy in adults) (Rutherford et al., 1999). In an incarcerated population, 15.5% of 78 inmate women met criteria for psychopathy (Salekin et al., 1998). These prevalence rates for psychopathy in females are lower than those generally reported for incarcerated men (25% to 30%) (Salekin et al., 1998).

Because the investigation of psychopathy in children and adolescents is just beginning (Frick et al., 1994; Rogers et al., 1997), gender differences in youth psychopathy are not well studied. In a study of 30 adolescents aged 14–17 years admitted to an inpatient psychiatry unit, 67% of the sample was female. Psychopathy was assessed with a modified version of the PCL-R. Results showed a significant difference in PCL-R scores by gender, with males scoring higher (more psychopathic features) than females (Myers et al., 1995). Studies of psychopathy in children have been completed on samples that are largely male; girls have constituted between 11% and 22% of these samples (Frick et al., 1994, 1999). In short, although psychopathy can be identified in female adults, adolescents, and children who are clinically referred or incarcerated, females have a lower prevalence of psychopathy than males at all developmental ages.

Correlates of female psychopathy have also been investigated. In children, preliminary analysis suggests that psychopathy is highly correlated with impulsive aggression and CD, and that these correlates appear similar for boys and girls meeting criteria for psychopathy (Frick et al., 1999). In adolescence, psychopathy in females remains highly correlated with aggressive conduct problems and delinquent behaviors (Myers et al., 1995). However, in studies of adult females with psychopathic features, gender differences emerge. Compared to psychopathic men, women who are psychopathic experience greater chronic unemployment, higher rates of marital separation, more dependency on social assistance programs, higher rates of telling lies, and more relationship difficulties (Salekin et al., 1998). They have lower rates of unlawful behaviors and are less likely to be violent than psychopathic men; in addition, they have higher rates of suicidality, somatization, histrionic personality disorder, depression, and anxiety than their male counterparts (Salekin et al., 1998).

In summary, psychopathy appears to be less pronounced in females than in males across the lifespan. A high degree of correlation with impulsive aggression and conduct problems is noted for females with psychopathic traits in childhood and adolescence. By adulthood, gender differences in interpersonal, legal, occupational, and comorbid psychiatric diagnostic domains emerge. Research suggests that psychopathic females account for a small proportion of those with childhood CD. It remains to be investigated whether biological variables such as autonomic nervous system (ANS) underarousal and psychological measures of reward dominance are similar in psychopathic females and males.

Delinquency

"Delinquency" is a legal term and is generally defined in terms of arrest rates, conviction, or adjudication of juveniles for acts that if committed by adults would be tried in criminal court (see Chapter 1). Delinquency includes serious crimes, as well as less serious illegal acts. Serious acts include aggravated assault, armed robbery, weapons carrying, drug trafficking, and rape. Juveniles also come to the attention of the courts because of "status offenses"; these are defined as acts that would be legal if committed by an adult, but come to the attention of authorities because of children's status as minors. Such status offenses include drinking alcohol; truancy from school; running away from home; and chronic disregard for parental, school, and societal rules (the so-called "ungovernable child" behaviors). Status offenses generally come to the attention of the family and probate court and are noncriminal acts (Rogers et al., 1997).

During the 1950s, most of the research on juvenile delinquency concentrated on males. Early theories of female juvenile delinquency emphasized early sexuality as either the cause or expression of it (Calhoun, Jurgens, & Chen, 1993; Hoyt & Scherer, 1998). For example, the supposedly "deceitful" nature of women (derived from practice at faking sexual arousal), combined with precocious biological maturity, was proposed to account for female delinquency (Pollak, 1950). Researchers began to document the prevalence of vague status offenses called "sex delinquencies" in females, such as incorrigibility or simply needing care and protection, as major differences between delinquent males and females (Cowie, Cowie, & Slater, 1968). Evidence suggesting that delinquent females ran away from home because of sexual and physical abuse and/or neglect and then broke laws to survive "on the streets" was ignored (Hoyt & Scherer, 1998). Female delinquency acquired a sexually charged stigma not associated with male delinquency. Historically, delinquent females were charged with immorality or status offenses because of concern about their sexual behavior and moral depravity (Schlossman & Wallach, 1978); they were subsequently treated more harshly by the juvenile courts than males who committed similar status offenses (Hoyt & Scherer, 1998).

Over the past 50 years, concern about the sexual and moral nature of female delinquency has been replaced by worry over the rising arrest rates of female juveniles for serious offenses. For example, between 1989 and 1993, the growth rate of female juvenile arrests was more than twice that of male juvenile arrests (Poe-Yamagata & Butts, 1996). From 1985 to 1994, violent crime arrest rates increased by 125% for females, as opposed to 67% for males; the female increase was mostly due to arrests for robbery and aggravated assault. Male juveniles do continue to exceed female juveniles in growth rates for homicide arrests (Hoyt & Scherer, 1998; Poe-Yamagata & Butts, 1996). Between 1989 and 1993, female arrests for property crimes climbed by 22%, whereas arrests of males for property crimes dropped by 3% (Poe-Yamagata & Butts, 1996). The growing similarities in male and female juvenile offenses are illustrated in Figure 9.1; it can be seen there that in 1992, the most common reasons for referral to juvenile court were almost identical for girls and boys. In a survey of 10,904 high school students from the 1995 Youth Risk Survey, female gender was significantly associated with carrying a weapon on school grounds (Simon, Crosby, & Dahlberg, 1999). Although arrest rates for all juveniles began to decrease toward the end of the 1990s, they remain considerably elevated over the rates of 30–40 years ago. Increasingly, female juveniles appear to be involved in serious delinquent acts and criminal offenses.

Female delinquency remains understudied; as a result, there exists little conclusive understanding of the important factors in its etiology. It is unclear whether delinquent female pursue a different developmental course or have different unique biosocial correlates as compared to delinquent males. Understanding and treatment of both female and male delinquency could be en-

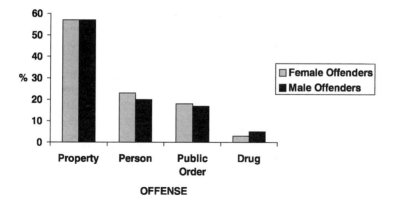

FIGURE 9.1. The most common reasons for referral to juvenile court in the United States by gender for 1992. Note that the gender rates for most offenses were nearly equal. Data from Butts et al. (1995).

hanced through the adoption of a gender-integrated theory of delinquency— one that is informed by further study of developmental, psychological, and social-ecological determinants in delinquent females (Hoyt & Scherer, 1998).

Deliberate Self-Harm

"Deliberate self-harm" (DSH) is a syndrome characterized by intentional, non-life-threatening, self-inflicted bodily harm of a socially unacceptable nature (Briere & Gil, 1998; Walsh & Rosen, 1988). The behaviors involved in DSH are of low lethality, can be chronic, and may be repetitive (Pattison & Kahan, 1983). They include self-inflicted trauma, which generally involves cutting the skin on the arms or legs, or burning the skin. Also included in the definition of DSH is nontherapeutic, nonlethal drug overdose (Taylor & Cameron, 1998). The definition of DSH is somewhat broader than the definition of "self-injurious behavior" or "self-mutilation," which is confined to the deliberate, direct destruction of bodily tissue without conscious suicidal intent, such as acts of cutting or burning (Favazza, 1998). This discussion uses the broader term of DSH.

The syndrome of DSH is distinct from suicidal behavior. The suicidal individual seeks to end all feeling by dying. In contrast, the individual with DSH seeks to regulate dysphoric, negative emotions and affects, or to reduce unbearable levels of internal tension and stress, by causing pain to the self (Briere & Gil, 1998; Favazza, 1998). As such, the syndrome of DSH represents a maladaptive coping mechanism in persons who are not intent on death (Herpertz, 1995; Winchel & Stanley, 1991).

Although the syndrome of DSH is associated with many negative feeling states, such as depression, loneliness, emptiness, guilt, and dissociation (Winchel & Stanley, 1991), there also exists a strong correlation with aggression and antisocial behavior (Simeon et al., 1992). DSH is highly prevalent in adults with character pathology (including borderline personality disorder or ASPD) relative to control subjects, and it is associated with greater lifetime histories of impulsive aggression, anger, and antisocial behaviors (Simeon et al., 1992). A study comparing 40 self-injurious prisoners to 40 non-self-injurious prisoners found a significantly higher rate of aggressive behaviors in those who also engaged in self-injury; these behaviors included higher rates of rage outbursts and of physical fighting and assault (Virkkunen, 1976). Higher levels of trait anger have been reported in adolescents admitted to psychiatric hospitalization because of repeated acts of DSH (Hawton, Kingsbury, Steinhardt, James, & Fagg, 1999). In a study of clinically referred adults, 21% of 390 subjects reported at least one incident of DSH. Of those subjects engaging in DSH, 71% reported DSH as a means of managing maladaptive anger and aggression directed at self or others (Briere & Gil, 1998). Psychiatric disorders of impulsive aggression (including intermittent explosive disorder) have been found to be related to DSH, independently of borderline personality disorder or ASPD; this had led some researchers to conceptualize DSH as a form of self-inflicted, impulsive aggression possibly associated with serotonin (5-HT) underfunctioning in the central nervous system (CNS) (Zlotnick, Mattia, & Zimmerman, 1999). Indeed, it appears that one form aggression may take is DSH.

There is evidence that female adolescents may be especially at risk for DSH. For example, a review of all cases of DSH in persons under 16 years of age presenting to a general hospital in Oxford, England, between 1976 and 1993 was completed (Hawton, Fagg, & Simkin, 1996). Behaviors included cutting, burning, and deliberate but nonsuicidal overdose of medication. There were 755 cases of DSH presenting to the hospital in children and adolescents in the 17 years of the study. Girls made up 85% of the sample. The overall female–male ratio in the study sample was 5.7:1. Based on their results, the authors estimated the sex ratio of DSH for the general population and found a female–male ratio of 9:1. Self-poisoning made up the majority of acts, and traumatic self-injury constituted a minority of the DSH behaviors. Boys engaged in self-injury more than girls, and girls engaged in overdose more than boys. Repeat episodes of DSH were more common in girls than in boys (Hawton et al., 1996).

Developmental trends in DSH are also evident (see Figure 9.2). Prior to age 12 years, DSH appears very uncommon for both boys and girls. Females appear to begin DSH at an earlier age than males. Beginning in early adolescence, female DSH rates rise much faster than male DSH rates. Gender differences appear maximal in midadolescence. By adulthood, rates of DSH have fallen, and the gender ratio is nearly 1:1 (Briere & Gil, 1998; Hawton et al., 1996).

Psychosocial and neurobiological correlates of DSH have been studied more frequently in adults than in children or adolescents. In adults, strong correlations with character pathology of the borderline or antisocial type have

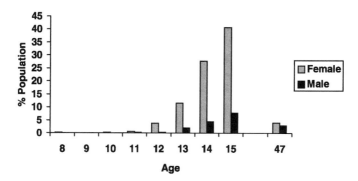

FIGURE 9.2. Developmental trends in deliberate self-harm by age and gender. Data from Briere and Gil (1998) and Hawton, Fagg, and Simkin (1996).

been documented (Simeon et al., 1992). Childhood histories of sexual and physical abuse are found more frequently in adults with DSH than in comparison groups (Santa Mina & Gallop, 1998). Psychiatric diagnoses of posttraumatic stress disorder (PTSD), depression, dissociative disorders, psychosis, mental retardation, and SUDs are also associated with DSH (Winchel & Stanley, 1991; Zlotnick et al., 1997, 1999). Dysregulation of CNS opiate, dopamine (DA), and 5-HT neurotransmitter systems have been associated with DSH in adults (Winchel & Stanley, 1991).

Correlates of DSH in youth are less well studied. Hawton et al. (1996) found each of several factors—relationship difficulties with family and friends, childhood sexual trauma, social isolation, and academic difficulties—to be present in more than 30% of their 755 subjects who came to the hospital with an episode of DSH. Another study has noted depression, hopelessness, impulsivity, anger, low self-esteem, and ineffective problem-solving strategies as important correlates of adolescent DSH (Hawton et al., 1999). In a population of psychiatrically hospitalized children and adolescents, a greater number of primary caretakers with whom patients had lived discriminated patients with self-directed aggression from those with other-directed aggression; youth who experienced frequent disruptions in caretaking were likely to engage in acts of self-injury during hospitalization (Vivona et al., 1995). This suggests a role for interpersonal attachment in the etiology of DSH for youth. Another important correlate of adolescent DSH is the phenomenon of "contagion." This refers to clusters of individuals engaging in DSH, generally in the immediate aftermath of a single individual engaging in such behavior (Taiminen, Kallio-Soukainen, Nokso-Koivisto, Kaljonen, & Helenius, 1998).

In summary, although DSH may be associated with a great many negative emotional internal states and psychiatric diagnoses, it can also be a maladaptive expression of anger and aggression. It remains distinct from suicide. The highest prevalence rates of DSH appear to occur in female adolescents.

Female adolescents appear to engage more frequently in overdose as a method of DSH, whereas males engage more in traumatic injury as a method of DSH. In adulthood, the rates of DSH drop, and the gender ratio becomes more nearly equal.

PREVALENCE AND STABILITY

Whether aggression is measured in terms of violent crime rates, arrest rates, CD, ASPD, personality dimensions of psychopathy, or continuous (dimensional) measures of overt and covert aggression in the population, males have elevated rates of such behaviors as compared to females. However, this does not mean that the prevalence rates of female aggression are negligible or unimportant. On the contrary, prevalence rates for relational and indirect forms of aggression are higher in females than in males and are associated with psychosocial adjustment difficulties in non-clinic-referred elementary school populations. Rates of covert aggression and antisocial behaviors have equal gender prevalence in adolescence. The arrest rate for female juvenile crime is rising. DSH, as a maladaptive expression of aggression, peaks in females during the adolescent years. CD is the second most prevalent psychiatric disorder and perhaps the most chronic psychiatric disorder in females, as noted above (Zoccolillo, 1993). Thus prevalence rates for female aggression and related behaviors are neither clinically insignificant, nor insignificant in terms of their impact on society.

A question of importance is the stability of aggression in females. Many studies have demonstrated the stability of aggression in males from the age of 8 years into adulthood (see Chapter 3). Olweus (1979) has reported that individual differences in male aggressiveness over age 8 years are virtually as stable as those in intelligence, with stability coefficients ranging between .79 and .81, depending on the method of observation. The stability of girls' aggressive behavior has been less well studied.

In a study of community elementary school children, Cairns and Cairns (1984) demonstrated that high-aggression girls showed as much stability as high-aggression boys from the fourth to the fifth grade. In a follow-up of the same sample, the stability of teacher-rated aggression from fourth to ninth grades was .40 to .56 for girls and .48 to .72 for boys (Cairns, Cairns, Neckerman, Ferguson, & Gariepy, 1989). The results show that the stability of aggression from the fourth to the eighth grade was as high for girls (.51) as it was for boys (.49). However, beginning in the ninth grade, girls' aggression correlated with earlier aggression less highly than boys' did (.13 and .36, respectively). Using a peer nomination instrument, Pulkkinen (1987) showed that aggressiveness was as stable for girls as for boys between the ages of 8 and 14 years (.37 for both boys and girls). However, in this same study, teacher ratings reported boys to be more stable than girls in their aggressive behaviors (.37 and .13, respectively) (Pulkkinen, 1992). These results suggest that in samples of non-clinic-referred students assessed in the community, aggression in girls demonstrates a fairly high stability during the elementary and middle school years, although reported stability rates vary as a function of the type of reporter used in the study design.

However, when other indices of aggressive outcome are used, a different picture emerges. Regarding antisocial behavior, arrest rates, and criminal convictions, stability coefficients for males exceed those for females. For example, in a study of individuals spanning 22 years, peer-nominated aggression at age 8 years correlated with criminal justice convictions at age 30 years much more highly for males (.24) than for females (.10) (Huesmann, Eron, Lefkowitz, & Walder, 1984). This finding was replicated by Pulkkinen (1987), who showed higher stability coefficients for males than for females between peer nominations of aggression in elementary school and later arrest rates. Thus males appear to have more stability in aggressive behaviors when criminal justice measures are used.

When longer study durations are examined, the stability of aggression for males also appears higher than for females. Aggressiveness stability coefficients from the ages of 8 to 30 years were .50 for males and .34 for females (Eron, 1992). Thus gender differences in stability coefficients vary according to the method of observation used (e.g., peer nomination, teacher rating scales, arrest rates), the manifestation of aggression one chooses to analyze (e.g., a spouse's rating of a subject's aggression, number of criminal convictions, violence of offenses committed, and/or punishment of one's own children), and the length of time of observation (stability coefficients for girls appear higher over shorter than over longer observation times). Despite these methodological differences, aggression in girls appears to demonstrate a fair amount of stability after 8 years of age (Eron, 1992).

CORRELATES

Research finds that the individual, family, and environmental correlates of aggression and antisocial behaviors are generally similar in males and females (Silverthorn & Frick, 1999; Webster-Stratton, 1996b; Zoccolillo, 1993). Although some differences exist, correlates of these behaviors are generally more similar than different across the two genders. This section reviews some correlates of female aggression and related behaviors.

Neuropsychology and Temperament

Various studies have demonstrated an association between diminished executive cognitive functions (ECFs) and aggressive/antisocial behaviors (Giancola, 1995). The neuropsychological abilities subsumed under the rubric of ECFs include attentional control, strategic goal planning, abstract reasoning, cognitive flexibility, hypothesis generation, response sequencing ordered in time, and the ability to organize and use information stored in working memory. These cognitive processes are crucial in organizing a behavioral response to solve a complex problem, and in planning, initiating, and regulating goal-directed behavior (Milner, 1995). The neuroanatomical sites that subserve ECFs are thought to involve the prefrontal cortex and aspects of its connections to striatal and limbic subcortical systems in the CNS (Fuster, 1997).

Most studies finding an association between low ECFs and aggressive/antisocial behaviors have studied males (see Chapter 6). However, a similar association between diminished ECFs and these behaviors has been found for adolescent females. In a study of 249 adolescent females aged 14–18 years, the group meeting psychiatric diagnostic criteria for CD demonstrated significantly poorer performance on neuropsychological tests assessing ECFs than did controls (Giancola, Mezzich, & Tarter, 1998a). This association could not be explained by the presence of comorbid attention-deficit/hyperactivity disorder (ADHD). This association was also found in a study of aggression in adolescent females meeting criteria for a diagnosis of psychoactive substance abuse (Giancola, Mezzich, & Tarter, 1998b). Deficits in ECFs appear more strongly related to overt aggression than to covert aggression in these studies.

Similarly to males, there appears to be a high rate of cognitive dysfunction in delinquent females. Longitudinal studies have shown that an IQ below 80 is a strong predictor ($r = .31$) of adolescent delinquency in females (Werner, 1987). Modest negative correlations ($r = -.21$) have been reported between girls' math achievement at age 10 years and aggressive behaviors at age 14 years (Tremblay, Masse, et al., 1992). These preliminary data suggest that girls with aggression and antisocial behavior may be characterized by high rates of cognitive dysfunction.

Deviations in temperament are also associated with these behaviors (see Chapter 5 for discussion). "Temperament" can be defined as a series of trait dimensions depicting individual differences in various types of behavioral, affective, and self-regulatory styles (Thomas & Chess, 1977). The term "difficult temperament" has been used to describe behaviors and affective states characterized by irritability, withdrawal from novel stimuli, negative mood, intense reactions to stimuli, low adaptability to change, distractibility, irregularities in biological rhythms, and poor attention span (Thomas & Chess, 1977). In boys, a difficult temperament is associated with more aggression and antisocial behavior than is an easy temperament (Kingston & Prior, 1995). This association has also been reported for adolescent females with CD (Giancola et al., 1998a). Difficult temperament is more strongly associated with covert aggression and nonaggressive antisocial behaviors than with overt aggression in females (Giancola et al., 1998a).

Social Skill and Social Role Deficits

Social skill deficits and deficiencies in the performance of social roles are common in youth with aggressive/antisocial behaviors (Riley, Ensminger, Green,

& Kang, 1998). Social roles for youth include role performance in the family and with peers, as well as academic performance and nonacademic activities at school (such as participation in extracurricular activities). In general, boys with conduct problems have poorer social role functioning than do girls with such problems (Riley et al., 1998). However, these girls demonstrate poorer social role functioning than healthy girls do. For example, girls with disruptive behavior disorders have poorer relationships with family and friends and participate in fewer social activities. They are also less well accepted by their peers than are non-behavior-disordered girls (Riley et al., 1998).

Girls with aggressive/antisocial behaviors have a high incidence of social communication and social information-processing difficulties. They appear less effective at communicating and behaving appropriately (Riley et al., 1998). Although they appear aware of the social conventions governing conversational interactions, they do not always display interactional behaviors with others consistent with their pragmatic awareness (Sanger, Hux, & Ritzman, 1999). Girls exhibiting relational forms of aggression tend to misattribute hostile intent to peers in social contexts that include an ambiguous (but not necessarily hostile) negative relational event (Crick & Werner, 1998). Aggressive girls tend to evaluate the social outcomes of aggressive behavior more positively than nonaggressive girls do (Crick & Werner, 1998); as a result, these girls are often impaired in their social role functioning. This type of social information-processing impairment may be frequently overlooked, because attention is more often focused on the girls' disruptive behaviors.

Youth with aggression and antisocial behaviors have also been shown to have academic difficulties and deficits in academic social role performance compared to children and adolescents without these behaviors (see Chapter 5). This appears equally true for females and males. Girls with disruptive behavior disorders, including CD and ADHD, are found to have poorer academic performance than healthy girls (Riley et al., 1998). Female adolescents self-reporting high levels of delinquent behavior are more likely to have poor classroom and school attendance than are nondelinquent females (Weist, Paskewitz, Jackson, & Jones, 1998).

Family Dysfunction

Aggressive/antisocial girls come from more adverse and dysfunctional family backgrounds than healthy girls do. Delinquent females tend to originate from nonintact families with a history of numerous parental changes (Calhoun et al., 1993). High rates of familial criminality and arrest in primary caregivers and relatives are found (Rosenbaum, 1989). Rates of parental mental illness are also high in families of antisocial girls. For example, one study reported higher rates of mothers with psychiatric illness among delinquent females than among matched nondelinquent controls (Offord, Abrams, Allen, & Poushinsky, 1979). High rates of alcoholism are reported in the biological fathers of females with juvenile offenses (Rosenbaum, 1989). These results suggest that rates of family dysfunction and familial psychopathology are similar in boys and girls with these problems (Webster-Stratton, 1996b).

Psychiatric Disorders and Mental Health Aspects

Females with aggression and related behaviors have many comorbid psychiatric and mental health conditions. These associated conditions are frequently overlooked in clinical treatment and juvenile justice settings, where attention is commonly focused on containing overt and covert aggression and antisocial behaviors. For example, in a study of 173 adolescents incarcerated for delinquency, the prevalence of a mental health disorder was 87% for females as opposed to 27% for males (Timmons-Mitchell et al., 1997). This section discusses common associated conditions found in girls with aggressive/antisocial behaviors.

Internalizing disorders such as depression and anxiety are more common in adolescent females than in adolescent males in the general population (Rutter, 1986). Adolescent females with CD also have high rates of emotional disorders (Zoccolillo & Rogers, 1991). The risk for developing an emotional disorder for girls with CD (relative to girls without CD) is 14.9 at ages 10–11 years, and 10.1 at ages 14–15 years (Zoccolillo, 1992). The presence of CD increases the likelihood that emotional disorders will co-occur (Flannery, Singer, & Wester, 2001; Zoccolillo, 1992). Generally the signs and symptoms of CD develop first, followed by the development of emotional disorders. A childhood psychiatric diagnosis of CD predicts the development of emotional disorders more strongly for adult women than for adult men (Robins, 1986). The longitudinal trend for females with CD appears to be an increasing prevalence of emotional disorders as they mature from preadolescence to adolescence and then into adulthood. In contrast, for males with CD, the highest prevalence of depression or emotional disorders is in preadolescence and decreases into adulthood (Zoccolillo, 1992). These data suggest that females with CD are at high risk for the co-occurrence of depression and anxiety.

PTSD is typically caused by an overwhelming event outside the range of ordinary human experience, such as experiencing child abuse, a shooting, or a rape. Symptoms include intrusive recollections, avoidant/numbing symptoms, and hyperarousal symptoms (see Chapter 4). Previous research has found that between 1% and 14% of the general population currently suffers from PTSD (American Psychiatric Association, 1994). In populations of juveniles convicted of offenses and characterized by high rates of CD, the prevalence of PTSD appears much higher. In a sample of incarcerated delinquent males, 32% met criteria for PTSD (Steiner, Garcia, & Matthews, 1997). Rates appear higher still for incarcerated delinquent females: In a study of 96 such females, 70% reported being exposed to traumatic experiences such as assault, shootings, or rape (Cauffman, Feldman, Waterman, & Steiner, 1998). Males have been found to be more likely to report witnessing a violent event (Steiner et al., 1997), and females to be more likely to directly experience a violent event (Cauffman et al., 1998). Cauffman and colleagues also found that 65% of their female sample had met criteria for PTSD at some point in their lifetimes. Delinquent females have six times higher rates of PTSD at some point in their lifetimes than are found for females in the general population, and are 50% more likely than delinquent males to exhibit symptoms of PTSD (Cauffman et al., 1998). Delinquent females meeting criteria for PTSD are found to have lower levels of behavioral restraint, more aggression, and lower impulse control than delinquent females not meeting these criteria (Cauffman et al., 1998).

In addition, high rates of sexual and physical abuse have been reported in female juvenile offender populations. For example, in one survey questionnaire study of offending adolescents, it was found that 64% of the females reported sexual abuse experiences, as contrasted with 13% of the males (D. Miller, Trapani, Fejes-Mendoza, Eggleston, & Dwiggins, 1995). Studies suggest that between 43% and 75% of antisocial girls have been sexually abused, compared to the general population rate of 12% (Calhoun et al., 1993). Physical abuse is also reported for 42% to 62% of such girls (Lewis et al., 1991).

ADHD is common in youth with aggression and antisocial behavior. Although this disorder is far more common among boys than girls (see Chapter 4), girls with ADHD are far more aggressive than girls without ADHD (Gaub & Carlson, 1997). Among psychiatrically referred youth, girls and boys with ADHD may have equal rates of aggression. However, in nonreferred samples of youth assessed in the community, girls with ADHD are less aggressive than boys with ADHD (Gaub & Carlson, 1997). The same is true for CD: Girls with ADHD have much higher rates of CD than girls without ADHD; however, they have only one-third the rate of CD found for boys with ADHD (Biederman, Faraone, Mick, et al., 1999). In addition, there appear to be high rates of internalizing disorders (depression and anxiety) in girls with ADHD (Biederman, Faraone, Mick, et al., 1999). This suggests that girls with aggressive/antisocial behaviors should be assessed for the presence of comorbid ADHD.

CD and SUDs frequently coexist in youth (Clark et al., 1997; Disney, Elkins, McGue, & Iacono, 1999; see Chapter 4). This association appears true for both male and female adolescents. For example, in a study of 626 pairs of 17-year-old twins, CD was found to increase the risk of SUDs in adolescence, independently of ADHD and regardless of gender (i.e., girls and boys with CD were at equal risk for developing SUDs) (Disney et al., 1999). In this study, odds ratios for the development of SUDs in the presence of CD or ADHD were calculated separately for males and females. By definition, odds ratios of greater than 1.0 demonstrate an association between an independent variable and a dependent variable. For male subjects, the odds ratio for the development of an SUD in the presence of ADHD was 1.30, and in the presence of CD was 4.61. For female subjects in this study, the odds ratio for the development of an SUD in the presence of ADHD was 2.11 and in the presence of CD was 6.16. In contrast to a diagnosis of ADHD, CD thus had an overwhelming influence on the development of SUDs for both genders (Disney et al., 1999).

The reverse association also appears to hold; that is, early-onset SUDs accelerate the pathway into CD for both males and females. For example, a 3-year longitudinal study of 1,212 urban children found that the early use of alcohol without parental permission was associated with higher levels of conduct problems by the ages of 10–12 years, and higher rates of growth of conduct problems during the transition from late childhood to early adolescence. Although the level of conduct problems was greater for boys than for girls, the association of early unsanctioned alcohol use and accelerating conduct problems was true for both genders (E. O. Johnson, Arria, Borges, Ialongo, & Anthony, 1995). Thus early-onset CD is associated with SUDs, and early-onset SUDs appear to be associated with escalating conduct problems for both boys and girls.

Research has linked eating disturbances with behavioral impulsivity in females (Wonderlich & Mitchell, 1997). The type of eating disturbance most associated with impulsivity is bulimia nervosa. Bulimia behaviors include binge eating and various methods of purging (e.g., self-induced vomiting or laxative use for weight control). Impulsive behaviors often associated with bulimia nervosa include affective undercontrol, suicidal gestures, shoplifting, SUDs, and sexual promiscuity (Wonderlich & Swift, 1990). Restrictive eating disorders such as anorexia nervosa appear less closely associated with impulsivity. Although not all studies agree (see Attie & Brooks-Gunn, 1989), an association between eating disturbances and aggression has been reported for late preadolescent and adolescent females. Girls who self-reported binge eating and purging or dietary restriction on a survey of 3,630 females in grades 6 through 12 had odds of aggressive behavior two to four times higher than girls who did not endorse these items (Thompson, Wonderlich, Crosby, & Mitchell, 1999). In this same study, the combination of female aggression and eating disturbance was also correlated with an increased rate of SUDs and suicide attempts.

Aggression and related behaviors are associated with increased rates of youth suicide as well (Brent et al., 1993; Garrison, McKweon, Valois, & Vincent, 1993). A history of antisocial behaviors or perpetrating assault during the adolescent years is a risk factor for female suicidal ideation, threats, and attempts (Flannery et al., 2001; Juon & Ensminger, 1997; Wannan & Fombonne, 1998). In females, depression interacts significantly with SUDs and CD to increase risk for suicidal behaviors (Wannan & Fombonne, 1998). Aggression toward others and aggression directed toward the self may not be opposite forms of aggressive expression. Both outward aggression and suicide attempts may reflect difficulties in impulse control (Cairns & Cairns, 1986). Given high rates of depression and SUDs, females with CD and outward expressions of aggression toward others are also at risk for suicidal behaviors.

Neurobiological Correlates

Neurobiological correlates of aggression and related behaviors are reviewed in Chapter 7. The majority of these previously reviewed studies investigate samples that are entirely or almost entirely male; much less is known about neurobiological correlates of aggression in girls. This section discusses what is known about the impact of menarcheal timing, testosterone, aggression, corticotropin-releasing hormone (CRH) and cortisol on female aggression and antisociality.

Menarcheal Timing

Differences in the timing of puberty have important implications for girls' development. Previous research has suggested that the experience of early-maturing girls differs from that of later-maturing girls (Grief & Ulman, 1982). In longitudinal studies from three different countries, increased rates of conduct problems, norm and rule violations, sexually precocious behavior, and disruptive behavior have been reported for early-maturing girls as compared to later-maturing girls (Caspi & Moffitt, 1991; Simmons & Blyth, 1987; Stattin & Magnusson, 1990). Early maturation may have negative consequences for the adolescent female because of increased social demands caused by her new sexual status, without the benefit of social and institutional social structures that smooth the way for later-maturing girls. Others may attribute greater social maturity to early-maturing girls than is warranted by their chronological age, with corresponding increases in social demands with which these girls are not yet ready to cope.

Later research has identified a biosocial interaction in early-maturing females that appears to heighten risk for conduct problems. This risk appears to be mediated by the school social environment. In a study of 297 non-clinic-referred girls assessed in their community school environments, early-maturing girls in mixed-gender school environments were more at risk for delinquency and conduct problems than early-maturing girls in all-girl school environments (Caspi, Lynam, Moffitt, & Silva, 1993). In this study, "early maturation" was defined as an age of menarche less than 12 years, 5 months (Caspi et al., 1993). Specifically, early-maturing females in mixed-gender environments as compared to all-girl environments had more familiarity with delinquent peers, engaged in more rule-violating behaviors, engaged in more delinquent activity, and persisted longer in their delinquent activity during the teenage years (Caspi et al., 1993). It may be that in mixed-sex school environments, delinquent behavior is more normative than in all-girl environments. Since boys are generally more delinquent and disruptive than girls, their presence in the school setting may provide girls with more delinquent role models and/or more social reinforcement for conduct problems.

Testosterone

Testosterone is produced by the testes of men, by the ovaries of women, and by the adrenal glands of both genders. *In utero*, testosterone masculinizes the fetus; in adults, it builds muscle and increases libido. The physiological effects of testosterone are similar in both males and females. However, absolute levels of testosterone are much lower in women than in men (Dabbs & Hargrove, 1997).

In males, testosterone appears linked to aggression in preclinical studies (Melloni, Connor, Xvan Hang, Harrison, & Ferris, 1997). In human males, testosterone also appears linked to aggression (see Chapter 7). The relationship of testosterone to aggression and antisocial behavior has been studied much less in females. In adult women who are incarcerated for crimes ranging from forgery to murder, testosterone as measured in the saliva has been found to be positively correlated with crimes of unprovoked violence (Dabbs, Ruback, Frady, Hopper, & Sgoutas, 1988). Salivary testosterone is also positively correlated with aggressive dominance over others among adult female prison inmates (Dabbs & Hargrove, 1997). In a laboratory study of non-clinic-referred adult volunteers, salivary testosterone levels were significantly related to feelings of anger and tension for both sexes (van Honk et al., 1999). These findings suggest that testosterone is related to aggression, anger, and violence in adult females, as has been reported for adult males.

The relationship between testosterone and aggression in adolescent females is much less clear. The two studies investigating this issue have both reported negative results. Susman et al. (1987) found no relationship between measures of testosterone and aggressiveness and delinquency in adolescent females. Brooks-Gunn and Warren (1989) found no correlation between aggressive affect and testosterone levels in girls aged 10–14 years. Thus the relationship between testosterone and aggressive/antisocial behaviors for adolescent females is much less clear than for incarcerated adult females with histories of violence.

CRH and Cortisol

The stress response in humans is mediated by a neuroendocrine system that includes the hypothalamic–pituitary–adrenal (HPA) axis and the stress hormone cortisol (see Chapter 7). In response to stress, the hypothalamus secretes CRH, which acts on the pituitary to release adrenocorticotropic hormone (ACTH). ACTH then acts at the level of the adrenal cortex to regulate the synthesis of cortisol, a stress hormone. Cortisol helps mobilize the individual to meet the physiological demands imposed by the need to respond to environmental stressors.

Cortisol and CRH are both linked to aggressive/antisocial behaviors in children, adolescents, and adults. Specifically, HPA underarousal and low cortisol concentrations have been associated with conduct problems and violence (Susman, Dorn, Inoff-Germain, Nottelmann, & Chrousos, 1997; Virkkunen, 1985). Overall, the evidence suggests that low HPA axis functioning is a correlate of such behaviors. The majority of studies have investigated this association in males (see Chapter 7). Very few studies have assessed cortisol or HPA axis functioning and its association with aggressive/antisocial behaviors in females. In 47 adolescent girls meeting diagnostic criteria for CD, morning plasma cortisol levels were significantly diminished compared to levels in 37 normal control girls (Pajer, Gardner, Rubin, Perel, & Neal, 2001). In a study of pregnant female adolescents aged 13–19 years old, Susman et al. (1999) found that lower concentrations of CRH were related to a greater number of CD symptoms in early pregnancy and in the postpartum period. In this study, no significant associations were found between plasma cortisol concentrations and CD symptoms. These findings are consistent with research showing hyporesponsivity of the stress system and antisocial behavior, and they extend this relationship to adolescent females.

Summary of Research on Correlates

In summary, females with aggression and related behaviors have many of the same correlates as males with these disorders. Neuropsychological deficits in cognition, impulse control, and ECFs are associated with female aggression, as they are in male aggression. Issues with difficult temperament are also related to aggressive/antisocial behaviors in girls. Social information-processing deficits (particularly attributing hostile intent to others in ambiguous social situations) have been described for girls with relational aggression, similar to boys with overt aggression. Aggressive girls have many social role deficits across multiple domains of daily life. Family dysfunction and parental and familial psychopathology are likewise common in the histories of antisocial girls. There appear to exist many mental health needs and comorbid psychiatric disorders in girls who meet criteria for CD and/or are incarcerated for juvenile offenses. Such girls, especially incarcerated girls, may have higher rates of comorbid PTSD than similar males. Delinquent females may experience higher lifetime rates of sexual and physical abuse than delinquent males. Girls with CD or other antisocial behaviors may have an earlier onset and higher rates of depression and anxiety than boys with CD; these rates of internalizing disorders may rise as girls progress into adolescence.

Much less research is available investigating the neurobiological correlates of aggression and related behaviors in female youth than in male youth. Current research supports a biosocial interaction between early menarcheal age and mixed-gender school environments in the development of conduct problems for girls. An association between conduct problems in adolescent females and underresponsiveness of the HPA axis is also suggested by the current literature. Little is known about CNS 5-HT, DA, and norepinephrine functioning or ANS underarousal in aggressive girls.

DEVELOPMENTAL PATHWAYS

The previous discussion serves to highlight several important points about aggressive and related behaviors in girls. First, although the forms of aggression may be different in girls versus boys (i.e., covert aggression or relational aggression vs. overt displays of aggression), during the adolescent years girls may exhibit a great deal of aggressive/antisocial behavior. Relative to the elementary school years, adolescent females increasingly engage in behavior that may qualify them for a psychiatric diagnosis of CD. Increasing numbers of females are also being arrested for criminal offenses in their adolescent years. Thus aggression and antisocial behaviors are not simply male problems; they cannot be ignored in girls.

Second, girls appear to develop these behaviors at a later age than boys. Boys are clearly more disruptive than girls during the elementary school years, but by adolescence the gender ratio for conduct problems narrows. Third, the risk factors for development of conduct problems in girls seem largely similar to those for the development of early-onset, chronic, and persistent aggressive/antisocial behavior in boys. Yet the prevalence rate of CD (for example) clearly favors boys over girls. That is, despite similar risk factors, the prevalence of CD is less in girls than in boys. Despite similar risk factors, therefore, girls develop aggressive/antisocial behaviors at a later age than boys with similar risk factors. How can the gender dissimilarities in prevalence rate and age of onset rates be explained?

The research suggests several possible answers to these questions. First, the answer may lie in part in measurement problems. As discussed earlier, one form that female aggression may take—relational aggression—may be less obvious to others and thus harder to measure in experimental designs. Next, it has been suggested that the symptoms of CD in girls are different from those in boys. Symptoms in girls may include increased acts of covert aggression and/or increased somatization complaints. If a researcher is only measuring overtly aggressive symptoms of CD, females with CD may be mistakenly underidentified.

However, a third possibility has been proposed. The developmental pathway to aggression and related behaviors may be different for girls than it is for boys. In the developmental psychopathology studies reviewed in Chapter 8, the vast majority of subjects have been males. What is true for the early development of conduct problems in boys may not be what is entirely true for the development of conduct problems in girls. After all, girls and boys have different biological constitutions. The early effects of neuroendocrine hormones such as testosterone on aggressive/antisocial behaviors are not the same for girls and boys. The timing of menarche—a physiological event not experienced by boys—may also have important implications for the development of such behaviors in girls. In addition, the socialization pressures on girls as they develop are very different from the socialization forces acting on boys. In most cultures, girls are not expected to engage in aggressive or antisocial behaviors, and are actively discouraged from behaving against societal norms (Eron, 1992). Girls are encouraged to exhibit more prosocial behaviors, and parents often encourage daughters' internalizing symptoms (e.g., deference toward others or shyness), whereas they encourage more assertive and externalizing behaviors in their sons (Keenan & Shaw, 1997). Physiological differences and socialization forces have not been accounted for in the predominantly male developmental psychopathology studies cited in Chapter 8, and may serve to alter the developmental progression of conduct problems in females.

Silverthorn and Frick (1999) propose a delayed-onset pathway for the development of antisocial behavior in girls. Although this pathway has many similarities to the developmental pathways for boys reviewed in Chapter 8, it also emphasizes factors specifically pertaining to biology and to socialization pressures, which alter the pathway to female antisocial behavior. The delayed-onset pathway for girls (which is schematically depicted in Figure 9.3) seeks to explain why, despite similar risk factors as in boys, antisocial behavior is less prevalent and occurs at a later age of onset in girls. Disruptive behavior can be equally prevalent across the two genders up to about age 5 years, but then boys clearly display more of it during the elementary school years. At puberty, there is a rise in female antisocial behaviors that can portend a poor outcome across multiple domains in adult life for adolescent females (Keenan & Shaw, 1997).

Similar to boys with early-onset antisocial behavior, girls in the delayed-onset pathway begin life with individual vulnerabilities. These may include a difficult temperament, poor impulse control, neurocognitive deficits, and the possible development of callous–unemotional personality traits (which serve to diminish empathy for others). These vulnerabilities interact with a difficult family environment (see Chapter 5 for discussion) to produce a series of failed parent–child interactions. As a result, preschool girls may show just as many

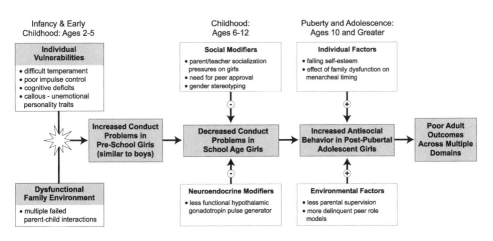

FIGURE 9.3. The delayed-onset developmental pathway to antisocial behavior in girls. Data from Silverthorn and Frick (1999).

problem behaviors as preschool boys. However, beginning with the elementary school years, boys with early-onset aggressive/antisocial behaviors become more entrenched in their behavior patterns, while girls in the delayed-onset pathway become less aggressive and antisocial. Why is this so?

It is possible that differences in prepubertal hormones and increased socialization pressures from parents, teachers, and peers to conform to stereotypically female behaviors may all serve to suppress the overt manifestations of antisocial behaviors for girls in childhood. There is evidence that the neuroendocrine milieu before puberty is different in males and females. Primate models suggest that the hypothalamic gonadotropin-releasing hormone (GnRH) generator, which facilitates secretion of sex hormones (gonadotropins), is capable of functioning at adult levels in males by infancy (Plant, 1994). However, there appears to be an active restraint system, such that the GnRH generator does not begin to produce adult levels of sex hormones in males until after puberty. In contrast, during infancy and childhood, females have an immature GnRH generator that is not capable of operating at adult levels until additional neurobiological maturational changes occur as a result of the initiation of puberty (Plant, 1994). During the prepubertal years, it takes less neurobiological restraint to constrain the production of sex hormones in girls than in boys, presumably because of the biological immaturity of the female GnRH generator. Thus, to the extent that gonadotropins influence disruptive behavior in childhood, boys may be more vulnerable to the expression of these behaviors than girls because of the existence of a fully operational yet restrained gonadotropin system (Plant, 1994; Silverthorn & Frick, 1999).

Several socialization processes that occur at the time girls enter elementary school may also help explain the decrease in female conduct problems relative to conduct problems in boys. As noted above, parents and teachers encourage girls to express their temperament and behavioral symptoms primarily through internalizing, not externalizing, symptoms (Keenan & Shaw, 1997). In contrast, boys are socially reinforced for aggressive behaviors, because these are generally seen by the culture as appropriately masculine (Eron, 1992). In addition, beginning at about 5 years of age and increasing throughout the elementary school years, peer relationships and peer approval become increasingly important—especially for girls. Beginning in kindergarten, children begin to adhere strongly and somewhat rigidly to gender stereotypes, identifying themselves as either "boys" or "girls," and engaging in school and play activities typical of their gender (Mann, 1994). They tend to have fairly inflexible sex-role definitions, which may contribute to children expecting that their same-gender peers will behave "like them" (i.e., in gender-appropriate ways). Thus increasing pressure from parents, teachers, and peers for children to conform to gender-stereotyped behaviors, and the increasing desire to seek approval from peers, may partially explain the childhood decrease in antisocial behaviors for girls and the increase in boys (Silverthorn & Frick, 1999).

At puberty and in the postpubertal adolescent years, there is a rise in antisocial behaviors for females. This increase narrows the prevalence rate in CD between males and females. This increase is primarily accounted for by increased symptoms of covert aggression in adolescent females. After diminishing conduct problems in the elementary school years, what can account for the increase in antisocial behaviors after puberty in females?

The delayed-onset model proposed by Silverthorn and Frick (1999) suggests that individual variables and environmental factors occurring at about the time of puberty serve to increase the risk for antisocial behavior in predisposed adolescent girls (i.e., those having individual vulnerabilities and growing up in a dysfunctional family environment)(see Figure 9.3). First, there is evidence that the myriad physical and psychological changes induced by puberty are viewed more negatively by females than by males (Petersen, Sarigiani, & Kennedy, 1991). Second, research suggests that the presence of psychosocial stressors during childhood, including family conflict and father absence, are associated with earlier menarche (Moffitt, Caspi, Belsky, & Silva, 1992). Third, there are psychological disruptions as girls move through puberty. Studies have suggested that although boys' self-esteem generally tends to increase throughout adolescence, girls' self-esteem may fall at puberty (Simmons & Blyth, 1987). Fourth, these physiological and psychological pubertal changes also occur at a time when parental supervision of adolescent females begins to diminish. This may allow for greater opportunities for at-risk girls to act in antisocial ways. Finally, during adolescence an increase occurs in the overall rate of antisocial behavior in the social milieu, since boys with both childhood-onset antisocial behavior and newly emerging, adolescent-onset antisocial behavior are committing more antisocial acts. The increase in antisocial behaviors in the environment may provide the at-risk girls with greater peer modeling and social reinforcement for antisocial behaviors. The physical and hormonal changes associated with puberty, the effects of earlier age of menarche on delinquent behavior, a negative self-image and falling self-esteem, and increased delinquent behaviors in the social milieu may thus all conspire to lead at-risk girls into more antisocial behaviors during adolescence (Silverthorn & Frick, 1999).

YOUNG ADULT OUTCOMES

Historically, it was generally believed that the adult outcomes for adolescent girls with aggressive/antisocial behaviors were relatively benign. They became involved in criminality much less frequently than similar adolescent boys as they grew into young adulthood. They were arrested less frequently than males. They married and conceived children, long considered indications of healthy adult adjustment for any female (Pajer, 1998). However, more recent research describes less optimistic outcomes for many adolescent females with aggression and related behaviors.

The concept of "homotypic continuity" is often used by developmental psychopathologists to describe a strong correlation between symptoms of a disorder at one point in time and the same symptoms at a later point in time. That is, a disorder with homotypic continuity evidences the same symptoms when a person is younger and at a later point in the individual's development. In contrast, the term "heterotypic continuity" describes the relationship between a disorder at one point in the life cycle and continued dysfunction at a later point in development, but with different signs and symptoms. Outcomes for adolescent females with aggressive/antisocial behaviors reveal evidence for both homotypic and heterotypic continuity.

Criminality

An example of homotypic continuity is the strong relationship between serious delinquent acts in adolescents with CD and continued criminality in these same individuals in adulthood. Homotypic continuity is robust for antisocial behavior among delinquent boys and continued criminal behavior among men (Pajer, 1998). Although homotypic continuity for antisocial acts and criminal behavior is much stronger for men than for women, there is evidence for similar continuity across adolescence and into young adulthood for females.

In a review of 16 studies of adult crime outcomes of delinquent adolescent girls (see Pajer, 1998), the crime rate in adulthood ranged from 10% to 96%, although rates clustered around 25% to 46% in the majority of reviewed studies. These studies were based on both arrest data and self-report of illegal activities. Rates were higher for girls incarcerated as adolescents and lower for girls in less restrictive settings. Adult crime rates were higher in all groups of antisocial girls than in comparison groups of either healthy control subjects or girls with other psychiatric problems. Higher rates of adult criminality are also found in follow-up studies of adolescent females incarcerated in their teenage years for crimes committed as juveniles, although rates are lower for females than for males. For example, in a study of 21 incarcerated 15-year-old delinquent females, 71% had adult arrest records at 7- to 12-year follow-up; this compared with an adult arrest rate of 95% at 7- to 12-year follow-up for age- and race-matched incarcerated adolescent males from the same study (Lewis et al., 1991). When adult incarcerated women are studied, they report high rates of youthful antisocial behaviors, including juvenile arrest rates ranging from 35% to 73% (Pajer, 1998). These data support the idea that many (although not all) teenage girls with CD and juvenile offenses demonstrate evidence of homotypic continuity and continue to be at risk for criminal activity and antisocial behavior as young adults when compared to healthy control subjects.

General Life Outcomes

Examples of heterotypic continuity are seen in the relationships between adolescent female CD and poor outcomes across multiple domains of adult life that are distinct from antisocial behavior. In other words, these outcomes do not include continued criminality or arrest rates (as would be the case for homotypic continuity), but rather poor functioning in such life areas as general health, interpersonal and relationship functioning, and education/occupational status. The generally poor adult outcomes for delinquent girls in these diverse domains belie the belief that their adult adjustment is typically benign.

General Health Status

Table 9.1 presents recent data on general health outcomes in young adulthood of adolescent girls with antisocial behavior in general and CD in particular.

TABLE 9.1. General Life Outcomes of Adolescent Females with Antisocial Behavior (ASB) and CD

Outcome	Girls with ASB/CD	Psychiatric controls	Healthy controls
General health outcomes			
Mortality (at 2- to 30-yr outcome)	6%–10%	5%	0.035%–10%
Lifetime # of sexual partners by age 21 yr	5–9	3–4	3–4
Contracted an STD[a] by age 21 yr	26%	10%–16%	16%
Pregnancy by age 21 yr	46%	23%–30%	18%
Psychiatric comorbidity (ASPD, histrionic personality disorder, mood/anxiety disorder)	14%–60%	NA[b]	0%–40%
Substance dependence	26%	9%–11%	7%
Nicotine dependence	28%	18%–36%	17%
Daily smoking	74%	41%	32%
Relationship outcomes			
Early marriage (<18 yr)	21%–33%	8%	9%
Unhappy in marriage (self-report)	100%	NA	14%
Education outcomes			
Stopping at high school	40%	NA	9%
Occupational outcomes			
Holding 10 or more jobs in the previous 10 yr	11%	1%	0%
Family functioning			
Family court involvement	8%–33%	NA	4%
Service utilization			
Social services	55%	35%	10%
Physician utilization	23%	0%	10%
Global young adult life adjustment			
Coping problems in ≥ 2 domains	42%–62%	26%	9%–12%

Note. Data from Pajer (1998) and Bardone et al. (1998).
[a]STD, sexually transmitted disease.
[b]NA, not available.

Comparisons to outcomes of girls with other psychiatric disorders and of healthy controls are also provided.

Mortality

Adult mortality rates of adolescent girls with CD have been compared to the mortality rates for adult females in the general population in four studies. Robins (1966) reported that 7% of a sample with CD had died at 30-year outcome, compared to a population-based death rate for women at the time of 7%. All deaths were reported as natural, nonviolent deaths. During this same time interval, 5% of nonantisocial psychiatric controls and 10% of healthy controls had also died. This study thus did not support increased mortality rates in adulthood for adolescent females with CD.

In contrast, three studies do support increased young adult death rates in adolescent girls with CD. In a study of all Swedish girls committed to state-run probationary schools, the 18-year mortality rate was 10%, compared to an expected death rate in the general population of 1.1% to 2.6%. Violent deaths were recorded in 77% of those who died (Rydelius, 1988). In a 2- to 4-year follow-up study of girls with CD who were initially admitted to an inpatient psychiatry unit, it was found that 6% of the girls had died violent deaths, as opposed to the age-matched normal population rate for violent deaths at the time of 0.034% (Zoccolillo & Rogers, 1991). In the Lewis et al. (1991) study, 21 incarcerated adolescent females were followed for 7–12 years. Over this time period, 19 of the 21 girls made suicide attempts; 1 died of completed suicide, and another of AIDS. The authors note that this death rate in their small sample was 180 times the expected death rate for females in the general population.

These data on adult mortality rates for adolescent females with CD are similar to adult mortality rates for delinquent boys. In a 50-year follow-up study of 1,000 delinquent and nondelinquent boys, Laub and Vaillant (2000) found that 13% of the delinquent males and only 6% of the nondelinquent males died of unnatural causes by age 65 years. Frequency of delinquency, misuse of alcohol, adult crime, dysfunctional home environment, and poor education were all statistically related to death, especially death by unnatural causes. Overall, the research suggests that, regardless of gender, adolescents with antisocial behavior and CD have increased adult mortality rates relative to the general population.

Reproductive Health

Research supports a link between female adolescent CD and adverse reproductive health outcomes. By age 21 years, girls with CD are found to have a higher number of sexual partners than either girls with other psychiatric disorders or healthy control girls (see Table 9.1). Girls with antisocial behavior engage in more frequent and more risky sexual behavior than healthy controls do (Booth & Zhang, 1997; Castillo Mezzich et al., 1997). They are also at higher risk for contracting a sexually transmitted disease (relative risk of 1.7, compared to depressed girls' relative risk of 0.6) (Bardone et al., 1998) and becoming pregnant by early adulthood (relative risk of 3.1 compared to healthy controls and 1.6 compared to depressed girls) (see Table 9.1; Bardone et al., 1998). Female CD is statistically associated with risk of teenage pregnancy, over and above the risk associated with depression (Kovacs, Krol, & Voti, 1994). These results suggest that access to reproductive health care is important for female adolescents with CD or other antisocial behavior.

Psychiatric Comorbidity

Young adult psychiatric comorbidity, defined as outcomes varying from commitment to an institution to formally diagnosed psychiatric disorders other than CD, is high in girls with CD. Adult psychiatric problems are more prevalent in adolescent females with antisocial behaviors than in healthy controls (see Table 9.1). Increased rates of adult personality, mood, anxiety, and other disorders have been found in teenage girls with CD as they mature into adulthood. For example, one study reported that 35% of girls with CD met criteria for ASPD as adults, compared to 0% of teenage girls without CD (Zoccolillo, Pickles, Quinton, & Rutter, 1992). Other studies have found that between 21% and 42% of girls with antisocial behavior develop hysterical and dramatic personality disorders as young adult women (Cloninger & Guze, 1970; Robins, 1966; Pajer, 1998). Rates of depression, anxiety disorders, and unexplained medical complaints (somatization) are much higher in teenage girls with CD as they grow up than in healthy controls (Flannery et al., 2001; Robins, 1986). Overall, reviews of the literature on psychiatric morbidity in females with antisocial behavior report psychiatric problems in between 14% and 60%, compared to psychiatric problems in healthy controls of between 0% and 40% (Pajer, 1998).

Longitudinal studies also report high rates of young adult substance dependence (including nicotine dependence) and daily smoking in teenage girls with CD. Adolescent CD significantly increases the risk for young adult substance dependence in general (Bardone et al., 1998). Although more girls with depression smoke tobacco than girls with CD, girls with either depression or CD are more nicotine-dependent as young adults than healthy control women (Bardone et al., 1998). By age 21 years, almost three-fourths of girls with teenage CD smoke daily—a much higher rate than that of either psychiatric or healthy control women (see Table 9.1; Bardone et al., 1998).

Relationship and Family Functioning

Most teenage girls with CD marry (Pajer, 1998). There is a trend for such girls to marry at under 18 years of age (Cloninger & Guze, 1970; Robins, 1966). Higher rates of marital difficulties, divorce, and extramarital sexual activity are reported for married teenage girls with CD than for other psychiatric patients and healthy controls (Pajer, 1998). Young adult outcomes of teenage girls with CD include high rates of marital violence. One study found that such girls are 3.9 times more likely to be involved in a mutually violent relationship than are normal or depressed control girls (Bardone, Moffitt, Caspi, Dickson, & Silva, 1996).

The adult family relations and parental functioning of adolescent girls with antisocial behavior are also problematic. In the longitudinal study of Robins (1966), 36% of the offspring of mothers with histories of CD were placed outside the home—a rate higher than that for either healthy control women or women with other psychiatric difficulties. Women with CD as teenagers have higher rates of involvement in family court than comparison women. In the Kauai Longitudinal Study, 33% of the women with delinquency in addition to other psychiatric problems had a family court history, compared to 8% of women with delinquency-only histories, but only 4% of healthy controls (Werner & Smith, 1992).

Education and Occupation

Academic and occupational underachievement is common for females with histories of delinquency or CD. Most studies report high rates of either dropping out of school before high school is completed, or failing to progress in education beyond high school (MacDonald & Achenbach, 1999). In the Kauai Longitudinal Study, Werner and Smith (1992) found that 40% of delinquent subjects did not progress beyond high school, compared to only 9% of the group without delinquency. Another study reported that girls with conduct problems were 3.8 times more likely to have no high school diploma than healthy control girls were (Bardone et al., 1996). A low level of maternal education is also a risk factor for the development of persistent aggression in male offspring—an example of risk across the generations (Nagin & Tremblay, 2001). Research on adult occupational status of girls with histories of antisocial behavior finds high rates of unstable job histories. In the Robins (1966) study, 11% of the antisocial group reported having 10 or more jobs in the previous 10 years, compared to 1% of psychiatric controls and 0% of healthy control subjects.

Service Utilization

"Service utilization" includes welfare use, involvement with other social service agencies, and medical care. Women with antisocial histories have higher rates of multiple service utilization than nonantisocial psychiatric controls or healthy comparison subjects (see Table 9.1). In the Dunedin Multidisciplinary Health and Development Study, a longitudinal study of a birth cohort in New Zealand, women with CD were 3.7 times more likely to use multiple sources of welfare than comparison women (Bardone et al., 1996). Rates of physician utilization are also higher for antisocial women than for controls (see Table 9.1).

Summary of Outcome Research

In summary, there is evidence to support both homotypic and heterotypic continuity in adult outcomes for teenage girls with CD or other forms of antisociality. Compared to women without such histories, these women have higher rates of criminality, higher mortality rates, a wide variety of psychiatric comorbid conditions, dysfunctional marriage and parenting relationships, poorer educational and employment outcomes, and a high rate of service utilization. As adults, therefore, they have higher rates of poor adjustment across multiple life functioning domains compared to control women. These data indicate that, contrary to the historical perception, the adult outcome for many adolescent girls with aggressive/antisocial behaviors is not benign.

CHAPTER SUMMARY

This chapter has reviewed issues in female aggression and related behaviors. As it becomes clearer that forms of female aggression may differ from male modes of aggression, the study of female aggression has developed in its own right. Although males tend to be more aggressive than females at all developmental ages throughout the lifespan, female aggression is neither uncommon, trivial, nor unimportant. Rates of CD are high for females, especially in adolescence, and rates of female juvenile crime in the population are rising. Psychopathy has been identified in females of all ages, is highly correlated with CD and other antisocial behavior, and is in need of continued research. DSH may be a maladaptive expression of anger and aggression, independent of suicide, that is most prevalent in samples of teenage girls. Stability rates of aggression for girls over time are less than for boys, but demonstrate modest correlations, especially when measured by observer rating scales or peer nomination techniques. Stability rates are clearly higher for males than for females when criminal justice indicators are used. Although the psychosocial correlates of aggression appear similar in boys and girls, there exist gender differences in age of onset and symptoms of CD. These may be explained in part by a different developmental pathway to adolescent CD in girls as opposed to boys—the delayed-onset pathway. Neurobiological correlates of aggression and CD remain poorly studied in females. Most importantly, the poor young adult outcomes of teenage girls with CD or other antisociality across multiple domains of life functioning bespeak a need for continuing research into this population.

Clinical Assessment, Case Formulation, and Treatment Planning

T he clinical assessment of youth with aggressive and antisocial behaviors generally occurs in mental health treatment settings. Although large numbers of such youth are seen in juvenile justice settings, the purpose of criminal justice is to adjudicate and contain youth who have broken laws. As society has begun to take a more punitive stance toward youthful offenders, rehabilitation may increasingly become a secondary goal to confinement and punishment (Grisso, 2000). Thus most clinical assessment of children and adolescents with aggression and related behaviors occurs in mental health treatment arenas, where their behaviors are usually defined in terms of conduct disorder (CD). Indeed, there is general agreement in the literature that CD is one of the most common forms of psychopathology in children (American Academy of Child and Adolescent Psychiatry [AACAP], 1997c). CD constitutes the most common reason for referral for psychiatric evaluation of children and adolescents, accounting for 30% to 50% of clinic referrals (Kazdin, 1996).

Since one goal of mental health professionals is to design and deliver effective clinical treatment interventions for children and adolescents with CD, it is critical to assess the factors clinically relevant to their behaviors. Assessment is crucial for several reasons. First, CD and related behaviors are complex forms of psychopathology, presenting with multiple deficits across a range of domains of daily life functioning. It is necessary for a clinician to clearly understand an individual youth's range of psychopathology and impairment, in order to develop a meaningful and comprehensive clinical treatment plan for that youth. Second, as previous chapters have discussed, multiple causal pathways to the development of CD exist. One size does not fit all, and different mechanisms operate in the development of problem behaviors for different individuals with CD. Third, CD in children and adolescents is highly comorbid with a number of other psychiatric diagnoses, which also need assessment and intervention. These conditions may include mood disorders; anxiety disorders, especially posttraumatic stress disorder (PTSD); substance use disorders (SUDs); specific disabilities in language, reading, or academic achievement, and attention-deficit/hyperactivity disorder (ADHD). Finally, multiple contextual/environmental and parenting/familial variables are relevant to the etiology of conduct problems in youth. A clinical assessment of these factors and their interactions is necessary so that a comprehensive and meaningful clinical treatment plan can be designed. By itself, the psychiatric diagnosis of CD provides very limited information for clinical treatment planning.

The main purposes of this chapter are (1) to present a general model of psychiatric assessment, case formulation, and treatment planning for youth with CD and related behaviors/disorders; and (2) to describe assessment tools useful in the evaluation of such youth. A brief look at forensic assessment (i.e., the determination of a youth's dangerousness to others) is also provided. But, first, a caveat is in order.

A CAVEAT: INCREASING RESOURCE LIMITATIONS IN CHILD AND ADOLESCENT MENTAL HEALTH TREATMENT

Because CD is a severe and complex form of psychopathology that affects multiple domains of individual functioning, mental health interventions can be successful only if they are carefully coordinated, aimed at multiple areas of individual dysfunction, and delivered over extended periods of time (AACAP, 1997c). However, economic trends in health care over the past two decades in the United States have been toward drastically reducing the availability of mental health resources, in order to contain mental health care and overall health care expenditures (HayGroup, 1998). This is being achieved both by reducing the actual number of mental health programs available, and by micromanaging mental health benefits through managed care "carve-out" contracts with insurance companies (Jellinek & Little, 1998; Iglehart, 1996). Not only private insurers, but also state Medicaid programs, are increasingly rationing mental health benefits through such "carve-out" contracts (Iglehart, 1996). The net results are fewer service providers and institutions; evershorter lengths of treatment for mental health patients; increasing fragmentation of mental health treatment care plans, wherein solitary, time-limited treatment interventions (with a primary emphasis on psychopharmacology) are supported for a strictly rationed number of treatment visits, in isolation from a comprehensive continuum of care; and an increasing loss of highly trained and experienced (but more expensive) mental health care providers, who are downsized for cost containment purposes in favor of less trained and experienced, but less expensive, clinicians (Jellinek & Little, 1998). In this economic reality, the comprehensive mental health care that youth with CD require is almost impossible to achieve in either routine community or private mental health care settings.

As an example of the increasing resource limitations in clinical mental health care, consider the following. The National Association of Psychiatric Health Systems, the Association of Behavioral Group Practices, and the National Alliance for the Mentally Ill commissioned the HayGroup (an actuarial and benefits consulting firm in Washington, DC) to analyze trends in the proportion of employer health care dollars spent on mental (behavioral) health care for the period 1988 through 1997. Using a statistical model, the Hay Group (1998) examined the values of benefits offered by more than 1,000 medium-sized and large employers in the United States for general health care, mental health care, and total health care.

Over the 10 years covered by the study, the total value of employer-provided health care benefits, in constant 1997 dollars, decreased by 10.2%. The value of general health care benefits decreased by 7.4%. Over the same time period, the value of mental health care benefits decreased by 54.1% (see Figure 10.1). In other words, $1 out of every $2 available for mental health care in 1988 was no longer available by 1997 to fund clinical services—a far greater decline than the decrease in general health care dollars. As a proportion of total health care costs, mental health care benefits decreased from 6.1% in 1988 to only 3.1% in 1997 (HayGroup, 1998).

Mental health care benefits have thus become increasingly limited since 1988. Day limits on inpatient psychiatric care, and visit limitations on ambulatory mental health care, have been imposed by more and more insurance

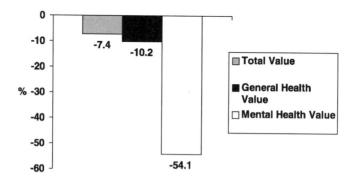

FIGURE 10.1. Percentages of change in health care benefits values, 1988–1997 (in constant 1997 dollars). Data from HayGroup (1998).

plans between 1988 through 1997 (see Figure 10.2). For example, at a time when outpatient general health care utilization increased by 27.4% between 1993 and 1996, mental health outpatient utilization decreased by 24.6% (HayGroup, 1998). In another example, a study examined patterns in utilization of psychiatric inpatient services by children and adolescents in general hospitals between 1988 and 1995 (Pottick, McAlpine, & Andelman, 2000). During the study period, there occurred a 44% decline in mean length of inpatient hospital stay and a 36% increase in hospital discharges for psychiatrically referred inpatient children and adolescents. The mean length of stay declined most for youth who were psychiatrically hospitalized in private facilities and those covered by private insurance, in contrast to public-funded state Medicaid.

The conclusions are clear: Mental health insurance benefits are increasingly "carved out" and micromanaged separately from general health care benefits; are increasingly harder to obtain; and, when obtained, are increasingly rationed and limited in the amount of mental health care they allow (Jellinek & Little, 1998; Iglehart, 1996).

Another problem facing clinicians attempting to develop comprehensive treatment plans for youth with CD is the growing number of uninsured children and adolescents in the United States. There is evidence that the growing emphasis on managed care as a way of reducing health care costs contributes to the rise in the number of uninsured people, especially children (Walsh, 1997). A recent study of health insurance coverage found 14.1% of youth aged 10–18 years, or 4.2 million youngsters, lacking any coverage at all in the United States for the year 1995 (Newacheck, Brindis,

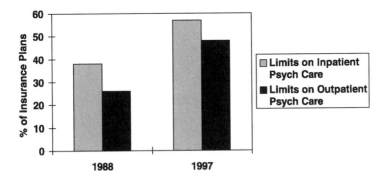

FIGURE 10.2. Evidence that mental health care benefits have become more limited since 1988: Percentages of insurance plans imposing day limits on psychiatric inpatient care and annual visit limits on outpatient psychiatric care, 1988–1997. Data from HayGroup (1998).

Cart, Marchi, & Irwin, 1999). Significantly more youth lacking insurance coverage were unable to get mental health care than youth with health insurance. The risk of being uninsured was higher for older adolescents, minorities, youth in low-income families, and youth living in single-parent households (Newacheck et al., 1999). These risk factors are similar to some of those found for CD (see Chapter 5). Thus the chances that health care insurance will not be available for mental health treatment planning are increased for youth with these risk factors.

In short, the caveat is that the very youth who need comprehensive, readily available, and long-duration mental health care for CD may not have enough (or any) mental health insurance coverage—and that mental health treatment without adequate funding is never satisfactory or effective. Into this harsh fiscal climate enter mental health clinicians who must attempt an inclusive assessment and treatment of youth with CD.

A GENERAL MODEL OF ASSESSMENT, CASE FORMULATION, AND TREATMENT PLANNING

Goals and Content Areas for Assessment

The current standard of care in the evaluation of children and adolescents requires an approach that employs multiple sources of information and multiple methods of data collection in various settings. At a minimum, assessment should include evaluation of a child/adolescent, parents, and family, and of the youth's behavior and performance at school (AACAP, 1995; Connor & Fisher, 1997). A listing of goals and specific content areas to be covered in assessment of youth with CD and related behaviors is presented in Table 10.1. It is evident from this table that information must be gathered about many aspects of a child's or adolescent's functioning, as well as many aspects of the family and psychosocial environment that the youth experiences on a day-to-day basis.

Completing the clinical assessment as outlined in Table 10.1 will leave a clinician with many data about various domains of functioning for a referred child or adolescent. However, this is only the first step in a more extensive process. The clinician must still understand how to use the collected data to create a rational and effective treatment plan within the currently available resource limitations for treatment. The data constitute only a static snapshot of various aspects of the referred youth's life. The challenge for the clinician in developing an effective, realistic, and individualized treatment plan is to understand how these various domains influence one another, to increase either risk for conduct problems or resilience. This is a much more demanding challenge for the clinician than simply collecting information. Its accomplishment, however, serves to distinguish realistic and effective treatment planning for an individual with CD from a sterile exercise in assessment—one that offers little actual hope for the referred youth and family.

TABLE 10.1. Goals and Specific Content Areas for the Assessment of Children and Adolescents with Conduct Disorder

Goal	Specific content
Child	
To assess a wide range of CD symptoms/behaviors	Overt–covert symptoms; aggressive–nonaggressive behaviors; behaviors committed alone or as part of a group; early-onset or adolescent-onset; acute or chronic time course
To assess a wide range of comorbid psychiatric disorders	Depression; bipolar disorder; psychotic disorders; anxiety disorders, including PTSD; ADHD; SUDs
To assess trauma history	Sexual abuse; physical abuse; neglect; witnessing violence
To assess cognitive development	Cognitive delay; learning disabilities (speech and language, reading, written expression); academic achievement
To assess biological development	Temperament; history of head injury, seizure, or CNS abnormality; *in utero* toxin exposure; birth complications
To assess interpersonal development	Attachment; capacity for empathy; quality of peer relationships; moral development; presence of callous–unemotional personality traits
To assess degree of impairment associated with the disorder	Impairment in school, family, interpersonal, and daily life activities
Family	
To assess family structure	Membership (genogram); connection or isolation from extended family and community support systems; single-parent status; non-traditional family structure
To assess parental psychopathology	Parental SUDs; mood disorders; somatization; antisocial personality disorder; adult ADHD
To assess the quality of parents' marital relationship	Divorce; marital conflict; domestic violence; marital satisfaction
To assess discipline and socialization practices used by parents	Low parental involvement with child; poor parental monitoring and supervision of child; harsh and inconsistent discipline practices; failure to utilize positive change strategies
Larger systems in the environment	
To assess the interaction between child/family and school environment	Safety; family involvement with child's school
To assess critical aspects of child's peer group	Antisocial or prosocial friends; isolated or with a number of available friendships
To assess the family social support network	Cultural/ethnic/religious identity; friendship networks; job/occupational network
To assess critical aspects of family social ecology	Safety; neighborhood violence and SUDs; socioeconomic status of family
To assess outside agencies' involvement with family	Human service providers; agencies of social control (protective services, legal system)
Resources available for clinical treatment	
To assess family's insurance status	Availability and adequacy of insurance (note that families of youth with CD may have no or little mental health insurance to support evaluation and treatment)
To assess treatment resources and expertise available in the clinical setting	Treatment setting (academic department of psychology/psychiatry, private office, community treatment center, emergency department); staffing levels; experience of available clinicians

Note. Data from Connor and Fisher (1997) and Frick (1998).

An Interactional Model of Child and Adolescent Mental Health Case Formulation

A colleague and I (Connor & Fisher, 1997) have described a general model of child and adolescent mental health case formulation that may be useful in the evaluation of youth with CD. Assessment is an open-ended, divergent process that must survey many domains of functioning (Table 10.1). For the resulting information to be used appropriately, it must be integrated into a more clinically useful form. The case formulation acts as a lens to define, focus, and prioritize the information gathered during assessment into a clinical understanding of the central issues leading the youth and family to seek help at this particular time. The individual case formulation as a convergent process is especially important in the clinical evaluation of a child or adolescent, given the amount of information from multiple sources that should be gathered during a comprehensive evaluation.

Shapiro (1989) identifies a number of commonly held misconceptions about the clinical case formulation: (1) that the case formulation is only useful for long-term treatment; (2) that the case formulation is only useful for psychodynamic therapy; (3) that the case formulation is primarily a training device and not helpful in actual clinical practice; and (4) that the case formulation must be all-inclusive, lengthy, and elaborate. However, since the case formulation represents the intermediate step between assessment (determining what is going on) and treatment planning (deciding what to do about what is going on), it seems essential regardless of the type of patient referred, the type of treatment offered, the therapeutic orientation and skills of the clinician, or the setting in which treatment takes place.

A model of juvenile mental health case formulation must satisfy several criteria (Connor & Fisher, 1997):

1. Case formulation should be *multitheoretical*, in order to encompass the variety of theories (behavioral, cognitive, neurobiological, pharmacological, family systems) utilized by practicing clinicians who evaluate and treat youth with CD and related behaviors.

2. Since the current state of knowledge in child/adolescent mental health does not endorse any one theory of causality, a model of case formulation must allow for *multicausality* (biological, psychological, social, and environmental causes) operating simultaneously across various system levels of a youngster's environment (youngster, parents, family, school, larger systems).

3. Because of the immature status of children and adolescents, clinical case formulation should emphasize a *developmental framework* that is sensitive to changes over time within a youngster's and family's behavior and experience.

4. The case formulation should allow a treatment plan to reflect the *current knowledge base* in the field.

5. Since youth are dependent on multiple systems for growth and development, child and adolescent clinical case formulation should emphasize *interactional patterns* among the youngster, family, and larger systems as powerful mechanisms in symptom onset and maintenance, and should acknowledge these as appropriate targets for therapeutic intervention.

6. A formulation must be *useful*; it need not be elaborate or lengthy, as long as it directs the clinician toward appropriate and realistic treatment options.

Steps in the Continuum from Assessment to Treatment Planning

In a time- and resource-limited mental health treatment environment, case formulation must consider assessment, case formulation, and treatment planning as part of a clinical continuum, in which each step is linked to all others. The steps in this continuum are outlined in Table 10.2 (Connor & Fisher, 1997).

TABLE 10.2. Steps in the Continuum of Assessment, Case Formulation, and Treatment Planning

- Assessment (see Table 10.1)

- Organization of information (by domain)
  Background of referral
  Child or adolescent
  Parents and family
  Larger systems

- Summarizing each domain
  Youth summary
  Parents/family summary
  Larger systems summary

- Case formulation proper
  Youth and parents/family
   Goodness of fit
   Circular interactions that maintain the clinical problems

  Parents/family and larger systems
   Goodness of fit
   Circular interactions that maintain the clinical problems

- Treatment planning
  Resources available for treatment, and resource limitations that constrain treatment options

  What do the youth, parents/family members, and/or larger systems want?

  Interrupting the circular interactions and improving goodness of fit among youth, parents/family, and larger systems

  Identifying the most effective level(s) of treatment (i.e., with whom to intervene): individual youth, parents/family, larger systems, some combination

Note. Data from Connor and Fisher (1997).

The case formulation actually begins at the second step—organization of information. The information collected during assessment must be organized in a meaningful fashion, so that it can be useful in constructing a case formulation. Clinical assessment data are first organized into information about the referral process. This includes the referred youngster's, each parent's, and the referral source's views of the problem, and what each party desires to accomplish by clinical referral. (Note that often a youth with CD desires nothing so much as to be left out of the clinical assessment process altogether!) The assessment data are next organized into three domains of information: child/adolescent, parents and family, and larger systems.

A summary statement is next developed for each of these three domains. The summary should not simply be a list of facts. Assessment data must be prioritized and integrated by the clinician in a meaningful fashion. On the basis of theory, research findings, and clinical experience, the clinician judges which are the most salient factors in each domain, and describes how they converge to produce the clinical picture observed. Table 10.3 presents the content to be covered in summary statements for each domain.

The summary statements are then used to develop a transactional case formulation that describes how the domains influence one another reciprocally to maintain conduct problems in the identified youngster. The identification of transactional elements serves to focus specific treatment interventions on interrupting maladaptive interactions across domains, and on helping restore the youth, parents, family, and larger systems to a more functional equilibrium. Two concepts are particularly useful in moving from the youth, par-

TABLE 10.3. Clinical Summary Statements in Three Domains

Youth summary statement

Description of presenting symptoms and problems; acute onset/chronicity of problems
Predisposing risk factors and individual vulnerabilities
Protective factors and individual strengths
Precipitating stressors (if any)
Impairment
Psychiatric diagnoses

Parents/family summary

The family as a system
Quality of parenting provided
Risk factors and vulnerabilities
Protective factors and strengths

Larger systems summary

Larger systems involved with the child/parents/family
Parents' support systems
Degree of isolation of the parents/family from support systems
Stresses that larger systems may cause parents/child/family

Note. Data from Connor and Fisher (1997).

ent, and larger systems summaries to the case formulation: "goodness of fit" and "circularity."

The concept of "goodness of fit" comes from the developmental psychopathology literature (Chess & Thomas, 1986). It refers to the idea that healthy functioning and development occur when there is a good match between the individual youth's capacities and the demands and expectations of the environment. "Poorness of fit," in which there is a mismatch between the youth's intrinsic capabilities and the expectations of the environment, results in increased risk of psychopathology. By identifying transactional elements among the three domains of functioning (child, parents and family, and larger systems), the case formulation seeks to clarify the goodness or poorness of fit. The notion of "fit" leads away from a focus on pathology and blame, and introduces a more normalizing framework. Implicit in the concept of goodness of fit is the idea of relationship. Good or poor fit is a result of the relationship between two entities, rather than the qualities of either one considered separately. A relationship implies bidirectional influence; each entity influences the other (Connor & Fisher, 1997).

In systems theory, a distinction is made between "circular" causality and "lineal" causality (Tomm, 1984). In lineal causality, influence is viewed as flowing in one direction, from prior cause to later effect. The concept of circularity encompasses interactional influences and patterns between the youth and parents, and between the youth/family and larger systems, that have the effect of maintaining problem behaviors or symptoms. For example, a parent's or family's responses to an individual child's or adolescent's problem behaviors help to sustain those behaviors, and the parent's or family's responses are sustained by the youngster's reactions to them. A circular case formulation should address not only how well the parents and family can meet the youth's needs but the extent to which the youth's needs and behaviors trigger conflicts in parents and family members. Likewise, circular interactions that serve to maintain problem behaviors should be identified between the parents/family and the larger systems in the youth's environment.

The end product of the case formulation step is a description of the interactive elements across the domains of youth, parents/family, and larger systems that serve to maintain the clinical problems currently being examined. This description should identify the goodness of fit among the identified youth, the family and environmental systems, and the circular patterns of interaction (interactive elements) across domains that serve to reinforce and perpetuate the problematic clinical picture (Connor & Fisher, 1997). This transactional approach to case formulation is illustrated in Figure 10.3.

Case formulation is useful only to the extent that it provides meaningful and individualized direction to treatment planning; otherwise, it remains a sterile academic exercise. When the formulation can identify circular patterns across domains (interactive elements A–F in Figure 10.3) that maintain problems, an obvious goal of treatment is to interrupt these patterns and improve the goodness of fit between the identified youth and other systems. Any effec-

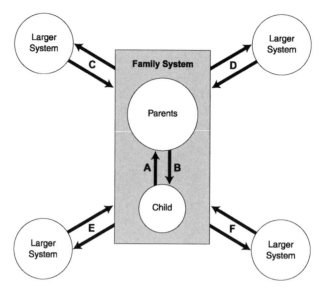

FIGURE 10.3. A transactional approach to clinical case formulation. Interactive elements (A–F) across the three domains of child, parents/family, and larger systems serve to maintain clinical problems via the mechanism of circular interactions. These interactive elements serve to define clinical interventions designed to disrupt maladaptive transactions and restore the system to a more functional equilibrium. Data from Connor and Fisher (1997).

tive intervention (e.g., behavior therapy, parenting assessment and interventions, assessment and treatment of parental psychopathology, social work, case management, psychopharmacology, school assessment and consultation, involvement of community systems of monitoring and care) directed at any level of the youth's social ecology singly or in combination (youth, parents, family, larger systems) that furthers this treatment goal should be considered by the clinical team.

The outcome of this process is a multimodal, multidisciplinary intervention that is consistent with the current standard of care for the assessment and treatment of CD in youth (AACAP, 1997c), ecologically valid for the referred youth with CD, and individualized for his or her specific circumstances. Even if treatment is interrupted—for example, because the family fails to return for treatment, because the youth with CD refuses treatment or is arrested, or because insurance limitations are exceeded—the case formulation and treatment plan will document what has already been accomplished and what still needs to be done if and when the patient and family do return to treatment. A treatment plan based on this model of case formulation also allows the clinician to appreciate the difference between an ideal plan (allowable if mental resources are plentiful) and a realistic yet limited plan within the current practice setting. If resources for treatment are not available or funded, the case formulation and treatment plan allow the clinician to understand what treatment interventions are missing but recommended, and to add these at a later date if they become available.

SPECIFIC ASSESSMENT TECHNIQUES AND TOOLS

As noted earlier, the current standard of care for youth with CD requires an assessment approach using multiple sources of information and multiple methods of data collection across various home, community, and school settings (AACAP, 1997c). Generally, information about a youth is gathered from the youth him- or herself, parents, and teachers. It is important to use multiple sources of information, because the youth's behavior may be different as reported by various observers in different settings, and the youth in question may have very different views of his or her behavior than parents or teachers may. Multiple techniques (such as structured diagnostic psychiatric interviews and behavior rating scales) are required, because any single source of information provides limited data about the construct to be evaluated. For example, diagnostic interviews provide reliable and valid information about the diagnosis of CD and any associated comorbid psychiatric diagnoses. But they provide little information about how severe a youngster's conduct problems are, or how this youngster's conduct problems compare to the behavior of same-age and same-gender peers (Kamphaus & Frick, 1996). In contrast, behavior rating scales completed by parents and teachers are excellent at providing information about severity of problem behaviors and comparisons with other youth, but are unable to provide diagnostic information (Frick, 1998).

Structured Diagnostic Interviews

Structured diagnostic interviews consist of standard questions that cover the symptom criteria sets for a variety of psychiatric diagnoses. Questions are asked of the youth or another informant (generally a parent) about his or her emotional and behavioral adjustment. In addition, questions are asked about onset, offset, and severity of psychiatric symptoms. A respondent's answers to questions are used to determine whether eligibility criteria for a psychiatric diagnosis are met. The clinical use of a structured diagnostic interview ensures that a uniform and systematic evaluation covering a multiplicity of psychiatric diagnoses is made of each patient. Structured diagnostic interviews usually inquire about the "current" episode, generally defined as symptoms occurring within the last 6–12 months. Some interviews also inquire about "lifetime" episodes (i.e., symptoms that may have occurred more than 6–12 prior to the present evaluation). Diagnostic interviews may be totally structured or semi-structured. Totally structured interviews are easily adapted to computers and require the interviewer to ask questions in exactly the same way for each evaluation. Because these interviews are scored for diagnoses algorithmically and require no clinical experience to administer, they can be given by nonprofessional interviewers. Semistructured interviews provide some freedom of choice as to how questions are asked, and allow the interviewer to pursue specific areas more thoroughly as the interview progresses; however, they require administration by a trained mental health professional and are not so easily adapted for computer use and scoring. There are several psychiatric diagnostic interviews (both semistructured and structured) available to assess behaviors associated with CD, as well as psychiatric disorders that often co-occur with CD. These interviews are listed in Table 10.4.

Structured interviews include the Diagnostic Interview Schedule for Children, Version IV (DISC-IV; Shaffer, Fisher, Lucas, Dulcan, & Schwab-Stone, 2000); the Child and Adolescent Psychiatric Assessment (CAPA; Angold & Costello, 2000), the Children's Interview for Psychiatric Syndromes (ChIPS; Weller, Weller, Fristad, Rooney, & Schecter, 2000), and the Dominic-R Pictorial Interview (Valla, Bergeron, & Smolla, 2000). As noted above, these can all be administered by personnel without professional training. Separate parent and child versions are generally available. All have computer versions for administration and algorithmic scoring either available or currently in development. Reliability and validity data are available on all, and are generally fair to good; validation is continuing on each of these interviews, so more normative data will be available in the future. Of particular interest is the Dominic-R (Valla et al., 2000), a computerized pictorial interview for young children. Pictures, rather than questions, are used in this interview because of the cognitive immaturity of 6- to 11-year-old children. If further validation data prove acceptable, this interviewing format may hold great promise for structured interviewing of youth with cognitive delays as well as young chronological age. Spanish versions of the DISC-IV, CAPA, and Dominic-R are available; the Dominic-R is also available in German and French.

Semistructured interviews include the Interview Schedule for Children and Adolescents (ISCA; Kovacs, 1985; Sherrill & Kovacs, 2000); the Schedule for Affective Disorders and Schizophrenia for School-Age Children (K-SADS; Chambers et al., 1985; Ambrosini, 2000; Orvaschel, Ambrosini, Rabinovich, 1993); and the Diagnostic Interview for Children and Adolescents (DICA; Reich, 2000). As described above, semistructured interviews allow for some freedom of choice and somewhat greater detail in questioning, but they require administration and scoring by a mental health professional who is familiar with psychiatric diagnosis. Therefore, semistructured interviews are rarely computer-assisted; they generally must be administered and scored by hand. The exception is the DICA, which was totally structured in earlier versions and has become more semistructured in later versions (Reich, 2000). A computer program is available for the DICA. As for the structured interviews, normative data are available on all these semistructured interviews, and are generally fair to good; again, too, ongoing validation is occurring, so more normative data will be available in the future. A Spanish version of the ISCA is currently available. Three different forms of the K-SADS currently exist (Ambrosini, 2000), and normative data are available on two of these. The

TABLE 10.4. Structured and Semistructured Diagnostic Interviews for Children and Adolescents

Reference	Interview	Format[a]	Informants	Age range	Computer version	Normative data available
Shaffer et al. (2000)	Diagnostic Interview Schedule for Children, Version IV (DISC-IV)	Structured	Parent, youth	6–17 9–17	Yes	Yes
Angold and Costello (2000)	Child and Adolescent Psychiatric Assessment (CAPA)	Structured	Parent, child	9–17	InD[b]	Yes
Weller et al. (2000)	Children's Interview for Psychiatric Syndromes (ChIPS)	Structured	Parent, child	6–18	InD	Yes
Valla et al. (2000)	Dominic-R Pictorial Interview	Structured	Child	6–11	Yes	Yes
Kovacs (1985); Sherrill and Kovacs (2000)	Interview Schedule for Children and Adolescents (ISCA)	Semistructured	Parent, child	8–17	No	Yes
Ambrosini (2000); Chambers et al. (1985); Orvaschel et al. (1993)	Schedule for Affective Disorders and Schizophrenia for School-Age Children (K-SADS)	Semistructured	Parent, child	6–18	No	Yes
Reich (2000)	Diagnostic Interview for Children and Adolescents (DICA)	Semistructured (formerly structured)	Parent, child, adolescent	6–17	Yes	Yes

[a]Structured interviews are designed for lay interviewers; semistructured interviews are designed to be administered by trained mental health professionals.
[b]InD, in development.

315

K-SADS-E (Orvaschel, 1995) is a dichotomous epidemiological version and assesses both current and lifetime rates of psychiatric diagnosis. Disorders are scored as present–absent. The K-SADS-PL (Kaufman et al., 1997) also assesses both present and lifetime diagnoses; however, it allows for graded scoring of symptoms as threshold, subthreshold, or none (absent).

Psychiatric diagnostic interviews generally require 60–90 minutes to complete in a face-to-face session. Length of time for completion is heavily dependent on the number of problems and symptoms exhibited by a child or adolescent, and therefore on the number of questions that must be asked. There are three main sources of variation across the diagnostic interviews presented in Table 10.4. As noted above, they differ in their structured versus semistructured construction, and thus different types of personnel are required to administer them. Second, interviews differ in whether they assess psychiatric disorders that were present at any point in a youth's lifetime, or whether they assess only disorders that are currently or recently present (past 6–12 months). Third, the answer formats of the interviews vary: Some interviews only allow categorical yes–no responses, and others allow for graded responses indicating symptom severity. Regardless of their differences, however, these diagnostic interviews all share the goal of obtaining a detailed description of a child's or adolescent's emotional and behavioral symptoms and functioning from multiple informants (Frick, 1998).

Behavior Rating Scales

Behavior rating scales are an important part of the clinical assessment of children and adolescents with CD and related behaviors/disorders for several reasons. First, behavior rating scales allow multiple informants—including a youth's parents, other adults or guardians in the youth's caretaking environment, and teachers—to rate the youth's behaviors and moods in a standardized manner. Some behavior rating scales have a self-report format, allowing the child or adolescent to report on his or her own emotions in a standardized fashion. Adolescent self-report scales may be especially useful in assessing internalizing symptoms (e.g., anxiety and depression), since these may not be readily observable to parents and teachers. Since behaviors may change in different settings during the day, information from multiple informants is necessary to assess the youngster's functioning across various environments in his or her daily life. Second, behavior rating scales are frequently used in research on youngsters with aggression and antisocial behaviors in general, and with diagnosed CD in particular. Perhaps the greatest strength of behavior rating scales is that many possess reliability and validity data for many different groups of youth and types of informants. This allows a child's or adolescent's moods or behaviors to be compared with those of specified reference groups, such as same-age or same-gender groups. The clinician can then confidently determine whether the youngster's scores as rated by self, parents, or teachers are elevated (and by how much), relative to those of peers. Finally, behavior rating scales are time- and resource-efficient. In an increasingly resource-scarce mental health treatment environment, the ability to evaluate multiple domains of a youth's moods and behaviors across home and school settings in a timely manner is most valuable.

Generalized Behavior Rating Scales

Generalized behavior rating scales used in the assessment of children and adolescents with CD and related behaviors are presented in Table 10.5. The scales are generalized because they address a number of areas of adjustment rather than a single domain of problems. The scales listed in the table have been chosen because they (1) have good to excellent normative data available (Frick, 1998;

TABLE 10.5. Selected Generalized Behavior Rating Scales

Scale/reference	Age range	Conduct domains	Other domains	Informants[a]
Behavior Assessment System for Children (BASC; Reynolds & Kamphaus, 1992)	4–18	Aggression, Conduct Problems	Adaptability, Anxiety, ADHD, Atypicality, Depression, Leadership, Learning Problems, Social Skills, Somatization, Study Skills, Withdrawal, Attitude to School and Teachers, Interpersonal Relations, Locus of Control, Relations with Parents, Self-Esteem, Self-Reliance, Sensation-Seeking, Sense of Inadequacy, Social Stress	P, T, C
Child Behavior Checklist (CBCL; Achenbach, 1991)	4–18	Aggressive Behavior, Delinquent Behavior	Withdrawn, Somatic Complaints, Anxious/ Depressed, Social Competence, Thought Problems, Attention Problems	P, T
Conners Rating Scales (Conners, 1997)	3–17	Oppositional Behavior, Fights, Anger Control Problems	Cognitive Problems, Anxious–Shy, Hyperactivity, Perfectionism, Social Problems, Psychosomatic, Family Problems	P, T, C
Personality Inventory for Children— Revised (PIC-R; Lachar & Gruber, 1991)	9–18	Delinquency	Achievement, Intellectual Screening, Development, Somatic Concerns, Depression, Family Relations, Withdrawal, Anxiety, Psychosis, Hyperactivity, Social Skills, Reality Distortion	P, C

[a]Informants: P, parent; T, teacher; C, child (or adolescent).

Kamphaus & Frick, 1996); (2) are commonly used in the assessment of youth with CD; and (3) are easily obtainable by the practicing clinician and efficient to use.

The Behavior Assessment System for Children (BASC; Reynolds & Kamphaus, 1992) has parent, teacher, and child forms available. It assesses a wide range of problem domains, including aggression and conduct problems, in youth 4–18 years of age. Normative data for the scale are very good, and the availability of an excellent standardization sample allows confident norm-referenced data interpretation. The BASC also includes a number of validity scales to help in detection of certain response patterns (such as social desirability or exaggeration of negative symptoms), which help the clinician in interpreting responses on the scale. Finally, the BASC includes a Relations with Parents subscale, which allows for assessment of parent–child relationship difficulties.

The Child Behavior Checklist (CBCL; Achenbach, 1991) is a comprehensive behavior rating scale commonly used in child and adolescent mental health practice and research. It assesses a wide range of problem behaviors, including internalizing, externalizing, and total symptoms. Among conduct problems, Aggressive Behavior and Delinquent Behavior (defined as overt and covert forms of aggression, respectively) are rated separately. A separate Social Competence scale is also included. The CBCL has been evaluated separately for different ages (i.e., 4–11 years and 12–18 years), for both genders, and for clinic and community (nonreferred) samples. Thus, with the CBCL, the clinician can evaluate an individual child's or adolescent's scores on all the symptom scales relative to same-age and same-gender peers who have not been referred for treatment. Parent and teacher forms are available for all ages, and a self-report form is available for youth aged 11–18 years.

The Conners Rating Scales (Conners, 1997) were recently revised and now include parent and teacher report forms for ages 3–17 years, and an adolescent report form for ages 12–17 years. A broad range of problem behaviors are assessed. Conduct problem subscales include Oppositional Behavior, Fights, and Anger Control Problems. The normative sample is extensive, and test–retest reliability and validity data are good. The Conners Rating Scales may be sensitive to medication effects and thus may be useful in monitoring response to pharmacological treatment.

The Personality Inventory for Children—Revised (PIC-R; Lachar & Gruber, 1991) has parent and child forms. Like other generalized behavior rating scales, it assesses a large number of problem domains. In terms of conduct problems, Delinquency (again defined as covert aggression) is assessed by this instrument, as opposed to physical aggression. Normative data are available for ages 9–18 years. Unlike other generalized scales, the PIC-R has a Family Relations subscale, which allows for assessment of a youth's family context.

Specific Behavior Rating Scales and a Measure of Global Functional Impairment

Specific selected behavior rating scales used in the assessment of children and adolescents with CD and related behaviors are presented in Table 10.6. These rating scales are specific because each assesses only one domain of behavior.

Because hyperactive–impulsive behavior is intimately connected to aggressive behavior in many youth, selected specific rating scales to assess both these behavior domains are presented. Finally, because youth with CD are generally impaired across multiple domains of daily functioning, it is important to include a measure of global functional impairment. One such measure is discussed.

Although numerous scales for assessing aggression, hostility, disruptive behavior, and conduct problems exist (see Furlong & Smith, 1994), the scales listed in Table 10.6 have been chosen because (1) they are commonly used in psychiatric practice; (2) some of the scales may be useful in efforts to define and subtype aggression more precisely (see Chapter 1); and (3) normative data are available on some of these scales. However, it should be noted that the quality of the normative data is generally less good on several of these specific rating scales than on the generalized behavior rating scales discussed above, and that a few specific scales have no such data at all. Therefore, some of these scales should be considered still in development. In addition to more normative data, additional information on internal consistency, reliability, and validity is required for some of these measures before they can be unequivocally recommended for use. A comprehensive review of specific rating scales, including available reliability and validity data, for the assessment of youth anger, hostility, and aggression can be found in Furlong and Smith (1994).

Specific Aggression Rating Scales. Seven specific aggression rating scales are listed in Table 10.6, along with their age range, domains of aggression covered, and types of informants. The New York Teacher Rating Scale for Disruptive and Antisocial Behavior (NYTRS; L. S. Miller et al., 1995) provides a broad measure of disruptive behavior. Four subscales of conduct problems include Defiance, Physical Aggression, Delinquent Aggression, and Peer Relations. Two composite scales may be derived from the four subscales, including Antisocial Behavior (Physical Aggression plus Delinquent Aggression plus four other items) and the Disruptive Behavior Scale (comprising all items in the NYTRS except those on the Peer Relations subscale). Normative data are provided from a large population of children in grades 1–10 from New York State. Validity data are good, scale internal consistency is moderate to excellent, and test–retest reliability is good. Interrater reliability is only fair (L. S. Miller et al., 1995). Overall, the NYTRS may be the best teacher scale available for assessing hostility and aggression in children and young adolescents.

The Peer Conflict Scale (Gadow, 1986) assesses physical and verbal aggression between the subject child and other peers. Informants include parents and teachers, who rate each of the 10 child's behaviors on a 4-point scale. Normative data are somewhat limited for the Peer Conflict Scale. Its correlation to direct observation of oppositional behavior is high, and test–retest reliability is moderately high. This scale may be sensitive to change with pharmacological treatment.

As its title indicates, the Predatory–Affective Aggression Questionnaire

TABLE 10.6. Selected Specific Behavior Rating Scales

Scale/reference	Age range	Conduct domains	Informants[a]
Aggression			
New York Teacher Rating Scale (NYTRS; L. S. Miller et al., 1995)	6–14	Defiance, Physical Aggression, Delinquent Aggression, Peer Relations	T
Peer Conflict Scale (Gadow, 1986)	6–12	Physical Aggression, Verbal Aggression	P, T
Predatory–Affective Aggression Questionnaire (Vitiello et al., 1990)	10–18	Predatory Aggression, Affective Aggression	O
Overt Aggression Scale (OAS; Yudofsky et al., 1986)	5–adult	Verbal Aggression, Physical Aggression Against Objects, Physical Aggression Against Self, Physical Aggression Against Other People	O
Proactive–Reactive Aggression Scale (Dodge & Coie, 1987)	5–18	Reactive Aggression, Proactive Aggression	P, T, O
Iowa Conners Teachers Rating Scale (Pelham et al., 1989)	5–10	Oppositional/Defiant, Inattention/Overactivity	T
Buss–Durkee Hostility Inventory—Children's Version (BDHI-C; Treiber et al., 1989)	7–10	Expressive Hostility, Experienced Anger	C
Hyperactivity–impulsivity			
Conners Global Index (Conners, 1997)	5–adult	Restless–Impulsive, Emotional Lability	P, T
Child Attention Problems (CAP) Scale (Edelbrock, 1978)	4–18	Inattention, Hyperactivity	T
ADHD Rating Scale—IV (DuPaul et al., 1998)	5–18	Inattention, Hyperactivity–Impulsivity	P, T
Global functional impairment			
Children's Global Assessment Scale (CGAS; Shaffer et al., 1983)	4–16	Severity of Disturbance	O

[a]Informants: P, parent; T, teacher; O, other (staff); C, child.

(Vitiello, Behar, Hunt, Stoff, & Ricciuti, 1990) distinguishes between "predatory" and "affective" aggression. Predatory aggression is similar to instrumental or proactive aggression, and affective aggression is similar to reactive, defensive, or impulsive aggression (see Table 1.3 in Chapter 1). This scale is designed to be completed by someone other than the target youth, such as a parent, teacher, or staff member on a mental health unit. The internal consistency of this scale is moderate (Cronbach's alpha = .73). Normative data for non-clinic-referred subjects do not exist for this scale.

The Overt Aggression Scale (OAS; Yudofsky, Silver, Jackson, Endicott, & Williams, 1986) is widely used for assessing the type and frequency of aggression in child and adult psychiatry. The OAS rates each episode of aggression on four subscales: (1) Verbal Aggression, (2) Physical Aggression Against Objects (property destruction), (3) Physical Aggression Against Self (self-injurious behavior), and (4) Physical Aggression Against Other People (assault). The type of staff intervention for each aggressive episode may also be rated. Within each category of aggression, there are weighted levels of severity and examples given as anchors for rating. Each incident is scored by adding the weighted scores from the most severe behaviors in each category and the most restrictive staff intervention for the incident. The OAS appears appropriate and feasible for use with children and adolescents (Kafantaris et al., 1996). Reliability of this scale is good, but data are limited. The Verbal Aggression subscale in children appears to have the lowest reliability (Yudofsky et al., 1986). The OAS may be sensitive to drug effects in both children and adults (Connor, Ozbayrak, Benjamin, Ma, & Fletcher, 1997; Kafantaris et al., 1996).

Two retrospective modifications of the OAS currently exist. The Modified Overt Aggression Scale (MOAS; Kay, Wolkenfeld, & Murrill, 1988) includes these four subscales: (1) Verbal Aggression, (2) Aggression Against Property, (3) Autoaggression, and (4) Physical Aggression. The informant is instructed to rate the most serious act of aggression committed by the patient during a specified time period (generally the past week or month). The MOAS refines the original OAS by upgrading the rating scale from a nominal scale to a 5-point interval scale that represents increasing levels of aggressive severity. The modification provides definitions for each category of aggression and a zero point for the absence of such behavior. The total aggression score is computed by multiplying the four individual scales by weights of 1, 2, 3, or 4 (reflecting increasing severity of aggression; the numerical order is as given above) and then summing the four weighted scores. The standardization data obtained for the MOAS support its internal, interrater, and longitudinal reliability (Kay et al., 1988).

A second modification of the OAS is confusingly also called the Modified Overt Aggression Scale (MOAS; Sorgi, Ratey, Knoedler, Markert, & Reichman, 1991). This instrument retrospectively rates aggressive behaviors occurring over the previous week. It modifies the original OAS by introducing a 5-point Likert scale to rate occurrence of aggression across the 16 scale items.

The four aggression categories of the original OAS are retained in this version of the MOAS. Although data are sparse, the internal consistency and interrater reliability of this version of the MOAS are good. It is most often used by ward staff to rate aggression in psychiatric inpatient settings. Normative data for non-clinic-referred subjects do not exist for the OAS or for either version of the MOAS.

In research examining social information-processing mechanisms (i.e., hostile attributional biases) in children, Dodge and Coie (1987) developed the Proactive–Reactive Aggression Scale, consisting of six items (three each for proactive and reactive aggression—see Table 1.1 in Chapter 1). The Proactive Aggression and Reactive Aggression subscales are found to be internally consistent, and factor analyses support convergent and discriminant validities. The scale may be completed by parents, teachers, or mental health staff.

The Iowa Conners Teachers Rating Scale (Pelham, Milich, Murphy, & Murphy, 1989) has two factors that assess Inattention/Overactivity and Oppositional/Defiant behavior as assessed by the child's classroom teacher. Normative data for this scale were obtained on a large group of children in kindergarten through fifth grade. The two subscales have been found to have test–retest reliability, internal consistency, and drug sensitivity. The scale is to be completed by a child's classroom teacher.

The Buss–Durkee Hostility Inventory—Children's Version (BDHI-C; Treiber et al., 1989) assesses the experience component of hostility and anger as self-reported by children. It is derived from the Buss–Durkee Hostility Inventory (Buss & Durkee, 1957). Internal consistency of the BDHI-C has not yet been reported (Furlong & Smith, 1994). Preliminary findings indicate a test–retest reliability of .57 (Treiber et al., 1989).

Specific Hyperactivity–Impulsivity Scales. Aggression in general and CD in particular are often accompanied by evidence of hyperactivity and/or impulsivity. Three selected hyperactivity–impulsivity scales that are reliable and valid include the Conners Global Index (Conners, 1997), the Child Attention Problems (CAP) Scale (Edelbrock, 1978), and the ADHD Rating Scale–IV (DuPaul, Power, Anastopoulos, & Reid, 1998). The Conners Global Index is a 10-item scale that was developed as a general measure of disruptive behavior; it includes subscales for Restless–Impulsive behavior and Emotional Lability. Normative data are available in the manual (Conners, 1997). The CAP Scale (Edelbrock, 1978) was derived from the Teacher Report Form (TRF) of the CBCL (Achenbach, 1991) by statistically extracting items that consistently loaded heavily on the Hyperactivity factor of the TRF and that were consistent with *Diagnostic and Statistical Manual of Mental Disorders,* third edition, revised (DSM-III-R) diagnostic criteria for ADHD. The CAP Scale has two subscales, Inattention and Hyperactivity. The psychometric characteristics of the scale support its reliability and validity. Normative data are available. It is completed by teachers and appears drug-sensitive. The ADHD Rating Scale—IV (DuPaul et al., 1998), which reflects DSM-IV diagnostic criteria, is an 18-item scale that has subscales for Inattention and Hyperactivity–Impulsivity. Parent and teacher versions are available. Normative data are extensive. The scale has good internal consistency, good test–retest reliability, and validity.

A Measure of Global Functional Impairment. Global scales of functional impairment attempt to provide a single, unidimensional measure of severity of disturbance and adequacy of social function in children and adolescents who are referred for mental health treatment. They are used as a summary statement of a patient's level of disturbance. Because youth with CD and related behaviors and are often impaired across multiple domains of life functioning, such a summary statement may be useful to the practicing clinician. The Children's Global Assessment Scale (CGAS; Shaffer et al., 1983) is one such scale. The CGAS is a 100-point scale, with scores above 70 essentially indicating normative functioning across all areas of family, school, and peers. Scores less than 70 indicate increasing severity and pervasiveness of daily life disturbance, and progressively poorer general daily life functioning. Anchor points are provided to help standardize assessment. Interrater reliability, test–retest reliability, and validity of the CGAS are supported (Shaffer et al., 1983).

Limitations of Behavior Rating Scales

Although many behavior rating scales possess good to excellent internal consistency, reliability, validity, and normative data, they have several limitations that require discussion. First, it is important to emphasize that psychiatric diagnoses cannot be made from behavior rating scales. Most rating scales assess psychopathology as a continuous dimension in the population, without a clear cutoff point beyond which pathology becomes evident. In contrast, psychiatric diagnoses are categorical; that is, if a certain number of symptoms are present and meet current diagnostic criteria, the diagnosis is assigned. Although this point appears self-evident, it is often confused in clinical practice. In the assessment of a youth with CD, psychiatric diagnostic interviews are often combined with behavior rating scales to obtain both psychiatric diagnoses and a picture of how frequent and severe the behaviors are, as rated by observers relative to the youth's same age and gender group.

Second, although many types of rating scales allow for different informants, the correlations across different observers using the same rating scale and rating the same youngster are often poor. In other words, parents and teachers often do not agree on a given youth's problem behaviors. One reason is that the different reports may reflect true situational variability in these behaviors. For example, covertly aggressive behaviors such as fire setting or vandalism may not be evident in the structured environment of school, but may be evident in the unmonitored community environment as rated by parents. Another source of discrepancy is rater bias. Parents and teachers completing behavior rating scales may be subject to several different types of bias. Ratings may be influenced by conscious attempts to make the ratings seem either more normal or more pathological for a given child or adolescent (Frick, 1998). An observer's ratings can also be influenced by more unconscious "response sets," such as a tendency to respond in a socially desirable manner (Kamphaus & Frick, 1996). The psychological adjustment of the informant may influence ratings as well. For example, a parent's level of depression or anxiety can influence his or her rating of a child (Kazdin, 1996). Finally, it is known that young children, prior to adolescence, are poor reporters of their own moods and behaviors. Self-reports from older children and adolescents may be more reliable and valid (Frick, 1998). Therefore, since any single informant has a different "window" on a child's or adolescent's behavior, any single source of information will be limited. A combination of sources is needed to provide the richest overall picture.

Direct Behavioral Observation

Direct observation of a youth's behavior is also important in the assessment of aggressive/antisocial behaviors in general and CD in particular, Direct observation is not subject to raters' biases or the perceptions of others in the youth's environment. Direct observation allows for a greater understanding of the environmental context in which aggression occurs. Children and adolescents may be observed in the natural setting of home or school. They may also be observed in an analogue setting, such as a behavioral laboratory classroom or playroom.

Standardized observational systems have been developed for use with children and adolescents (see Frick, 1998, for a discussion). These systems clearly define the behaviors that are to be observed, the setting in which the behaviors are to be observed, the method for recording observations, and the person who is to conduct the observation (e.g., research assistant, parent, teacher).

Behavioral systems of observation can provide valuable information about a youngster's conduct problems that complements information obtained from psychiatric diagnostic interviewing and behavioral rating scales. However, they are very expensive in terms of time and effort required. In an increasingly resource-scarce clinical environment, behavioral observations play a secondary role to diagnostic interviewing and behavior rating scales in the assessment of youth with CD.

FORENSIC ASSESSMENT: ASSESSING RISK OF HARM TO OTHERS

A special case of clinical assessment of youth with CD is the mental health evaluation of a juvenile's potential for future assaultive or other violent behavior that may harm others. This is a question that mental health clinicians are often asked to answer, especially while consulting to juvenile court settings, court mental health clinics, psychiatric emergency rooms, and community mental health crisis teams.

There has been very little research on the accuracy of clinical prediction of violence with children and adolescents. The extant literature identifies serious limitations to our ability to predict who will and who will not engage in future violent acts. Prediction is limited because of low base rates of violent behaviors in certain populations (which increase false-positive errors), as well as our inability to identify unforeseeable circumstances that will arise to stimulate an individual's violence. More is known about risk assessment in adults than in juveniles, in adolescents than in prepubertal children, and in males than in females (Grisso, 1998).

When mental health clinicians are asked to assess a youngster's violence

TABLE 10.7. Risk and Resilience Factors in a Forensic Evaluation of Dangerousness to Others

Risk factors (↑ risk)	Resilience factors (↓ risk)

Past violent behavior
    Chronicity
    Early onset (< 11 years)
    Frequency
    Severity
    Context
	Committed to school
	
	Doing well in school
	
	Intent to continue education
	
	Attachment to parents

Substance use	Association with conventional peers
Association with violent groups	Association with conventional community institutions

Family conflict and aggression
    Antisocial families as models of
        aggression
    Victim of abuse/neglect
    Aggression as coping strategy for solving
        problems	

Social stressors	

Personality traits
    Anger
    Impulsivity
    Lack of empathy	

Co-occurring psychiatric disorders
    Depression
    Bipolar disorder
    PTSD
    ADHD
    Psychosis	

Opportunity
    Specific target individual identified
    Availability of weapons	

Note. Data from Grisso (1998).

potential, they should approach the task by using a set of risk factors known empirically to be related to future violence. None of these risk factors are powerful enough alone or in combination to produce individual predictions with great accuracy. However, they do provide a structure for systematic inquiry into variables known to be associated with risk for aggression and violence. The assessment of dangerousness needs to evaluate individual, familial, and contextual/environmental risk factors, as well as factors contributing to resilience. Risk and resilience factors are presented in Table 10.7.

The aim of a forensic evaluation of risk to harm others is to offer a risk estimate, rather than an absolute statement of whether a given adolescent will or will not engage in aggressive and violent behavior. In a risk estimate approach, information is gathered about the youth on a set of risk factors. The clinician notes whether the degree of risk is increased or decreased by the information on each factor; he or she then combines, carefully weighs, and evaluates the information, and arrives at a conclusion about the degree of risk that the youngster poses in relation to some comparison group (e.g., youth in general of the same age and gender, youth seen in the same emergency room).

CHAPTER SUMMARY

This chapter presents methods for assessing a child or adolescent with CD in the clinical setting. A general scheme for combining assessment information from multiple informants and multiple systems into an organized case formulation to arrive at an ecologically meaningful treatment plan for the individual child and family is presented. Specific assessment tools and their strengths and limitations are then discussed. The need for such a systematic approach to the assessment of youth with CD in the clinical treatment setting is made ever greater by the increasing resource constraints on mental health treatment. Finally, an approach to the forensic assessment of dangerousness to others is discussed.

CHAPTER 11

Psychosocial Interventions

In the last two decades, research reviews of what may be accomplished by clinical interventions to reduce chronic aggression and related behaviors in youth have taken a turn toward guarded optimism. Previously, there was a decidedly pessimistic (indeed, almost nihilistic) view of what treatment might achieve. Reviews of research conducted in the 1960s and 1970s documented a lack of treatment efficacy; some even explicitly wondered whether it was at all possible to intervene effectively for children and adolescents diagnosed with conduct disorder (CD) (Romig, 1978; Shamsie, 1981). This view has now been replaced by a cautious and tempered degree of encouragement about treatment. Although most clinicians and researchers in the mental health field would agree that effective treatments are still lacking for CD and other forms of aggressive/antisocial behaviors in the young, such behaviors may indeed be partly modifiable (Rutter, Giller, & Hagell, 1998). This change has been driven by several advances in the field over the last 20 years.

First, there has been tremendous growth in knowledge concerning the developmental psychopathology of early-onset CD. By clarifying the developmental trajectory that these children may follow, by identifying various risk and protective factors that may modify this trajectory, and by becoming more skilled in understanding the complex interplay between developmental and contextual forces in the etiology of CD, therapists and treatment outcome researchers have acquired a conceptual model that can facilitate both assessment and the design and selection of treatment interventions (McMahon & Wells, 1998). Second, research has consistently pointed out the failure of single-component treatment interventions to alter the course of aggressive/antisocial behaviors in the young. This has allowed the development and evaluation of multimodal, multicomponent interventions to address the multiple individual and social systems affecting youngsters with such behaviors (Kazdin, 1996, 1997). Third, recent research is evaluating interventions with the most difficult-to-treat subtypes of youth with conduct problems: chronically (i.e., multiply offending) delinquent adolescents (Borduin, 1999). Finally, important advances in designing and evaluating community-based prevention efforts are documenting that early intervention programs can indeed have long-term preventive effects on aggressive/antisocial behaviors (Yoshikawa, 1994; Zigler, Taussig, & Black, 1992). These developments have clarified that partially effective clinical treatments for conduct problems in youngsters can be achieved. However, meaningful treatments are difficult to accomplish. They require comprehensive interventions that simultaneously target multiple domains and areas of dysfunction in a youngster's life, and are delivered over a long period of time (generally more than several years). Furthermore, early recognition of a child at risk for CD is important. Although the symptoms of CD remain modifiable in the young child, early interventions may be more effective than those implemented later, when the stability of conduct problems has become greater.

Despite these advances, treatment gains are limited and remain modest. Youth with aggressive and antisocial behaviors who undergo comprehensive treatment remain more deviant than children who do not have such problems to begin with. As such, even "successful" treatment does not normalize these youth. The effects of such treatment are on the order of a 12% to 25% reduction in onset or in existing symptoms, compared with rates of control groups; there is considerable variation across treatment studies and among individuals (Elliot & Tolan, 1999; Rutter et al., 1998). These figures may seem small, yet they are far from trivial. On an epidemiological level, youth under the age of 18 years account for approximately 30% of all arrests for index offenses, including 19% of violent crimes and 35% of property crimes (Federal Bureau of Investigation, 1996). On a social level, juvenile aggressive/antisocial behaviors consume much of the resources of child mental health, juvenile justice, and special education systems (Borduin, 1999). Treatments that may reduce those behaviors or their onset rates by even a small amount may translate into significant societal savings in social services, educational assets, and legal resources.

Of all treatment modalities for conduct problems in youngsters, psychosocial treatments have been the most well researched (Kazdin, 1997; Mcmahon & Wells, 1998; Rutter et al., 1998). The purpose of this chapter is to review psychosocial treatments with empirical evidence of efficacy for aggression and related behaviors in youth. The treatments included in this chapter have been selected because they each have two or more methodologically controlled, group design studies demonstrating their efficacy in comparison to either a placebo condition, a waiting-list control group, or another treatment. Requiring replication of effectiveness from two or more studies protects us against drawing hopeful yet false conclusions about efficacy from new, unreplicated treatments. First, treatment outcome research findings about variables with important clinical implications are examined. Family interventions for both preadolescent children and adolescents are next reviewed, followed by cognitive-behavioral strategies and community prevention efforts. A brief look at some treatments that seem ineffective concludes the chapter.

VARIABLES WITH IMPORTANT CLINICAL IMPLICATIONS

Age

In all psychosocial treatments for conduct problems, age appears to be an important modifier of clinical outcome. In general, the greatest degree of improvement is found in the treatment of children under 8 years of age (Frick, 1998; Kazdin, 1996; McMahon & Wells, 1998). As children grow older, treatments for aggressive and antisocial behaviors usually become less effective. An important implication of this finding is that a major focus of intervention for youth with such behaviors should be on prevention and early intervention. Given what we now know of antecedents and risk factors for the development of severe conduct problems, early and comprehensive treatment of at-risk young children is important to prevent the later development of more severe behavior problems.

Generalization of Treatment Effects

"Generalization" refers to the extension of treatment effects outside the therapeutic setting. Four major types of generalization are recognized (Forehand & Atkeson, 1977; McMahon & Wells, 1998). "Setting generalization" means the transfer of treatment effects to settings in which treatment did not take place (e.g., from the therapist's office to home or school). "Temporal generalization" refers to the maintenance of treatment effects over time following termination of treatment. "Sibling generalization" pertains to the transfer of newly acquired skills to untreated siblings in the family, and improvement in the siblings' behaviors. "Behavioral generalization" means that targeted changes in specific problem behaviors are accompanied by improvements in other nontargeted behaviors (e.g., in a youth with multiple conduct problems, if oppositional behavior is the therapeutic target and improves, stealing also diminishes in frequency).

With the notable exception of family interventions for preadolescent children, the overall generalization of treatment effects is poor. First, setting generalization is limited: Improvements obtained in youngsters' problem behaviors in one setting (such as the treatment clinic) generally do not carry over into other settings (such as home and school). Second, research on temporal generalization has typically studied the maintenance of treatment gains over only short time periods, such as 6 months to 1 year (Frick, 1998); many of these studies have demonstrated continued treatment efficacy over a duration of several months, but the few studies that have examined longer periods generally do not indicate continued treatment efficacy over many years' time. Finally, with the notable exception of research on family interventions for preadolescent children, studies have usually not found evidence of sibling or behavioral generalization.

The limited generalization of psychosocial treatments has several important clinical implications. First, given limited setting generalization, effective interventions for aggressive and antisocial behaviors in youth need to target multiple arenas in these youngster's lives, both internal and external. Internal arenas include social problem solving, attributions, and impulse control. External arenas include risk factors in parents/families, neighborhoods, and schools. Second, given limited temporal generalization, CD and other forms of aggressive/antisocial behavior should be viewed within a chronic disease model (Frick, 1998; Kazdin, 1987, 1996). The conventional method of administering time- and treatment-visit-limited clinical interventions, often within a highly managed and rationed managed care model of mental health service delivery, simply does not work for CD and related problems in young people. Such problems should be considered chronic conditions that require continued intervention, monitoring, and outcome evaluation over the entire course of the lifespan (Kazdin, 1987). Finally, clinical treatments that focus on single psychosocial processes believed to be important in the development and maintenance of aggressive/antisocial behaviors are doomed to be ineffective. Given that multiple, interacting processes lead to the development and continuation of these behaviors, and given that subgroups of children with these behaviors may have differing types of processes, the success of focused psychosocial interventions will be limited.

Severity and Pervasiveness of Symptoms

Other major modifiers of treatment outcome in this population include symptom severity in youth and families, as well as the pervasiveness of symptoms across multiple settings (e.g., home, school, community). Generally, psychosocial treatments for CD and other forms of aggressive/antisocial behaviors have the best outcome for youngsters and families with less severe problems. More severe risk factors that predict early-onset CD and a poor longitudinal prognosis over the course of development also predict poor response to treatment (Kazdin, 1997). As a therapeutic rule, less severely disturbed patients get better more frequently than more severely disturbed ones do. One possible exception to this is found in the work of Henggeler and Borduin (1990) and their multisystemic approach to severely recidivistic antisocial teenagers (see below). This approach addresses the clinical needs of this most difficult group and has some documented therapeutic benefits.

FAMILY INTERVENTIONS

Family Interventions for Preadolescent Children

Family-oriented approaches to the psychosocial treatment of preadolescent children with conduct problems have typically been based on a social learning model of behavioral intervention with parents (McMahon & Wells, 1998; Miller & Prinz, 1990). Although many different types of parent management training (PMT) exist, the underlying rationale for all programs is based on the general view that conduct problems are inadvertently developed and sustained in the home by maladaptive parent–child interactions (Kazdin, 1987). These maladaptive interchanges have been termed "coercive interaction patterns," and are thought to play a central role in promoting and maintaining aggressive and oppositional child behaviors (Patterson, 1982, 1986). Patterson's theory of coercive family process has been described in Chapters 5 and 8 of this book.

PMT refers to procedures in which parents are trained to interact differently with their children; it is designed to alter the pattern of parent–child interchanges to promote prosocial rather than coercive behavior within a family. Parenting behaviors such as establishing clear and consistent rules for a child to follow, providing positive reinforcement for appropriate and prosocial behaviors, delivering mild forms of punishment to suppress aversive behavior, and negotiating compromises are emphasized. All PMT programs share several common elements. First, treatment is conducted primarily with the parent or parents, who directly implement new procedures in the home. The therapist has little direct intervention with the child. Second, parents are helped to refocus from a preoccupation with conduct problems to an emphasis on prosocial goals. Third, treatment sessions cover social learning principles and the procedures that follow from them. These procedures include defining, monitoring, and tracking child behavior; forms of positive reinforcement, such as praise and positive parent attention; forms of extinction and mild punishment, including ignoring negative behaviors, response cost, and time-out procedures; giving clear and consistent commands; and problem-solving strategies. Fourth, there is extensive use of didactic instruction, modeling, role playing, behavioral rehearsal, and structured homework exercises (Kazdin, 1997).

Of all the psychosocial treatments for youth with conduct problems, PMT is the best researched and has the most empirical support in controlled outcome trials of its efficacy (Kazdin, 1997). PMT interventions have been successfully utilized in both clinic and home settings, and have been implemented both with individual families and with groups of families. Controlled outcome studies support efficacy across a variety of parent and teacher outcome measures, direct observation measures, and school and police records. Gains may be maintained over 1–4 years after treatment (Kazdin, 1997; McMahon & Wells, 1998). The first PMT programs were developed by Hanf (1969) and Patterson (1976), and such programs have been subsequently modified and developed by several independent groups of clinical researchers. Selected PMT programs with empirical research support for their efficacy are presented in Table 11.1.

The Helping the Noncompliant Child program for parents of children 3–8 years of age employs a controlled learning environment in which a parent is taught to change maladaptive interaction patterns with a child (Forehand & McMahon, 1981). Sessions are typically conducted in a clinic setting with individual families. The treatment program consists of two phases. During the differential-attention phase of treatment (Phase I), a parent learns to break the

TABLE 11.1. PMT Programs for Preadolescents

Program (reference)	Age range	Behavior target	Evidence for efficacy in comparison trials	Evidence for generalization
Helping the Noncompliant Child (Forehand & McMahon, 1981)	3–8	Noncompliance	+	Setting Temporal (1 to 4.5 yr) Sibling Behavioral
BASIC (Webster-Stratton, 1996)	3–8	Conduct problems	+	Setting Temporal (1 to 3 yr) Behavioral
Oregon Social Learning Center (OSLC) program (Patterson, 1975)	3–12	Conduct problems	+	Setting Temporal (1 to 2 yr) Sibling Behavioral
Defiant Children (Barkley, 1997b)	2–12	Oppositional defiant behavior	+	Setting Behavioral

cycle of coercive interchanges by learning new skills whose goal is to establish a more positive, mutually reinforcing relationship with the child. The parent is first taught to attend to and describe the child's appropriate behavior while eliminating commands, questions, and criticisms. The parent is next taught to use verbal and physical attention contingent upon compliance and other appropriate behaviors. Phase II of the treatment program consists of teaching the parent to use appropriate commands and a time-out procedure to decrease the child's noncompliant behavior. The parent then works toward implementing the program outside the clinic.

The Helping the Noncompliant Child program has been extensively evaluated in terms of its short-term effectiveness, generalization, and social validity (see McMahon & Wells, 1998). Short-term effectiveness and setting generalization from the clinic to the home have been demonstrated. Follow-up assessments have shown temporal generalization up to 4.5 years after treatment (Forehand & Long, 1988). Sibling generalization, in which untreated siblings in the home environment become more compliant to maternal directives, has also been demonstrated (Humphreys, Forehand, McMahon, & Roberts, 1978). Finally, improvement in child compliance has been accompanied by decreases in other conduct symptoms such as aggression and tantrums, thereby supporting the behavioral generalization of the program (Wells, Forehand, & Griest, 1980).

A second PMT program for 3- to 8-year-old children, called BASIC (Webster-Stratton, 1996a), has been developed from the original work of Hanf (1969) and uses components of the Forehand and McMahon (1981) program. BASIC refers to basic PMT skills, as contrasted with ADVANCE, another PMT program teaching more advanced skills. BASIC is unique in that it uses a videotape modeling/group discussion format. A standard package of 10 videotape programs of parent skills is shown by a therapist to groups of parents. There are approximately 250 videotape vignettes, each lasting about 2 minutes. These include examples of parents interacting with their children in both appropriate and inappropriate ways. After each vignette, the therapist leads a discussion with parents of the relevant parent–child interactions. Parents are then given homework assignments to practice various parenting skills with their children outside the clinic setting. The BASIC program has recently been expanded to include more advanced parenting skills and to include a videotape program for children, focusing on child social skills (see McMahon & Wells, 1998; Webster-Stratton, 1996a).

Outcome studies support both the immediate and longer-term effects of the BASIC PMT program (Brestan & Eyberg, 1998; Webster-Stratton, Kolpacoff, & Hollingsworth, 1988; Webster-Stratton, Hollinsworth, & Kolpacoff, 1989). Positive changes in mothers' and children's behaviors, and in maternal perceptions of the children's adjustment at posttreatment compared to a waiting-list control group, are documented. Equal efficacy for the videotape BASIC program and for an individual PMT curriculum has been reported, despite the individual PMT sessions' requiring up to five times as much therapist time as BASIC (McMahon & Wells, 1998). Setting generalization occurs from clinic to home, and temporal generalization up to 3 years after treatment has been documented for BASIC. Behavioral generalization to child conflict management and problem-solving skills with peers has also been found (McMahon & Wells, 1998).

The Oregon Social Learning Center (OSLC) program for children 3–12 years of age is based upon the work of Patterson and his associates (Patterson, 1975). The OSLC program first emphasizes reading assignments to help parents acquire the necessary background for further skills training. Parents are next taught to specify and track children's problem behaviors. They are then assisted in developing a positive reinforcement system based upon social learning principles, and a consequence (mild punishment) program for noncompliance or aggressive behavior. As parents progress in treatment, they become increasingly responsible for designing and implementing behavior management programs at home for a variety of child problem behaviors. Finally, problem-solving and negotiating strategies are taught to parents.

The OSLC PMT program has been extensively evaluated in both clinic and community settings (Breston & Eyberg, 1998; McMahon & Wells, 1998). Improvements in mothers' perceptions of their children's adjustment have been reported, and there is evidence of generalization across setting, across time (up to 2 years after treatment), to other behaviors, and to the siblings of children with conduct problems. The OSLC program has been shown to have comparable effects for families with older (6.5- to 12.5-year-old) and younger (2.5- to 6.5-year-old) children, although dropout rates from treatment were higher among families of older children (McMahon & Wells, 1998).

Barkley (1987, 1997b) has developed and tested a PMT program for oppositional defiant behavior in 2- to 12-year-old children that uses some of the original components of Hanf (1969) and Forehand and McMahon (1981). Barkley's Defiant Children program is an expansion and modification of a two-stage PMT program originally developed by Hanf over 30 years ago, and consists of two core procedures designed to teach parents more effective ways of dealing with child noncompliance. In the first procedure, parents are taught an effective method of attending positively to ongoing appropriate child behaviors (particularly compliance with requests) while ignoring inappropriate behaviors. In the second procedure, parents are instructed in the immediate use of time-out procedures following child noncompliance with a command (Barkley, 1997b). The current program consists of 10 steps taught to parents individually or in groups. The steps emphasize parent training and skill building in child management concepts. These include instruction in making positive or negative consequences immediate upon a child's behaviors; making consequences consistent across settings, over time, and between parents; establishing incentive reward programs for appropriate behaviors before the introduction of punishment for child aversive behaviors; anticipating and planning for child misbehaviors; and recognizing that interactions between family members are reciprocal, with each member of an interchange playing a role (Barkley, 1997b).

Outcome research has shown the Defiant Children PMT program to be effective in improving parental selective attending skills, parental delivery of commands, children's solitary play behavior, and parental use of effective discipline practices. Setting generalization has been shown from clinic to home, and some behavioral generalization also occurs when children's impulsive behavior improves following PMT training for oppositional defiant behavior (Barkley, 1997b).

Family Interventions for Adolescents

A recent advance in the psychosocial treatment of youth with aggressive and antisocial behaviors is the increased attention paid to developing and evaluating interventions with seriously antisocial adolescents. Adolescents with recurrent, multiple offenses, some of which may be violent, represent the most difficult-to-treat segment of this general population. Closely allied with this advance are the development and evaluation of multimodal, multicomponent interventions to address the multiple social needs of these adolescents. Since these interventions are more recent developments than the evaluation of PMT programs for preadolescent children with conduct problems, much less research on them is currently available. In addition, the treatment effects for adolescents with antisocial behaviors are much less than for younger children, because of increased rates of treatment dropout and more pervasive and serious problems (Kazdin, 1997). Nevertheless, the three programs shown in Table 11.2 and discussed below all have empirical research to support their efficacy in controlled outcome studies.

TABLE 11.2. **Family Interventions for Adolescents**

Program (reference)	Behavior target	Evidence for efficacy in comparison trials	Evidence for generalization
Oregon Social Learning Center (OSLC) program (Forgatch & Patterson, 1989)	Delinquency	+	Setting Temporal (1 to 3 yr)
Functional family therapy (FFT; Alexander & Parsons, 1982)	Delinquency, multiple offenses, previous incarceration	+	Temporal (1 to 2.5 yr) Sibling
Multisystemic therapy (MST; Henggeler & Borduin, 1990)	Delinquency, multiple offenses, often violent	+	Temporal (1 to 4 yr) Behavioral

Patterson and colleagues have modified their OSLC parent training intervention for use in families of adolescents with conduct problems (Forgatch & Patterson, 1989; Patterson & Forgatch, 1987). Specific changes include (1) expanding the list of targeted behaviors for parental monitoring and tracking to include any activities that put an adolescent at risk for further delinquency (e.g., school truancy, curfew violations, substance misuse); (2) a strong emphasis on parental monitoring and supervision of the teenager; (3) more age-appropriate forms of punishment, including work details, restriction of free time and activities, and restitution of stolen/damaged property; (4) asking parents to report legal offenses to juvenile authorities and then to act as advocates for the adolescent in court (as a way of decreasing the risk of the youth's removal from home); and (5) greater involvement of the adolescent in treatment (McMahon & Wells, 1998). The efficacy of this treatment approach has been compared to that of a treatment-as-usual condition in a study of chronically delinquent adolescent boys with an average of eight previous offenses (Bank, Marlowe, Reid, Patterson, & Weinrott, 1991). The comparison condition consisted of behavioral–family systems therapy, group treatment for the adolescents, and (for many adolescents) drug counseling. Some treatment gains were noted during 1 year of treatment, including a reduction in offense rates in the adolescents receiving the OSLC treatment relative to the treatment-as-usual condition. However, by 1-year follow-up the offense rates of the two groups were equal, and remained that way over the next 2 years of follow-up. Adolescents in the OSLC parent training condition did spend less time in institutions than teenagers in the comparison group over the first and second years of follow-up. Some evidence of setting generalizability is also reported from clinic to home and community. Despite these positive findings, therapist burnout is reported as high, given the extreme distress and multiple problems of these families (McMahon & Wells, 1998).

Functional family therapy (FFT) is a family intervention for adolescents with antisocial behaviors that reflects an integrative approach to treatment and relies on systems, behavioral, and cognitive views of dysfunction (Alexander & Parsons, 1982). Clinical problems are conceptualized from the standpoint of the functions they serve for the family as a system, as well as for individual family members. The underlying rationale is that an adolescent's problem behavior is the only way some interpersonal function, such as intimacy, distance, or support, can be met among family members. Maladaptive interactions within the family are thought to preclude more direct means of fulfilling these interpersonal functions. The goal of FFT is to alter interaction and communication patterns in such a way as to foster more adaptive functioning (Kazdin, 1997). In its current form, FFT consists of five components (Alexander, Waldron, Newberry, & Liddle, 1988). The introduction/impression phase is concerned with family members' expectations prior to therapy. In the assessment phase, the therapist identifies the behavioral, cognitive, and emotional expectations of each family member, as well as the family processes in need of change. Inappropriate attributions and expectations among family members are modified in the induction/therapy phase. In the behavior change/education phase, various behavioral techniques are employed, including communication skills training, behavioral contracting, and contingency management. In the generalization/termination phase, the clinician's task is to facilitate maintenance of therapeutic gains while fostering family independence and gradual disengagement from the therapeutic context.

Most of the initial empirical research on the efficacy of FFT was conducted in the 1970s and focused on the families of delinquent adolescents with relatively minor status offenses. These studies demonstrated improved family communication and lower recidivism rates in adolescents receiving FFT therapy as opposed to psychodynamic counseling or a no-treatment control (see McMahon & Wells, 1998). Temporal generalization was demonstrated up to 2.5 years after treatment (Alexander & Parsons, 1973). The siblings of adolescents in FFT showed a decreased probability of court involvement over time, supporting the treatment's sibling generalization (Klein, Alexander, & Parsons, 1977). More recently, FFT has been shown to be effective with multiply offending, previously incarcerated delinquent adolescents. Such adolescents participating in FFT were less likely to be charged with committing an offense in a 15-month follow-up period than were such adolescents placed in group homes (60% vs. 93%) (Barton, Alexander, Waldron, Turner, & Warburton, 1985). These results have been replicated in a sample of 27 disadvantaged rural families of delinquent and multiply offending adolescents (Gordon, Graves, & Arbuthnot, 1995). These results support the ability of FFT to alter conduct problems among some seriously delinquent youth.

Multisystemic therapy (MST) is a family systems approach to treating adolescents with conduct problems that emphasizes both the interactional nature of adolescent psychopathology and the role of multiple systems in which an adolescent is embedded, including family, school, and peer group (Henggeler & Borduin, 1990). Like FFT, MST maintains the view that clinical problems of the adolescent emerge within the context of the family. Unlike other family approaches, MST considers the family as just one (albeit a very important one) of a number of systems that affect the teenager. These other systems include peers, schools, and neighborhoods (Kazdin, 1997). In MST, treatment is expanded to include the interactions of the teenager with the family and with these larger systems. Because multiple influences are targeted by the focus of MST, many different treatment techniques are used. Thus MST is a package of interventions that are flexibly deployed with adolescents and their families.

Several family therapy techniques are used in MST to identify problems, facilitate communication, build family cohesion, and alter maladaptive family interactional patterns. MST also includes other domains within its therapeutic purview, such as marital difficulties, unemployment, and/or school difficulties. Therapists are guided by a set of treatment principles (e.g., "Focus on systemic strengths," "Interventions should be developmentally appropriate") that serve to integrate the disparate treatment elements into a coherent approach that is individualized for each family. As such, MST is more that a mere amalgamation of different therapy techniques. The focus of MST remains on how interrelated systems affect the adolescent and each other (Kazdin, 1997; McMahon & Wells, 1998).

A strength of MST is that several outcome studies have evaluated efficacy with seriously antisocial youth, many with arrest and incarceration histories including violent crime. Thus MST has been evaluated in the most difficult-to-treat population of young people with conduct problems. MST has been compared with alternative mental health treatment conditions in studies of offending adolescents; it has been shown to reduce adolescent problem behaviors, arrest rates, incarceration rates, and peer aggression, and to increase family cohesion, in comparison to these other treatments (Henggeler et al., 1986; Henggeler, Melton, & Smith, 1992). In a follow-up study, the superiority of MST over other treatments was maintained up to 2.4 years (Heneggler, Melton, Smith, Schoenwald, & Hanley, 1993). MST has also been shown to be effective with other problem behaviors, supporting the treatment's behavioral generalization. Lower rates of alcohol and cannabis use, and lower rates of substance-use-related arrests have been demonstrated for youth who receive MST than for youth in comparison treatment conditions (Heneggler et al., 1992). A strength of the outcome studies of MST is that many of the treated youth are severely impaired. Another strength is the conceptualization of conduct problems at multiple levels of dysfunction in relationship to the individual adolescent (Borduin, 1999).

Limitations of Family Interventions

Although all of the above-described family interventions for youth with aggressive/antisocial behaviors have been found effective in controlled outcome studies, several limitations can be identified. First, some families may not respond to or be able to make use of PMT. PMT makes several demands on parents, such as mastering educational materials, understanding the principles of social learning, systematically observing child behavior, consistently implementing specific procedures at home, and attending weekly therapy sessions. Parents with low socioeconomic status (SES), low intelligence, less than a high school education, marital conflict, or serious forms of psychopathology may not benefit from or have the means to participate in treatment (Barkley, 1997b; Kazdin, 1997). Age is also a modifier of outcome in PMT programs: As a child with conduct problems grows older, PMT's effectiveness diminishes. Thus PMT programs are less effective in adolescence—the developmental period where serious conduct problems peak. This is illustrated for one PMT program in Figure 11.1: The percentage of responders to PMT declines as youth enter adolescence.

There is evidence that inexperienced therapists do not appear as effective as more experienced therapists in maintaining parents in PMT programs (Frankel & Simmons, 1992). Clinicians working with families of severely antisocial youth often encounter parental resistance to PMT, which increases the risk of family dropout from treatment. More highly trained and experienced clinicians appear to do better at motivating, confronting, and supporting parents as they progress through PMT (Barkley, 1997b; McMahon & Wells, 1998). However, this finding runs counter to the current cost-cutting economic trends in clinical mental health care delivery systems. Currently, the managed care insurance industry appears to support the use of the least expensive clinicians in real-world mental health settings (see Chapter 10). Since these are often beginning therapists with little experience, PMT's effectiveness in the real world may be much less than it could be if support for experienced and highly trained therapists was valued among mental health insurance payers.

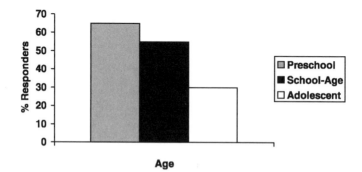

FIGURE 11.1. Percentage of responders by age for youth in one PMT program. As children become older, the number of responders to PMT decreases. Data from Barkley, Guevremont, Anastopoulos, and Fletcher (1993) and Barkley (1997b).

In regard to family interventions for adolescents in particular, other limitations exist. As the severity, frequency, and intensity of psychopathology deepen in the adolescent and family system, response rates diminish, and dropout rates from treatment increase (Kazdin, 1997). The temporal generalization of treatment effects after therapy has been completed appears less robust for adolescents than for children (McMahon & Wells, 1998). So, even though family interventions for conduct problems in children and adolescents have made remarkable gains over the past 30 years, their limitations (especially for adolescents) must be understood.

COGNITIVE-BEHAVIORAL SKILLS TRAINING

Research has found that traditional relationship-based psychosocial therapies grounded on the principles of psychodynamic therapy, whose goal is to help the individual develop insight into his or her behavior by utilizing the patient–therapist relationship as an agent of change, are largely ineffective in the treatment of conduct problems (Kazdin, 2000). Although family-based interventions have proven effective in treating youth with aggressive/antisocial behaviors, families of such youth often drop out of treatment or are otherwise unable or unwilling to participate. This has led to the conceptualization, development, and evaluation of other types of therapies that more directly involve these youth in treatment.

It has long been recognized that young persons with aggressive/antisocial behaviors have deficient social skills. They have poor peer relations, exhibit faulty social judgment, and experience peer rejection as a result. They also often display poor impulse control, especially when comorbid attention-deficit/hyperactivity disorder (ADHD) is present. Research has documented that distortions and deficits in social cognition underlie these skill deficiencies. These cognitive process distortions are not merely reflections of intellectual functioning; rather, they contribute independently to maladaptive behavioral adjustment and problematic social demeanor (Kazdin, 1997).

Various cognitive processes have been studied in aggressive and antisocial young people. These include overattribution of hostile, aggressive intent to others, especially in social situations where the cues of actual intent are ambiguous (Crick & Dodge, 1994). If social cues are perceived as threatening and hostile, these youth are more likely to react aggressively toward others. Deficits, distortions, and dysfunctions in other cognitive processes—such as generating alternative solutions to interpersonal problems, identifying the means to obtain specific ends (such as making a friend), making attributions to others of the motivation of their actions, perceiving how others feel, and predicting the effects of one's own actions upon others—have also been found to relate to disruptive behaviors and overt aggression (Kazdin, 1996; Lochman & Dodge, 1994).

Cognitive-behavioral therapy (CBT) for aggressive/antisocial youth refers to a broad class of psychosocial treatments that have been developed specifically to target the various deficiencies thought to contribute to conduct problems. Unlike psychodynamic therapies, whose goal is to help an individual develop insight into his or her maladaptive thoughts and behaviors, CBT seeks directly to help a child or adolescent develop and use specific skills to change these cognitions and behaviors. As such, CBT is a skills-building type of intervention. Another key component of all forms of CBT is a focus on practicing the use of these new skills in interpersonal situations, including rehearsal in real-life situations.

Behavioral Social Skills Training Approaches

Early CBT interventions for youth with conduct problems focused on maladaptive overt behaviors, such as poor social skills. The underlying rationale for social skills training in these youngsters has been that youth who display problematic social skills in interpersonal interactions often do so to secure rewards from the environment; therefore, direct training in more adaptive skills to get what one desires should be a potentially viable treatment method for such youth. Behavioral social skills training typically involves modeling appropriate skills, coaching, role playing, practice, feedback, and positive reinforcement.

These social skills training approaches for young people with conduct problems have been evaluated in comparison to other treatments and no-treatment control conditions. In a study of male delinquents aged 10–16 years, who were randomly assigned to a social skills training group, an attention placebo group, or a no-treatment group for 12 treatment sessions lasting 1 hour each, results indicated specific improvements in many individual social skills at outcome for the social skills training group relative to the other two conditions. Improvements were maintained at a 3-month follow-up (Spence & Marzillier, 1981). Michelson et al. (1983) studied a clinical population of 61 boys aged 8–12 years, and compared social skills training, interpersonal problem solving, and a nondirective control condition. The two active treatment conditions resulted in significant changes on parent, teacher, and self-report rating scales relative to the nondirective control condition. The social skills training group continued to show behavioral improvement over a 1-year follow-up, while the other two conditions failed to show evidence of temporal generalization. Although these controlled studies showed efficacy for social skills training in youngsters with conduct problems, more recent research has shown limited results from single-component programs (McMahon & Wells, 1998). A meta-analytic review of 79 controlled studies of children's social skills training found only moderate short-term effectiveness. More importantly, subjects with internalizing disorders were found to benefit more than aggressive subjects from social skills training (Schneider, 1992). As a result, skills training programs for youngsters with aggressive and antisocial behaviors have more recently emphasized a cognitive model of psychopathology.

Approaches Based on a Cognitive Model

An essential assumption of the cognitive model is that when youth with conduct problems encounter an anger- or frustration-arousing event, their emotional, physiological, and behavioral reactions are largely determined by their cognitive perceptions and appraisals of the event, rather than by the event itself (Coie & Dodge, 1998; Kendall, 1985; McMahon & Wells, 1998). Treatment interventions focused on these cognitive processes and distortions may then be effective in changing behavior. Several CBT programs based on this model have been developed and evaluated.

Coping Power is a 33-session, school-based program developed to teach cognitive skills associated with each stage of social information processing (Lochman, Lampron, Gemmer, & Garris, 1987; Lochman & Wells, 1996). Elementary-school-age children meet once weekly in a group format at school. Children practice reviewing examples of social encounters and discussing social cues and motivations of others in social encounters. They then practice skills that include identifying interpersonal problems, generating alternative solutions to these problems, and evaluating the solutions according to prosocial judgment criteria. Skills for managing anger arousal are also addressed. Outcome studies have evaluated the effects of the Coping Power program and found it more effective in reducing disruptive and aggressive behavior in the classroom than either a no-treatment or a goal-setting-alone comparison condition (Lochman, Burch, Curry, & Lampron, 1984). Evidence of temporal generalization was found at a 7-month follow-up (Lochman & Lampron, 1988). Behavioral generalization of the program has also been supported: Lower rates of substance misuse at a 3-year follow-up were found in boys with conduct problems who completed the program (Lochman, 1992).

Problem-solving skills training (PSST) has been developed to teach cognitive skills for problem identification, solution generation and evaluation, solution selection, and solution enactment (Kazdin, 1996, 1997). PSST is administered over 20 sessions to preadolescent children with conduct problems. Children receive training and practice in problem-solving skills, and then learn to apply the skills to interpersonal and academic tasks. PSST has been extensively evaluated in both inpatient and outpatient clinically referred youth. Outcomes have been compared with those for traditional relationship-based psychotherapies and with attention placebo control conditions; PSST demonstrates clear superiority over these other conditions at treatment end and at 1-year follow-up (Kazdin, Esveldt-Dawson, French, & Unis, 1987; Kazdin & Wassell, 2000). PSST produces improvements in children with serious aggressive conduct problems, as well as in children with mild to moderate conduct problems, in both inpatient and outpatient settings.

A 20-session CBT treatment program for 6- to 13-year-old clinically referred youth with CD has been developed and evaluated by Kendall and colleagues (Kendall & Braswell, 1985; Kendall, Reber, McLeer, Epps, & Ronan, 1990). CBT was compared to supportive and insight-oriented psychotherapy.

Results indicated the superiority of CBT on teacher measures of self-control and prosocial behavior, and on self-reports of perceived social competence. The percentage of children who improved from deviant to within the nondeviant range of behavior was significantly higher for the CBT program, supporting the efficacy of this treatment.

Limitations of Cognitive-Behavioral Skills Training

CBT skills training interventions for young people have demonstrated efficacy in reducing aggressive and antisocial behaviors. This group of therapies provides a means for engaging the individual child or adolescent in treatment when family-based approaches are not possible. However, CBT too has several limitations.

First, children's stage of cognitive development is a modifier of clinical response to CBT. In a meta-analysis of CBT for children with maladaptive behaviors, the treatment effect of CBT is almost twice as large for children functioning at a formal operational level of cognitive development (ages 11–13 years) than it is for youth at the less advanced preoperational and concrete operational stages (ages 5–7 years and 7–11 years, respectively) (Durlak, Fuhrman, & Lampman, 1991). In other words, as children become more cognitively sophisticated with development, the benefits of CBT appear to increase. This is illustrated in Figure 11.2, where "effect size" (a measure of treatment efficacy in units of standard deviation) is plotted for children at different levels of cognitive development. Suggested effect sizes are 0.80 for a large effect, 0.50 for a medium effect, and 0.20 for a small effect (Cohen, 1988).

The pervasiveness and severity of individual and family dysfunction also appear to modify the effectiveness of CBT. The number of risk factors for on-

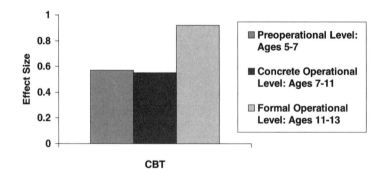

FIGURE 11.2. The effect size of CBT varies by level of cognitive development. As children develop more sophisticated cognitive abilities, CBT appears to become more effective. Data from Durlak, Fuhrman, and Lampman (1991).

set of CD, and the poor long-term prognosis associated with a greater number of factors, predict a poor response to CBT (Kazdin, 1997). Research has shown that although youth with multiple individual, family, and environmental risk factors for CD still improve with CBT, the magnitude of change is not as great as that achieved for cases with fewer risk factors (Kazdin, 1997).

Duration of CBT appears to influence behavioral outcomes as well. Brief or time-limited CBT programs (i.e., those with fewer than 10 hours/sessions) are less likely to show benefits with clinical populations. More durable effects are achieved with longer or time-unlimited programs extending up to 50–60 treatment sessions (Kazdin, 1997). In addition, evidence suggests that the quality of therapist training, skill, and experience are associated with the magnitude and durability of therapeutic changes. As is the case for family interventions, there is evidence that more highly skilled and experienced therapists achieve more effective results with CBT programs than beginning clinicians do (Kazdin, 2000). Given the current economic pressures from the managed health care insurance industry to limit the number of outpatient mental health visits and to encourage less trained and experienced (and therefore less costly) clinicians to provide the majority of psychosocial mental health care (see above and Chapter 10), the effectiveness of CBT programs as actually delivered in the community to patients in the real world may be much less than it could be.

PREVENTION PROGRAMS

Prevention programs are designed to keep a problem from occurring. "Primary prevention" consists of those interventions designed to prevent the development of disorder and to promote the health and development of persons who are as yet unaffected by dysfunction. "Secondary prevention" focuses on those persons who already show early (yet mild) signs of dysfunction, or who are at risk for developing the clinical problem. Primary prevention efforts target a population as a whole and often require broad-based legislative, political, economic, and popular support to be implemented. Examples include gun control and universal seat-belt laws for children. Truly primary prevention efforts targeting aggression and related behaviors in youth are uncommon. Most prevention efforts for young people with such problems are secondary prevention efforts in populations of at-risk children and families.

Preventing aggressive/antisocial behaviors from developing is very attractive, because these behaviors are so costly to society and so difficult to treat once they become chronic and entrenched within an individual. Moreover, such behaviors are well suited to prevention efforts. Conduct problems develop slowly over time, with different types of individual, familial, and environmental risk factors gradually accumulating over many years before overt violence or delinquency emerges (Group for the Advancement of Psychiatry, 1999; Kazdin, 1996). This offers multiple opportunities to reduce the number of risk factors and to increase the number of protective factors for an at-risk child, within the parent–child environment, and within the child's wider social ecology.

The prevention of conduct problems has received increasing attention over the past two decades. There are several reasons for this interest. First, advances have occurred in clarifying developmental pathways to early-onset antisocial behavior. This progress has helped delineate specific risk and protective factors at various stages within these developmental pathways. In turn, risk factors provide rational targets for prevention efforts to reduce aggressive/antisocial behaviors in youth. Second, the limitations of treatment for these behaviors after they become stabilized within a youngster are increasingly appreciated. Treatments for CD, including psychiatric hospitalization and psychotherapy, are expensive and inefficient. For many young people with CD, multiple interventions are likely to be needed over the course of their development, further increasing treatment costs to society and burdening already strained mental health care delivery systems. Furthermore, psychiatric treatments are often given too late in development, after a youth has engaged in many years of aggressive/antisocial behavior, and fail to demonstrate much efficacy or durability of therapeutic gains. Third, mental health treatments must be given to individuals or small groups of individuals. Thus these interventions can reach only a small portion of those in need—a problem exacerbated by the continued rationing of mental health insurance in the United States. Finally, punitive juvenile justice interventions, although currently politically popular, also fail to demonstrate effects over time. Incarceration of convicted children and adolescents does not appear helpful in ameliorating their aggression or related behaviors, and the costs of juvenile justice detention and incarceration are rising (Kazdin, 1997; Rutter et al., 1998).

Prevention programs all share a broad goal of building social competence and resilience in youth. As such, the focus of prevention programs differs from the focus of treatment programs. Mental health interventions focus on problems, whereas prevention programs focus on promoting adaptive social functioning (Kazdin, 1996). Promoting broad social competence may help avert a multiplicity of problems. Thus prevention programs have more comprehensive goals than treatment programs.

Two classes of prevention interventions are applicable to youth with conduct problems: early intervention programs, and programs that specifically target the prevention of these problems. Early intervention programs are not focused on conduct problems per se. These prevention programs have as a goal providing an array of early education and family support to families of infants and preschool-age children who are at risk for maladaptive developmental outcomes because of various factors, including poverty or single-parent status. Other prevention programs are more specifically focused on preventing conduct problems. The following sections provide a brief review of selected programs.

Early Intervention Programs

There are many different programs whose goal is to promote social adaptive functioning by providing a range of emotional, informational, instrumental, and/or educational support to families of children from infancy to 5 years of age. As noted above, these programs do not have the prevention of conduct problems as their stated goal; rather, they combine the goals of economic self-sufficiency with those of family support and preschool education. They provide a mix of child care, family support, parental educational and job training, parent child-rearing education and PMT, and preschool education to high-risk families. There is evidence that broad early intervention programs may have long-term effects on reducing the occurrence of conduct problems (Yoshikawa, 1994, 1995; McMahon & Wells, 1998; Zigler et al., 1992). These long-term effects have been noted later in childhood and adolescence, and in at least one program into adulthood (Schweinhart, Barnes, & Weikart, 1993). This is of particular interest, because the prevention of such problems has not been the stated goal of early intervention programs.

A review identified 40 early education or family support programs that had been developed as of the late 1980s (Yoshikawa, 1995). Of these programs, four have provided longitudinal outcome data on conduct problems. These four early intervention programs are presented in Table 11.3. Four common elements have been identified in these interventions: (1) Each program includes both family support and early childhood education components; (2) the intervention is implemented during a child's first 5 years of life; (3) the duration of the intervention is at least 2 years (range 2–5 years); and (4) the intervention has short- to long-term effects on risk factors known to be associated with conduct problems (McMahon & Wells, 1998; Yoshikawa, 1995).

The High/Scope Perry Preschool Program was designed for preschoolers deemed at risk for delayed intellectual functioning and eventual academic and school failure. It was conducted from 1962 through 1967 with some 123 African American children aged 3–4 years in Ypsilanti, Michigan (Berrueta-Clement, Schweinhart, Barnett, Epstein, & Weikart, 1984; Schweinhart et al., 1993). Children were randomly assigned to intervention or control conditions. The preschool intervention consisted of high-quality, cognitively oriented, early childhood education for 1–2 academic years. Teachers conducted frequent home visits to keep parents involved with their children's academic activities and progress. Monthly parent small-group sessions provided opportunities for parent support in child rearing.

Longitudinal data on children up to age 19 revealed a number of positive outcomes indicative of improved social competence in program attendees. Compared with control children, those who received the intervention condition showed better attitudes toward school, had lower rates of grade retention and placement in special education services, and showed better academic

TABLE 11.3. Early Intervention Programs with Long-Term Effects on Conduct Problems

Reference	Program	Intervention components	Comparison group	Duration	Outcomes
Berrueta-Clement et al. (1984)	High/Scope Perry Preschool Program	Educational component Teacher–parent home visits Parent group meetings	Random assignment to control group	30 mo	At 10-yr follow-up, reduced rates of delinquency, improved classroom performance. At 23-yr follow-up, reduced rates of adult criminality and improved employment rates.
Lally et al. (1988)	Syracuse Univ. Family Development Research Program	Home visits Parent ed. Day care Human service resources	Matched control group	5 yr	At 10-yr follow-up, reduced antisocial behaviors and arrests.
Provence and Naylor (1983)	Yale Child Welfare Research Program	Home visits Parent ed. Pediatric and development checkups Day care	Matched control group	2 yr	At 10-yr follow-up, more families self-supporting, fewer children, reduced aggression in children.
Johnson (1988)	Houston Parent–Child Development Center	Home visits Child ed. Parent ed. Entire-family focus	Random assignment to control group	2 yr	At 1- to 8-yr follow-up, decreased special ed. services, classroom conduct problems, aggression. At 7- to 15-yr follow-up, intervention and comparison groups equal on aggression.

achievement. Moreover, reduced rates of delinquent behaviors occurred in adolescence for those who received the program: Decreased rates of self-reported delinquency were reported at age 14 years, and reduced official chronic delinquency occurred at age 19 years (Berrueta-Clement, Schweinhart, Barnett, & Weikart, 1987). At age 27 years, reduced rates of adult criminality were found in those who received the intervention, compared to those who received the control condition (Schweinhart et al., 1993).

The effects of the High/Scope Perry Preschool Program have been evaluated in several different ways. One way of assessing the magnitude of the effects of program or treatment interventions involves calculating an effect size. The effect size is a statistic that translates the results of different studies using different methodologies into a common metric utilizing the standard deviation. As mentioned above, in the social sciences an effect size of 0.20 is considered small, 0.50 is moderate, and 0.80 or greater is large. The Perry Preschool Program has an effect size of 0.42 for delinquent and other antisocial behavior (Yoshikawa, 1994, 1995). Another way of estimating the magnitude of a program's effects is to calculate the costs and benefits of the program in constant dollar amounts. Monetary values are estimated for the program costs, as well as for benefits in such areas as education, employment, public welfare assistance, delinquency, and crime. Results indicate that the High/Scope Perry Preschool Program, which cost roughly $12,356 per family, yielded benefits totaling $108,002 per family—a net program benefit value per family of $95,646 (in constant 1993 dollars). Most of the dollar benefits were due to savings in the criminal justice system and to savings for crime victims (Schweinhart et al., 1993; Yoshikawa, 1995).

The Syracuse University Family Development Research Program attempted to bolster family and child functioning in an economically disadvantaged population (Lally, Mangione, & Honig, 1988). Low-SES women were recruited into the program during their last trimester of pregnancy. They were mostly young, single parents with less than a high school education and poor employment histories. Many had histories of arrest or appearance in court. A matched control group was later established. Interventions consisted of paraprofessionals' working with target families on a weekly basis in the home. Parent education about nutrition, sound mother–child relationships, and support for the development of human service contacts were provided. The educational component consisted of 4.5 continuous years of high-quality child care at Syracuse University Children's Center.

Longitudinal follow-up data revealed a number of positive outcomes. When children were between 13 and 16 years of age, significant reductions in rates of delinquency and arrest compared to control children were documented (Lally et al., 1988). The severity of offenses and the degree of chronicity were much higher in the control group. The effect size for the Syracuse program on delinquent and other antisocial behaviors was 0.48 (Yoshikawa, 1995). Averaged across the entire sample, the costs for court and penal procedures were $186 for each child in the intervention group and

$1,985 for each of the children in the matching no-intervention control condition (Zigler et al., 1992).

The Yale Child Welfare Research Program focused its intervention efforts primarily on mothers raising young children in high-risk environments (Provence & Naylor, 1983). The goal was to alleviate some of the stresses of poverty and provide supports, so that the mothers could devote more of their time and energy to parenting their children (Zigler et al., 1992). Women entered the program during their pregnancies, and services were provided until the children were 30 months of age. Intervention components consisted of home visits by clinical and health professionals who provided parental education on solving practical problems, as well as on making parenting decisions about children's future education, family goals, and career goals. Program workers interacted with human service agencies to help secure additional assistance for the families. Pediatric visits were made available on a regular basis to monitor the children's health, growth, and development. Child care was provided between 2 and 28 months of age. After the program ended, a matched control group was identified.

At a 10-year follow-up, intervention mothers had obtained more education than control group mothers and had largely become self-supporting by the time their firstborns were 12.5 years old. Intervention mothers also had fewer children and spaced their births more widely (Seitz, Rosenbaum, & Apfel, 1985). Although delinquent behaviors were not targeted, reductions in aggression were noted in intervention children compared to control children (Zigler et al., 1992). The calculated effect size of this program on delinquent behavior, 1.13, was large (Yoshikawa, 1995). Because children of mothers who received the intervention appeared to be more socially competent across a variety of outcomes, they required fewer remedial and supportive services (including court hearings) than did control children. The dollar benefit was estimated at an average savings of $1,120 per intervention child per year (Seitz et al., 1985; Zigler et al., 1992).

The Houston Parent–Child Development Center was designed to promote social and intellectual competence in children from low-income Mexican American families (Johnson, 1988). The program was carried out between 1970 and 1977. At 1 year of age, children were randomly assigned to the intervention or control groups. The program lasted 2 years, and its emphasis was on mother–child interaction in the family setting. During the first year, mothers received 25 home visits from paraprofessionals. Mothers were provided information on baby care, education concerning child development, advice on handling stress, and guidance in creating a stimulating home environment. Weekend workshop sessions were designed to involve fathers and siblings in the program. In the second year, children attended morning nursery school while mothers participated in child management and homemaker classes.

At a follow-up when the children were aged 4–7 years, results showed that boys in the control group were more destructive, more overactive, and less emotionally sensitive than children in the intervention group (Johnson & Breckenridge, 1982). At 5–8 years after program completion, intervention children showed fewer aggressive, hostile, and acting-out behaviors (Johnson & Walker, 1987). However, 7–15 years after program completion (when children were in grades 4 through 11), the earlier differences between groups in aggressive behavior were no longer apparent. Positive program effects remained for intervention children in domains measuring a supportive home environment (Johnson, 1989). These results indicate that the 2-year Houston program decreased children's aggressive/antisocial behavior as rated by parents and teachers over 1–8 years following program completion. However, effects began to disappear when children entered adolescence. The effect size for the Houston Parent–Child Development Center's impact on delinquent and other conduct problem behaviors was 0.48 (Yoshikawa, 1995).

In summary, longitudinal evidence from all four of these early intervention programs gives some indication that juvenile delinquency and predelinquent behaviors may be reduced (Yoshikawa, 1994; Zigler et al., 1992). This is noteworthy, for these programs did not have reductions in conduct problems as their stated goal. These programs may alleviate some of the risk factors known to be specifically associated with aggressive/antisocial behaviors, such as academic failure, poor parenting skills, and child cognitive deficiencies.

Prevention Programs Specifically Focused on Conduct Problems

Several prevention programs have been designed and implemented with the specific goal of preventing conduct problems in young people. There are two generations of such interventions. The first-generation programs began in the 1980s and reported their longitudinal findings in the 1990s; the second-generation programs are still in progress. These second-generation programs tend to provide more comprehensive intervention components and to implement the interventions for a longer period of time than the earlier intervention trials did (McMahon & Wells, 1998). Two examples of first-generation programs, and one example of a second-generation program, are included in Table 11.4 and described below.

The Seattle Social Development Project was a first-generation intervention program for elementary school children. It was based on a social development model and sought to enhance prosocial development, reduce aggressive/antisocial behaviors, and reduce the risk for delinquency and substance misuse by promoting in families and school classrooms conditions hypothesized to be necessary for social bonding (Hawkins & Weis, 1985; Hawkins, Von Cleve, & Catalano, 1991). According to the Seattle social development model, conduct problems are inhibited by high levels of social bonding to prosocial others, institutions, and values (O'Donnell, Hawkins, & Abbott, 1995). The components of bonding include positive relationships with others, commitment to a valued program of action, and beliefs about what is right and

TABLE 11.4. Selected Prevention Programs Specifically Focused on Conduct Problems

Reference	Program	Intervention components	Comparison group	Duration	Outcomes
First-generation interventions					
Hawkins et al. (1991)	Seattle Social Development Project	Classroom Social PST[a] Assertiveness training PMT	Random assignment to control group	2 yr	At 5-yr follow-up, reduced rates of substance use in girls and delinquency in boys.
Tremblay et al. (1995)	Montreal Longitudinal Experimental Study	PMT SST[b]	Random assignment to attention control or no treatment control	2 yr	At 6-yr follow-up, reduced rates of arrest, delinquency, substance misuse, and gang involvement. No difference in school adjustment.
Second-generation interventions					
Conduct Problems Prevention Research Group (1999a, 1999b)	Families and Schools Together (FAST) Track program	PMT Home visits/case mgt. CBST[c] Academic tutoring Classroom interventions	Random assignment to control group	10 yr (intensive, grades 1–2 and 5–6)	At 1-yr follow-up, reduced aggression, enhanced parenting, improved reading.

[a]PST, problem-solving training.
[b]SST, social skills training.
[c]CBST, cognitive-behavioral skills training.

wrong. The conditions thought necessary for social bonding include opportunities for involvement in conventional activities, skills for successful involvement, and rewards for conventional behavior. The model hypothesizes that the levels of opportunities, and the skills and rewards, available in families and schools affect youth's degree of attachment to family and school, their degree of commitment to conventional lines of action within these settings, and their belief in the conventional moral and legal order of society (Hawkins et al., 1991).

The Seattle Social Development Project was initiated in the first grade, with elements of intervention implemented at various points between first and sixth grades. Children were randomly assigned to the intervention or a no-treatment control group. Program classroom components included teacher training in the use of proactive classroom management methods, cognitive social skills training, interactive teaching methods, and cooperative learning strategies. Children received a social problem-solving curriculum in first grade and training in refusal skills in sixth grade. A parent training component sought to teach parents effective family management skills. The program was initiated in 1981, and the core elements lasted 2 years (Hawkins et al., 1991). Outcome was evaluated when children were in the sixth grade. Girls who completed the intervention had lower rates of substance use initiation, and boys who completed the program demonstrated lower rates of involvement with antisocial peers and less initiation of delinquency, compared to children in the control condition (O'Donnell, Hawkins, Catalano, Abbott, & Day, 1995).

Another first-generation intervention program specifically designed to prevent conduct problems was the Montreal Longitudinal Experimental Study (Tremblay, Vitaro, et al., 1992; Tremblay, Pagani-Kurtz, Masse, Vitaro, & Phil, 1995). The program was implemented in the second and third grades with high-risk aggressive boys initially identified in kindergarten during the 1984 school year. Boys were randomly assigned to an intervention group, an attention placebo group, and a no-intervention control group. The intervention program combined a parent training component with child social skills training.

As of 1994, annual assessments had been conducted in the Montreal study from ages 10 through 15 years. During elementary school, boys who completed the intervention condition were less likely to be described by teachers and peers as having serious difficulties, were more likely to have a positive peer group, and were less likely to have engaged in delinquent behaviors than boys in the control conditions (Tremblay, Vitaro, et al., 1992). During early adolescence, boys who received the intervention were less likely to be involved with gangs, were less involved with delinquent behavior, were less likely to be arrested, and engaged in substance misuse less frequently than boys in the comparison conditions (Tremblay et al., 1995). However, the earlier positive effects of the program on school adjustment found during the elementary school years were not maintained into adolescence. Despite the program's failure to show continued good academic adjustment, the Montreal study has presented some of the most encouraging findings to date about the long-term maintenance effects of interventions that focus specifically on the prevention of conduct problems in young persons (McMahon & Wells, 1998).

The Family and Schools Together (FAST) Track program is an example of a second-generation prevention intervention for conduct problems. As noted above, second-generation programs are more comprehensive than earlier prevention interventions and tend to implement their interventions over a longer period of time. FAST Track is a comprehensive multisite intervention intended to prevent severe and chronic conduct problems in a sample of children identified as high-risk at school entry. The FAST Track model of intervention is based upon interrupting known child and family risk factors for CD, specifically identified from developmental psychopathology pathways that lead to early-onset conduct problems (Conduct Problems Prevention Research Group, 1992). School entry is the chosen point of intervention because (1) at this time there are identifiable markers of the child and family variables that predict high risk for severe CD; and (2) school entry marks a significant developmental transition for both children and their families, which may make them more responsive to reorganization and change (Conduct Problems Prevention Research Group, 1992; Frick, 1998).

The components of the FAST Track intervention are designed to target specific processes known from previous research to be implicated in the development of conduct problems. The program takes a multicomponent and comprehensive approach to treatment, in recognition of the multidetermined etiology of CD. First, 22 sessions of PMT are conducted in a group format. Standard PMT techniques as well as enhanced interventions, including cognitive-behavioral skills training, are included. Second, a home visitor/case manager is provided biweekly, to help parents practice skills and respond to problems in the home environment. Third, the program provides a cognitive-behavioral skills training component to children; this focuses on anger coping strategies, interpersonal problem-solving skills, and friendship and play skill activities. Children practice their newly learned skills in weekly 30-minute guided play sessions with a classroom peer. Fourth, an academic tutoring component emphasizing reading skills is provided. The tutoring takes place three times a week, and at least once a week the children's parents are present to participate in the children's academic progress. Fifth, the program includes a universal classroom intervention for all students that the teachers implement. The classroom intervention is designed to facilitate emotional awareness, self-control, and interpersonal problem-solving skills. Teachers are helped in developing contingency management behavioral interventions to manage disruptive behavior effectively in the classroom. The FAST Track program is intensive and includes summertime interventions.

The FAST Track collaborative study is currently following a high-risk sample of almost 900 children who have been identified by both teachers and parents as displaying high rates of conduct problems during kindergarten. A representative sample from the same schools as the high-risk children serves as a comparison group. About 30% of the sample are girls, so it will be possible to compare gender differences both in developmental course and in the effects of interventions. Half of the high-risk children are participating in the intensive and long-term intervention, which begins in grade 1 and continues to grade 10, with two periods of more intensive intervention at school entry (grades 1–2) and the transition to middle school (grades 5–6).

Initial results for the first year of FAST Track are available. Results are reported for 891 high-risk kindergarten children and controls from four sites in the United States: Durham, North Carolina; Nashville, Tennessee; Seattle, Washington; and a rural region of central Pennsylvania. Results show modest positive effects on children's social, emotional, and academic skills; children's peer interactions and social status; parenting practices; and child conduct problems. There is little evidence of differential intervention effects across child gender, race, site, or cohort (Conduct Problems Prevention Group, 1999a, 1999b).

These generally positive results in a high-risk sample are encouraging. However, a closer inspection of the data reveals many areas that did not improve and some difficulties with treatment delivery in these families, despite the comprehensiveness of the FAST Track intervention program. For example, whereas 6 of 8 variables measuring high-risk children's social cognition and reading improved, only 2 of 5 variables measuring the children's peer relations and social competence improved with the intervention. Only 5 of 11 variables measuring positive parenting behaviors improved, and only 4 of 12 measures of child aggressive/disruptive behavior improved over the first year of intervention. Parents attended, on average, only 56.3% of the parent group sessions offered (Orrell-Valentine, Pinderhughes, Valente, Laird, & Conduct Problems Prevention Research Group, 1999). These results underscore how difficult it is to engage high-risk families in treatment, and how daunting a task it is to make a meaningful impact on such families even with comprehensive, multidisciplinary, and long-term psychoeducational interventions delivered early in their high-risk children's lives (Conduct Problems Prevention Group, 1999a, 1999b).

The FAST Track program is a model example of a second-generation comprehensive treatment approach to conduct problem behaviors. First it is prevention-oriented, being designed to prevent the blossoming of CD in children known to be at high risk. Second, the interventions are comprehensive and focus on psychosocial mechanisms identified by research as associated with the development of CD. Third, the FAST Track program is community-based and implemented through local schools. This allows the program to reach a large number of children and families who might be unwilling or unable to access mental health services. As a result of its school-based location, many children with subthreshold conduct problems (i.e., problems not yet severe enough to come to the attention of mental health care providers or juvenile justice authorities) can receive interventions (Frick, 1998). Although the results after 1 year of intervention are modest, they are encouraging.

Not all comprehensive, multimodal, long-term, community-based treatment programs have demonstrated positive outcomes. An example is the Fort Bragg Evaluation Project (FBEP; Bickman, Lambert, Andrade, & Penaloza, 2000). This was a demonstration project designed to improve mental health outcomes for children and adolescents who were referred for mental health treatment. The FBEP provided a broad continuum of mental health services, including outpatient therapy, day treatment, in-home counseling, therapeutic foster homes, specialized group homes, 24-hour crisis management services, and (if necessary) acute hospitalization. Individual case managers and interdisciplinary treatment teams worked with children who were assigned to more intensive services, to integrate and fit services to the needs of each individual child. Treatment plans used the least-restrictive-service options, and services were community-based. Data were collected over seven waves, comparing 574 children receiving FBEP demonstration services with 410 children receiving mental health services as usual (Bickman, 1997; Bickman et al., 2000).

Initially, there was great hope that the FBEP's continuum-of-care model would produce better clinical outcomes for youth with mental health needs at lower cost. Unfortunately, this has not proven to be the case. Results at 12 months (Bickman et al., 1995), 18 months (Hamner, Lambert, & Bickman, 1997), and 5 years (Bickman et al., 2000) have shown no differences in clinical outcomes between children treated in the FBEP and children who received mental health services as usual. In addition, costs were significantly higher for children in the FBEP than for control children (Bickman et al., 2000). This series of studies illustrates the difficulties in intervening effectively with youth who have mental health difficulties, including CD.

Summary of Prevention Programs

In summary, both early intervention programs and specific intervention programs for conduct problems generally (but not universally) appear to have long-term benefits on diminishing rates of delinquency and other antisocial behaviors, CD, substance use initiation, and aggression over follow-up periods lasting from 1 to 27 years. As measured by effect size, the magnitude of their benefits is medium to large. However, not all programs demonstrate effectiveness. Those programs that do show significantly positive results also reveal that many important variables do not improve with comprehensive interventions. Moreover, the obstacles to treatment are large. Despite these caveats, the results are largely encouraging. Substantial savings are demonstrated to accrue to society largely from diminished judicial and crime costs for families who complete these prevention programs relative to control groups.

The characteristics of successful programs include (1) multimodal interventions that target family supports and early childhood education (interventions with only a single focus are much less effective); (2) interventions of sufficient intensity delivered on a daily to weekly basis; (3) sufficient duration of intervention (at least 2 years and often longer); (4) use of interventions shown to be effective in ameliorating known psychosocial mechanisms that increase risk for CD; (5) interventions that begin early in a child's life (between ages 0 and 6 years); and (6) collaboration among community, school, and mental health professionals. Prevention programs that have these characteristics appear to reduce CD during a child's development.

These empirically tested and moderately effective prevention and intervention models stand in stark contrast to the current delivery of services for youth at risk for CD. Under mental health service delivery systems characterized by managed care, interventions are supported in piecemeal fashion for a limited number of visits (generally fewer than 10). This focus on single interventions for brief time periods is known to be insufficient in intensity and duration to have appreciable effects on young persons with conduct problems; however, this focus is what is generally supported through carve-out mental health managed care insurance systems. Effective prevention and intervention models for youth with aggressive/antisocial behaviors requires cooperation across many different disciplines. These include collaborations involving financial structures, physical space accommodations, and personnel across mental health disciplines, schools, community agencies, and often juvenile justice institutions. This multidisciplinary collaborative model does not fit easily into traditional psychiatric service delivery structures largely funded by state or private managed care insurance systems. In the clinical arena, systems of care remain largely fragmented and isolated from one another. The models of prevention described above are encouraging not only because they appear effective in the prevention of CD, but because they provide a blueprint for a new type of collaborative structure effective in the prevention and treatment of conduct problems in children and adolescents.

TREATMENTS THAT APPEAR NOT TO WORK

Currently there are over 230 documented psychotherapies available for children and adolescents (Kazdin, 2000). The vast majority of these interventions have not yet been empirically evaluated. Thus there is no accumulated body of scientific evidence in which treatments have empirically emerged as consistently ineffective for conduct problems in young persons (Kazdin, 1997). From such a limited data base, it remains premature to conclude that untested treatments are indeed ineffective for aggression and related behaviors in youth. However, there is some evidence that certain psychotherapy interventions are less effective for CD than those discussed above.

The efficacy of psychoanalysis for children with disruptive behavior disorders has been examined (Fonagy & Target, 1994). In a retrospective chart review of 763 cases of child psychoanalysis and psychotherapy treated at the Anna Freud Centre in the United Kingdom, 135 children with a principal diagnosis of a disruptive behavior disorder (ADHD, CD, or oppositional defiant disorder) were individually matched with others suffering from emotional disorders (anxiety and depression). Improvement rates were significantly higher for the emotional group than for the disruptive group. Early termination from treatment was observed for 31% of the children within 1 year. This result supports previous research that has found relationship-based psychotherapies less effective than family interventions or CBT for conduct problems in youth (Kazdin, 1996).

Some evidence has emerged that placing aggressive/antisocial youth together in group therapy formats may be less than useful. When youngsters with CD are placed together in groups, in the absence of any prosocial youngsters without CD, peer bonding to deviant group members may occur and reinforce antisocial attitudes, values, and behaviors (Feldman, Caplinger, & Wodarski, 1983). Current treatments for aggressive/antisocial youngsters in such settings as schools, hospitals, juvenile corrections facilities, and ambulatory clinics often emphasize group therapy for CD. This intervention, whether conducted alone or in combination with PMT, can be associated with increases in behavioral problems and substance use among group members (Dishion & Andrews, 1995).

CHAPTER SUMMARY

This chapter has discussed psychosocial treatments with empirical evidence for effectiveness in young persons with CD and other forms of aggressive/antisocial behavior. In contrast to earlier views, a cautious, tempered opinion is emerging that CD in youngsters can be partially modified. Although the magnitude of effects is not large (15% to 25%), even small improvements in rates of CD onset or sequelae (such as juvenile crime, juvenile justice costs, crime victim costs, teenage pregnancy, and substance misuse) are not trivial for society.

Advances in research have clarified the risk and protective factors that appear salient concerning vulnerabilities for early-starter developmental psychopathology pathways to CD. Child variables (such as social information-processing and other cognitive distortions), parenting variables (such as coercive parent–child interactions and child supervision failures), and systems variables (such as the roles of neighborhoods, schools, and peers in facilitating risk) are better understood now as a result of this research. This understanding has facilitated the development and evaluation of psychosocial treatment interventions specifically designed to address known risk factors. Family interventions based on PMT programs for young children, family interventions for adolescents, and forms of CBT for skill building have been demonstrated to be effective for youth with aggressive/antisocial behaviors. Prevention programs, whether nonspecific early intervention programs or specific projects to prevent these behaviors, have shown promise in ameliorating conduct problems and delinquency in at-risk children and families.

Research has also identified program components necessary for interventions to be effective. These include (1) interventions designed to target known risk factors for CD; (2) multicomponent programs that address child, family, and school elements; (3) early intervention before conduct problems become stabilized in adolescence; and (4) interventions that are delivered with sufficient frequency and intensity (generally daily to weekly over a minimum of at least 2 years). It is noted that these components of effective interventions stand in contrast to the interventions for CD currently supported by the managed care insurance industry, which are generally delivered in piecemeal fashion over brief time periods.

This review also highlights areas in need of further research. First, comprehensive, reliable, and valid treatment selection guidelines for youth with conduct problems need to be developed. We need more information on what specific treatments for what particular child in what specific family and at what developmental period are most effective. Second, research on the impact of comorbid psychiatric conditions (such as mood disorders, ADHD, and substance use disorders) on the longitudinal and treatment outcomes of youth with CD would advance clinical care. Third, studies on the impact of subtypes of aggressive/antisocial behavior on outcome, service utilization, and treatment efficacy are needed. For example, do overtly aggressive symptoms predict the same longitudinal outcome and response to treatment as covertly aggressive symptoms? Do girls and boys with conduct problems respond similarly or differently to treatment? Finally, further research is needed to explore the benefits and costs of combined pharmacotherapeutic–psychosocial treatments in subsets of aggressive/antisocial youth with comorbid conditions such as ADHD that predict response to medication.

◈ CHAPTER 12

Psychopharmacological Treatments

T here has been substantial progress in pediatric psychopharmacology over the past three decades. Recent research has contributed to significant advances in the development of new drugs for juvenile psychiatric illnesses, new indications for existing medications, and increasing knowledge about drug safety and efficacy (Campbell & Cueva, 1995a, 1995b; Gadow, 1991; Klein et al., 1994; Simeon, 1989). Given the growing clinical use of psychiatric medication for children and adolescents, a recent report of the U.S. Surgeon General emphasizes a need for more research in pediatric psychopharmacology (Satcher, 2000). Scientific progress in neuropharmacology, biochemistry, and noninvasive brain imaging, as well as methodological advances in research, have offered investigators new approaches in developing treatments for psychiatric illnesses in youth. Progress has also been made in the development of clinical drug trials in the pediatric age range, and ethical issues and other challenges in the biological treatment of youth are being defined more clearly (Campbell & Cueva, 1995a; Klein et al., 1994).

Clinically, maladaptive aggression is a problem with multiple, complex causes; its heterogeneous etiology generally requires a multidisciplinary psychoeducational and community approach to treatment. Since both preclinical and clinical research have begun to reveal the underlying neurobiological mechanisms that subserve aggression, increased interest has been generated in the possibilities of adjunctive pharmacological treatment of maladaptive aggression in psychiatrically referred children and adolescents (Connor & Steingard, 1996). This is not occurring without controversy, however. Opponents of biomedical aggression research and treatment are quick to point out that many psychosocial correlates and causes of maladaptive aggression exist for youth, and that these issues—not narrowly defined investigations into the neurobiology of aggression—are in urgent need of national and community attention and resources.

This debate should not be framed as an either–or proposition. As presented in Chapters 6 and 7, psychobiology and neurobiology are clearly important in the etiology of maladaptive aggression and antisociality in youth, and may be rational targets for biological interventions as part of a comprehensive treatment plan. The issue for future aggression research is not social versus biological causation; the issue is to understand how the interaction of biological vulnerabilities with problematic social environments during the developing years results in the expression of treatment-resistant maladaptive aggression and related behaviors. The next issue to understand is how both biological and psychosocial treatment interventions might be helpful in ameliorating these behaviors. Psychosocial interventions have been reviewed in Chapter 11; this chapter reviews issues in pharmacological treatment.

RATIONALE FOR PSYCHOTROPIC TREATMENT OF MALADAPTIVE AGGRESSION

Since aggression is mediated through biological mechanisms, it is possible that psychotropic interventions could attenuate aggressive/antisocial behaviors in the early years, resulting in less problematic development as a child matures into adulthood. The pharmacological down-regulation of these behaviors might also help the child make better use of accompanying psychoeducational and community interventions.

A problem facing both clinicians and health care policy makers is what types of aggression may require adjunctive psychiatric medication treatment and what types of aggression may require exclusively psychosocial and psychoeducational intervention. Current research has begun to identify types of aggression that may respond to two psychopharmacological approaches:

1. *Target symptom approach.* Aggression that has an early age of onset in the childhood years; is chronic, severe, and frequently occurring; is not connected to identifiable social cues in the environment; and causes impairment to the child and those around him or her may constitute one form of medication-responsive maladaptive aggression. This type of aggression often has an impulsive, hyperactive, explosive, hostile, irritable, or rageful component (Campbell, Gonzalez, & Silva, 1992), and it occurs in many different psychiatric disorders, not just conduct disorder (CD). There is pharmacological evidence that this type of impulsive aggression may respond to a variety of psychiatric medications, regardless of the actual psychiatric diagnosis. This target symptom approach to the pharmacological treatment of maladaptive aggression is analogous to the palliative medical treatment of excessive pain or fever with analgesic or antipyretic medication, in a patient where an underlying medical or surgical illness is not treatable or curable.

2. *Primary illness approach.* Aggression occurring as an associated symptom of an identifiable psychiatric illness that is itself amenable to pharmaco-

logical treatment may be another type of medication-responsive aggression. Research in pediatric psychopharmacology over the past three decades has identified a number of juvenile psychiatric syndromes that are responsive to pharmacotherapy (Campbell & Cueva, 1995a, 1995b). For example, aggression occurring in the context of a psychotic, mood, or disruptive behavior disorder may respond as the underlying syndrome is treated by medication (Connor & Steingard, 1996). The treatment of maladaptive aggression with psychiatric medication in the primary illness approach is analogous to the medical treatment of fever or pain that accompanies infectious disease. The fever or pain is a physiological mechanism associated with the underlying medical condition. As treatment alleviates the medical illness, the fever and pain subside. Treatment is not palliative, but directed at the underlying condition.

Research has also begun to define what types of aggression in children and adolescents may respond to psychosocial interventions. For example, in one study 44 children with CD admitted to an inpatient psychiatry unit for severe and intractable aggressive behaviors were randomly assigned under double-blind conditions to placebo or lithium treatment (Malone et al., 1997). Of those admitted to the hospital and given placebo, almost 50% responded with diminished aggression. This suggests that many severely aggressive children and adolescents do not require medication and may respond to psychosocial treatments in structured therapeutic environments. Another point of this study is that nonresponse to milieu treatment was associated with chronicity, severity, and frequency of aggression; associated hyperactivity; and a lack of acute social stressors as precipitants for aggressive behaviors. These associated symptoms that predict nonresponse to psychosocial treatments for aggression suggest the possibility of underlying neurobiological etiologies for aggressive behaviors. They further suggest the possibility of adjunctive medication therapy for these youth as discussed above (Malone et al., 1997; Sanchez, Armenteros, Small, Campbell, & Adams, 1994).

There is another type of aggression that may not respond to pharmacological treatments. The instrumental or predatory subtype of aggression is aggressive behavior that is used to obtain needed resources from the environment (e.g., the premeditated holdup of a liquor store to obtain money). Predatory aggression is associated with low levels of autonomic nervous system (ANS) arousal, is planned and premeditated, and does not appear responsive to biological interventions (Eichelman, 1988).

PHARMACOEPIDEMIOLOGY OF AGGRESSION IN CLINICALLY REFERRED YOUTH

"Pharmacoepidemiology" is defined as the application of epidemiological knowledge, methods, and reasoning to the study of the beneficial and adverse effects and uses of drugs in human populations (Zito & Riddle, 1995). Epidemiological research methods are used to increase knowledge about specific human populations in three areas: (1) drug safety, (2) efficacy of drug treatments for disease, and (3) drug treatment prevalence. Recent pharmacoepidemiological studies of the prevalence of psychiatric medication interventions for children and adolescents suggests that such interventions are growing in the United States. Children as young as 3 years of age may receive psychiatric medications for a variety of behavioral and affective disorders (Zito et al., 2000).

Preliminary pharmacoepidemiological investigations of drug treatment prevalence in specific populations of clinically referred, seriously emotionally disturbed children and adolescents reveal that psychiatric medication treatment for aggression is very common (Connor, Ozbayrak, Harrison, & Melloni, 1998; Connor, Ozbayrak, Kusiak, Caponi, & Melloni, 1997). In one study, 83 children and adolescents consecutively admitted to acute residential treatment over 17 months were assessed for the prevalence and patterns of use of psychotropic medications, particularly anticonvulsants. At admission, 76% of these youth were receiving psychiatric pharmacotherapy, 40% were receiving two or more drugs concurrently, and 15% were taking a combination of anticonvulsant and other psychiatric medications. Results showed that neuroleptic medications were prescribed in the study population at rates greatly exceeding their psychiatric diagnostic indications (i.e., psychotic disorders, tic disorders, bipolar disorders, autism), and that their use was statistically correlated with aggressive behavior, independently of psychiatric diagnosis. Stimulants and antidepressants were underprescribed relevant to their diagnostic indications (i.e., attention-deficit/hyperactivity disorder [ADHD], depression, anxiety) in these 83 youth (Connor, Ozbayrak, et al., 1998). In a second study of the same patient population, lifetime histories of aggression were associated with combined pharmacotherapy use (i.e., the concurrent use of two or more psychiatric medications), independently of psychiatric diagnosis (Connor, Ozbayrak, Kusiak, et al., 1997). These studies are limited because of their small sample size and nonrepresentative study population. Nevertheless, they suggest that medication treatment for chronic maladaptive aggression is common among seriously emotionally disturbed youth who are clinically referred. Furthermore, the results suggest the need to establish more definitely the safety and efficacy of medication interventions for such youth.

PRINCIPLES OF CLINICAL MEDICATION MANAGEMENT

The use of adjunctive medications in the treatment of aggressive youth can easily fail if it is not carried out systematically (Eichelman, 1988). Indeed, there is a very real risk that nonmethodically conducted medication trials may result in the exposure of aggressive youth to multiple ineffective medications, each with the potential for adverse side effects or drug–drug pharmacological interactions that may impair the youngsters' quality of life. A rational, systematic approach to the clinical medication management of aggressive children and adolescents is presented in Table 12.1.

To begin with, psychotropic treatment for maladaptive aggression should be considered only after a thorough psychiatric assessment has been completed. Assessment needs to consider psychosocial, educational, and community aspects of aggression first. Medication should be used as an adjunct to a comprehensive psychosocial and psychoeducational treatment plan. If maladaptive aggression continues despite such a plan, and if it has the qualities (e.g., chronicity, severity, frequency, associated impulsivity–hyperactivity) that suggest a target symptom approach, adjunctive medication therapy for aggression may be considered after psychosocial and psychoeducational interventions have been instituted. If aggression occurs as an associated symptom of a medication-responsive psychiatric illness, such as a psychotic disorder, depression, or ADHD (the primary illness approach), the clinician may wish to begin a medication trial earlier in treatment—perhaps at the same time as

---

TABLE 12.1. Principles of Medication Management for Clinically Referred Aggressive Children and Adolescents

1. Use a medication-responsive psychiatric diagnosis or a behavioral–biological rationale as the basis for prescribing medication for aggression, and only after conducting a complete diagnostic assessment.

2. Only use medication for aggression adjunctively within a coordinated multidisciplinary psychoeducational treatment plan.

3. Obtain written informed consent from the child's legal guardian, and oral assent from children 7 years of age or older, for all medication trials.

4. When considering a medication trial for maladaptive aggression, attempt to treat the underlying psychiatric syndrome first.

5. When beginning empirical treatment for an aggressive child or adolescent, use the most benign interventions first.

6. When beginning medication treatment for aggression, have some quantifiable means of assessing drug safety and efficacy.
   a. Define the objective behaviors and quality-of-life measures to be tracked.
   b. Use empirical methods (validated, treatment-sensitive rating scales).
   c. Obtain off-drug baseline data and on-drug treatment data for comparison.
   d. Obtain data at regular intervals during drug treatment.

7. Institute medication trials for aggressive behavior systematically.
   a. Whenever possible, medication should be introduced as a single variable into treatment.
   b. Medication trials for aggressive behavior should be introduced for preplanned periods of time that have clear beginnings and endings, so that drug efficacy can be assessed.
   c. Explore the full dose range of a single medicine for an adequate length of time (generally several weeks) before switching to a different drug or adding medicines.
   d. Avoid polypharmacy with multiple drugs all given at subtherapeutic doses.
   e. Follow drug serum levels where available.

other interventions, since research supports the efficacy of medication therapies for these conditions (Campbell & Cueva, 1995a, 1995b; Connor & Steingard, 1996).

When clinical medication trials for maladaptive aggression are instituted, they should be done so systematically. Written informed consent from a youth's parent or legal guardian, and oral assent of the child or adolescent, are necessary before any medication trial may begin. Either the target symptom approach or the primary illness approach to the medication treatment of aggression needs to be explained. Next, the objective behaviors and quality-of-life measures that will be used to track medications response over time need to be defined. Baseline data should be collected prior to drug treatment, using reliable and valid rating scales or observational strategies for the target behaviors; these findings should be compared to on-drug data. If possible, individual-patient, treatment-reversal, single-trial designs are recommended. These are on–off–on or off–on–off designs in which medication is periodically removed and restarted, in order to test its safety and efficacy in relation to the target behaviors. A medication should be introduced as a single variable into treatment—not introduced with a variety of other treatment changes at the same time—so that both its effects on target behaviors and its side effects are more clearly discernible. The full dose range of a single drug should be explored for an adequate length of time at each dose level (generally several weeks) before the medication is clinically abandoned and another or additional medications are begun. The danger of ineffective polypharmacy, in which multiple drugs each given at subtherapeutic doses for indeterminate lengths of time, is very real in the pharmacological treatment of aggressive youth. Finally, medications should be introduced into treatment for preplanned periods of time that have clear beginnings and endings. Medication should not be given to aggressive youngsters for indeterminate and lengthy periods of time without periodic reassessment of the proposed treatment plan's clinical risks and benefits. If these systematic principles for psychotropic treatment of aggression in children and adolescents are followed, the clinical use of such drugs becomes much more rational, with an increased probability of establishing efficacy and minimizing adverse side effects.

The next several sections review selected studies investigating the pharmacological treatment of aggression and related behaviors in children and adolescents since 1980. For the purposes of this chapter, these behaviors are defined (unless otherwise indicated) as behaviors within the overt spectrum, such as physical assault, threats of violence, impulsive property destruction, temper outbursts, rage attacks, oppositional defiant behavior, conduct problems, hostility, irritability, and/or impulsive violence. Premeditated, planned, or instrumental aggression is not included in this chapter's definition of aggression and related behaviors. Neuroleptics and atypical antipsychotics are first reviewed, followed by stimulants, antidepressants, mood stabilizers, and

adrenergic agents. Inclusion criteria for this review include (1) methodologically controlled or open studies investigating drug efficacy for aggression and
related behaviors, and (2) use in the child or adolescent age range. Exclusion
criteria include (1) case reports and (2) studies not reporting outcomes for aggression and related behaviors.

NEUROLEPTICS AND ANTIPSYCHOTICS

Neuroleptics and antipsychotic drugs form a large group of psychoactive medications mainly known for their antipsychotic clinical properties. The older
drugs in this class were originally called "neuroleptics" because of their ability
to mimic neurological syndromes, such as Parkinson's disease and acute dys-
tonia. Presently, this group of psychiatric medications is divided into two subgroups: the older typical neuroleptics and the newer atypical antipsychotics.
Examples of typical neuroleptics include chlorpromazine, molindone, fluphenazine, and haloperidol. In the central nervous system (CNS), these agents
pharmacologically block postsynaptic dopamine (DA) receptors in the meso-
limbic system and in the basal ganglia. Typical neuroleptics are defined by the
neurological side effects they cause, including tardive dyskinesia, acute dystonic reactions, and extrapyramidal side effects. The newer atypical antipsychotics were developed in an effort to treat psychotic symptoms without
the side effects of the typical neuroleptics. They are characterized by antago-
nism of serotonin (5-HT) neurotransmission as well as DA neurotransmission.
This property may be one mechanism that causes the lower side effect rates in
these newer drugs. Examples of atypical antipsychotics include clozapine,
risperidone, olanzepine, ziprasidone, and quetiapine.

In children and adolescents, neuroleptics and atypical antipsychotics are
used in clinical practice to treat psychotic disorders and symptoms, such as
childhood-onset schizophrenia and juvenile mania; Tourette's disorder and
chronic motor or vocal tic disorders; and behavioral disturbances in autism
and in persons with mental retardation (Campbell, Rapoport, & Simpson,
1999). They are also used in the adjunctive treatment of CD and of severe,
chronic, and refractory impulsive aggression (Toren, Laor, & Weizman,
1998). Neuroleptic and antipsychotic use in the treatment of ADHD has diminished because of the efficacy of stimulant medications for this disorder.
Neuroleptics and atypical antipsychotics are the psychiatric medications most
often used for nonspecific but severe aggression and related behaviors, independently of psychiatric diagnosis, in seriously emotionally disturbed children
and adolescents (Connor, Ozbayrak, et al., 1998).

Overt aggression in CD is a common target symptom for which neuroleptics and atypical antipsychotics are prescribed for clinically referred youth.
Since 1980, four randomized controlled clinical trials of these drugs for juvenile CD have been completed; these are described in Table 12.2. Across all
four controlled trials, a total of 127 youngsters aged between 5 and 15 years

TABLE 12.2. Neuroleptic and Antipsychotic Medications for CD in Youth

Reference	Sample size	Age	Design	Medication	Trial duration	Total dose	Response
Findling et al. (2000)	20	5–15	RCT[a]	Risperidone	10 wk	0.75–1.5 mg/d	Drug sig. superior to placebo
Greenhill et al. (1985)	31	6–11	RCT	Molindone or thioridazine	8 wk	Molindone avg. dose, 27 mg/d; thioridazine avg. dose, 170 mg/d	Both drugs sig. superior to placebo
Campbell et al. (1984)	61	5–12	RCT	Haloperidol	6 wk	1–6 mg/d	Drug sig. superior to placebo, and equal to lithium
Campbell et al. (1982)	15	6–11	RCT	Haloperidol or chlorpromazine	6 wk	Haloperidol, 4–16 mg/d; chlorpromazine, 100–200 mg/d	Both drugs sig. superior to placebo
Total	127	5–15	4 RCTs	Risperidone, molindone, thioridazine, haloperidol, chlorpromazine	6–10 wk	Variable	All RCTs show sig. superiority for drug in CD

Note. Risperidone is an atypical antipsychotic; molindone, thioridazine, haloperidol, and chlorpromazine are typical neuroleptics.
[a]RCT, randomized controlled trial (in this and subsequent tables).

have been investigated. These trials have been short, generally 6–10 weeks in length. Most trials for CD have used typical neuroleptics, including molindone, thioridazine, haloperidol, or chlorpromazine; only one such trial has used a newer atypical antipsychotic, risperidone. Remarkably, all four randomized controlled trials of neuroleptics or atypical antipsychotics for CD have shown significant statistical superiority over placebo (see Table 12.2).

Maladaptive aggression and related behaviors in children and adolescents with autism, other pervasive developmental disorders, or mental retardation have also been targets for neuroleptic/antipsychotic treatment. Since 1980, a total of 280 children and adolescents aged between 2 and 18 years have been studied in five controlled and seven open trials; these are presented in Table 12.3. Older typical neuroleptics used in these trials have included haloperidol, chlorpromazine, and fluphenazine; the only newer atypical antipsychotic that has been investigated in this population is risperidone. Clinical trials have lasted from 2 weeks to 1 year. All five randomized controlled trials have reported statistically significant drug superiority over placebo, and all seven open trials have reported reductions in aggression and related behaviors in youngsters with developmental disorders.

Psychotic disorders in youth include childhood-onset schizophrenia; juvenile mania and depression with psychotic symptoms are also often viewed and treated as psychotic disorders, although mania and depression are episodes of mood disorders, strictly speaking (Campbell et al., 1999). Psychotic symptoms include hallucinations, delusions, and formal thought disorder and can be found in a variety of other psychiatric diagnoses, including severe posttraumatic stress disorder (PTSD) and mental retardation (Toren et al., 1998). Table 12.4 lists studies since 1980 assessing the efficacy of neuroleptics and atypical antipsychotics for aggression and related behaviors in youngsters with psychotic disorders and symptoms.

Two randomized controlled studies have been completed assessing the efficacy of clozapine and/or haloperidol in childhood-onset schizophrenia (see Table 12.4). Spencer and Campbell (1994) found haloperidol statistically superior to placebo in the treatment of aggression and related behaviors in this disorder. Kumra et al. (1996) compared clozapine, an atypical antipsychotic, with haloperidol, a typical neuroleptic, in youth with schizophrenia and found a trend favoring clozapine over haloperidol for aggressive behaviors. Seven of eight open trials, using a variety of atypical antipsychotics, have reported drug efficacy for aggression and related behaviors. Clozapine may be more efficacious than olanzepine in this population (Kumra et al., 1998). A total of 161 psychotic youth have been investigated in clinical drug trials lasting from 1 to 136 weeks. A wider variety of atypical antipsychotics have been investigated in juvenile psychotic disorders and symptoms than in CD or developmental disorders.

Aggression as a target symptom for atypical antipsychotic drug treatment, regardless of psychiatric diagnosis, has been investigated in two open trials using risperidone (Mandoki, 1995; Simeon, Carrey, Wiggins, Milin, &

TABLE 12.3. Neuroleptic and Antipsychotic Medications for Aggression and Related Behaviors in Youth with Developmental Disorders

Reference	Sample size	Age	Medication	Trial duration	Total dose	Response
RCTs						
Aman et al. (1991)	30	4–16	Chlorpromazine	3 wk	1.75 mg/kg/d	Drug sig. superior to placebo
Anderson et al. (1989)	45	2–7	Haloperidol	14 wk	0.25–4.0 mg/d	Drug sig. superior to placebo
Perry et al. (1989)	60	2–7	Haloperidol	26 wk	0.5–4.0 mg/d	Continued drug benefits over 6 mo
Anderson et al. (1984)	40	2–7	Haloperidol	6 wk	0.5–3.0 mg/d	Drug sig. superior to placebo
Van Bellinghen and De Troch (2001)	13	6–14	Risperidone	4 wk	0.03–0.06 mg/kg/d	Drug sig. superior to placebo
Open trials						
Buitelaar (2000)	26	10–18	Risperidone	8–52 wk	0.5–4.0 mg/d	92% reduction in aggression and related behaviors
Nicolson et al. (1998)	10	4–10	Risperidone	12 wk	1.0–2.5 mg/d	80% response rate
Perry et al. (1997)	6	7–14	Risperidone	4–32 wk	1–6 mg/d	Reduced anger and hyperactivity
McDougle et al. (1997)	18	5–18	Risperidone	12 wk	1–4 mg/d	67% response rate
Findling et al. (1997)	6	5–9	Risperidone	8 wk	0.75–1.5 mg/d	Sig. improvement in aggression and related behaviors
Fisman and Steele (1996)	14	9–17	Risperidone	4–40 wk	0.75–1.5 mg/d	92% response rate in aggression and related behaviors
Joshi et al. (1988)	12	7–11	Haloperidol or fluphenazine	2–7 wk	0.5–4.0 mg/d	Sig. improvement in aggression and related behaviors
Total	280[a]	2–18	Risperidone, haloperidol, chlorpromazine, fluphenazine	2–52 wk	Variable	All 5 RCTs report drug sig. superior to placebo; all 7 open trials report variable reductions in aggression and related behaviors

Note. Risperidone is an atypical antipsychotic; haloperidol, chlorpromazine, and fluphenazine are typical neuroleptics.
[a] 188 in 5 RCTs; 92 in 7 open trials.

TABLE 12.4. Neuroleptic and Antipsychotic Medications for Aggression and Related Behaviors in Youth with Psychotic Disorders/Symptoms

Reference	Sample size	Age	Medication	Trial duration	Total dose	Diagnosis	Response
RCTs							
Kumra et al. (1996)	21	Avg. 14.0	Clozapine or haloperidol	6 wk	Clozapine, 25–525 mg/d; haloperidol, 7–27 mg/d	COS[a]	Trend toward behavioral improvement on clozapine > haloperidol
Spencer and Campbell (1994)	16	5–11	Haloperidol	10 wk	0.5–3.0 mg/d	COS	Drug sig. superior to placebo
Open studies							
McConville et al. (2000)	10	12–15	Quetiapine	3 wk	200–800 mg/d	Mixed	Sig. improvement in symptoms
Frazier et al. (1999)	28	4–17	Risperidone	1–136 wk	1.7 mg/d	JM[b]	82% response rate in aggression and related behaviors
Kumra et al. (1998)	8	10–18	Olanzepine	8 wk	12.5–20 mg/d	COS	17% improvement; olanzepine less effective than clozapine
Armenteros et al. (1997)	10	11–18	Risperidone	6 wk	4–10 mg/d	COS	Sig. improvement in aggression and related behaviors
Turetz et al. (1997)	11	9–13	Clozapine	16 wk	200–300 mg/d	COS	70% response rate in aggression and related behaviors
Kowatch et al. (1995)	10	6–15	Clozapine	6 wk	75–225 mg/d	Mixed	42% response rate in aggression and related behaviors
Frazier et al. (1994)	11	11–17	Clozapine	6 wk	125–825 mg/d	COS	58% improvement rate
Remschmidt et al. (1994)	36	18.3	Clozapine	22 wk	50–800 mg/d	COS	75% response rate in aggression and related behaviors
Total	161[c]	4–18	Clozapine, risperidone, olanzepine, quetiapine, haloperidol	1–136 wk	Variable	COS, JM	1 RCT shows trend toward behavioral improvement; 7 of 8 open trials report efficacy for aggression and related behaviors; clozapine may be more effective than olanzepine or haloperidol

Note. Clozapine, olanzepine, and risperidone are atypical antipsychotics; haloperidol is a typical neuroleptic.
[a]COS, childhood-onset schizophrenia.
[b]JM, juvenile mania.
[c]37 in 2 RCTs; 124 in 8 open trials.

Hosenbocus, 1995). These studies are described in Table 12.5; they have reported 85% to 100% improvement rates in aggression and related behaviors in 17 youngsters with heterogeneous psychiatric diagnoses.

In summary, post-1980 studies of typical neuroleptics and atypical antipsychotics have investigated the treatment of aggression and related behaviors in a variety of psychiatric diagnoses, including CD, developmental disorders, psychotic disorders and symptoms, and heterogeneous disorders where aggression is problematic and resistant to other forms of intervention. The majority of both controlled and open studies have reported improvement in aggression, either relative to placebo or relative to the patients' baseline condition. The findings suggest that these medications are effective in the treatment of problematic aggression in youngsters meeting clinical criteria for these psychiatric diagnoses.

Before these results can be uncritically accepted, however, several caveats are in order. First, most of the studies reviewed did not precisely define or specifically investigate aggression and related behaviors; these were among many symptoms that appeared to improve in these clinical trials. Clinical trials investigating the possible efficacy of neuroleptics or atypical antipsychotics on carefully defined subtypes of aggression remain needed. Second, it remains unclear whether neuroleptics and atypical antipsychotics have an effect on the specific neurobiological mechanisms that subserve aggressive behaviors in humans, or whether they simply suppress a wide variety of behaviors, including aggression. Finally, the class of antipsychotic medications has many side effects. Side effects of the typical neuroleptics include tardive dyskinesia, acute dystonic reactions, parkinsonian symptoms, akathisia, increased prolactin release, anticholinergic symptoms, sedation, and a lowering of the seizure threshold in susceptible patients. Side effects of the newer atypical antipsychotics are less, but include weight gain, sedation, hyperprolactinemia with

TABLE 12.5. Neuroleptic and Antipsychotic Medications for Aggression and Related Behaviors in Youth, Regardless of Diagnosis

Reference	Sample size	Age	Medication	Trial duration	Total dose	Response
Simeon et al. (1995)	7	11–17	Risperidone	3–60 wk	1–4 mg/d	85% response rate in aggression and related behaviors
Mandoki (1995)	10	7–17	Risperidone	6–12 wk	2–6 mg/d	100% improvement rate
Total	17	7–17	Risperidone	3–60 wk	Variable	Both studies report improvement in aggression and related behaviors

Note. Both studies were open trials.

resultant galactorrhea, menstrual irregularities, impotence, and breast enlargement. Since maladaptive aggression may be episodic and intermittent, yet chronically recurring over many years, careful clinical consideration must be given to use of this medication class for aggression and related behaviors in developing children and adolescents.

STIMULANTS

The stimulants are a class of psychoactive medications in clinical use primarily for the treatment of ADHD in children and adolescents. They are also used in neurology to treat the sleep attacks of narcolepsy. The stimulants are referred to as such because of their ability to increase the level of activity, arousal, or alertness of the CNS. Chemically, they are structurally similar to the catecholamines DA and norepinephrine (NE), and they may mimic the actions of these neurotransmitters in the CNS. Increasing intrasynaptic DA may enhance the functioning of executive cognitive functions mediated by the prefrontal cortex, overcoming the deficits in inhibitory control and working memory reported in youth with ADHD (Barkley, DuPaul, & Connor, 1999; Greenhill, Halperin, & Abikoff, 1999).

Currently, there are four marketed immediate-release stimulant medications: methylphenidate, dextroamphetamine, Adderall®, and pemoline. (Pemoline's use has been curtailed because of concerns over its potential for hepatic toxicity. Adderall® is a mixed amphetamine and dextroamphetamine product.) Studies of the short-term efficacy of stimulant medications on the symptoms of ADHD constitute the largest body of treatment literature on any childhood-onset psychiatric disorder (Greenhill et al., 1999; Spencer et al., 1996). Improvements in ADHD symptoms have been noted in between 65% and 75% of the 5,899 patients assigned to stimulant treatment in research studies, compared to between 4% and 30% of patients assigned to placebo (Greenhill et al., 1999). The stimulant medications are the psychotropic drugs most commonly employed with children and adolescents for the symptoms of moderate to severe ADHD (Barkley et al., 1999).

Although the presence of aggression is not required for the diagnosis of ADHD, aggression is frequently observed in children and adolescents with ADHD (Hinshaw, 1987). Substantial data indicate differences between children with and without aggression in this population. Whereas the ADHD symptoms of inattention and distractibility predict academic difficulties, comorbid aggression and conduct problems predict a far worse outcome, including risk for substance use disorders, antisocial personality disorder, depression, and continuing aggression (Paternite, Loney, Salisbury, & Whaley, 1999). Indeed, studies have demonstrated that childhood ADHD co-occurs with CD in between 40% and 80% of clinically referred cases (Biederman, Newcorn, & Sprich, 1991). Because of the overlap between ADHD and aggression in some youth, and because of the poor outcomes for these individuals, studies have investigated the efficacy of stimulant medication for treating aggression in children and adolescents with disruptive behavior disorders.

Eighteen methodologically controlled clinical trials of stimulant treatment for aggression in ADHD and/or CD completed since 1980 are summarized in Table 12.6. A total of 429 children and adolescents receiving treatment with stimulant medications for aggression in the context of these disorders have been studied in 15 randomized controlled trials and 3 trials with double-blind methodology. Studies have used various measurement techniques to assess aggression, including direct observation, rating scales, and laboratory paradigms in which children are assessed during verbal provocation tasks. Results are in remarkable agreement: Significant stimulant effects for treating aggression in the context of ADHD and/or CD have been reported in 16 of the 18 controlled trials (see Table 12.6). Both of the studies reporting no significant differences used verbal provocation paradigms in laboratory settings, suggesting that stimulant treatment effects on aggression may vary by how aggression is measured (Murphy, Pelham, & Lang, 1992). Covert forms of aggression such as property destruction and stealing may respond to stimulant treatment as well as the more overt forms, when they occur in the context of the disruptive behavior disorders (Hinshaw, Heller, & McHale, 1992). Stimulants may also ameliorate aggressive behaviors in children with CD, independently of comorbid ADHD (Klein et al., 1997). There appear to be linear effects of methylphenidate on decreasing aggression in ADHD, with increasing efficacy up to 0.6 mg/kg/dose (Hinshaw, Henker, Whalen, Erhardt, & Dunnington, 1989). These research studies suggest that aggression occurring within the context of the disruptive behavior disorders may be a robust target for stimulant drug treatment within the context of a multidisciplinary psychoeducational treatment plan.

Few studies have investigated the effects of dextroamphetamine on aggressive behaviors in youth with ADHD. There is a suggestion that dextroamphetamine may have a greater effect than methylphenidate on such symptoms as aggression, irritability, explosiveness, and oppositional defiant behaviors (Arnold, 2000). Effect sizes of dextroamphetamine on aggression and related behaviors in ADHD are about 0.45 (Arnold, 2000). As such, future studies should more thoroughly investigate dextroamphetamine's efficacy for these behaviors within the context of ADHD and CD.

This review suggests other areas for future research. First, the investigation of stimulant drug efficacy in the disruptive behavior disorders by subtype of aggression is important. Although most research has studied overtly aggressive behaviors, some research suggests that covert types of aggression may respond to stimulants as well. Second, although most studies have investigated boys, girls too may meet the criteria for ADHD and CD. Stimulants' effects on aggression as they may vary by gender need further study. Finally, few of the studies reviewed have assess teenagers; most have studied elementary school children and early adolescents. More studies are needed assessing stimulant effects on aggression in ADHD during middle to late adolescence.

TABLE 12.6. Stimulants for Aggression and Related Behaviors in Youth with Disruptive Behavior Disorders (ADHD and CD)

Reference	Sample size	Age	Design	Medication	Trial duration	Total dose	Response
Connor et al. (2000)*	8	6–16	RCT	MPH[a]	12 wk	Avg. 32.5 mg/d	Sig. improvement on drug relative to baseline
Kent et al. (1999)	50	4–14	RCT (n of 1)	MPH	2–52 wk	0.3–0.6 mg/kg/dose	n of 1 design (each subject as own control); sig. improvement
Kolko et al. (1999)	22	7–13	RCT	MPH	6 wk	0.3–0.6 mg/kg/dose	Sig. improvement
Bukstein and Kolko (1998)	18	6–12	RCT	MPH	3 wk	0.3–0.6 mg/kg/dose	Sig. improvement
Klein et al. (1997)*	84	6–15	RCT	MPH	5 wk	Avg. 41 mg/d	Sig. improvement in CD independently of ADHD
Casat et al. (1995)	6	8–11	DB[b]	MPH	Lab paradigm	0.6 mg/kg/dose	Sig. improvement
Matier et al. (1992)	14	6–12	DB	MPH	Lab paradigm	0.1–0.2 mg/kg/dose	Sig. improvement
Hinshaw et al. (1992)	22	6–12	RCT	MPH	Lab paradigm	0.3 mg/kg/dose	Response to MPH seen in covert aggression
Murphy et al. (1992)	26	6–11	RCT	MPH	5 wk	0.3 mg/kg/dose	Sig. improvements in aggression on direct observation; NSD[c] on lab provocation task

Study	N	Age	Design	Drug	Duration	Dose	Result
Pelham et al. (1991)	20	7–11	RCT	MPH	Lab paradigm	0.3 mg/kg/dose	NSD on lab provocation task
Kaplan et al. (1990)	6	13–16	DB	MPH	7 wk	0.6 mg/kg/dose	Sig. improvement
Gadow et al. (1990)	11	5–11	RCT	MPH	2 wk	0.3–0.6 mg/kg/dose	Sig. improvement
Barkley et al. (1989)	37	6–13	RCT	MPH	3 wk	0.3–0.5 mg/kg/dose	Aggressive ADHD responded as well as nonaggressive ADHD to drug
Hinshaw, Buhrmester, et al. (1989)	24	6–12	RCT	MPH	Lab paradigm	0.6 mg/kg/dose	Sig. improvements on verbal provocation task
Hinshaw, Henker, et al. (1989)	25	6–12	RCT	MPH	3 wk	0.3–0.6 mg/kg/dose	Sig. improvement
Klorman et al. (1988)	24	6–12	RCT	MPH	2 wk	0.3 mg/kg/dose	Sig. improvement
Amery et al. (1984)	10	avg. 9.6	RCT	dAMP[d]	2 wk	Avg. 0.75 mg/kg/d	Sig. improvement
Hinshaw et al. (1984)	22	8–13	RCT	MPH	Lab paradigm	0.15–1.15 mg/kg/d	NSD on lab provocation task
Total	429[e]	4–16	15 RCTs, 3 DBs	17 MPH, 1 dAMP	Variable	Variable	16 controlled trials, sig. superiority for drug in ADHD and/or CD; 2 RCTs, NSD on lab provocation tasks

*Diagnosis = ADHD + CD, otherwise all diagnoses are ADHD.
[a]MPH, methylphenidate (in this and Table 12.7).
[b]DB, double-blind trial.
[c]NSD, no significant difference (in this and subsequent tables).
[d]dAMP, d-amphetamine.
[e]26 in 3 DB trials, 403 in 15 RCTs.

ANTIDEPRESSANTS

There are several different types of antidepressants in clinical use for children and adolescents with psychiatric disorders. The oldest types are monoamine oxidase inhibitors and tricyclic antidepressants (TCAs). Examples of TCAs include imipramine, desipramine, amitriptyline, and nortriptyline. Newer antidepressants have safer side effect profiles and include the selective serotonin reuptake inhibitors (SSRIs), such as fluoxetine, paroxetine, sertraline, fluvoxamine, and citalopram. A number of other antidepressants have different chemical configurations; these include venlafaxine, nefazodone, trazodone, mirtazapine, and bupropion.

Although research in antidepressants in the pediatric age range has lagged behind studies in adults, a growing body of evidence attests to the efficacy of these medicines for a variety of disorders in children and adolescents. TCAs have been found effective for childhood anxiety disorders, such as school phobia, separation anxiety, and obsessive–compulsive disorder (OCD); ADHD; and nocturnal enuresis (bedwetting). Efficacy for child or adolescent depression has yet to be demonstrated for the TCAs, however (Geller, Reising, Leonard, Riddle, & Walsh, 1999). In addition, because of clinical concern over their cardiovascular safety profile, TCAs are no longer considered first-line antidepressants in child psychiatry (Geller et al., 1999). Monoamine oxidase inhibitors are rarely if ever used in child psychiatry, because of their adverse safety profile and risk for hypertensive reactions when mixed with tyramine-containing foods. SSRIs are increasingly used in juvenile psychiatric disorders because of efficacy equal to that of the TCAs and a better safety profile. Use in depression and OCD is well established for the SSRIs in the pediatric age range (Emslie, Walkup, Pliszka, & Ernst, 1999). Selective mutism, school phobia, and separation anxiety probably respond to SSRIs (Birmaher et al., 1994). No efficacy for ADHD has been established with the SSRIs (Emslie et al., 1999). Of the other antidepressants, there exists solid evidence that bupropion is effective in the treatment of ADHD (Emslie et al., 1999). Research into the efficacy of venlafaxine, nefazodone, and mirtazapine is just beginning, and studies are presently ongoing in the child and adolescent age range.

The first rationale for considering antidepressant treatment for aggression and related behaviors in clinically referred youth comes from 5-HT research investigating aggression in preclinical animal studies and treatment studies of aggressive adults. For example, animal models investigating neurobiological mechanisms of aggressive behaviors in the CNS find that the neurohormone arginine vasopressin facilitates aggression, whereas 5-HT inhibits aggressive behavior by blocking the activity of vasopressin in the anterior hypothalamus (Ferris, 2000). SSRIs such as fluoxetine have been shown to down-regulate aggressive behaviors in humans, nonhuman primates, and smaller laboratory animals, suggesting an antiaggressive effect for SSRIs (Fuller, 1996, Sanchez & Meier, 1997). Impulsive aggression in adults with personality disorders has been shown to respond to fluoxetine (Coccaro, Kavoussi, & Hauger, 1997). These findings raise the question of whether impulsive aggression in psychiatrically referred youth might also respond to SSRIs.

A second rationale comes from research showing that anger attacks may occur in 30% to 40% of depressed adult patients (Fava & Rosenbaum, 1999). Depressed adults with rage and anger attacks may have greater CNS 5-HT dysregulation than depressed adults without such attacks (Fava et al., 2000). Since impulsivity, irritability, and hostility can be prominent symptoms of depression in children and adolescents, these youth may exhibit similar CNS 5-HT deficits and thus may respond to SSRIs.

A third rationale for considering antidepressant treatment for aggression and related behaviors in clinically referred youth comes from reports of the efficacy of TCAs and bupropion in the treatment of ADHD. Since ADHD is often highly comorbid with aggression and CD, effective treatment of ADHD with these antidepressants might also ameliorate aggression and related behaviors in the disruptive behavior disorders (Emslie et al., 1999; Geller et al., 1999).

Twelve post-1980 studies assessing the efficacy of antidepressant treatment for aggression and related behaviors in various juvenile psychiatric disorders are described in Table 12.7. Such treatment has been assessed most thoroughly in the disruptive behavior disorders, with only a few studies assessing outcomes in anxiety, depressive, and autistic disorders. In the disruptive behavior disorders, three randomized controlled trials assessing 117 youth, and two open trials assessing a further 30 youth, have provided solid support for the use of bupropion in treating comorbid aggression and CD within the context of ADHD (see Table 12.7). One randomized trial and one open chart review (assessing a total of 89 youth) have furnished some support for the use of TCAs in this same context (Biederman, Baldessarini, Wright, Keenan, & Faraone, 1993; Wilens, Biederman, Geist, Steingard, & Spencer, 1993). Trazodone, an older antidepressant with some selective action on 5-HT, was found effective for aggression in one open trial of 22 youngsters with disruptive behavior disorders (Zubieta & Alessi, 1992).

Despite the strong theoretical rationale from preclinical animal and adult treatment studies for inhibiting aggression by increasing CNS 5-HT functioning with SSRIs, the literature on SSRIs in child psychiatry is surprisingly thin and mixed in its results. Only one randomized trial with a very small number of children ($n = 6$) suffering from selective mutism examined the use of fluoxetine in aggression and related behaviors, and it found no significant difference between the drug treatment and baseline conditions (Black & Uhde, 1994). Open studies using paroxetine for the treatment of rage attacks in Tourette's disorder, and a small study of fluoxetine in autistic children and young adults, have reported improvement rates for aggressive behaviors varying between 21% and 76% (Bruun & Budman, 1998; Fatemi, Realmuto, Khan, & Thuras, 1998). In an open study of depressed youth that specifically

TABLE 12.7. Antidepressants for Aggression and Related Behaviors in Youth

Reference	Sample size	Age	Design	Medication	Trial duration	Total dose	Diagnosis	Response
TCAs								
Biederman et al. (1993)	31	6–17	RCT	DMI[a]	6 wk	4–5 mg/kg/d	DBD[b]	Response in ADHD + CD equal to response in ADHD – CD
Wilens et al. (1993)	58	7–18	Open	NTP[c]	2–232 wk	Avg. 2 mg/kg/d	DBD	Sig. improvement
Trazodone								
Zubieta and Alessi (1992)	22	5–12	Open	—	12–56 wk	Avg. 4.8 mg/kg/d	DBD	70% improvement
Bupropion								
Riggs et al. (1998)	13	14–17	Open	—	5 wk	300 mg/d	DBD	Sig. improvement
Conners et al. (1996)	72	6–12	RCT	—	6 wk	3–6 mg/kg/d	DBD	Sig. improvement
Barrickman et al. (1995)	15	7–16	RCT	—	6 wk	1.4–5.7 mg/kg/d	DBD	Sig. improvement; equal to MPH
Casat et al. (1987)	30	6–12	RCT	—	6 wk	150–250 mg/d	DBD	Sig. improvement
Simeon et al. (1986)	17	7–13	Open	—	8 wk	50–150 mg/d	DBD	71% response rate

SSRIs

Study								
Bruun and Budman (1998)	45	Avg. 16	Open	Paroxetine	8 wk	Avg. 33 mg/d	TD[d]	76% improvement
Fatemi et al. (1998)	7	9–20	Open	Fluoxetine	5–128 wk	20–80 mg/d	Autism	21% improvement
Constantino, Liberman, et al. (1997)	19	13–17	Open	Fluoxetine, paroxetine, sertraline	5 wk	10–40 mg/d	Depression	NSD
Black and Uhde (1994)	6	5–16	RCT	Fluoxetine	12 wk	12–27 mg/d	Elective mutism	NSD
Total	335[f]	6–20[e]		Desipramine, nortriptyline, bupropion, fluoxetine, paroxetine, sertraline	2–232 wk	Variable		Strongest data for bupropion in DBD

[a] DMI, desipramine.
[b] DBD, disruptive behavioral disorders (in this and subsequent tables).
[c] NTP, nortriptyline.
[d] TD, Tourette's disorder (in this and subsequent tables).
[e] 4 RCTs in DBD, 1 in elective mutism; 7 open trials—4 in DBD, 1 each in depression, autism, TD.
[f] 154 in 5 RCTs; 181 in 7 open trials.

examined SSRI treatment of aggressive behaviors, no significant differences were found between on-drug behaviors and baseline levels of aggression (Constantino, Liberman, & Kincaid, 1997).

In summary, this review of antidepressants in children and adolescents finds support for the efficacy of these drugs in the treatment of aggression and related behaviors primarily within the context of the disruptive behavior disorders, particularly ADHD. Little evidence to date suggests that SSRIs are effective for aggression in the context of depression, anxiety disorders, or developmental disorders in children and adolescents. Most studies on the drug treatment of childhood mood disorders have not specifically examined effects on aggression and related behaviors; thus the hypothesis that enhancing CNS 5-HT functioning will down-regulate such behaviors in psychiatrically referred young persons has not yet been adequately tested.

MOOD STABILIZERS

Mood stabilizers include lithium, as well as the anticonvulsants divalproex sodium and carbamazepine. These medicines are increasingly used in child and adolescent psychiatry to treat bipolar illness in adolescents; manic-like symptoms in children, which may include affective lability, irritability, poor judgment, and expansive mood; and severe aggression and rage attacks in clinically referred youngsters (Biederman et al., 1998; Ryan, Bhatara, & Perel, 1999).

Lithium

Lithium is a naturally occurring alkali metal, found in various mineral deposits and in seawater. The preparations used in psychiatry are the lithium salts, primarily lithium carbonate or citrate. Lithium has physiological effects on electrolytes, CNS neurotransmitters, and cellular transport mechanisms. The CNS effects of lithium are thought to be caused by altered neuronal membrane transport mechanisms related to effects on the distribution of sodium, calcium, and magnesium, and on glucose metabolism. Lithium has been noted to inhibit release of NE and DA, and may enhance 5-HT release in neurons. These effects have been suggested as possible causes of lithium's mood-stabilizing and antiaggressive qualities, although its mechanisms of action in the CNS are not fully understood (Viesselman, 1999).

It has been demonstrated both in laboratory animals and in adult psychiatric patients that lithium has antiaggressive properties (Eichelman, 1992; Sheard, Marini, Bridges, & Wagner, 1976). This finding—together with the fact that explosive aggression and CD are so common, are so difficult to treat, and cause such impairment among psychiatrically referred youth—provides the rationale for investigating lithium's antiaggressive effects in children and adolescents. Post-1980 studies of lithium's efficacy for aggression and related behaviors in referred youth are presented in Table 12.8. These studies have investigated a total of 170 youngsters in five randomized controlled and four open research protocols. The findings are decidedly mixed. Among the five randomized controlled trials, three studies have found a statistically significant difference favoring lithium over placebo, and the other two have found no significant drug–placebo differences (Campbell et al., 1984; Campbell, Adams, et al., 1995; Klein, 1991; Malone, Delaney, Luebbert, Cater, & Campbell, 2000; Rifkin et al., 1997). These studies have generally been short (2–6 weeks) and have reported no correlation between lithium serum levels and antiaggressive response in psychiatrically referred youth with CD and/or explosive, affective aggression.

Aggression subtypes may be important in determining the efficacy of lithium. Open studies have found that explosive aggression with a hostile affective component may respond better to lithium than "pure" CD does (DeLong & Aldershof, 1987). Randomized studies have also reported that aggression with a reactive, explosive component responds to lithium much better than premeditated, instrumental aggression does (Campbell, Adams, et al., 1995).

A considerable amount of information has been accumulated about the safety and short-term adverse effects of lithium in the pediatric age group. Common side effects of lithium administration include vomiting, stomachaches, nausea, hand tremor, enuresis, and headaches (Campbell, Kafantaris, & Cueva, 1995). Generally, children aged 5–12 years report more side effects on lithium than teenagers do (Campbell, Kafantaris, et al., 1995). Information about the long-term safety of lithium in the pediatric age group remains limited, because of the short duration of most lithium studies in youth. In the only long-term study reported to date, DeLong and Aldershof (1987) treated a large number of children and adolescents with lithium over 10 years. They reported that only one child developed mild goiter without hypothyroidism after 4 years. However, the long-term safety of lithium use in the pediatric age range has not yet been established.

Divalproex Sodium (Valproate)

Divalproex sodium (valproate) is an anticonvulsant in clinical use for treating simple and complex absence seizures, migraine headache, and bipolar illness in adults (Davanzo & McCracken, 2000). Use of divalproex sodium for juvenile bipolar illness is beginning; however, its use for this condition in youth is not yet approved by the U.S. Food and Drug Administration (Kowatch et al., 2000). Hypotheses on the mechanisms of action include its interaction with neuronal voltage-sensitive sodium channels and its enhancement of gamma-aminobutyric acid concentrations, a major inhibitory neurotransmitter in the CNS (Davanzo & McCracken, 2000).

In adults, another clinical indication for divalproex sodium is in the treat-

TABLE 12.8. Lithium for Aggression and Related Behaviors in Youth

Reference	Sample size	Age	Design	Trial duration	Dose and serum level	Diagnosis	Response
Malone et al. (2000)	20	10–17	RCT	6 wk	900–2,100 mg/d 0.78–1.55 mEq/L	CD	Drug sig. superior to placebo
Rifkin et al. (1997)	14	12–17	RCT	2 wk	NR[a] 0.6–1.25 mEq/L	CD	NSD
Campbell, Adams, et al. (1995)	25	5–12	RCT	6 wk	600–1,800 mg/d 0.53–1.79 mEq/L	CD	Drug sig. superior to placebo
Klein (1991)	17	6–15	RCT	5 wk	NR 0.6–1.2 mEq/L	CD	NSD
Campbell et al. (1984)	21	5–12	RCT	4 wk	500–2,000 mg/d 0.32–1.51 mEq/L	CD	Drug sig. superior to placebo
DeLong and Aldershof (1987)	33	5–17	Open	56–120 wk	NR	CD	15% response rate
DeLong and Aldershof (1987)	9	6–16	Open	36–200 wk	NR	Explosive/ affective aggression	56% response rate
Vetro et al. (1985)	17	3–12	Open	24 wk	Avg. 26 mg/kg/d 0.68 mEq/L	CD	76% response rate
Siassi (1982)	14	7–13	Open	12 wk	900–2,100 mg/d 1.0–1.6 mEq/L	CD	Sig. reduction in aggression in drug group
Total	170[b]	3–17	5 RCTs, 4 open	2–200 wk	600–2,100 mg/d 0.32–1.79 mEq/L		Mixed: 3 RCTs support and 2 RCTs do not support lithium efficacy; 3 open trials support and 1 does not support lithium efficacy

[a]NR, not reported.
[b]97 in 5 RCTs; 73 in 4 open trials.

ment of nonbipolar patients exhibiting violent and other aggressive behaviors within a variety of psychiatric conditions (Lindenmayer & Kotsaftis, 2000). In children and adolescents, manic-like symptoms may appear clinically as chronic and extreme irritability, hostility, disruptive behaviors, rage attacks, moodiness, low frustration tolerance, and explosive aggression. Nosologically, these symptoms draw youth with the diagnoses of CD, oppositional defiant disorder (ODD), and intermittent explosive disorder into the spectrum of youngsters who might be considered for treatment with divalproex sodium (Biederman et al., 1998). Table 12.9 lists the only two studies available to date investigating divalproex sodium for aggressive behavior in youngsters. One randomized controlled study and one open study from the same research group have assessed a total of 30 youth. Divalproex sodium was found to be significantly superior to placebo in reducing rage and temper outbursts in juveniles with ODD or CD (Donovan et al., 2000).

Carbamazepine

Carbamazepine is an anticonvulsant chemically related to the TCAs. It is currently used in neurology to treat simple and complex partial seizures, generalized seizures, and some pain syndromes (e.g., trigeminal and glossopharyngeal neuralgias). It has been found helpful in treating mania in adults, and is now being studied for similar use in juvenile manic-like symptoms and explosive aggression in children and adolescents (Viesselman, 1999). A meta-analysis of 29 reports found some support for the usefulness of carbamazepine in ADHD (Silva, Munoz, & Alpert, 1996), although it is not widely prescribed for this condition in the United States. Carbamazepine exerts its anticonvulsant effects by blocking the repetitive firing of neuronal action potentials (Viesselman, 1999). Its antimanic and antiaggressive effects remain poorly understood.

Carbamazepine has been found effective in reducing aggression in adults with psychiatric disorders (Tariot et al., 1998). Because of this finding, and (again) because aggression and CD in youth can be difficult to treat and severely impairing, carbamazepine has been investigated in the pharmacological treatment of CD. At present, only one open study and one randomized controlled trial assessing the efficacy of carbamazepine for CD in 32 children and adolescents have been completed (see Table 12.9). Whereas the open trial supported efficacy, the randomized trial found no significant difference between carbamazepine and placebo (Cueva et al., 1996).

Summary of Mood Stabilizer Research

In summary, this review of the mood stabilizers finds some support for the efficacy of lithium and divalproex sodium in the pharmacological treatment of aggression and related behaviors in youth. Little evidence to date supports the use of carbamazepine in this context. The findings of efficacy from randomized controlled trials of lithium and divalproex sodium suggest that further re-

TABLE 12.9. Anticonvulsants for Aggression and Related Behaviors in Youth

Reference	Sample size	Age	Design	Trial duration	Dose and serum level	Diagnosis	Response
Divalproex sodium							
Donovan et al. (2000)	20	10–18	RCT	6 wk	750–1,500 mg/d Avg. 82.2 µg/ml	ODD/CD	Drug sig. superior to placebo
Donovan et al. (1997)	10	15–18	Open	5 wk	1,000 mg/d 45–113 µg/ml	ODD/CD	Sig. decrease in aggression at end of study
Carbamazepine							
Cueva et al. (1996)	22	5–11	RCT	6 wk	400–800 mg/d 5–9.1 µg/ml	CD	NSD
Kafantaris et al. (1992)	10	5–11	Open	3 wk	600–800 mg/d 4.8–10.4 µg/ml	CD	90% improved
Total	62[a]	5–18	2 RCTs, 2 open	3–6 wk	Variable		RCTs support divalproex > carbamazepine

[a] 30 on divalproex; 32 on carbamazepine.

search should explore the use of these agents in clinically referred children and adolescents with severe aggression accompanied by juvenile manic-like symptoms.

ADRENERGIC AGENTS

Psychotropic medications that down-regulate adrenergic tone in the peripheral nervous system and diminish adrenergic neurotransmission in the CNS have been used adjunctively to treat aggression and related behaviors in psychiatric patients. These medications include clonidine, guanfacine, and beta-adrenergic blockers ("beta-blockers" for short), such as propranolol, nadolol, and pindolol. Since impulsive explosive aggression in clinically referred patients is often accompanied by overarousal of the ANS and by increased CNS epinephrine and NE activity, a rationale for the use of this class of medication in the pharmacological treatment of aggression is to diminish catecholamine activity both peripherally and in the CNS. Reduction of adrenergic activity may be accompanied by reduced frequency and intensity of aggressive outbursts in psychiatric patients (Connor, 1993).

Clonidine

Clonidine was first synthesized in 1962, and its primary clinical use is to treat hypertension in adults. In pediatric psychiatry, clonidine was first used to treat tics in children with Tourette's disorder. Since then, the use of clonidine (both alone and in combination with other psychiatric medications) to treat impulsive, aggressive, and overaroused behaviors in tic disorders, ADHD, and other psychiatric disorders has grown rapidly (Connor, Fletcher, & Swanson, 1999). Clonidine is a presynaptic alpha$_2$-adrenergic agonist that acts in the CNS at the level of the locus coeruleus in the midbrain to down-regulate overall NE tone. Because NE mechanisms have been implicated in explosive aggression, clonidine has been studied "off-label" in children and adolescents with CD and aggression (Connor, Barkley, & Davis, 2000).

Post-1980 investigations of clonidine in the adjunctive pharmacological treatment of aggression in various juvenile psychiatric disorders are presented in Table 12.10. These seven studies included a total of 114 juveniles with ADHD, CD, PTSD, and Tourette's disorder. Four randomized controlled trials and three open trials are reviewed. These studies suggest that clonidine in divided doses ranging from 0.1 to 0.4 mg/day may be effective in the adjunctive treatment of aggression in referred youth. The four randomized controlled trials suggest that the effects of clonidine may be more robust for aggression occurring within the disruptive behavior disorders than within Tourette's disorder. However, because the sample sizes in these studies were small, the results remain suggestive rather than definitive; further methodologically controlled investigations with larger sample sizes are required.

TABLE 12.10. Clonidine and Guanfacine for Aggression and Related Behaviors in Youth

Reference	Sample size	Age	Design	Trial duration	Total dose	Diagnosis	Response
Clonidine							
Connor et al. (2000)	8	Avg. 9.3	RCT	12 wk	0.1–0.3 mg/d	ADHD + CD	Sig. benefit on drug compared to baseline
Harmon and Riggs (1996)	7	3–6	Open	4 wk	0.05–0.2 mg/d	PTSD	100% improvement rate
Schvehla et al. (1994)	18	6–12	Open	3 wk	0.15–0.4 mg/d	ADHD + CD	61% improvement rate
Kemph et al. (1993)	17	5–15	Open	4–72 wk	0.15–0.4 mg/d	CD	88% improvement rate
Leckman et al. (1991)	24	Avg. 15.6	RCT	12 wk	0.1–0.2 mg/d	TD	NSD
Goetz et al. (1987)	30	Avg. 19.2	RCT	12 wk	0.0075–0.015 mg/kg/d	TD	NSD
Hunt et al. (1985)	10	8–13	RCT	8 wk	0.05–0.2 mg/d	ADHD	Sig. benefit on drug compared to placebo
Total	114[a]	3–19	4 RCTs, 3 open	3–72 wk	0.1–0.4 mg/d		Clonidine effects on aggression and related behaviors appear stronger in DBD than in TD
Guanfacine							
Scahill et al. (2001)	34	7–15	RCT	8 wk	1.5–3.0 mg/d	ADHD + TD	Sig. improvement compared to placebo
Horrigan and Barnhill (1995)	15	7–17	Open	5–10 wk	0.5–3.0 mg/d	ADHD	60% improvement rate
Chappell et al. (1995)	10	8–16	Open	4–20 wk	0.75–3.0 mg/d	ADHD + TD	40% improvement rate
Hunt et al. (1995)	13	4–20	Open	4 wk	0.5–4.0 mg/d	ADHD	NSD between baseline and drug
Total	72[b]	4–20	3 open, 1 RCT	4–20 wk	0.5–4.0 mg/d	ADHD ± TD	Open studies suggest less efficacy for guanfacine than for clonidine; RCT suggests sig. improvement

[a] 72 in 4 RCTs; 42 in 3 open trials.
[b] 34 in 1 RCT; 38 in 3 open trials.

Guanfacine

Guanfacine is a newer alpha$_2$-adrenergic agonist that differs from clonidine in several ways. Guanfacine has a more specific receptor-binding profile; it appears to bind preferentially to alpha$_2$-adrenergic receptors in prefrontal cortical regions of the CNS, as opposed to the subcortical binding site of clonidine at the level of the locus coeruleus. As a result, guanfacine has fewer sedating and hypotensive side effects than clonidine, and possibly a more specific mechanism of action on neuropsychological processes serving attention span, vigilance, and impulse control. Guanfacine also has a longer pharmacokinetic half-life than clonidine, allowing for longer therapeutic effects and less frequent daily dosing (Chappell et al., 1995; Hunt, Arnsten, & Asbell, 1995; Scahill et al., 2001).

Three open studies and one controlled study investigating the efficacy of guanfacine in 72 children and adolescents with ADHD and Tourette's disorder are presented in Table 12.10. The open studies suggest that guanfacine may have positive treatment effects on aggression and related behaviors in clinically referred youngsters. The controlled study demonstrated statistically significant effects for guanfacine compared to placebo on teacher-rated hyperactive–impulsive behaviors in 7- to 15-year-old children with ADHD and tic disorders.

Beta-Blockers

Beta-blockers are competitive antagonists of NE and epinephrine action at beta-adrenergic receptor sites. These receptors are found in both the CNS and the peripheral nervous system. In the periphery, beta$_1$-adrenergic receptors mediate cardiac chonotropic and inotropic effects, and beta$_2$-adrenergic receptors modulate pulmonary bronchodilation and peripheral vasodilation. These receptors are ubiquitous in the CNS, where they help modulate arousal and anxiety (Connor, Ozbayrak, Benjamin, Ma, & Fletcher, 1997).

Beta-blocking drugs include propranolol, nadolol, pindolol, metoprolol, and atenolol. These agents differ in their selectivity for beta-adrenergic receptors and in their lipid solubility (which determines peripheral or CNS site of action). For example, propranolol and nadolol are nonselective beta-blockers acting on both beta$_1$- and beta$_2$-adrenergic receptors. Atenolol and metoprolol are selective beta$_1$-blockers. Propranolol is very lipid-soluble and readily enters the brain, exerting effects both centrally and peripherally. Nadolol and atenolol cross the blood–brain barrier in only small amounts and thus act primarily in the periphery. Other beta-blockers have intermediate degrees of lipid solubility.

In adults, beta-blockers such as propranolol, nadolol, and pindolol have been found in controlled studies to be effective in reducing impulsive and explosive aggression and rage attacks in patients with autism, mental retardation, and organic brain damage such as dementia (Connor, 1993). Because signs and symptoms of adrenergic overarousal often accompany these behaviors in clinically referred patients, beta-blocking agents have been investigated in the adjunctive pharmacological treatment of excessive aggression in such patients. Studies since 1980 investigating beta-blockers for aggression in referred children and adolescents are presented in Table 12.11. These studies include four open and one randomized controlled trial investigating a total of 101 children, adolescents, and young adults with a variety of psychiatric syndromes who were treated with nadolol, pindolol, or propranolol. The four open trials have reported improvement rates varying between 63% and 91%. The one randomized controlled trial investigated 32 children receiving either pindolol or methylphenidate in a crossover design (Buitelaar, van der Gaag, Swaab-Barneveld, & Kuiper, 1996). Pindolol was given in doses of 20–40 mg/day. Although it was effective for conduct problems compared to placebo, it was not superior to methylphenidate in this study sample. Furthermore, a high rate of side effects, including nightmares, hallucinations, and paraesthesias caused many aggressive youth to discontinue pindolol treatment. While open trials suggest that beta-blockers may be effective in reducing aggression in a variety of psychiatric diagnoses, the lack of randomized controlled trials with agents other than pindolol prevents firm conclusions supporting their use for this purpose from being drawn in the pediatric age range.

OTHER MEDICATIONS

Benzodiazepines are anxiolytic medications that include lorazepam, clonazepam, diazepam, chlordiazepoxide, and oxazepam. Evidence in adult psychiatry indicates that lorazepam and clonazepam often decrease hostility, irritability, and aggression in patients with psychotic and manic agitation. However, in roughly 1% of these patients, use of benzodiazepines may result in disinhibition and worsening of aggressive dyscontrol (Dietch & Jennings, 1988). In addition, psychological dependence and drug withdrawal reactions may occur upon medication discontinuation after long-term use of benzodiazepines. For these reasons, benzodiazepines are rarely used in the pharmacological treatment of aggression in children and adolescents.

Buspirone is a nonbenzodiazepine anxiolytic that exerts effects on the 5-HT neurotransmitter system by acting as an agonist at 5-HT_{1A} presynaptic receptors and as a partial agonist at postsynaptic 5-HT_{1A} receptors. Buspirone has little risk of disinhibition and few or no addicting or withdrawal effects (Sussman, 1994). Buspirone use for aggression in hospitalized psychiatric children in doses up to 50 mg/day has been investigated, but few therapeutic effects were reported (Pfeffer, Jiang, & Domeshek, 1997). Thus the use of benzodiazepine and nonbenzodiazepine anxiolytics in the treatment of aggression in clinically referred youth is not supported by the available scientific literature at present.

TABLE 12.11. Beta-Blockers for Aggression and Related Behaviors in Youth

Reference	Sample size	Age[a]	Design	Medication	Duration	Dose	Diagnosis	Response
Connor, Ozbayrak, Benjamin, et al. (1997)	12	9–24	Open	Nadolol	16 wk	30–220 mg/d	DD[b]	83% improvement rate
Buitelaar et al. (1996)	32	7–13	RCT	Pindolol	4 wk	20–40 mg/d	ADHD	Sig. improvement on drug compared to placebo; many side effects on pindolol
Famularo et al. (1988)	11	6–12	Open	Propranolol	4 wk	2.5 mg/kg/d	PTSD	91% response rate
Kuperman and Stewart (1987)	16	4–24	Open	Propranolol	12 wk	80–280 mg/d	Mixed	63% response rate
Williams et al. (1982)	30	7–35	Open	Propranolol	8–120 wk	50–1,600 mg/d	Organic[c]	80% response rate
Total	101[d]	4–35	1 RCT, 4 open	Nadolol, pindolol, propranolol	4–120 wk	Variable	Variable	Open studies report 63%–91% response rate for aggression and related behaviors

[a]Mean age of study subjects < 18 years.
[b]DD, developmental disorders.
[c]Organic, organic brain disease.
[d]32 in 1 RCT; 69 in 4 open trials.

THE USE OF AS-NEEDED (P.R.N.) MEDICATION

The administration of "as-needed" (in Latin, *pro re nata*, or "p.r.n.") sedative psychotropic medication to aggressive children and adolescents is a common practice in inpatient treatment settings (Vitiello et al., 1991). Up to 86% of long-term child psychiatry inpatients may receive p.r.n. medications, mainly for episodes of acute disruptive behavior (Vitiello, Ricciuti, & Behar, 1987). Despite this widespread clinical practice, very little research has been conducted to support the use of p.r.n. medications for acute aggression in psychiatrically referred youth.

In adult psychiatric inpatients, no significant association has been found between psychiatric diagnosis and whether a patient received p.r.n. drugs; moreover, no correlation has been found between the type of p.r.n. medication given (e.g., antipsychotics, anxiolytics) and patient diagnosis (Walker, 1991). In the only randomized controlled trial of p.r.n. medications in child psychiatry, each of 21 children (5–13 years old) received either oral or intramuscular doses of diphenhydramine, a sedative–hypnotic ($n = 9$), or placebo ($n = 12$) (Vitiello et al., 1991). Results showed no drug–placebo difference in acute disruptive behavior. However, there was a significant difference in acute behaviors by method of drug delivery; children receiving intramuscular injections calmed down significantly more than children receiving oral p.r.n. medication. The conclusion is fairly clear: Acutely disruptive children wish to avoid "the needle." In this study, therefore, pharmacological p.r.n. efficacy for aggressive behaviors was determined by a route effect (essentially aversive behavioral conditioning) and not a drug effect.

Other types of medications commonly given for acute aggression on inpatient child psychiatry units include neuroleptic and antipsychotic drugs. These have not yet been studied to determine whether p.r.n. drug use is effective independently of the route of administration. Despite widespread clinical practice, the available scientific literature does not support the use of p.r.n. medications for acute aggressive and disruptive behaviors in child psychiatry.

WHICH MEDICINE TO USE?

Although many different medications have some efficacy in the adjunctive treatment of aggression, in clinical practice guidance is needed to select an appropriate drug for an individual patient. An algorithm to help guide clinical practice, based on a primary illness approach to the pharmacological treatment of aggression, is presented in Figure 12.1. As a clinical rule, therapy with a single agent should be tried before combined pharmacotherapy is attempted. Each drug should be tried in low, medium, and high doses for an adequate length of time at each dose before the next agent is tried. This algorithm will change in the future as more controlled studies of pharmacological efficacy for aggression in the context of psychiatric illness become available.

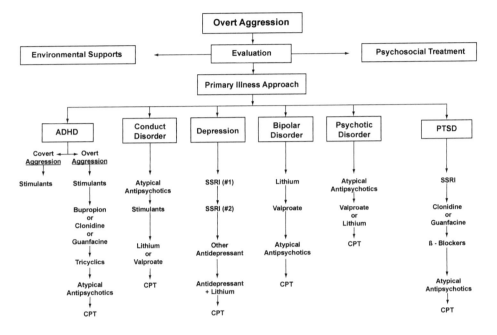

FIGURE 12.1. An algorithm to guide clinical practice, based on a primary illness approach to the use of psychiatric medications for aggression. Note that a careful clinical evaluation and consideration of environmental supports and psychosocial treatments should occur before medication is prescribed. This figure does not depict a medication algorithm to treat aggression in the context of traumatic brain injury or epilepsy. The psychopharmacological treatment of PTSD will vary, depending on the nature of the presenting symptoms. For mood symptoms SSRIs are used initially, and for psychotic symptoms antipsychotics may be considered. CPT, combined pharmacotherapy.

For explosive, rageful, impulsive aggression that occurs in the context of an unclear primary psychiatric illness, a target symptom approach is used. In such an approach, the most benign interventions are used first, and clear behavioral and side effect outcomes are tracked. An algorithm based on a target symptom approach to the pharmacological management of aggression is presented in Figure 12.2.

CHAPTER SUMMARY

Over the past three decades, the research data base in pediatric psychopharmacology has grown much larger. As part of an overall multidisciplinary psychoeducational treatment plan, psychiatric medication interventions for youth with disruptive behavior disorders, mood disorders, developmental disorders, and psychotic disorders and symptoms are becoming more widely accepted.

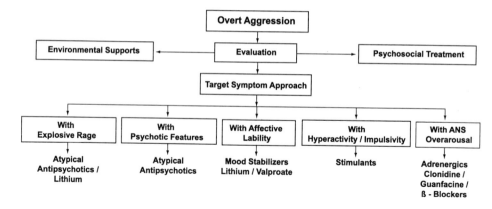

FIGURE 12.2. An algorithm to guide clinical practice, based on a target symptom approach to the use of psychiatric medications for aggression. The research does not yet support the recommendation of one of these medications as clearly superior over the others for explosive aggression. Note that a careful clinical evaluation and consideration of environmental supports and psychosocial treatments should occur before prescribing medication. The psychopharmacological treatment of aggression in the context of traumatic brain injury or epilepsy is not discussed here.

Because excessive, inappropriate aggression is a common problem in clinically referred children and adolescents, may be refractory to psychosocial interventions, and can cause severe impairment, increasing interest has focused on the possibility of finding effective medications for these youth. This interest has been encouraged by a developing research base on the neurobiological mechanisms of aggression in animal models and in adult psychiatric patients.

Not every aggressive psychiatrically referred youth requires a medication intervention. A substantial number of such children and adolescents may respond to psychosocial therapeutic interventions, monitoring, and environmental structure. Aggression precipitated by clear environmental and social stressors, such as dangerous neighborhoods or family violence, may greatly improve without medication interventions. However, when aggression is chronic, frequent, and severe; occurs in the absence of identifiable psychosocial precipitants; has an explosive quality; is accompanied by impulsivity, hostility, or irritability; and does not respond to behavioral and family treatment interventions, further psychiatric evaluation to assess the possibility of medication treatment may be warranted.

When medication is used to treat aggression, a systematic approach is best utilized to maximize benefits and minimize side effects. Empirical methods of data collection must be used to track effects on target behaviors and to monitor safety and possible side effects. Either a target symptom approach or a primary illness approach to the pharmacological treatment of aggression in clinically referred children and adolescents must be clarified.

This chapter's review of the pediatric psychopharmacology literature since 1980 finds support for several psychiatric medications as possibly effective in the adjunctive treatment of juvenile aggression within the context of various psychiatric diagnoses. Strong support from more than one randomized controlled clinical trial is found for the use of neuroleptics for aggression and related behaviors in CD, developmental disorders, and psychotic disorders and symptoms. Multiple methodologically controlled studies support the efficacy of stimulant medications in the adjunctive clinical treatment of aggression within the disruptive behavior disorders, including ADHD and (to a lesser extent), CD. Multiple controlled trials strongly support the efficacy of the atypical antidepressant bupropion, and (to a lesser extent) the TCA desipramine, for aggression occurring within the context of ADHD. Some support is found for the clinical use of lithium and divalproex sodium for aggression in CD, especially in youth with manic-like symptoms. Clonidine and beta-blockers deserve more research attention in this population; little support is found for the use of carbamazepine. The use of SSRI antidepressants as antiaggression strategies remains unproven in pediatric psychiatry.

Further research is needed to address several issues. First, regardless of psychiatric diagnosis, the subtype of aggression may be important in defining pharmacological response. There is emerging evidence that aggression with explosive, impulsive, hyperactive, or manic-like qualities may respond to a variety of psychiatric medications. Instrumental or predatory aggression does not appear to respond to medication interventions. Further studies are needed that investigate the efficacy of specific drug types for more carefully defined aggression subtypes within various psychiatric diagnoses. Second, the specific neurobiological mechanisms that subserve aggression need to be defined more precisely. These may provide more specific targets for psychiatric medication interventions in the future. Such research offers hope of greater therapeutic precision and efficacy with minimal side effects. Lastly, combined psychosocial and medication interventions for clinically referred youth with excessive, inappropriate aggression need to be compared to psychosocial interventions given alone, in order to clarify which aggressive youngsters might benefit from adjunctive medication intervention.

The issue for future research on aggression and its treatment is to better understand how the interaction of biological vulnerabilities with problematic social environments during the developing years may result in the development of chronic, severe, frequent, and impairing aggression and related behaviors for some children and adolescents. The next issue is to clarify how biological and psychosocial treatment interventions, alone or in combination, may be helpful in ameliorating maladaptive aggression in these youth.

References

Aarons, G. A., Brown, S. A., Hough, R. L., Garland, A. F., & Wood, P. A. (2001). Prevalence of adolescent substance use disorders across five sectors of care. *Journal of the American Academy of Child and Adolescent Psychiatry, 40*, 419–426.

Achenbach, T. M. (1991). *Manual for the Child Behavior Checklist/4–18 and 1991 profile*. Burlington, VT: University of Vermont, Department of Psychiatry.

Achenbach, T. M., Conners, C. K., Quay, H. C., Verhulst, F. C., & Howell, C. T. (1989). Replications of empirically derived syndromes as a basis for taxonomy of child/adolescent psychopathology. *Journal of Abnormal Child Psychology, 17*, 299–323.

Achenbach, T. M., & Edelbrock, C. S. (1978). The classification of child psychopathology: A review and analysis of empirical efforts. *Psychological Bulletin, 85*, 1275–1301.

Achenbach, T. M., & Edelbrock, C. S. (1983). *Manual for the Child Behavior Checklist and revised Child Behavior Profile*. Burlington: University of Vermont, Department of Psychiatry.

Achenbach, T. M., Howell, C. T., McConaughy, S. H., & Stanger, C. (1995a). Six-year predictors of problems in a national sample of children and youth: I. Cross-informant syndromes. *Journal of the American Academy of Child and Adolescent Psychiatry, 34*, 336–347.

Achenbach, T. M., Howell, C. T., McConaughy, S. H., & Stanger, C. (1995b). Six-year predictors of problems in a national sample of children and youth: III. Transitions to young adult syndromes. *Journal of the American Academy of Child and Adolescent Psychiatry, 34*, 658–669.

Adams, D. A., & Victor, M. (1981). *Principles of neurology* (2nd ed.). New York: McGraw-Hill.

af Klinteberg, B. (1996). Biology, norms, and personality: A developmental perspective. *Neuropsychobiology, 34*, 146–154.

Afifi, A. K., & Uc, E. Y. (1998). Cortical–subcortical circuitry for movement, cognition, and behavior. In C. E. Coffey & R. A. Brumback (Eds.), *Textbook of pediatric neuropsychiatry* (pp. 65–100). Washington, DC: American Psychiatric Press.

Akiskal, H. S. (1995). Developmental pathways to bipolarity: Are juvenile-onset depressions pre-bipolar? *Journal of the American Academy of Child and Adolescent Psychiatry, 34*, 754–763.

Albert, D. J., & Walsh, M. L. (1984). Neural systems and the inhibitory modulation of agnostic behavior: A comparison of mammalian species. *Neuroscience and Biobehavioral Reviews, 8,* 5–24.

Albert, D. J., Walsh, M. L., & Jonik, R. H. (1993). Aggression in humans: What is its biological foundation? *Neuroscience and Biobehavioral Reviews, 17,* 405–425.

Alexander, J. F., & Parsons, B. V. (1973). Short-term behavioral intervention with delinquent families: Impact on family process and recidivism. *Journal of Abnormal Psychology, 81,* 219–225.

Alexander, J. F., & Parsons, B. V. (1982). *Functional family therapy.* Monterey, CA: Brooks/Cole.

Alexander, J. F., Waldron, H. B., Newberry, A. M., & Liddle, N. (1988). Family approaches to treating delinquents. In E. W. Nunnally, C. S. Chilman, & F. M. Cox (Eds.), *Mental illness, delinquency, addictions, and neglect* (pp. 128–146). Newbury Park, CA: Sage.

Allen, J. P., Hauser, S. T., & Borman-Spurrell, E. (1996). Attachment theory as a framework for understanding sequelae of severe adolescent psychopathology: An 11–year follow-up study. *Journal of Consulting and Clinical Psychology, 64,* 254–263.

Allen, T. J., Moeller, F. G., Rhoades, H. M., & Cherek, D. R. (1997). Subjects with a history of drug dependence are more aggressive than subjects with no drug use history. *Drug and Alcohol Dependence, 46,* 95–103.

Alm, P. O., af Klinteberg, B., Humble, K., Leppert, J., Sorensen, S., Thorell, L.-H., Lidberg, L., & Oreland, L. (1996). Psychopathy, platelet MAO activity and criminality among former juvenile delinquents. *Acta Psychiatrica Scandinavica, 94,* 105–111.

Alm, P. O., Alm, M., Humble, K., Leppert, J., Sorensen, S., Lidberg, L., & Oreland, L. (1994). Criminality and platelet monoamine oxidase activity in former juvenile delinquents as adults. *Acta Psychiatrica Scandinavica, 89,* 41–45.

Aman, M. G., Marks, R. E., Turbott, S. H., Wilsher, C. P., & Merry, S. N. (1991). Clinical effects of methylphenidate and thioridazine in intellectually subaverage children. *Journal of the American Academy of Child and Adolescent Psychiatry, 30,* 246–256.

Amato, P. R., & Keith, B. (1991). Parental divorce and the well-being of children: A meta-analysis. *Psychological Bulletin, 110,* 26–46.

Ambrosini, P. J. (2000). Historical development and present status of the Schedule for Affective Disorders and Schizophrenia for School-Age Children (K-SADS). *Journal of the American Academy of Child and Adolescent Psychiatry, 39,* 49–58.

American Academy of Child and Adolescent Psychiatry (AACAP), Work Group on Quality Issues. (1995). Practice parameters for the psychiatric assessment of children and adolescents. *Journal of the American Academy of Child and Adolescent Psychiatry, 34,* 1386–1402.

American Academy of Child and Adolescent Psychiatry (AACAP), Work Group on Quality Issues. (1997a). Practice parameters for the assessment and treatment of children and adolescents with bipolar disorder. *Journal of the American Academy of Child and Adolescent Psychiatry, 36,* 138–157.

American Academy of Child and Adolescent Psychiatry (AACAP), Work Group on Quality Issues. (1997b). Practice parameters for the assessment and treatment of children and adolescents with substance use disorders. *Journal of the American Academy of Child and Adolescent Psychiatry, 36*(10, Suppl.), 140S–156S.

American Academy of Child and Adolescent Psychiatry (AACAP), Work Group on Quality Issues (1997c). Practice parameters for the assessment and treatment of children and adolescents with conduct disorder. *Journal of the American Academy of Child and Adolescent Psychiatry, 36*(10, Suppl.), 122S–139S.

American Academy of Child and Adolescent Psychiatry (AACAP), Work Group on Quality Issues. (1998a). Practice parameters for the assessment and treatment of children and adolescents with depressive disorders. *Journal of the American Academy of Child and Adolescent Psychiatry, 37*(10, Supp.), 63S–83S.

American Academy of Child and Adolescent Psychiatry (AACAP), Work Group on Quality Issues. (1998b). Practice parameters for the assessment and treatment of children and adolescents with posttraumatic stress disorder. *Journal of the American Academy of Child and Adolescent Psychiatry, 37*(10, Suppl.), 4S–26S.

American Psychiatric Association (APA). (1968). *Diagnostic and statistical manual of mental disorders* (2nd ed.). Washington, DC: Author.

American Psychiatric Association (APA). (1980). *Diagnostic and statistical manual of mental disorders* (3rd ed.). Washington DC: Author.

American Psychiatric Association (APA). (1987). *Diagnostic and statistical manual of mental disorders* (3rd ed., rev.). Washington, DC: Author.

American Psychiatric Association (APA). (1994). *Diagnostic and statistical manual of mental disorders* (4th ed.). Washington, DC: Author.

American Psychiatric Association (APA). (1998). *Fact sheet: Violence and mental illness.* Washington, DC: Author.

American Psychiatric Association (APA), Psychiatric Services Resource Center. (1997). *Violent behavior and mental illness: A compendium of articles from Psychiatric Services and Hospital and Community Psychiatry.* Washington, DC: Author.

American Psychological Association, Commission on Violence and Youth. (1993). *Violence and youth: Psychology's response.* Washington, DC: Public Interest Directorate, American Psychological Association.

Amery, B., Minichiello, M. D., & Brown, G. L. (1984). Aggression in hyperactive boys: Response to *d*-amphetamine. *Journal of the American Academy of Child Psychiatry, 23,* 291–294.

Anderson, J. C., Williams, S., McGee, R., & Silva, P. A. (1987). DSM-III disorders in preadolescent children. *Archives of General Psychiatry, 44,* 69–76.

Anderson, L. T., Campbell, M., Adams, P., Small, A. M., Perry, R., & Shell, J. (1989). The effects of haloperidol on discrimination learning and behavioral symptoms in autistic children. *Journal of Autism and Developmental Disorders, 19,* 227–239.

Anderson, L. T., Campbell, M., Grega, D. M., Perry, R., Small, A. M., & Green, W. H. (1984). Haloperidol in the treatment of infantile autism: Effects on learning and behavioral symptoms. *American Journal of Psychiatry, 141,* 1195–1202.

Andrews, G., Slade, T., & Peters, L. (1999). Classification in psychiatry: ICD-10 versus DSM-IV. *British Journal of Psychiatry, 174,* 3–5.

Angold, A., & Costello, E. J. (1992). Comorbidity in children and adolescents with depression. *Child and Adolescent Psychiatric Clinics of North America, 1,* 31–51.

Angold, A., & Costello, E. J. (2000). The Child and Adolescent Psychiatric Assessment (CAPA). *Journal of the American Academy of Child and Adolescent Psychiatry, 39,* 39–48.

Anthony, J., & Scott, P. (1960). Manic–depressive psychosis in childhood. *Journal of Child Psychology and Psychiatry, 1,* 53–72.

Appelbaum, P. S., Robbins, P. C., & Monahan, J. (2000). Violence and delusions: Data from the MacArthur Violence Risk Assessment Study. *American Journal of Psychiatry, 157,* 566–572.

Archer, J. (1991). The influence of testosterone on human aggression. *British Journal of Psychology, 82,* 1–28.

Armenteros, J. L., Whitaker, A. H., Welikson, M., Stedge, D. J., & Gorman, J. (1997). Risperidone in adolescents with schizophrenia: An open pilot study. *Journal of the American Academy of Child and Adolescent Psychiatry, 36,* 694–700.

Armsworth, M. W., & Holaday, M. (1993). The effects of psychological trauma on children and adolescents. *Journal of Counseling and Development, 72,* 49–56.

Arnold, L. E. (2000). Methylphenidate vs. amphetamine: Comparative review. *Journal of Attention Disorders, 3,* 200–211.

Arnsten, A. F. T. (1999). Development of the cerebral cortex: XIV. Stress impairs prefrontal cortical function. *Journal of the American Academy of Child and Adolescent Psychiatry, 38,* 220–222.

Arnsten, A. F. T., & Goldman-Rakic, P. S. (1998). Noise stress impairs prefrontal cortical cognitive function in monkeys. *Archives of General Psychiatry, 55,* 362–368.

Arora, R. C., Fitchner, C. G., & O'Connor, F. (1993). Paroxetine binding in the blood platelets of posttraumatic stress disordered patients. *Life Sciences, 53,* 919–928.

Arredondo, D. E., & Butler, S. F. (1994). Affective comorbidity in psychiatrically hospitalized adolescents with conduct disorder or oppositional defiant disorder: Should conduct disorder be treated with mood stabilizers? *Journal of Child and Adolescent Psychopharmacology, 4,* 151–158.

Arseneault, L., Moffitt, T. E., Caspi, A., Taylor, P. J., & Silva, P. A. (2000). Mental disorders and violence in a total birth cohort. *Archives of General Psychiatry, 57,* 979–986.

Arseneault, L., Tremblay, R. E., Boulerice, B., Seguin, J. R., & Saucier, J.-F. (2000). Minor physical anomalies and family adversity as risk factors for violent delinquency in adolescence. *American Journal of Psychiatry, 157,* 917–923.

Asarnow, J. R., & Asarnow, R. F. (1996). Childhood-onset schizophrenia. In E. J. Mash & R. A. Barkley (Eds.), *Child psychopathology* (pp. 340–361). New York: Guilford Press.

Atkins, M. S., & Stoff, D. M. (1993). Instrumental and hostile aggression in childhood disruptive behavior disorders. *Journal of Abnormal Child Psychology, 21,* 165–178.

Atkins, M. S., Stoff, D. M., Osborne, M. L., & Brown, K. (1993). Distinguishing instrumental and hostile aggression: Does it make a difference? *Journal of Abnormal Child Psychology, 21,* 355–365.

Attie, I., & Brooks-Gunn, J. (1989). The development of eating problems in adolescent girls: A longitudinal study. *Developmental Psychology, 25,* 70–79.

August, G. J., Realmuto, G. M., Joyce, T., & Hektner, J. M. (1999). Persistence and desistance of oppositional defiant disorder in a community sample of children with ADHD. *Journal of the American Academy of Child and Adolescent Psychiatry, 38,* 1262–1270.

August, G. J., Stewart, M. A., & Holmes, C. S. (1983). A four-year follow-up of hyperactive boys with and without conduct disorder. *British Journal of Psychiatry, 143,* 192–198.

Babinski, L. M., Hartsough, C. S., & Lambert, N. M. (1999). Childhood conduct problems, hyperactivity–impulsivity, and inattention as predictors of adult criminal activity. *Journal of Child Psychology and Psychiatry, 40*, 347–355.

Bada, H. S., Bauer, C. R., Shankaran, S., Lester, B., Wright, L. L., Verter, J., Smeriglio, V. L., Finnegan, L. P., & Maza, P. L. (1998). Central and autonomic nervous systems; signs associated with *in utero* exposure to cocaine/opiates. *Annals of the New York Academy of Sciences, 846*, 431–434.

Bagley, C. (1992). Maternal smoking and deviant behavior in 16–year-olds: A personality hypothesis. *Personality and Individual Differences, 13*, 377–378.

Bandura, A. (1973). *Aggression: A social learning analysis.* Englewood Cliffs, NJ: Prentice-Hall.

Bank, L., Marlow, J. H., Reid, J. B., Patterson, G. R., & Weinrott, M. R. (1991). A comparative evaluation of parent training interventions for families of chronic delinquents. *Journal of Abnormal Child Psychology, 19*, 15–33.

Banks, T., & Dabbs, J. M. (1996). Salivary testosterone and cortisol in a delinquent and violent urban subculture. *Journal of Social Psychology, 136*, 49–56.

Bardone, A. M., Moffitt, T. E., Caspi, A., Dickson, N., & Silva, P. A. (1996). Adult mental health and social outcomes of adolescent girls with depression and conduct disorder. *Developmental Psychopathology, 8*, 811–829.

Bardone, A. M., Moffitt, T. E., Caspi, A., Dickson, N., Stanton, W. R., & Silva, P. (1998). Adult physical health outcomes of adolescent girls with conduct disorder, depression, and anxiety. *Journal of the American Academy of Child and Adolescent Psychiatry, 37*, 594–601.

Barkley, R. A. (1987). *Defiant children: A clinician's manual for parent training.* New York: Guilford Press.

Barkley, R. A. (1996). Attention-deficit hyperactivity disorder. In E. J. Mash & R. A. Barkley (Eds.), *Child psychopathology* (pp. 63–112). New York: Guilford Press.

Barkley, R. A. (1997a). Behavioral inhibition, sustained attention, and executive functions: Constructing a unifying theory of ADHD. *Psychological Bulletin, 121*, 65–94.

Barkley, R. A. (1997b). *Defiant children: A clinician's manual for assessment and parent training* (2nd ed.). New York: Guilford Press.

Barkley, R. A. (1998). *Attention-deficit hyperactivity disorder: A handbook for diagnosis and treatment* (2nd ed.). New York: Guilford Press.

Barkley, R. A., DuPaul, G. J., & Connor, D. F. (1999). Stimulants. In J. S. Werry & M. G. Aman (Eds.), *Practitioner's guide to psychoactive drugs for children and adolescents* (2nd ed., pp. 213–247). New York: Plenum Press.

Barkley, R. A., Fischer, M., Edelbrock, C. S., & Smallish, L. (1990). The adolescent outcome of hyperactive children diagnosed by research criteria: I. An 8 year prospective follow-up study. *Journal of the American Academy of Child and Adolescent Psychiatry, 29*, 546–557.

Barkley, R. A., Guevremont, D. C., Anastopoulos, A. D., & Fletcher, K. E. (1993). A comparison of three family therapy programs for treating family conflicts in adolescents with attention-deficit hyperactivity disorder. *Journal of Consulting and Clinical Psychology, 60*, 450–462.

Barkley, R. A., McMurray, M. B., Edelbrock, C. S., & Robbins, K. (1989). The response of aggressive and nonaggressive ADHD children to two doses of methylphenidate. *Journal of the American Academy of Child and Adolescent Psychiatry, 28*, 873–881.

Barrickman, L. L., Perry, P. J., Allen, A. J., Kuperman, S., Arndt, S. V., Herrmann, K. J., & Schumacher, E. (1995). Bupropion versus methylphenidate in the treatment of attention-deficit hyperactivity disorder. *Journal of the American Academy of Child and Adolescent Psychiatry, 34,* 649–657.

Barton, C., Alexander, J. F., Waldron, H., Turner, C. W., & Warburton, J. (1985). Generalizing treatment effect of functional family therapy: Three replications. *American Journal of Family Therapy, 13,* 16–26.

Bartusch, D. R. J., Lynam, D. R., Moffitt, T. E., & Silva, P. A. (1997). Is age important?: Testing a general versus developmental theory of antisocial behavior. *Criminology, 35,* 13–48.

Bates, J. E., Pettit, G. S., Dodge, K. A., & Ridge, B. (1998). Interaction of temperamental resistance to control and restrictive parenting in the development of externalizing behavior. *Developmental Psychology, 34,* 982–995.

Bauer, L. O., & Hesselbrock, V. M. (1999). P300 decrements in teenagers with conduct problems: Implications for substance abuse risk and brain development. *Biological Psychiatry, 46,* 263–272.

Bauermeister, J. J., Canino, G., & Bird, H. (1994). Epidemiology of disruptive behavior disorders. *Child and Adolescent Psychiatric Clinics of North America, 3,* 177–194.

Beaumont, J. G. (1983). *Introduction to neuropsychology.* New York: Guilford Press.

Becker, D. F., Grilo, C. M., Morey, L. C., Walker, M. L., Edell, W. S., & McGlashan, T. H. (1999). Applicability of personality disorder criteria to hospitalized adolescents: Evaluation of internal consistency and criterion overlap. *Journal of the American Academy of Child and Adolescent Psychiatry, 38,* 200–205.

Behnke, M., Davis Eyler, F., Conlon, M., Wobie, K., Stewart Woods, N., & Cumming, W. (1998). Incidence and description of structural brain abnormalities in newborns exposed to cocaine. *Journal of Pediatrics, 132,* 291–294.

Bellinger, D. C. (1995). Interpreting the literature on lead and child development: The neglected role of the "experimental system." *Neurotoxicology and Teratology, 17,* 201–212.

Bellinger, D. C., & Dietrich, K. N. (1994). Low-level lead exposure and cognitive function in children. *Pediatric Annals, 23,* 600–605.

Bellinger, D. C., Leviton, A., Allred, E., & Rabinowitz, M. (1994). Pre- and postnatal lead exposure and behavior problems in school-aged children. *Environmental Research, 66,* 12–30.

Benjamin, S. (1999). A neuropsychiatric approach to aggressive behavior. In F. Ovsiew (Ed.), *Neuropsychiatry and mental health services* (pp. 149–196). Washington, DC: American Psychiatric Press.

Benton, A. L. (1991). Prefrontal injury and behavior in children. *Developmental Neuropsychology, 7,* 275–281.

Berenbaum, S. A., & Resnick, S. M. (1997). Early androgen effects on aggression in children and adults with congenital adrenal hyperplasia. *Psychoneuroendocrinology, 22,* 505–515.

Berkowitz, L. (1993). *Aggression: Its causes, consequences and control.* New York: Academic Press.

Berkowitz, L. (1994). Guns and youth. In L. D. Eron, J. H. Gentry, & P. Schlegel (Eds.), *Reason to hope: A psychosocial perspective on violence and youth* (pp. 251–279). Washington, DC: American Psychological Association.

Berman, S. L., Kurtines, W. M., Silverman, W. K., & Serafini, L. T. (1996). The impact of exposure to crime and violence on urban youth. *American Journal of Ortho-psychiatry, 66,* 329–336.

Bernstein, D. P., Cohen, P., Skodol, A., Bezirganian, S., & Brook, J. S. (1996). Childhood antecedents of adolescent personality disorders. *American Journal of Psychiatry, 153,* 907–913.

Bernstein, D. P., Cohen, P., Velez, C. N., Schwab-Stone, M., Siever, L. J., & Shinsato, L. (1993). Prevalence and stability of the DSM-III-R personality disorders in a community-based survey of adolescents. *American Journal of Psychiatry, 150,* 1237–1243.

Bernstein, G. A., & Borchardt, C. M. (1991). Anxiety disorders in childhood and adolescence: A critical review. *Journal of the American Academy of Child and Adolescent Psychiatry, 30,* 519–532.

Bernstein, G. A., Borchardt, C. M., & Perwien, A. R. (1996). Anxiety disorders in children and adolescents: A review of the past 10 years. *Journal of the American Academy of Child and Adolescent Psychiatry, 35,* 1110–1119.

Berrueta-Clement, J. R., Schweinhart, L. J., Barnett, W. S., Epstein, A. S., & Weikart, D. P. (1984). *Changed lives: The effects of the Perry Preschool Program on youths through age 19.* Ypsilanti, MI: High/Scope Press.

Berrueta-Clement, J. R., Schweinhart, L. J., Barnett, W. S., & Weikart, D. P. (1987). The effects of early educational intervention on crime and delinquency in adolescence and early adulthood. In J. D. Burchard & S. N. Burchard (Eds.), *Primary prevention of psychopathology: Vol. 10. Prevention of delinquent behavior* (pp. 220–240). Newbury Park, CA: Sage.

Bickman, L. (1997). Resolving issues raised by the Fort Bragg evaluation: New directions for mental health services research. *American Psychologist, 52,* 562–565.

Bickman, L., Guthrie, P. R., Foster, E. M., Lambert, E. W., Summerfelt, W. T., Breda, C. S., & Heflinger, C. A. (1995). *Evaluating managed mental health services: The Fort Bragg experiment.* New York: Plenum Press.

Bickman, L., Lambert, W., Andrade, A. R., & Penaloza, R. V. (2000). The Fort Bragg continuum of care for children and adolescents: Mental health outcomes over 5 years. *Journal of Consulting and Clinical Psychology, 68,* 710–716.

Biederman, J., Baldessarini, R. J., Wright, V., Keenan, K., & Faraone, S. (1993). A double-blind placebo controlled study of desipramine in the treatment of ADD: III. Lack of impact of comorbidity and family history factors on clinical response. *Journal of the American Academy of Child and Adolescent Psychiatry, 32,* 199–204.

Biederman, J., Faraone, S., Mick, E., & Lelon, E. (1995). Psychiatric comorbidity among referred juveniles with major depression: Fact or artifact? *Journal of the American Academy of Child and Adolescent Psychiatry, 34,* 579–590.

Biederman, J., Faraone, S. V., & Lapey, K. (1992). Comorbidity of diagnosis in attention-deficit hyperactivity disorder. *Child and Adolescent Psychiatric Clinics of North America, 2,* 335–360.

Biederman, J., Faraone, S. V., Chu, M. P., & Wozniak, J. (1999). Further evidence of a bidirectional overlap between juvenile mania and conduct disorder in children. *Journal of the American Academy of Child and Adolescent Psychiatry, 38,* 468–476.

Biederman, J., Faraone, S. V., Mick, E., Williamson, S., Wilens, T. E., Spencer, T. J., Weber, W., Jetton, J., Kraus, I., Pert, J., & Zallen, B. (1999). Clinical correlates of ADHD in females: Findings from a large group of girls ascertained from pediatric and psychiatric referral sources. *Journal of the American Academy of Child and Adolescent Psychiatry, 38,* 966–975.

Biederman, J., Mick, E., Bostic, J. Q., Prince, J., Daly, J., Wilens, T. E., Spencer, T., Garcia-Jetton, J., Russell, R., Wozniak, J., & Faraone, S. V. (1998). The naturalistic course of pharmacologic treatment of children with maniclike symptoms: A systematic chart review. *Journal of Clinical Psychiatry, 59,* 628–637.

Biederman, J., Mick, E., Faraone, S. V., & Burback, M. (2001). Patterns of remission and symptom decline in conduct disorder: A four-year prospective study of an ADHD sample. *Journal of the American Academy of Child and Adolescent Psychiatry, 40,* 290–298.

Biederman, J., Newcorn, J., & Sprich, S. (1991). Comorbidity of attention deficit hyperactivity disorder with conduct, depressive, anxiety, and other disorders. *American Journal of Psychiatry, 148,* 564–577.

Biederman, J., & Spencer, T. (1999). Depressive disorders in childhood and adolescence: A clinical perspective. *Journal of Child and Adolescent Psychopharmacology, 9,* 233–237.

Bird, H. R., Canino, G., Rubio-Stipec, M., Gould, M. S., Ribera, J., Sesman, M., Woodbury, M., Huertas-Goldman, S., Pagan, A., Sanchez-Lacay, A., Moscoso, M. (1988). Estimates of the prevalence of childhood maladjustment in a community survey in Puerto Rico. *Archives of General Psychiatry, 45,* 1120–1126.

Birmaher, B., Ryan, N. D., Williamson, D. E., Brent, D. A., Kaufman, J., Dahl, R. E., Perel, J., & Nelson, B. (1996). Childhood and adolescent depression: A review of the past 10 years. Part I. *Journal of the American Academy of Child and Adolescent Psychiatry, 35,* 1427–1439.

Birmaher, B., Stanley, M., Greenhill, L., Twomey, J., Gavrilescu, A., & Rabinovich, H. (1990). Platelet imipramine binding in children and adolescents with impulsive behavior. *Journal of the American Academy of Child and Adolescent Psychiatry, 29,* 914–918.

Birmaher, B., Waterman, G. S., Ryan, N., Cully, M., Balach, L., Ingram, J., & Brodsky, M. (1994). Fluoxetine for childhood anxiety disorders. *Journal of the American Academy of Child and Adolescent Psychiatry, 33,* 993–999.

Bjorkqvist, K., Osterman, K., & Kaukiainen, A. (1992). The development of direct and indirect aggressive strategies in males and females. In K. Bjorkqvist & P. Niemela (Eds.), *Of mice and women: Aspects of female aggression* (pp. 51–64). San Diego, CA: Academic Press.

Black, B., & Uhde, T. W. (1994). Treatment of elective mutism with fluoxetine: A double-blind, placebo-controlled study. *Journal of the American Academy of Child and Adolescent Psychiatry, 33,* 1000–1006.

Blais, M. A., Hilsenroth, M. J., & Castlebury, F. D. (1997). Content validity of the DSM-IV borderline and narcissistic personality disorder criteria sets. *Comprehensive Psychiatry, 38,* 31–37.

Blanchard, R. J., & Blanchard, D. C. (1984). Affect and aggression: An animal model applied to human behavior. In R. J. Blanchard & D. C. Blanchard (Eds.), *Advances in the study of aggression* (pp. 1–62). New York: Academic Press.

Block, J. H., Block, J., & Gjerde, P. F. (1986). The personality of children prior to divorce. *Child Development, 57,* 827–840.

Blumberg, S. H., & Izard, C. E. (1985). Affective and cognitive characteristics of depression in 10- and 11-year-old children. *Journal of Personality and Social Psychology, 49,* 194–202.

Blumensohn, R., Ratzoni, G., Weizman, A., Israeli, M., Greuner, N., Apter, A., Tyano, S., & Biegon, A. (1995). Reduction in serotonin 5HT$_2$ receptor binding on platelets of delinquent adolescents. *Psychopharmacology, 118,* 354–356.

Bohman, M. (1996). Predisposition to criminality: Swedish adoption studies in retrospect. In G. R. Brock & J. A. Goode (Eds.), *Ciba Foundation Symposium No. 194: Genetics of criminal and antisocial behavior* (pp. 99–114). Chichester, England: Wiley.

Boll, T. J., Williams, M. A., Kashden, J. L., & Putzke, J. D. (1998). Examination: III. Neuropsychological testing. In C. E. Coffey & R. A. Brumback (Eds.), *Textbook of pediatric neuropsychiatry* (pp. 221–252). Washington, DC: American Psychiatric Press.

Booth, R. E., & Zhang, Y. (1996). Severe aggression and related conduct problems among runaway and homeless adolescents. *Psychiatric Services, 47,* 75–80.

Booth, R. E., & Zhang, Y. (1997). Conduct disorder and HIV risk behaviors among runaway and homeless adolescents. *Drug and Alcohol Dependence, 48,* 69–76.

Borduin, C. M. (1999). Multisystemic treatment of criminality and violence in adolescents. *Journal of the American Academy of Child and Adolescent Psychiatry, 38,* 242–249.

Bowden, C. L., Deutsch, C. K., & Swanson, J. M. (1988). Plasma dopamine-ß-hydroxylase and platelet monoamine oxidase in attention deficit disorder and conduct disorder. *Journal of the American Academy of Child and Adolescent Psychiatry, 27,* 171–174.

Bowlby, J. (1969). *Attachment and loss: Vol. 1. Attachment.* New York: Basic Books.

Bowring, M. A., & Kovacs, M. (1992). Difficulties in diagnosing manic disorders among children and adolescents. *Journal of the American Academy of Child and Adolescent Psychiatry, 31,* 611–614.

Brady, K. T., Myrick, H., & McElroy, S. (1998). The relationship between substance use disorders, impulse control disorders, and pathological aggression. *American Journal on Addictions, 7,* 221–230.

Bremner, J. D., Randall, P., Vermetten, E., Staib, L., Bronen, R. A., Mazure, C., Capelli, S., McCarthy, G., Innis, R. B., & Charney, D. S. (1997). Magnetic resonance imaging-based measurement of hippocampal volume in posttraumatic stress disorder related to childhood physical and sexual abuse: A preliminary report. *Biological Psychiatry, 41,* 23–32.

Brener, N. D., Simon, T. R., Krug, E. G., & Lowry, R. (1999). Recent trends in violence-related behaviors among high school students in the United States. *Journal of the American Medical Association, 282,* 440–446.

Brennan, P. A., Grekin, E. R., & Mednick, S. A. (1999). Maternal smoking during pregnancy and adult male criminal outcomes. *Archives of General Psychiatry, 56,* 215–219.

Brennan, P. A., Mednick, S. A., & Hodgins, S. (2000). Major mental disorders and criminal violence in a Danish birth cohort. *Archives of General Psychiatry, 57,* 494–500.

Brennan, P. A., & Raine, A. (1997). Biosocial bases of antisocial behavior: Psychophysiological, neurological, and cognitive factors. *Clinical Psychology Review, 17,* 589–604.

Brennan, P. A., Raine, A., Schulsinger, F., Kirkegaard-Sorensen, L., Knop, J., Hutchings, B., Rosenberg, R., & Mednick, S. A. (1997). Psychophysiological protective factors for male subjects at high risk for criminal behavior. *American Journal of Psychiatry, 154,* 853–855.

Brent, D. A., Johnson, B., Bartle, S., Bridge, J., Rather, C., Matta, J., Connolly, J., & Constantine, D. (1993). Personality disorder, tendency to impulsive violence, and suicidal behavior in adolescents. *Journal of the American Academy of Child and Adolescent Psychiatry, 32,* 65–79.

Brent, D. A., Johnson, B. A., Perper, J., Connolly, J., Bridge, J., Bartle, S., & Rather, C. (1994). Personality disorder, personality traits, impulsive violence, and completed suicide in adolescents. *Journal of the American Academy of Child and Adolescent Psychiatry, 33,* 1080–1086.

Brent, D. A., Perper, J. A., & Allman, C. J. (1987). Alcohol, firearms, and suicide among youth: Temporal trends in Allegheny County, Pennsylvania 1960 to 1983. *Journal of the American Medical Association, 257,* 3369–3372.

Brent, D. A., Perper, J. A., Moritz, G., Baugher, M., Schweers, J., & Roth, C. (1994). Suicide in affectively ill adolescents: A case–control study. *Journal of Affective Disorders, 31,* 193–202.

Breslau, N., Davis, G. C., & Andreski, P. (1995). Risk factors for PTSD-related traumatic events: A prospective analysis. *American Journal of Psychiatry, 152,* 529–535.

Brestan, E. V., & Eyberg, S. M. (1998). Effective psychosocial treatments of conduct-disordered children and adolescents: 29 years, 82 studies, and 5,272 kids. *Journal of Clinical Child Psychology, 27,* 180–189.

Brier, N. (1995). Predicting antisocial behavior in youngsters displaying poor academic achievement: A review of risk factors. *Journal of Developmental and Behavioral Pediatrics, 16,* 271–276.

Briere, J., & Gil, E. (1998). Self-mutilation in clinical and general population samples: Prevalence, correlates, and functions. *American Journal of Orthopsychiatry, 68,* 609–620.

Brodsky, B. S., Malone, K. M., Ellis, S. P., Dulit, R. A., & Mann, J. J. (1997). Characteristics of borderline personality disorder associated with suicidal behavior. *American Journal of Psychiatry, 154,* 1715–1719.

Brook, J. S., Whiteman, M., & Finch, S. (1993). Role of mutual attachment in drug use: A longitudinal study. *Journal of the American Academy of Child and Adolescent Psychiatry, 32,* 982–989.

Brook, J. S., Whiteman, M., Finch, S., & Cohen, P. (1995). Aggression, intrapsychic distress, and drug use: Antecedent and intervening processes. *Journal of the American Academy of Child and Adolescent Psychiatry, 34,* 1076–1084.

Brook, J. S., Whiteman, M., Finch, S. J., & Cohen, P. (1996). Young adult drug use and delinquency: Childhood antecedents and adolescent mediators. *Journal of the American Academy of Child and Adolescent Psychiatry, 35,* 1584–1592.

Brooks, J. H., & Reddon, J. R. (1996). Serum testosterone in violent and nonviolent young offenders. *Journal of Clinical Psychology, 52,* 475–483.

Brooks-Gunn, J., & Warren, M. P. (1989). Biological and social contributions to negative affect in young adolescent girls. *Child Development, 60,* 40–55.

Brown, G., Chadwick, O., Shaffer, D., Rutter, M., & Traub, M. (1981). A prospective study of children with head injuries: III. Psychiatric sequelae. *Psychological Medicine, 11,* 63–78.

Brown, G. L., Ebert, M. H., Goyer, P. F., Jimerson, D. C., Klein, W. J., Bunney, W. E., & Goodwin, F. K. (1982). Aggression, suicide, and serotonin: Relationships to CSF amine metabolites. *American Journal of Psychiatry, 139,* 741–746.

Brown, K., Atkins, M. S., Osborne, M. L., & Milnamow, M. (1996). A revised teacher rating scale for reactive and proactive aggression. *Journal of Abnormal Child Psychology, 24,* 473–480.

Brown, S. A., Gleghorn, A., Schuckit, M., Myers, M. G., & Mott, M. A. (1996). Conduct disorder among adolescent substance abusers. *Journal of Studies on Alcohol, 57,* 314–324.

Brunner, H. G., Nelen, M., Breakefield, X. O., Ropers, H. H., & van Oost, B. A. (1993). Abnormal behavior associated with a point mutation in the structural gene for monoamine oxidase A. *Science, 262,* 578.

Bruun, R. D., & Budman, C. L. (1998). Paroxetine treatment of episodic rages associated with Tourette's disorder. *Journal of Clinical Psychiatry, 59,* 581–584.

Buitelaar, J. K. (2000). Open-label treatment with risperidone of 26 psychiatrically-hospitalized children and adolescents with mixed diagnoses and aggressive behavior. *Journal of Child and Adolescent Psychopharmacology, 10,* 19–26.

Buitelaar, J. K., van der Gaag, J., Swaab-Barneveld, H., & Kuiper, M. (1996). Pindolol and methylphenidate in children with attention-deficit hyperactivity disorder: Clinical efficacy and side-effects. *Journal of Child Psychology and Psychiatry, 37,* 587–595.

Bukstein, O. G. (1996). Aggression, violence, and substance abuse in adolescents. *Child and Adolescent Psychiatric Clinics of North America, 5,* 93–109.

Bukstein, O. G., Brent, D. A., & Kaminer, Y. (1989). Comorbidity of substance abuse and other psychiatric disorders in adolescents. *American Journal of Psychiatry, 146,* 1131–1141.

Bukstein, O. G., Glancy, L. J., & Kaminer, Y. (1992). Patterns of affective comorbidity in a clinical population of dually diagnosed adolescent substance abusers. *Journal of the American Academy of Child and Adolescent Psychiatry, 31,* 1041–1045.

Bukstein, O. G., & Kolko, D. J. (1998). Effects of methylphenidate on aggressive urban children with attention deficit hyperactivity disorder. *Journal of Clinical Child Psychology, 27,* 340–351.

Bureau of Justice Statistics. (2000). *Criminal victimization in the United States, 1997.* Washington, DC: U. S. Department of Justice.

Burns, J. M., Baghurst, P. A., Sawyer, M. G., McMichael, A. J., & Tong, S. (1999). Lifetime low-level exposure to environmental lead and children's emotional and behavioral development at ages 11–13 years. *American Journal of Epidemiology, 149,* 740–749.

Buss, A. H., & Durkee, A. (1957). An inventory for assessing different kinds of hostility. *Journal of Consulting Psychology, 21,* 343–349.

Butts, J. A., Snyder, H. N., Finnegan, T. A., Augheobaugh, A. L., Tierney, J. J., Sullivan, D. P., & Poole, R. S. (1995). *Juvenile court statistics: 1992.* Washington, DC: Office of Juvenile Justice and Delinquency Prevention.

Caceres, C., & Burns, J. W. (1997). Cardiovascular reactivity to psychological stress may enhance subsequent pain sensitivity. *Pain, 69,* 237–244.

Cadoret, R. J., Cain, C. A., & Crowe, R. R. (1983). Evidence for gene–environment interaction in the development of adolescent antisocial behavior. *Behavior Genetics, 13,* 301–310.

Cadoret, R. J., Yates, W. R., Troughton, E., Woodworth, G., & Stewart, M. A. (1995). Genetic–environmental interaction in the genesis of aggressivity and conduct disorders. *Archives of General Psychiatry, 52,* 916–924.

Cairns, R. B., & Cairns, B. D. (1984). Predicting aggressive patterns in girls and boys: A developmental study. *Aggressive Behavior, 10,* 227–242.

Cairns, R. B., & Cairns, B. D. (1986). The developmental–interactional view of social behavior: Four issues of adolescent aggression. In D. Olweus, J. Block, & M. Radke-Yarrow (Eds.), *Development of antisocial and prosocial behavior: Research, theories, and issues* (pp. 315–342). New York: Academic Press.

Cairns, R. B., Cairns, B. D., Neckerman, H. J., Ferguson, L. L., & Gariepy, L. -L. (1989). Growth and aggression: 1. Childhood to early adolescence. *Developmental Psychology, 25,* 320–330.

Calhoun, G., Jurgens, J., & Chen, F. (1993). The neophyte female delinquent: A review of the literature. *Adolescence, 28,* 461–471.

Campbell, M., Adams, P. B., Small, A. M., Kafantaris, V., Silva, R. R., Shell, J., Perry, R., Overall, J. E. (1995). Lithium in hospitalized aggressive children with conduct disorder: A double-blind and placebo-controlled study. *Journal of the American Academy of Child and Adolescent Psychiatry, 34,* 445–453.

Campbell, M., & Cueva, J. E. (1995a). Psychopharmacology in child and adolescent psychiatry: A review of the past seven years. Part I. *Journal of the American Academy of Child and Adolescent Psychiatry, 34,* 1124–1132.

Campbell, M., & Cueva, J. E. (1995b). Psychopharmacology in child and adolescent psychiatry: A review of the past seven years. Part II. *Journal of the American Academy of Child and Adolescent Psychiatry, 34,* 1262–1272.

Campbell, M., Gonzalez, N. M., & Silva, R. R. (1992). The pharmacologic treatment of conduct disorders and rage outbursts. *Psychiatric Clinics of North America, 15,* 69–85.

Campbell, M., Gonzalez, N. M., Ernst, M., Silva, R. R., & Werry, J. S. (1993). Antipsychotics (neuroleptics). In J. S. Werry & M. G. Aman (Eds.), *Practitioner's guide to psychoactive drugs for children and adolescents* (pp. 269–296). New York: Plenum Press.

Campbell, M., Kafantaris, V., & Cueva, J. E. (1995). An update on the use of lithium carbonate in aggressive children and adolescents with conduct disorder. *Psychopharmacology Bulletin, 31,* 93–102.

Campbell, M., Rapoport, J. L., & Simpson, G. M. (1999). Antipsychotics in children and adolescents. *Journal of the American Academy of Child and Adolescent Psychiatry, 38,* 537–545.

Campbell, M., Small, A. M., Green, W. H., Jennings, S. J., Perry, R., Bennett, W. G., & Anderson, L. (1984). Behavioral efficacy of haloperidol and lithium carbonate. *Archives of General Psychiatry, 41,* 650–656.

Campbell, M., Small, A. M., Green, W. H., Jennings, S. J., Perry, R., Bennett, W. G., Padron-Gayol, M., & Anderson, L. (1982). Lithium and haloperidol in hospitalized aggressive children. *Psychopharmacology Bulletin, 18,* 126–130.

Campbell, S. B. (1991). Longitudinal studies of active and aggressive preschoolers: Individual differences in early behavior and outcome. In D. Cicchetti & S. L. Toth (Eds.), *Rochester Symposium on Developmental Psychopathology: Vol. 2. Internalizing and externalizing expressions of dysfunction* (pp. 57–90). Hillsdale, NJ: Erlbaum.

Campbell, S. B., & Ewing, L. J. (1990). Follow-up of hard-to-manage preschoolers: Adjustment at age 9 and predictors of continuing symptoms. *Journal of Child Psychology and Psychiatry, 31,* 871–889.

Campbell, S. B., Breaux, A. M., Ewing, L. J., & Szumowski, E. K. (1986). Correlates and predictors of hyperactivity and aggression: A longitudinal study of parent-referred problem preschoolers. *Journal of Abnormal Child Psychology, 14,* 217–234.

Cantor, J. (2000). Media violence. *Journal of Adolescent Health, 27*(Suppl.), 30–34.

Cantwell, D. P., & Baker, L. (1984). Parental mental illness and psychiatric disorders in "at risk" children. *Journal of Clinical Psychiatry, 45*, 503–507.

Capaldi, D. M., & Patterson, G. R. (1994). Interrelated influences of contextual factors on antisocial behavior in childhood and adolescence for males. In D. C. Fowles, P. Sutker, & S. H. Goodman (Eds.), *Progress in experimental personality and psychopathology research* (pp. 165–198). New York: Springer.

Caplan, R. (1994). Thought disorder in childhood. *Journal of the American Academy of Child and Adolescent Psychiatry, 33*, 605–615.

Caplan, R., Arabelle, S., Guthrie, D., Komo, S., Shields, W. D., Hansen, R., & Chayasirisobhon, S. (1997). Formal thought disorder and psychopathology in pediatric primary generalized and complex partial epilepsy. *Journal of the American Academy of Child and Adolescent Psychiatry, 36*, 1286–1294.

Caplan, R., Guthrie, D., Fish, B., Tanguay, P. E., & David-Lando, G. (1989). The Kiddie Formal Thought Disorder Rating Scale (K-FTDS): Clinical assessment, reliability, and validity. *Journal of the American Academy of Child and Adolescent Psychiatry, 28*, 208–216.

Caplan, R., Guthrie, D., Tang, B., Komo, S., & Asarnow, R. F. (2000). Thought disorder in childhood schizophrenia: Replication and update of concept. *Journal of the American Academy of Child and Adolescent Psychiatry, 39*, 771–778.

Caplan, R., Perdue, S., Tanguay, P. E., & Fish, B. (1990). Formal thought disorder in childhood onset schizophrenia and schizotypal personality disorder. *Journal of Child Psychology and Psychiatry, 31*, 169–177.

Caplan, R., & Tanguay, P. E. (1991). Development of psychotic thinking in children. In M. Lewis (Ed.), *Child and adolescent psychiatry: A comprehensive textbook* (pp. 310–330). Baltimore: Williams & Wilkins.

Carlson, E. A. (1998). A prospective longitudinal study of attachment disorganization/disorientation. *Child Development, 69*, 1107–1128.

Carlson, G. A. (1990). Child and adolescent mania: Diagnostic considerations. *Journal of Child Psychology and Psychiatry, 31*, 331–342.

Caron, C., & Rutter, M. (1991). Comorbidity in child psychopathology: Concepts, issues, and research strategies. *Journal of Child Psychology and Psychiatry, 32*, 1063–1080.

Casat, C. D., Pearson, D. A., Van Davelaar, M. J., & Cherek, D. R. (1995). Methylphenidate effects on a laboratory aggression measure in children with ADHD. *Psychopharmacology Bulletin, 31*, 353–356.

Casat, C. D., Pleasants, D. Z., & Van Wyck Fleet, J. (1987). A double-blind trial of bupropion in children with attention deficit disorder. *Psychopharmacology Bulletin, 23*, 120–122.

Caspi, A., Henry, B., McGee, R. O., Moffitt, T. E., & Silva, P. A. (1995). Temperamental origins of child and adolescent behavior problems: From age three to age fifteen. *Child Development, 66*, 55–68.

Caspi, A., Lynam, D., Moffitt, T. E., & Silva, P. A. (1993). Unraveling girls' delinquency: Biological, dispositional, and contextual contributions to adolescent misbehavior. *Developmental Psychology, 29*, 19–30.

Caspi, A., & Moffitt, T. E. (1991). Individual differences are accentuated during periods of social change: The sample case of girls at puberty. *Journal of Personality and Social Psychology, 61*, 157–168.

Caspi, A., Moffitt, T. E., Newman, D. L., & Silva, P. A. (1996). Behavioral observations at age 3 years predict adult psychiatric disorders. Longitudinal evidence from a birth cohort. *Archives of General Psychiatry, 53*, 1033–1039.

Caspi, A., & Silva, P. A. (1995). Temperamental qualities at age three predict personality traits in young adulthood: Longitudinal evidence from a birth cohort. *Child Development, 66*, 486–498.

Castellanos, F. X., Elia, J., Kruesi, M. J. P., Gulotta, C. S., Mefford, I. N., Potter, W. Z., Ritchie, G. F., & Rapoport, J. L. (1994). Cerebrospinal fluid monoamine metabolites in boys with attention-deficit hyperactivity disorder. *Psychiatry Research, 52*, 305–316.

Castellanos, F. X., Giedd, J. N., Berquin, P. C., Walther, J. M., Sharp, W., Tran, T., Vaituzis, A. C., Blumenthal, J. D., Nelson, J., Bastain, T. M., Zijdenbos, A., Evans, A. C., & Rapoport, J. L. (2001). Quantitative brain magnetic resonance imaging in girls with attention-deficit/hyperactivity disorder. *Archives of General Psychiatry, 58*, 289–295.

Castillo Mezzich, A., Tarter, R. E., Giancola, P. R., Lu, S., Kirisci, L., & Parks, S. (1997). Substance use and risky sexual behavior in female adolescents. *Drug and Alcohol Dependence, 44*, 157–166.

Cauffman, E., Feldman, S., Waterman, J., & Steiner, H. (1998). Posttraumatic stress disorder among female juvenile offenders. *Journal of the American Academy of Child and Adolescent Psychiatry, 37*, 1209–1216.

Centers for Disease Control (CDC). (1991). *Preventing lead poisoning in young children: A statement by the Centers for Disease Control.* Atlanta, GA: Author.

Centers for Disease Control (CDC). (1996a). Population-based prevalence of perinatal exposure to cocaine—Georgia, 1994. *Morbidity and Mortality Weekly Report, 45*, 887–891.

Centers for Disease Control and Prevention (CDC). (1996b). Youth risk behavior surveillance system, 1995. *Morbidity and Mortality Weekly Report, 45*(SS-4), 29–41.

Chambers, W. J., Puig-Antich, J., Hirsch, M., Paez, P., Ambrosini, P. J., Tabrizi, M. A., & Davies, M. (1985). The assessment of affective disorders in children and adolescents by semi-structured interview: Test–retest reliability of the Schedule for Affective Disorders and Schizophrenia for School-Aged Children, Present Episode. *Archives of General Psychiatry, 42*, 696–702.

Chappell, P. B., Riddle, M. A., Scahill, L., Lynch, K. A., Schultz, R., Arnsten, A., Leckman, J. F., & Cohen, D. J. (1995). Guanfacine treatment of comorbid attention-deficit hyperactivity disorder and Tourette's syndrome: Preliminary clinical experience. *Journal of the American Academy of Child and Adolescent Psychiatry, 34*, 1140–1146.

Charney, D. S., Deutch, A. Y., Krystal, J. H., Southwick, S. M., & Davis, M. (1993). Psychobiological mechanisms of posttraumatic stress disorder. *Archives of General Psychiatry, 50*, 294–305.

Charney, D. S., Grillon, C., & Bremner, J. D. (1998). The neurobiological basis of anxiety and fear: Circuits, mechanisms, and neurochemical interactions (Part I). *The Neuroscientist, 1*, 35–44.

Chasnoff, I. J., Anson, A., Hatcher, R., Stenson, H., Iaukea, K., & Randolph, L. A. (1998). Prenatal exposure to cocaine and other drugs: Outcome at four to six years. *Annals of the New York Academy of Sciences, 846*, 314–328.

Chermack, S. T., & Giancola, P. R. (1997). The relation between alcohol and aggression: An integrated biopsychosocial conceptualization. *Clinical Psychology Review, 17*, 621–649.

Chess, S., & Thomas, A. (1986). *Temperament in clinical practice*. New York: Guilford Press.

Chiriboga, C. A. (1998). Neurological correlates of fetal cocaine exposure. *Annals of the New York Academy of Sciences, 846,* 109–125.

Chiriboga, C. A., Brust, J. C., Bateman, D., & Hauser, W. A. (1999). Dose–response effect of fetal cocaine exposure on newborn neurologic function. *Pediatrics, 103,* 79–85.

Choquet, M., Menke, H., & Manfredi, R. (1991). Interpersonal aggressive behavior and alcohol consumption among young urban adolescents in France. *Alcohol and Alcoholism: International Journal of the Medical Council on Alcoholism, 26,* 381–390.

Christian, R. E., Frick, P. J., Hill, N. L., Tyler, L., & Frazier, D. R. (1997). Psychopathy and conduct problems in children: II. Implications for subtyping children with conduct problems. *Journal of the American Academy of Child and Adolescent Psychiatry, 36,* 233–241.

Christoffel, K. K. (1997). Firearm injuries affecting U. S. children and adolescents. In J. D. Osofsky (Ed.), *Children in a violent society* (pp. 42–71). New York: Guilford Press.

Cicchetti, D. (1984). The emergence of developmental psychopathology. *Child Development, 55,* 1–7.

Cicchetti, D., & Lynch, M. (1993). Toward an ecological/transactional model of community violence and child maltreatment: Consequences for children's development. In D. Reiss, J. E. Richters, M. Radke-Yarrow, & D. Scharff (Eds.), *Children and violence* (pp. 96–118). New York: Guilford Press.

Clark, D. B., Pollock, N., Bukstein, O. G., Mezzich, A. C., Bromberger, J. T., & Donovan, J. E. (1997). Gender and comorbid psychopathology in adolescents with alcohol dependence. *Journal of the American Academy of Child and Adolescent Psychiatry, 36,* 1195–1203.

Clark, L. A., Watson, D., & Reynolds, S. (1995). Diagnosis and classification of psychopathology: Challenges to the current system and future directions. *Annual Review of Psychology, 46,* 121–153.

Clarke, R. A., Murphy, D. L., & Constantino, J. N. (1999). Serotonin and externalizing behavior in young children. *Psychiatry Research, 86,* 29–40.

Cleckley, H. (1941). *The mask of sanity*. St. Louis, MO: Mosby.

Cleckley, H. (1950). *The mask of sanity* (2nd ed.). St. Louis, MO: Mosby.

Cleckley, H. (1976). *The mask of sanity* (5th ed.). St. Louis, MO: Mosby.

Cloninger, C. R. (1978). The antisocial personality. *Hospital Practice, 13,* 97–106.

Cloninger, C. R. (1987a). Neurogenetic adaptive mechanisms in alcoholism. *Science, 236,* 410–416.

Cloninger, C. R. (1987b). A systematic method for clinical description and classification of personality variants: A proposal. *Archives of General Psychiatry, 44,* 573–588.

Cloninger, C. R., & Gottesman, I. I. (1987). Genetic and environmental factors in antisocial behavior disorders. In S. A. Mednick, T. E. Moffitt, & S. Stack (Eds.), *The causes of crime: New biological approaches* (pp. 92–109). Cambridge, England: Cambridge University Press.

Cloninger, C. R., & Guze, S. B. (1970). Psychiatric illness and female criminality: The role of sociopathy and hysteria in the antisocial woman. *American Journal of Psychiatry, 127,* 303–311.

Coble, P. A., Taska, L. S., Kupfer, D. J., Kazdin, A. E., Unis, A., & French, N. (1984).

EEG sleep "abnormalities" in preadolescent boys with a diagnosis of conduct disorder. *Journal of the American Academy of Child Psychiatry, 23,* 438–447.

Coccaro, E. F., Kavoussi, R. J., & Hauger, R. L. (1997). Serotonin function and antiaggressive response to fluoxetine: A pilot study. *Biological Psychiatry, 42,* 546–552.

Coccaro, E. F., Kavoussi, R. J., Sheline, Y. I., Berman, M. E., & Csernansky, J. G. (1997). Impulsive aggression in personality disorder correlates with platelet 5–HT2a receptor binding. *Neuropsychopharmacology, 1,* 211–216.

Coccaro, E. F., Siever, L. J., Klar, H. M., Maurer, G., Cochrane, K., Cooper, T. B., Mohs, R. C., & Davis, K. L. (1989). Serotonergic studies in patients with affective and personality disorders. *Archives of General Psychiatry, 46,* 587–599.

Cohen, D., Nisbett, R. E., Bowdle, B. F., & Schwarz, N. (1996). Insult, aggression, and the Southern culture of honor: An "experimental ethnography." *Journal of Personality and Social Psychology, 70,* 945–960.

Cohen, J. (1988). *Statistical power analysis for the behavioral sciences* (2nd ed.). Hillsdale, NJ: Erlbaum.

Cohen, P., Cohen, J., Kasen, S., Velez, C. N., Hartmark, C., Johnson, J., Rojas, M., Brook, J., & Streuning, E. L. (1993). An epidemiological study of disorders in late childhood and adolescence: I. Age and gender-specific prevalence. *Journal of Child Psychiatry and Psychology, 34,* 851–867.

Cohen, P., Velez, N., Kohn, M., Schwab-Stone, M., & Johnson, J. (1987). Child psychiatric diagnosis by computer algorithm: Theoretical issues and empirical tests. *Journal of the American Academy of Child and Adolescent Psychiatry, 26,* 631–638.

Coie, J. D., & Dodge, K. A. (1998). Aggression and antisocial behavior. In W. Damon (Series Ed.) & N. Eisenberg (Vol. Ed.), *Handbook of child psychology* (5th ed.): *Vol. 3. Social, emotional, and personality development* (pp. 779–862). New York: Wiley.

Coie, J. D., Dodge, K. A., & Kupersmidt, J. B. (1990). Peer group behavior and social status. In S. R. Asher & J. D. Coie (Eds.), *Peer rejection in childhood* (pp. 17–59). Cambridge, England: Cambridge University Press.

Commission on Classification and Terminology of the International League Against Epilepsy. (1981). Proposal for revised electroencephalographic classification of epileptic seizures. *Epilepsia, 22,* 489.

Comstock, G. A., & Paik, H. (1994). The effects of television violence on antisocial behavior: A meta-analysis. *Communication Research, 21,* 516–546.

Conduct Problems Prevention Research Group. (1992). A developmental and clinical model for the prevention of conduct disorder: The FAST Track program. *Development and Psychopathology, 4,* 509–527.

Conduct Problems Prevention Research Group. (1999a). Initial impact of the FAST Track prevention trial for conduct problems: I. The high-risk sample. *Journal of Consulting and Clinical Psychology, 67,* 631–647.

Conduct Problems Prevention Research Group. (1999b). Initial impact of the FAST Track prevention trial for conduct problems: II. Classroom effects. *Journal of Consulting and Clinical Psychology, 67,* 648–657.

Conner, K. R., Cox, C., Duberstein, P. R., Tian, L., Nisbet, P. A., & Conwell, Y. (2001). Violence, alcohol, and completed suicide: A case-control study. *American Journal of Psychiatry, 158,* 1701–1705.

Conners, C. K. (1997). *Conners Rating Scales—Revised: Technical manual.* North Tonawanda, NY: Multi-Health Systems.

Conners, C. K., Casat, C. D., Gualtieri, C. T., Weller, E., Reader, M., Reiss, A., Weller, R. A., Khayrallah, M., & Ascher, J. (1996). Bupropion hydrochloride in attention deficit disorder with hyperactivity. *Journal of the American Academy of Child and Adolescent Psychiatry, 35*, 1314–1321.

Connor, D. F. (1993). Beta blockers for aggression: A review of the pediatric experience. *Journal of Child and Adolescent Psychopharmacology, 3*, 99–114.

Connor, D. F., Barkley, R. A., & Davis, H. T. (2000). A pilot study of methylphenidate, clonidine, or the combination in ADHD comorbid with aggressive oppositional defiant or conduct disorder. *Clinical Pediatrics, 39*, 15–25.

Connor, D. F., & Fisher, S. G. (1997). An interactional model of child and adolescent mental health clinical case formulation. *Clinical Child Psychology and Psychiatry, 2*, 353–368.

Connor, D. F., Fletcher, K. E., & Swanson, J. M. (1999). A meta-analysis of clonidine for symptoms of attention-deficit hyperactivity disorder. *Journal of the American Academy of Child and Adolescent Psychiatry, 38*, 1551–1559.

Connor, D. F., Melloni, R. H., Jr., & Harrison, R. J. (1998). Overt categorical aggression in referred children and adolescents. *Journal of the American Academy of Child and Adolescent Psychiatry, 37*, 66–73.

Connor, D. F., Ozbayrak, K. R., Benjamin, S., Ma, Y., & Fletcher, K. E. (1997). A pilot study of nadolol for overt aggression in developmentally delayed individuals. *Journal of the American Academy of Child and Adolescent Psychiatry, 36*, 826–834.

Connor, D. F., Ozbayrak, K. R., Harrison, R. J., & Melloni, R. H., Jr. (1998). Prevalence and patterns of psychotropic and anticonvulsant medication use in children and adolescents referred to residential treatment. *Journal of Child and Adolescent Psychopharmacology, 8*, 27–38.

Connor, D. F., Ozbayrak, K. R., Kusiak, K. A., Caponi, A. B., & Melloni, R. H., Jr. (1997). Combined pharmacotherapy in children and adolescents in a residential treatment center. *Journal of the American Academy of Child and Adolescent Psychiatry, 36*, 248–254.

Connor, D. F., & Steingard, R. J. (1996). A clinical approach to the pharmacotherapy of aggression in children and adolescents. *Annals of the New York Academy of Sciences, 794*, 290–307.

Constantino, J. N. (1995). Early relationships and the development of aggression in children. *Harvard Review of Psychiatry, 2*, 259–273.

Constantino, J. N. (1998). Dominance and aggression over the life course: Timing and direction of causal influences. *Behavioral and Brain Sciences, 21*, 369.

Constantino, J. N., Grosz, D., Saenger, P., Chandler, D. W., Nandi, R., & Earls, F. J. (1993). Testosterone and aggression in children. *Journal of the American Academy of Child and Adolescent Psychiatry, 32*, 1217–1222.

Constantino, J. N., Liberman, M., & Kincaid, M. (1997). Effects of serotonin reuptake inhibitors on aggressive behavior in psychiatrically hospitalized adolescents: Results of an open trial. *Journal of Child and Adolescent Psychopharmacology, 7*, 31–44.

Constantino, J. N., Morris, J. A., & Murphy, D. L. (1997). CSF 5–HIAA and family history of antisocial personality disorder in newborns. *American Journal of Psychiatry, 154*, 1771–1773.

Cook, E. H., Stein, M. A., Ellison, T, Unis, A. S., & Leventhal, B. L. (1995). Attention deficit hyperactivity disorder and whole-blood serotonin levels: Effects of comorbidity. *Psychiatry Research, 57*, 13–20.

Cook, P. J., Lawrence, B. A., Ludwig, J., & Miller, T. R. (1999). The medical costs of gunshot injuries in the United States. *Journal of the American Medical Association, 282,* 447–454.

Cooper, J. R., Bloom, F. E., & Roth, R. H. (1986). *The biochemical basis of neuro-pharmacology* (5th ed.). New York: Oxford University Press.

Cooper, J. R., Bloom, F. E., & Roth, R. H. (1991). *The biochemical basis of neuro-pharmacology* (6th ed.). New York: Oxford University Press.

Cornell, D. G., Warren, J., Hawk, G., Stafford, E., Oram, G., & Pine, D. (1996). Psychopathy in instrumental and reactive violent offenders. *Journal of Consulting and Clinical Psychology, 64,* 783–790.

Costello, E. J., Costello, A. J., Edelbrock, C., Burns, B. J., Dulcan, M. K., Brent, D., & Janiszewski, S. (1988). Psychiatric disorders in pediatric primary care. *Archives of General Psychiatry, 45,* 1107–1116.

Cowie, J., Cowie, V., & Slater, E. (1968). *Delinquency in girls.* London: Heinemann.

Crick, N. R., & Bigbee, M. A. (1998). Relational and overt forms of peer victimization: A multiinformant approach. *Journal of Consulting and Clinical Psychology, 66,* 337–347.

Crick, N. R., Bigbee, M. A., & Howes, C. (1996). Gender differences in children's normative beliefs about aggression: How do I hurt thee? Let me count the ways. *Child Development, 67,* 1003–1014.

Crick, N. R., & Dodge, K. A. (1994). A review and reformulation of social information-processing mechanisms in children's social adjustment. *Psychological Bulletin, 115,* 74–101.

Crick, N. R., & Dodge, K. A. (1996). Social information-processing mechanisms in reactive and proactive aggression. *Child Development, 67,* 993–1002.

Crick, N. R., & Grotpeter, J. K. (1995). Relational aggression, gender, and social-psychological adjustment. *Child Development, 66,* 710–722.

Crick, N. R., & Werner, N. E. (1998). Response decision processes in relational and overt aggression. *Child Development, 69,* 1630–1639.

Crijnen, A. A. M., Achenbach, T. M., & Verhulst, F. C. (1999). Problems reported by parents of children in multiple cultures: The Child Behavior Checklist syndrome constructs. *American Journal of Psychiatry, 156,* 569–574.

Crowe, R. R. (1974). An adoption study of antisocial personality. *Archives of General Psychiatry, 31,* 785–791.

Cryanowski, J. M., Frank, E., Young, E., & Shear, K. (2000). Adolescent onset of the gender difference in lifetime rates of major depression. *Archives of General Psychiatry, 57,* 21–27.

Cueva, J. E., Overall, J. E., Small, A. M., Armenteros, J. L., Perry, R., & Campbell, M. (1996). Carbamazepine in aggressive children with conduct disorder: A double-blind and placebo-controlled study. *Journal of the American Academy of Child and Adolescent Psychiatry, 35,* 480–490.

Cunningham, M. D., & Reidy, T. J. (1998). Antisocial personality disorder and psychopathy: Diagnostic dilemmas in classifying patterns of antisocial behavior in sentencing evaluations. *Behavioral Sciences and the Law, 16,* 333–351.

Dabbs, J. M., Jr., & Hargrove, M. F. (1997). Age, testosterone, and behavior among female prison inmates. *Psychosomatic Medicine, 59,* 477–480.

Dabbs, J. M., Jurkovic, G. J., & Frady, R. L. (1991). Salivary testosterone and cortisol among late adolescent male offenders. *Journal of Abnormal Child Psychology, 19,* 469–478.

Dabbs, J. M., Ruback, R. B., Frady, R. L., Hopper, C. H., & Sgoutas, D. S. (1988). Saliva testosterone and criminal violence among women. *Personality and Individual Differences, 9*, 269–275.

Damasio, A. R. (1994). *Descartes' error: Emotion, reason, and the human brain.* New York: Avon Books.

Daugherty, T. K., & Quay, H. C. (1991). Response perseveration and delayed responding in childhood behavior disorders. *Journal of Child Psychology and Psychiatry, 32*, 453–461.

Davanzo, P. A., & McCracken, J. T. (2000). Mood stabilizers in the treatment of juvenile bipolar disorder. *Child and Adolescent Psychiatric Clinics of North America, 9*, 159–182.

Davidson, M., Giordani, A. B., Mohs, R. C., Mykytyn, V. V., Platt, S., Aryan, Z. S., & Davis, K. L. (1987). Control of exogenous factors affecting plasma homovanillic acid concentration. *Psychiatry Research, 20*, 307–312.

Davis, T. C., Byrd, R. S., Arnold, C. L., Auinger, P., & Bocchini, Jr., J. A. (1999). Low literacy and violence among adolescents in a summer sports program. *Journal of Adolescent Health, 24*, 403–411.

Dawe, H. C. (1934). An analysis of two hundred quarrels of preschool children. *Child Development, 5*, 139–157.

Dawson, M. E. (1990). Psychophysiology at the interface of clinical science, cognitive science, and neuroscience. *Psychophysiology, 27*, 243–255.

Day, R., & Wong, S. (1996). Anomalous perceptual asymmetries for negative emotional stimuli in the psychopath. *Journal of Abnormal Psychology, 105*, 648–652.

Deb, S., Lyons, I., Koutzoukis, C., Ali, I., & McCarthy, G. (1999). Rate of psychiatric illness 1 year after traumatic brain injury. *American Journal of Psychiatry, 156*, 374–378.

DeBellis, M. D., Lefter, L., Trickett, P. K., & Putnam, F. W. (1994). Urine catecholamine excretion in sexually abused girls. *Journal of the American Academy of Child and Adolescent Psychiatry, 33*, 320–327.

de Chateau, P. (1990). Mortality and aggressiveness in a 30–year follow-up study in child guidance clinics in Stockholm. *Acta Psychiatrica Scandinavica, 81*, 472–476.

Delamater, A. M., & Lahey, B. B. (1983). Physiological correlates of conduct problems and anxiety in hyperactive and learning-disabled children. *Journal of Abnormal Child Psychology, 11*, 85–100.

Delaney-Black, V., Covington, C., Ostrea, E., Jr., Romero, A., Baker, D., Tagle, M. T., Nordstrom-Klee, B., Silvestre, M. A., Angelilli, M. L., Hack, C., & Long, J. (1996). Prenatal cocaine and neonatal outcome: Evaluation of dose–response relationship. *Pediatrics, 98*, 735–740.

Delaney-Black, V., Covington, C., Templin, T., Ager, J., Martier, S., & Sokol, R. (1998). Prenatal cocaine exposure and child behavior. *Pediatrics, 102*, 945–950.

Delga, I., Heinssen, R. K., Fritsch, R. C., Goodrich, W., & Yates, B. T. (1989). Psychosis, aggression, and self-destructive behavior in hospitalized adolescents. *American Journal of Psychiatry, 146*, 521–525.

Delgado-Escueta, A., Mattson, R. H., King, L., Goldensohn, E. S., Spiegel, H., Madsen, J., Crandall, P., Dreifuss, F., & Porter, R. J. (1981). The nature of aggression during epileptic seizures. *New England Journal of Medicine, 305*, 711–716.

DeLong, G. R., & Aldershof, A. L. (1987). Long-term experience with lithium treatment in childhood: Correlation with clinical diagnosis. *Journal of the American Academy of Child and Adolescent Psychiatry, 26*, 389–394.

Dery, M., Toupin, J., Pauze, R., Mercier, H., & Fortin, L. (1999). Neuropsychological characteristics of adolescents with conduct disorder: Association with attention-deficit-hyperactivity and aggression. *Journal of Abnormal Child Psychology, 27,* 225–236.

Deutsch, D. (1997). *The fabric of reality: The science of parallel universes—and its implications.* New York: Penguin.

Devinsky, O., Morrell, M. J., & Vogt, B. A. (1995). Contributions of anterior cingulate cortex to behavior. *Brain, 118,* 279–306.

Dierker, L. C., Merikangas, K. R., & Szatmari, P. (1999). Influence of parental concordance for psychiatric disorders on psychopathology in offspring. *Journal of the American Academy of Child and Adolescent Psychiatry, 38,* 280–288.

Dietch, J. T., & Jennings, R. K. (1988). Aggressive dyscontrol in patients treated with benzodiazepines. *Journal of Clinical Psychiatry, 49,* 184–188.

Dishion, T. J., & Andrews, D. W. (1995). Preventing escalation in problem behaviors with high-risk young adolescents: Immediate and 1–year outcomes. *Journal of Consulting and Clinical Psychology, 63,* 538–548.

Disney, E. R., Elkins, I. J., McGue, M., & Iacono, W. G. (1999). Effects of ADHD, conduct disorder, and gender on substance use and abuse in adolescence. *American Journal of Psychiatry, 156,* 1515–1521.

Dodge, K. A. (1986). A social information processing model of social competence in children. In M. Perlmutter (Ed.), *Minnesota Symposium on Child Psychology* (Vol. 18, pp. 77–125). Hillsdale, NJ: Erlbaum.

Dodge, K. A. (1991). The structure and function of reactive and proactive aggression. In D. J. Pepler & K. H. Rubin (Eds.), *The development and treatment of childhood aggression* (pp. 201–218). Hillsdale, NJ: Erlbaum.

Dodge, K. A., Bates, J., & Pettit, G. S. (1990). Mechanisms in the cycle of violence. *Science, 250,* 1678–1683.

Dodge, K. A., & Coie, J. D. (1987). Social information processing factors in reactive and proactive aggression in children's peer groups. *Journal of Personality and Social Psychology, 53,* 1146–1158.

Dodge, K. A., & Frame, C. L. (1982). Social cognitive biases and deficits in aggressive boys. *Child Development, 53,* 620–635.

Dodge, K. A., Lochman, J. E., Harnish, J. D., Bates, J. E., & Pettit, G. S. (1997). Reactive and proactive aggression in school children and psychiatrically impaired chronically assaultive youth. *Journal of Abnormal Psychology, 106,* 37–51.

Dodge, K. A., & Newman, J. P. (1981). Biased decision-making processes in aggressive boys. *Journal of Abnormal Psychology, 90,* 375–379.

Dodge, K. A., Pettit, G. S., & Bates, J. E. (1994). Socialization mediators of the relation between socioeconomic status and child conduct problems. *Child Development, 65,* 649–665.

Dodge, K. A., Pettit, G. S., Bates, J. E., & Valente, E. (1995). Social information-processing patterns partially mediate the effect of early physical abuse on later conduct problems. *Journal of Abnormal Psychology, 104,* 632–643.

Dolan, M. (1994). Psychopathy—a neurobiological perspective. *British Journal of Psychiatry, 165,* 151–159.

Dollard, J., Doob, C. W., Miller, N. E., Mowrer, O. H., & Sears, R. R. (1939). *Frustration and aggression.* New Haven, CT: Yale University Press.

Donnerstein, E., Slaby, R. G., & Eron, L. D. (1994). The mass media and youth aggression. In L. D. Eron, J. H. Gentry, & P. Schlegel (Eds.), *Reason to hope: A psychosocial perspective on violence and youth* (pp. 219–250). Washington, DC: American Psychological Association.

Donovan, A.-M., Halperin, J. M., Newcorn, J. H., & Sharma, V. (1999). Thermal response to serotonergic challenge and aggression in attention deficit hyperactivity disorder children. *Journal of Child and Adolescent Psychopharmacology, 9*, 85–91.

Donovan, S. J., Stewart, J. W., Nunes, E. V., Quitkin, F. M., Parides, M., Daniel, W., Susser, E., & Klein, D. F. (2000). Divalproex treatment of youth with explosive temper and mood lability: A double-blind, placebo-controlled crossover design. *American Journal of Psychiatry, 157*, 818–820.

Donovan, S. J., Susser, E. S., Nunes, E. V., Stewart, J. W., Quitkin, F. M., & Klein, D. F. (1997). Divalproex treatment of disruptive adolescents: A report of 10 cases. *Journal of Clinical Psychiatry, 58*, 12–15.

DuPaul, G. J., Power, T. J., Anastopoulos, A. D., & Reid, R. (1998). *ADHD Rating Scale—IV: Checklists, norms, and clinical interpretation.* New York: Guilford Press.

Durlak, J. A., Fuhrman, T., & Lampman, C. (1991). Effectiveness of cognitive-behavior therapy for maladapting children: A meta-analysis. *Psychological Bulletin, 110*, 204–214.

Dwivedi, K. N., Beaumont, G., & Brandon, S. (1984). Electrophysiological responses in high and low aggressive young adolescent boys. *Acta Paedopsychiatrica, 50*, 179–190.

Eagly, A. H., & Steffen, V. J. (1986). Gender and aggressive behavior: A meta-analytic review of the social psychological literature. *Psychological Bulletin, 100*, 309–330.

Earls, F., Reich, W., Jung, K. G., & Cloninger, C. R. (1988). Psychopathology in children of alcoholic and antisocial parents. *Alcoholism: Clinical and Experimental Research, 12*, 481–487.

Eaves, L. J., Silberg, J. L., Meyer, J. M., Maes, H. H., Simonoff, E., Pickles, A., Rutter, M., Neale, M. C., Reynolds, C. A., Erikson, M. T., Heath, A. C., Loeber, R., Truett, K. R., & Hewitt, J. K. (1997). Genetics and developmental psychopathology: 2. The main effects of genes and environment on behavioral problems in the Virginia Twin Study of Adolescent Behavioral Development. *Journal of Child Psychology and Psychiatry, 38*, 965–980.

Edelbrock, C. (1978). *Childhood Attention Problems (CAP) scale.* University Park: Pennsylvania State University.

Edelbrock, C., Rende, R., Plomin, R., & Thompson, L. A. (1995). A twin study of competence and problem behavior in childhood and early adolescence. *Journal of Child Psychology and Psychiatry, 36*, 775–785.

Egeland, B., Pianta, R., & O'Brien, M. A. (1993). Maternal intrusiveness in infancy and child maladaptation in early school years. *Development and Psychopathology, 5*, 359–370.

Eichelman, B. (1987). Neurochemical and psychopharmacologic aspects of aggressive behavior. In H. Y. Meltzer (Ed.), *Psychopharmacology: The third generation of progress* (pp. 697–704). New York: Raven Press.

Eichelman, B. (1988). Toward a rational pharmacotherapy for aggressive and violent behavior. *Hospital and Community Psychiatry, 39*, 31–39.

Eichelman, B. (1992). Aggressive behavior: From laboratory to clinic. *Quo vadit? Archives of General Psychiatry, 49*, 488–492.

Elliot, D. S., & Tolan, P. H. (1999). Youth violence prevention, intervention, and social policy. In D. J. Flannery & C. R. Huff (Eds.), *Youth violence: Prevention, intervention, and social policy* (pp. 3–46). Washington, DC: American Psychiatric Press.

Elliott, F. A. (1987). Neuroanatomy and neurology of aggression. *Psychiatric Annals, 17,* 385–388.

Ellis, G. T., & Sekyra, F. (1972). The effect of aggressive cartoons on behavior of first grade children. *Journal of Psychology, 81,* 37–43.

Ellis, L. (1988). The victimful–victimless crime distinction, and seven universal demographic correlates of victimful criminal behavior. *Personality and Individual Differences, 9,* 525–548.

el-Sheikh, M. (1994). Children's emotional and physiological responses to interadult angry behavior: The role of history of interparental hostility. *Journal of Abnormal Child Psychology, 22,* 661–678.

Emery, R. E., & Laumann-Billings, L. (1998). An overview of the nature, causes, and consequences of abusive family relationships. *American Psychologist, 53,* 121–135.

Emslie, G. J., Walkup, J. T., Pliszka, S. R., & Ernst, M. (1999). Nontricyclic antidepressants: Current trends in children and adolescents. *Journal of the American Academy of Child and Adolescent Psychiatry, 38,* 517–528.

Eppright, T. D., Kashani, J. H., Robison, B. D., & Reid, J. C. (1993). Comorbidity of conduct disorder and personality disorders in an incarcerated juvenile population. *American Journal of Psychiatry, 150,* 1233–1236.

Eron, L. D. (1992). Gender differences in violence: Biology and/or socialization? In K. Bjorkqvist & P. Niemela (Eds.), *Of mice and women: Aspects of female aggression* (pp. 89–97). San Diego, CA: Academic Press.

Esser, G., Schmidt, M. H., & Woerner, W. (1990). Epidemiology and course of psychiatric disorders in school-age children-results of a longitudinal study. *Journal of Child Psychology and Psychiatry, 31,* 243–263.

Eyler, F. D., Behnke, M., Conlon, M., Woods, N. S., & Wobie, K. (1998a). Birth outcome from a prospective, matched study of prenatal crack/cocaine use: I. Interactive and dose effects on health and growth. *Pediatrics, 101,* 229–237.

Eyler, F. D., Behnke, M., Conlon, M., Woods, N. S., & Wobie, K. (1998b). Birth outcome from a prospective, matched study of prenatal crack/cocaine use: II. Interactive and dose effects on neurobehavioral assessment. *Pediatrics, 101,* 237–241.

Eysenck, H. J. (1964). *Crime and personality.* London: Methuen.

Fagot, B. I., & Kavanaugh, K. (1990). The prediction of antisocial behavior from avoidant attachment classifications. *Child Development, 61,* 864–873.

Famularo, R., Fenton, T., Kinscherff, R., & Augustyn, M. (1996). Psychiatric comorbidity in childhood posttraumatic stress disorder. *Child Abuse and Neglect, 20,* 953–961.

Famularo, R., Kinscherff, R., & Fenton, T. (1988). Propranolol treatment for childhood posttraumatic stress disorder, acute type. *American Journal of Diseases of Children, 142,* 1244–1247.

Faraone, S. V., Biederman, J., Keenan, K., & Tsuang, M. T. (1991). Separation of DSM-III attention deficit disorder and conduct disorder: Evidence from a family genetic study of American child psychiatry patients. *Psychological Medicine, 21,* 109–121.

Faraone, S. V., Biederman, J., Wozniak, J., Mundy, E., Mennin, D., & O'Donnell, D. (1997). Is comorbidity with ADHD a marker for juvenile-onset mania? *Journal of the American Academy of Child and Adolescent Psychiatry, 36,* 1046–1055.

Farrington, D. P. (1989). Early predictors of adolescent aggression and adult violence. *Victims and Violence, 4,* 79–100.

Farrington, D. P. (1991). Childhood aggression and adult violence: Early precursors and later-life outcomes. In D. J. Pepler & K. H. Rubin (Eds.), *The development and treatment of childhood aggression* (pp. 5–29). Hillsdale, NJ: Erlbaum.

Farrington, D. P. (1995). The development of offending and antisocial behaviour from childhood: Key findings from the Cambridge study on delinquent development. *Journal of Child Psychology and Psychiatry, 36*, 929–964.

Farrington, D. P. (1997). The relationship between low resting heart rate and violence. In A. Raine, P. A. Brennan, D. P. Farrington, & S. A. Mednick (Eds.), *Biosocial bases of violence* (pp. 89–105). New York: Plenum Press.

Fast, D. K., Conry, J., & Loock, C. A. (1999). Identifying fetal alcohol syndrome among youth in the criminal justice system. *Journal of Developmental and Behavioral Pediatrics, 20*, 370–372.

Fatemi, S. H., Realmuto, G. M., Khan, L., & Thuras, P. (1998). Fluoxetine in treatment of adolescent patients with autism: A longitudinal open trial. *Journal of Autism and Developmental Disorders, 28*, 303–307.

Fava, M., & Rosenbaum, J. F. (1999). Anger attacks in patients with depression. *Journal of Clinical Psychiatry, 60*(Suppl. 15), 21–24.

Fava, M., Rosenbaum, J. F., Pava, J. A., McCarthy, M. K., Steingard, R. J., & Bouffides, E. (1993). Anger attacks in unipolar depression: Part I. Clinical correlates and response to fluoxetine treatment. *American Journal of Psychiatry, 150*, 1158–1163.

Fava, M., Vuolo, R. D., Wright, E. C., Nierenberg, A. A., Alpert, J. E., & Rosenbaum, J. F. (2000). Fenfluramine challenge in unipolar depression with and without anger attacks. *Psychiatry Research, 94*, 9–18.

Favazza, A. R. (1998). The coming of age of self-mutilation. *Journal of Nervous and Mental Disease, 186*, 259–268.

Federal Bureau of Investigation. (1994). *Crime in the United States, 1994*. Washington, DC: U.S. Government Printing Office.

Federal Bureau of Investigation (1996). *Uniform crime reports*. Washington, DC: U.S. Government Printing Office.

Feehan, M., Stanton, W. R., McGee, R., Silva, P. A., & Moffitt, T. E. (1990). Is there an association between lateral preference and delinquent behavior? *Journal of Abnormal Psychology, 99*, 198–201.

Feingold, A. (1994). Gender differences in personality: A meta-analysis. *Psychological Bulletin, 116*, 429–456.

Feldman, R. A., Caplinger, T. E., & Wodarski, J. S. (1983). *The St. Louis conundrum: The effective treatment of antisocial youths*. Englewood Cliffs, NJ: Prentice-Hall.

Fenwick, P. (1993). Aggression and epilepsy. In C. Thompson & P. Cohen (Eds.), *Violence: Basic and clinical science* (pp. 76–98). London: Butterworth–Heinemann.

Ferdinand, R. F., & Verhulst, F. C. (1995). Psychopathology from adolescence into young adulthood: An 8–year follow-up study. *American Journal of Psychiatry, 152*, 1586–1594.

Fergusson, D. M., & Lynskey, M. T. (1996). Adolescent resiliency to family adversity. *Journal of Child Psychology and Psychiatry, 37*, 281–292.

Ferris, C. F. (2000). Adolescent stress and neural plasticity in hamsters: A vasopressin/serotonin model of inappropriate aggressive behavior. *Experimental Physiology, 85*, 85S–90S.

Feshbach, S. (1970). Aggression. In P. Mussen (Ed.), *Carmichael's manual of child psychology* (Vol. 2, pp. 159–259). New York: Wiley.

Filion, D. L., Dawson, M. E., Schell, A. M., & Hazlett, E. A. (1991). The relationship between skin conductance orienting and the allocation of processing resources. *Psychophysiology, 28,* 410–424.

Fils-Aime, M.-L., Eckardt, M. J., George, D. T., Brown, G. L., Mefford, I., & Linnoila, M. (1996). Early-onset alcoholics have lower cerebrospinal fluid 5–hydroxyindoleacetic acid levels than late-onset alcoholics. *Archives of General Psychiatry, 53,* 211–216.

Findling, R. L., Maxwell, K., & Wiznitzer, M. (1997). An open clinical trial of risperidone monotherapy in young children with autistic disorder. *Psychopharmacology Bulletin, 33,* 155–159.

Findling, R. L., McNamara, N. K., Branicky, L. A., Schluchter, M. D., Lemon, E., & Blumer, J. L. (2000). A double-blind pilot study of risperidone in the treatment of conduct disorder. *Journal of the American Academy of Child and Adolescent Psychiatry, 39,* 509–516.

Fingerhut, L. A. (1993). *Firearm mortality among children, youths, and young adults 1–34 years of age: Trends and current status. United States 1985–1990* (Advance Data from Vital and Health Statistics, No. 231). Hyattsville, MD: National Center for Health Statistics.

Fingerhut, L. A., Jones, C., & Makuc, D. (1994). *Firearm and motor vehicle injury mortality—variations by state, race, and ethnicity (1990–91): United States* (Advance Data from Vital and Health Statistics, No. 242). Hyattsville, MD: National Center for Health Statistics.

Finkelhor, D., & Berliner, L. (1995). Research on the treatment of sexually abused children: A review and recommendations. *Journal of the American Academy of Child and Adolescent Psychiatry, 34,* 1408–1423.

Finkelstein, J. W., Susman, E. J., Chinchilli, V. M., Kunselman, S. J., D'Arcangelo, M. R., Schwab, J., Demers, L. M., Liben, L. S., Lookingbill, G., & Kulin, H. E. (1997). Estrogen or testosterone increases self-reported aggressive behaviors in hypogonadal adolescents. *Journal of Clinical Endocrinology and Metabolism, 82,* 2433–2438.

Fischer, M., Barkley, R. A., Fletcher, K. E., & Smallish, L. (1993a). The stability of dimensions of behavior in ADHD and normal children over an 8–year follow-up. *Journal of Abnormal Child Psychology, 21,* 315–337.

Fischer, M., Barkley, R. A., Fletcher, K. E., & Smallish, L. (1993b). The adolescent outcome of hyperactive children: Predictors of psychiatric, academic, social, and emotional adjustment. *Journal of the American Academy of Child and Adolescent Psychiatry, 32,* 324–332.

Fisher, L., & Blair, R. J. R. (1998). Cognitive impairment and its relationship to psychopathic tendencies in children with emotional and behavioral difficulties. *Journal of Abnormal Child Psychology, 26,* 511–519.

Fisman, S., & Steele, M. (1996). Use of risperidone in pervasive developmental disorders: A case series. *Journal of Child and Adolescent Psychopharmacology, 6,* 177–190.

Flannery, D. J., Singer, M. I., & Wester, K. (2001). Violence exposure, psychological trauma, and suicide risk in a community sample of dangerously violent adolescents. *Journal of the American Academy of Child and Adolescent Psychiatry, 40,* 435–442.

Fleming, J. E., & Offord, D. R. (1990). Epidemiology of childhood depressive disorders: A critical review. *Journal of the American Academy of Child and Adolescent Psychiatry, 29,* 571–580.

Fletcher, K. E. (1996). Childhood posttraumatic stress disorder. In E. J. Mash & R. A. Barkley (Eds.), *Child psychopathology* (pp. 242–276). New York: Guilford Press.

Flisher, A. J., Kramer, R. A., Hoven, C. W., Greenwald, S., Alegria, M., Bird, H. R., Canino, G., Connell, R., & Moore, R. E. (1997). Psychosocial characteristics of physically abused children and adolescents. *Journal of the American Academy of Child and Adolescent Psychiatry, 26,* 123–131.

Fonagy, P., & Target, M. (1994). The efficacy of psychoanalysis for children with disruptive disorders. *Journal of the American Academy of Child and Adolescent Psychiatry, 33,* 45–55.

Forehand, R., & Atkeson, B. M. (1977). Generality of treatment effects with parents as therapists: A review of assessment and implementation procedures. *Behavior Therapy, 8,* 575–593.

Forehand, R., & Long, N. (1988). Outpatient treatment of the acting out child: Procedures, long term follow-up data, and clinical problems. *Advances in Behaviour Research and Therapy, 10,* 129–177.

Forehand, R., & McMahon, R. J. (1981). *Helping the noncompliant child: A clinician's guide to parent training.* New York: Guilford Press.

Forgatch, M. S., & Patterson, G. R. (1989). *Parents and adolescents living together: Part 2. Family problem solving.* Eugene, OR: Castalia.

Forth, A. E., Kosson, D. S., & Hare, R. D. (1997). *The Psychopathy Checklist: Youth Version.* Toronto: Multi-Health Systems.

Fowles, D. C. (1988). Psychophysiology and psychopathology: A motivational approach. *Psychophysiology, 25,* 373–391.

Fowles, D. C. (1994). A motivational theory of psychopathology. In R. Dienstbier & W. D. Spaulding (Eds.), *Nebraska Symposium on Motivation* (Vol. 41, pp. 181–238). Lincoln: University of Nebraska Press.

Frankel, F., & Simmons, J. Q., III. (1992). Parent behavioral training: Why and when some parents drop out. *Journal of Clinical Child Psychology, 21,* 322–330.

Frazier, J. A., Gordon, C. T., McKenna, K., Lenane, M. C., Jih, D., & Rapoport, J. L. (1994). An open trial of clozapine in 11 adolescents with childhood-onset schizophrenia. *Journal of the American Academy of Child and Adolescent Psychiatry, 33,* 658–663.

Frazier, J. A., Meyer, M. C., Biederman, J., Wozniak, J., Wilens, T. E., Spencer, T. J., Kim, G. S., & Shapiro, S. (1999). Risperidone treatment for juvenile bipolar disorder: A retrospective chart review. *Journal of the American Academy of Child and Adolescent Psychiatry, 38,* 960–965.

Frick, P. J. (1998). *Conduct disorders and severe antisocial behavior.* New York: Plenum Press.

Frick, P. J., Kamphaus, R. W., Lahey, B. B., Christ, M. A. G., Hart, E. L., & Tannenbaum, T. E. (1991). Academic underachievement and the disruptive behavior disorders. *Journal of Consulting and Clinical Psychology, 59,* 289–294.

Frick, P. J., Kuper, K., Silverthorn, P., & Cotter, M. (1995). Antisocial behavior, somatization, and sensation-seeking behavior in mothers of clinic-referred children. *Journal of the American Academy of Child and Adolescent Psychiatry, 34,* 805–812.

Frick, P. J., Lahey, B. B., Loeber, R., Tannenbaum, L., Van Horn, Y., Christ, M. A. G., Hart, E. A., & Hanson, K. (1993). Oppositional defiant disorder and conduct disorder: A meta-analytic review of factor analyses and cross-validation in a clinical sample. *Clinical Psychology Review, 13,* 319–340.

Frick, P. J., Lilienfeld, S. O., Ellis, M., Loney, B., & Silverthorn, P. (1999). The association between anxiety and psychopathy dimensions in children. *Journal of Abnormal Child Psychology, 27,* 383–392.

Frick, P. J., O'Brien, B. S., Wootton, J. M., & McBurnett, K. (1994). Psychopathy and conduct problems in children. *Journal of Abnormal Psychology, 103*, 700–707.

Fried, I. (1995). Mellansjo School–Home: Psychopathic children admitted 1928–1940, their social adaptation over 30 years. A longitudinal prospective follow-up. *Acta Paediatrica,* (Suppl. 408), 1–42.

Fried, P. A., Watkinson, B., & Gray, R. (1992). A follow-up study of attentional behavior in 6–year-old children exposed prenatally to marijuana, cigarettes, and alcohol. *Neurotoxicology and Teratology, 14*, 299–311.

Fristad, M. A., Weller, E. B., & Weller, R. A. (1992). Bipolar disorders in children and adolescents. *Child and Adolescent Psychiatric Clinics of North America, 1*, 13–29.

Fritsch, R. C., Heinessen, R. K., Delga, I., Goodrich, W., & Yates, B. T. (1992). Predicting hospital adjustment by adolescent inpatients. *Hospital and Community Psychiatry, 43*, 49–53.

Frodi, A., Macaulay, J., & Thome, P. R. (1977). Are women always less aggressive than men?: A review of the experimental literature. *Psychological Bulletin, 84*, 634–660.

Frost, L. A., Moffitt, T. E., & McGee, R. (1989). Neuropsychological correlates of psychopathology in an unselected cohort of young adolescents. *Journal of Abnormal Psychology, 98*, 307–313.

Fuller, R. W. (1996). The influence of fluoxetine on aggressive behavior. *Neuropsychopharmacology, 14*, 77–81.

Furlong, M. J., & Smith, D. C. (1994). Assessment of youths' anger, hostility, and aggression using self-report and rating scales. In M. Furlong & D. Smith (Eds.), *Anger, hostility, and aggression: Assessment, prevention, and intervention strategies for youth* (pp. 167–244). Brandon, VT: Clinical Psychology.

Fuster, J. M. (1997). *The prefrontal cortex: Anatomy, physiology, and neuropsychology of the frontal lobe* (3rd ed.). Philadelphia: Lippincott–Raven.

Gabel, S., & Shindledecker, R. (1991). Aggressive behavior in youth: Characteristics, outcome, and psychiatric diagnoses. *Journal of the American Academy of Child and Adolescent Psychiatry, 30*, 982–988.

Gabel, S., Stadler, J., Bjorn, J., Shindledecker, R., & Bowden, C. L. (1993a). Biodevelopmental aspects of conduct disorder in boys. *Child Psychiatry and Human Development, 24*, 125–141.

Gabel, S., Stadler, J., Bjorn, J., Shindledecker, R., & Bowden, C. L. (1993b). Dopamine-beta-hydroxylase in behaviorally disturbed youth. *Biological Psychiatry, 34*, 434–442.

Gabel, S., Stadler, J., Bjorn, J., Shindledecker, R., & Bowden, C. L. (1994). Sensation seeking in psychiatrically disturbed youth: Relationship to biochemical parameters and behavior problems. *Journal of the American Academy of Child and Adolescent Psychiatry, 33*, 123–129.

Gabel, S., Stadler, J., Bjorn, J., Shindledecker, R., & Bowden, C. L. (1995). Homovanillic acid and monoamine oxidase in sons of substance-abusing fathers: Relationship to conduct disorder. *Journal of Studies on Alcohol, 56*, 135–139.

Gabrielli, W. F., & Mednick, S. A. (1980). Sinistrality and delinquency. *Journal of Abnormal Psychology, 89*, 654–661.

Gadow, K. D. (1986). *Peer Conflict Scale.* Unpublished manuscript, State University of New York at Stony Brook.

Gadow, K. D. (1991). Clinical issues in child and adolescent psychopharmacology. *Journal of Consulting and Clinical Psychology, 59*, 842–852.

Gadow, K. D., Nolan, E. E., Sverd, J., Sprafkin, J., & Paolicelli, L. (1990). Methylphenidate in aggressive–hyperactive boys: I. Effects on peer aggression in public school settings. *Journal of the American Academy of Child and Adolescent Psychiatry, 29,* 710–718.

Gadow, K. D., & Sprafkin, J. (1993). Television "violence" and children with emotional and behavioral disorders. *Journal of Emotional and Behavioral Disorders, 1,* 54–63.

Galvin, M., Shekhar, A., Simon, J., Stilwell, B., Ten Eyck, R., Laite, G., Karwisch, G., & Blix, S. (1991). Low dopamine-beta-hydroxylase: A biological sequela of abuse and neglect? *Psychiatry Research, 39,* 1–11.

Garmezy, N., Masten, A., & Tellegen, A. (1984). The study of stress and competence in children. *Child Development, 55,* 97–111.

Garnet, K. E., Levy, K. N., Mattanah, J. J. F., Edell, W. S., & McGlashan, T. H. (1994). Borderline personality disorder in adolescents: Ubiquitous or specific? *American Journal of Psychiatry, 151,* 1380–1382.

Garralda, M. E., Connell, J., & Taylor, D. C. (1990). Peripheral psychophysiological reactivity to mental tasks in children with psychiatric disorders. *European Archives of Psychiatry and Clinical Neuroscience, 240,* 44–47.

Garralda, M. E., Connell, J., & Taylor, D. C. (1991). Psychophysiological anomalies in children with emotional and conduct disorders. *Psychological Medicine, 21,* 947–957.

Garrison, C. Z., McKweon, R. E., Valois, R. F., & Vincent, M. L. (1993). Aggression, substance use, and suicidal behaviors in high school students. *American Journal of Public Health, 83,* 179–184.

Garrison, W. T., Ecker, B., Friedman, M., Davidoff, R., Haeberle, K., & Wagner, M. (1990). Aggression and counteraggression during child psychiatric hospitalization. *Journal of the American Academy of Child and Adolescent Psychiatry, 29,* 242–250.

Gaub, M., & Carlson, C. L. (1997). Gender differences in ADHD: A meta-analysis and critical review. *Journal of the American Academy of Child and Adolescent Psychiatry, 36,* 1036–1045.

Geller, B. (1997, March). *Double-blind placebo-controlled study of lithium for adolescents with comorbid bipolar and substance dependency disorders.* Paper presented at the *Annual Mid-Year Institute of the American Academy of Child and Adolescent Psychiatry,* Hamilton, Bermuda.

Geller, B., Fox, L. W., & Clark, K. A. (1994). Rate and predictors of prepubertal bipolarity during follow-up of 6- to 12–year-old depressed children. *Journal of the American Academy of Child and Adolescent Psychiatry, 33,* 461–468.

Geller, B., & Luby, J. (1997). Child and adolescent bipolar disorder: A review of the past 10 years. *Journal of the American Academy of Child and Adolescent Psychiatry, 36,* 1168–1176.

Geller, B., Reising, D., Leonard, H. L., Riddle, M. A., & Walsh, B. T. (1999). Critical review of tricyclic antidepressant use in children and adolescents. *Journal of the American Academy of Child and Adolescent Psychiatry, 38,* 513–516.

Geller, B., Sun, K., Zimerman, B., Luby, J., Frazier, J., & Williams, M. (1995). Complex and rapid-cycling in bipolar children and adolescents: A preliminary study. *Journal of Affective Disorders, 34,* 259–268.

Gerbner, G., & Signorielli, N. (1990). *Violence profile, 1967 through 1988–89: Enduring patterns.* Unpublished manuscript, Annenberg School of Communication, University of Pennsylvania.

Gerra, G., Zaimovic, A., Avanzini, P., Chittolini, B., Giucastro, G., Caccavari, R., Palladino, M., Maestri, D., Monica, C., Delsignore, R., Brambilla, F. (1997). Neurotransmitter–neuroendocrine responses to experimentally induced aggression in humans: Influence of personality variable. *Psychiatry Research, 66,* 33–43.

Gerra, G., Zaimovic, A., Giucastro, G., Folli, F., Maestri, D., Tessoni, A., Avanzini, P., Caccavari, R., Bernasconi, S., & Brambilla, F. (1998). Neurotransmitter–hormonal responses to psychological stress in peripubertal subjects: Relationship to aggressive behavior. *Life Sciences, 62,* 617–625.

Gerring, J. P., Brady, K. D., Chen, A., Vasa, R., Grados, M., Bandeen-Roche, K. J., Bryan, R. N., & Denckla, M. B. (1998). Premorbid prevalence of ADHD and development of secondary ADHD after closed head injury. *Journal of the American Academy of Child and Adolescent Psychiatry, 37,* 647–654.

Gershon, E. S., Hamovit, J. H., Gurnoff, J. J., & Nurnberger, J. I. (1987). Birth-cohort changes in manic and depressive disorders in relatives of bipolar and schizoaffective patients. *Archives of General Psychiatry, 44,* 314–319.

Gerstle, J. E., Mathias, C. W., & Stanford, M. S. (1998). Auditory P300 and self-reported impulsive aggression. *Progress in Neuropsychopharmacology and Biological Psychiatry, 22,* 575–583.

Giaconia, R. M., Reinherz, H. Z., Silverman, A. B., Pakiz, B., Frost, A. K., & Cohen, E. (1995). Traumas and posttraumatic stress disorder in a community population of older adolescents. *Journal of the American Academy of Child and Adolescent Psychiatry, 34,* 1369–1380.

Giancola, P. R. (1995). Evidence for dorsolateral and orbital prefrontal cortical involvement in the expression of aggressive behavior. *Aggressive Behavior, 21,* 431–450.

Giancola, P. R., Martin, C. S., Tarter, R. E., Pelham, W. E., & Moss, H. B. (1996). Executive cognitive functioning and aggressive behavior in preadolescent boys at high risk for substance abuse/dependence. *Journal of Studies on Alcohol, 57,* 352–359.

Giancola, P. R., Mezzich, A. C., & Tarter, R. E. (1998a). Executive cognitive functioning, temperament, and antisocial behavior in conduct-disordered adolescent females. *Journal of Abnormal Psychology, 107,* 629–641.

Giancola, P. R., Mezzich, A. C., & Tarter, R. E. (1998b). Disruptive, delinquent and aggressive behavior in female adolescents with a psychoactive substance use disorder: Relation to executive cognitive functioning. *Journal of Studies on Alcohol, 59,* 560–567.

Giancola, P. R., Moss, H. B., Martin, C. S., Kirisci, L., & Tarter, R. E. (1996). Executive cognitive functioning predicts reactive aggression in boys at high risk for substance abuse: A prospective study. *Alcoholism: Clinical and Experimental Research, 20,* 740–744.

Gjone, H., & Stevenson, J. (1997). A longitudinal twin study of temperament and behavior problems: Common genetic or environmental influences? *Journal of the American Academy of Child and Adolescent Psychiatry, 36,* 1448–1456.

Glick, P. C. (1989). Remarried families, stepfamilies, and stepchildren: Brief demographic profile. *Family Relations, 38,* 24–27.

Glod, C. A., & Teicher, M. H. (1996). Relationship between early abuse, posttraumatic stress disorder, and activity levels in prepubertal children. *Journal of the American Academy of Child and Adolescent Psychiatry, 35,* 1384–1393.

Goetz, C. G., Tanner, C. M., Wilson, R. S., Carroll, S., Como, P. G., & Shannon, K. M. (1987). Clonidine and Gilles de la Tourette's syndrome: Double-blind study using objective rating methods. *Annals of Neurology, 21,* 307–310.

Goldberg, S. (1991). Recent developments in attachment theory and research. *Canadian Journal of Psychiatry, 36,* 393–400.

Goodenough, F. L. (1931). *Anger in young children.* Minneapolis: University of Minnesota Press.

Goodman, R. (1995). The relationship between normal variation in IQ and common childhood psychopathology: A clinical study. *European Child and Adolescent Psychiatry, 4,* 187–196.

Goodman, R., Simonoff, E., & Stevenson, J. (1995). The impact of child IQ, parent IQ and sibling IQ on child behavioural deviance scores. *Journal of Child Psychology and Psychiatry, 36,* 409–425.

Goodwin, F., & Jamison, K. (1990). *Manic–depressive illness.* New York: Oxford University Press.

Goodyear, I., & Cooper, P. (1993). A community study of depression in adolescent girls: II. The clinical features of identified disorder. *British Journal of Psychiatry, 163,* 374–380.

Gordon, D. A., Graves, K., & Arbuthnot, J. (1995). The effect of functional family therapy for delinquents on adult criminal behavior. *Criminal Justice and Behavior, 22,* 60–73.

Gottfredson, M. R., & Hirschi, T. (1990). *A general theory of crime.* Stanford, CA: Stanford University Press.

Gowers, W. R. (1881). *Epilepsy and other chronic convulsive diseases, their causes and symptoms.* London: Churchill.

Granger, D. A., Weisz, J. R., & Kauneckis, D. (1994). Neuroendocrine reactivity, internalizing behavior problems, and control-related cognitions in clinic-referred children and adolescents. *Journal of Abnormal Psychology, 103,* 267–276.

Grann, M., Langstrom, N., Tengstrom, A., & Kullgren, G. (1999). Psychopathy (PCL-R) predicts violent recidivism among criminal offenders with personality disorders in Sweden. *Law and Human Behavior, 23,* 205–217.

Gray, J. A. (1982). *The neuropsychology of anxiety: An enquiry into the functions of the septohippocampal system.* Oxford: Oxford University Press.

Gray, J. A. (1987). *The psychology of fear and stress* (2nd ed.). Cambridge, England: Cambridge University Press.

Greenhill, L. L., Halperin, J. M., & Abikoff, H. (1999). Stimulant medications. *Journal of the American Academy of Child and Adolescent Psychiatry, 38,* 503–512.

Greenhill, L. L., Solomon, M., Pleak, R., & Ambrosini, P. (1985). Molindone hydrochloride treatment of hospitalized children with conduct disorder. *Journal of Clinical Psychiatry, 46,* 20–25.

Grief, E. B., & Ulman, K. J. (1982). Psychological impact of menarche on early adolescent females: A review of the literature. *Child Development, 53,* 1413–1430.

Grimes, T., Cathers, T., & Vernberg, E. (1996). *Emotionally disturbed children's reaction to violent media segments.* Unpublished manuscript, School of Journalism and Mass Communication, Kansas State University.

Grisso, T. (1998). *Forensic evaluation of juveniles.* Sarasota, FL: Professional Resources Press.

Grisso, T. (2000). The changing face of juvenile justice. *Psychiatric Services, 51,* 425–427.

Group for the Advancement of Psychiatry, Committee on Preventive Psychiatry. (1999). Violent behavior in children and youth: Preventive intervention from a psychiatric perspective. *Journal of the American Academy of Child and Adolescent Psychiatry,* 38, 235–241.

Guerra, N. G., Huesmann, L. R., Tolan, P. H., Van Acker, R., & Eron, L. D. (1995). Stressful events and individual beliefs as correlates of economic disadvantage and aggression among urban children. *Journal of Consulting and Clinical Psychology,* 63, 518–528.

Guerri, C. (1998). Neuroanatomical and neurophysiological mechanisms involved in central nervous system dysfunctions induced by prenatal alcohol exposure. *Alcoholism: Clinical and Experimental Research,* 22, 304–312.

Guthrie, E., Mast, J., Richards, P., McQuaid, M., & Pavlakis, S. (1999). Traumatic brain injury in children and adolescents. *Child and Adolescent Psychiatric Clinics of North America,* 8, 807–826.

Guzder, J., Paris, J., Zelkowitz, P., & Feldman, R. (1999). Psychological risk factors for borderline pathology in school-age children. *Journal of the American Academy of Child and Adolescent Psychiatry,* 38, 206–212.

Guzder, J., Paris, J., Zelkowitz, P., & Marchessault, K. (1996). Risk factors of borderline pathology in children. *Journal of the American Academy of Child and Adolescent Psychiatry,* 35, 26–33.

Haapasalo, J., & Tremblay, R. E. (1994). Physically aggressive boys from age 6 to 12: Family background, parenting behavior, and prediction of delinquency. *Journal of Consulting and Clinical Psychology,* 62, 1044–1052.

Halperin, J. M., Newcorn, J. H., Kopstein, I., McKay, K. D., Schwartz, S. T., Siever, L. J., & Sharma, V. (1997). Serotonin, aggression, and parental psychopathology in children with attention-deficit hyperactivity disorder. *Journal of the American Academy of Child and Adolescent Psychiatry,* 36, 1391–1398.

Halperin, J. M., Newcorn, J. H., Schwartz, S. T., Sharma, V., Siever, L. J., Koda, V. H., & Gabriel, S. (1997). Age-related changes in the association between serotonergic function and aggression in boys with ADHD. *Biological Psychiatry,* 41, 682–689.

Halperin, J. M., Sharma, V., Siever, L. J., Schwartz, S. T., Matier, K., Wornell, G., & Newcorn, J. H. (1994). Serotonergic function in aggressive and nonaggressive boys with attention deficit hyperactivity disorder. *American Journal of Psychiatry,* 151, 243–248.

Halpern, C. T., Udry, J. R., Campbell, B., & Suchindran, C. (1993). Relationships between aggression and pubertal increases in testosterone: A panel analysis of adolescent males. *Social Biology,* 40, 8–24.

Hammen, C., & Rudolph, K. D. (1996). Childhood depression. In E. J. Mash & R. A. Barkley (Eds.), *Child psychopathology* (pp. 153–195). New York: Guilford Press.

Hamner, K. M., Lambert, E. W., & Bickman, L. (1997). Children's mental health in a continuum of care: Clinical outcomes at 18 months for the Fort Bragg demonstration. *Journal of Mental Health Administration,* 24, 465–471.

Hanf, C. (1969). *A two-stage program for modifying maternal controlling during mother–child (M-C) interaction.* Paper presented at the meeting of the Western Psychological Association, Vancouver, British Columbia, Canada.

Hann, D. M., Castino, R. J., Jarosinski, J., & Britton, H. (1991, April). Relating mother–toddler negotiation patterns to infant attachment and maternal depression with an adolescent mother sample. In J. Osofsky & L. Hubbs-Tait (Chairs), *Consequences of adolescent parenting: Predicting behavior problems in toddlers and preschoolers.* Symposium conducted at the biennial meeting of the Society for Research in Child Development, Seattle, WA.

Hanna, G. L., Yuwiler, A., & Coates, J. K. (1995). Whole blood serotonin and disruptive behaviors in juvenile obsessive–compulsive disorder. *Journal of the American Academy of Child and Adolescent Psychiatry, 34*, 28–35.

Harden, P. W., & Pihl, R. O. (1995). Cognitive function, cardiovascular reactivity, and behavior in boys at high risk for alcoholism. *Journal of Abnormal Psychology, 104*, 94–103.

Hare, R. D. (1980). A research scale for the assessment of psychopathy in criminal populations. *Personality and Individual Differences, 1*, 111–119.

Hare, R. D. (1985). Comparison of procedures for the assessment of psychopathy. *Journal of Consulting and Clinical Psychology, 53*, 7–16.

Hare, R. D. (1991). *The Hare Psychopathy Checklist—Revised.* Toronto: Multi-Health Systems.

Hare, R. D., Hart, S. D., & Harpur, T. J. (1991). Psychopathy and the DSM-IV criteria for antisocial personality disorder. *Journal of Abnormal Psychology, 100*, 391–398.

Harmon, R. J., & Riggs, P. D. (1996). Clonidine for posttraumatic stress disorder in preschool children. *Journal of the American Academy of Child and Adolescent Psychiatry, 35*, 1247–1249.

Harnish, J. D., Dodge, K. A., & Valente, E. (1995). Mother–child interaction quality as a partial mediator of the roles of maternal depressive symptomatology and socioeconomic status in the development of child behavior problems: Conduct Problems Prevention Research Group. *Child Development, 66*, 739–753.

Harpur, T. J., & Hare, R. D. (1994). Assessment of psychopathy as a function of age. *Journal of Abnormal Psychology, 103*, 604–609.

Harpur, T. J., Hare, R. D., & Hakstian, A. R. (1989). Two-factor conceptualization of psychopathy: Construct validity and assessment implications. *Psychological Assessment: A Journal of Consulting and Clinical Psychology, 1*, 6–17.

Harrington, R., Fudge, H., Rutter, M., Pickles, A., & Hill, J. (1990). Adult outcomes of childhood and adolescent depression. *Archives of General Psychiatry, 47*, 465–473.

Harris, G. T., Rice, M. E., & Quinsey, V. L. (1994). Psychopathy as a taxon: Evidence that psychopaths are a discrete class. *Journal of Consulting and Clinical Psychology, 62*, 387–397.

Harris, J. C. (1995). Neuropsychological testing: Assessing the mechanisms of cognition and behavioral functioning. In J. C. Harris (Ed.), *Developmental neuropsychiatry: Vol. 2. Assessment, diagnosis, and treatment of developmental disorders* (pp. 20–54). New York: Oxford University Press.

Hart, D., Hofmann, V., Edelstein, W., & Keller, M. (1997). The relation of childhood personality types to adolescent behavior and development: A longitudinal study of Icelandic children. *Developmental Psychology, 33*, 195–205.

Hart, E. L., Lahey, B. B., Loeber, R., & Hanson, K. S. (1994). Criterion validity of informants in the diagnosis of disruptive behavior disorders in children: A preliminary study. *Journal of Consulting and Clinical Psychology, 62*, 410–414.

Hart, S. D., & Hare, R. D. (1989). Discriminant validity of the psychopathy checklist in a forensic psychiatric population. *Psychological Assessment: A Journal of Consulting and Clinical Psychology, 1*, 211–218.

Hartup, W. W. (1974). Aggression in childhood: Developmental perspectives. *American Psychologist, 29*, 336–341.

Hartup, W. W., & de Wit, J. (1974). The development of aggression: Problems and perspectives. In J. de Wit & W. Hartup (Eds.), *Determinants and origins of aggressive behavior* (pp. 595–620). The Hague: Mouton.

Hauser, W. A. (1995). Epidemiology of epilepsy in children. In P. D. Adelson & P. M. Black (Eds.), *Surgical treatment of epilepsy in children* (pp. 419–429). Philadelphia: Saunders.

Hawkins, J. D., Von Cleve, E., & Catalano, Jr., R. F. (1991). Reducing early childhood aggression: Results of a primary prevention program. *Journal of the American Academy of Child and Adolescent Psychiatry, 30,* 208–217.

Hawkins, J. D., & Weis, J. G. (1985). The social developmental model: An integrated approach to delinquency prevention. *Journal of Primary Prevention, 6,* 73–97.

Hawton, K., Fagg, J., & Simkin, S. (1996). Deliberate self-poisoning and self-injury in children and adolescents under 16 years of age in Oxford, 1976–1993. *British Journal of Psychiatry, 169,* 202–208.

Hawton, K., Kingsbury, S., Steinhardt, K., James, A., & Fagg, J. (1999). Repetition of deliberate self-harm by adolescents: The role of psychological factors. *Journal of Adolescence, 22,* 369–378.

Hay, D. F., & Ross, H. S. (1982). The social nature of early conflict. *Child Development, 53,* 105–113.

HayGroup. (1998). *Health care plan design and cost trends—1988 through 1997.* Report prepared for the National Association of Psychiatric Health Systems, the Association of Behavioral Group Practices, and the National Alliance for the Mentally Ill. (Available from HayGroup, 1500 K Street NW, Suite 1000, Washington, DC 20005)

Hechtman, L., Weiss, G., & Perlman, T. (1984). Young adult outcome of hyperactive children who received long-term stimulant treatment. *Journal of the American Academy of Child Psychiatry, 23,* 261–269.

Heim, C., Newport, D. J., Heit, S., Graham, Y. P., Wilcox, M., Bansall, R., Miller, A. H., & Nemeroff, C. B. (2000). Pituitary–adrenal and autonomic responses to stress in women after sexual and physical abuse in childhood. *Journal of the American Medical Association, 284,* 592–597.

Hellgren, L., Gillberg, I. C., Bagenholm, A., & Gillberg, C. (1994). Children with deficits in attention, motor control, and perception (DAMP) almost grown up: Psychiatric and personality disorders at age 16 years. *Journal of Child Psychology and Psychiatry, 35,* 1255–1271.

Hendren, R. L., De Backer, I., & Pandina, G. J. (2000). Review of neuroimaging studies of child and adolescent psychiatric disorders from the past 10 years. *Journal of the American Academy of Child and Adolescent Psychiatry, 39,* 815–828.

Henggeler, S. W. (1989). *Delinquency in adolescence.* Newbury Park, CA: Sage.

Henggeler, S. W., & Borduin, C. M. (1990). *Family therapy and beyond: A multisystemic approach to treating the behavior problems of children and adolescents.* Pacific Grove, CA: Brooks/Cole.

Henggeler, S. W., Melton, G. B., & Smith, L. A. (1992). Family preservation using multisystemic therapy: An effective alternative to incarcerating serious juvenile offenders. *Journal of Consulting and Clinical Psychology, 60,* 953–961.

Henggeler, S. W., Melton, G. B., Smith, L. A., Schoenwald, S. K., & Hanley, J. H. (1993). Family preservation using multisystemic treatment: Long-term follow-up to a clinical trial with serious juvenile offenders. *Journal of Child and Family Studies, 4,* 283–293.

Henggeler, S. W., Rodick, J. D., Borduin, C. M., Hanson, C. L., Watson, S. M., & Urey, J.

R. (1986). Multisystemic treatment of juvenile offenders: Effects on adolescent behavior and family interaction. *Developmental Psychopathology, 22,* 132–141.

Henry, B., Moffitt, T. E., Robins, L. N., Earls, F., & Silva, P. A. (1993). Early family predictors of child and adolescent antisocial behavior: Who are the mothers of delinquents? *Criminal Behavior and Mental Health, 3,* 97–118.

Herning, R. I., Hickey, J. E., Pickworth, W. B., & Jaffe, J. H. (1989). Auditory event-related potentials in adolescents at risk for drug abuse. *Biological Psychiatry, 25,* 598–609.

Herpertz, S. (1995). Self-injurious behaviour: Psychopathological and nosological characteristics in subtypes of self-injurers. *Acta Psychiatrica Scandinavica, 91,* 57–68.

Herrenkohl, T. I., Maguin, E., Hill, K. G., Hawkins, J. D., Abbott, R. D., & Catalaño, R. F. (2000). Developmental risk factors for youth violence. *Journal of Adolescent Health, 26,* 176–186.

Herzberg, J. L., & Fenwick, P. B. C. (1988). The aetiology of aggression in temporal-lobe epilepsy. *British Journal of Psychiatry, 153,* 50–55.

Hetherington, E. M., & Stanley-Hagan, M. (1999). The adjustment of children with divorced parents: A risk and resiliency perspective. *Journal of Child Psychology and Psychiatry, 40,* 129–140.

Hewitt, J. K., Silberg, J. L., Rutter, M., Simonoff, E., Meyer, J. M., Maes, H., Pickles, A., Neale, M. C., Loeber, R., Erickson, M. T., Kendler, K. S., Heath, A. C., Truett, K. R., Reynolds, C. A., & Eaves, L. J. (1997). Genetics and developmental psychopathology: 1. Phenotypic assessment in the Virginia Twin Study of Adolescent Behavioral Development. *Journal of Child Psychology and Psychiatry, 38,* 943–963.

Hill, S. Y., & Hruska, D. R. (1992). Childhood psychopathology in families with multigenerational alcoholism. *Journal of the American Academy of Child and Adolescent Psychiatry, 31,* 1024–1030.

Hill, S. Y., & Muka, D. (1996). Childhood psychopathology in children from families of alcoholic female probands. *Journal of the American Academy of Child and Adolescent Psychiatry, 35,* 725–733.

Hinshaw, S. P. (1987). On the distinction between attentional deficits/hyperactivity and conduct problems/aggression in child psychopathology. *Psychological Bulletin, 101,* 443–463.

Hinshaw, S. P. (1992). Externalizing behavior problems and academic underachievement in childhood and adolescence: Causal relationships and underlying mechanisms. *Psychological Bulletin, 111,* 127–155.

Hinshaw, S. P., & Anderson, C. A. (1996). Conduct and oppositional defiant disorders. In E. J. Mash & R. A. Barkley (Eds.), *Child psychopathology* (pp. 113–149). New York: Guilford Press.

Hinshaw, S. P., Buhrmester, & Heller, T. (1989). Anger control in response to verbal provocation: Effects of stimulant medication for boys with ADHD. *Journal of Abnormal Child Psychology, 17,* 393–407.

Hinshaw, S. P., Heller, T., & McHale, J. P. (1992). Covert antisocial behavior in boys with attention-deficit hyperactivity disorder: External validation and effects of methylphenidate. *Journal of Consulting and Clinical Psychology, 60,* 274–281.

Hinshaw, S. P., Henker, B., & Whalen, C. K. (1984). Self-control in hyperactive boys in anger-inducing situations: Effects of cognitive-behavioral training and of methylphenidate. *Journal of Abnormal Child Psychology, 12,* 55–77.

Hinshaw, S. P., Henker, B., Whalen, C. K., Erhardt, D., & Dunnington, R. E., Jr. (1989). Aggressive, prosocial, and nonsocial behavior in hyperactive boys: Dose effects of methylphenidate in naturalistic settings. *Journal of Consulting and Clinical Psychology, 57,* 636–643.

Hinshaw, S. P., Simmel, C., & Heller, T. L. (1995). Multimethod assessment of covert antisocial behavior in children: Laboratory observations, adult ratings, and child self-report. *Psychological Assessment, 7,* 209–219.

Hofstra, M. B., van der Ende, J., & Verhulst, F. C. (2000). Continuity and change of psychopathology from childhood into adulthood: A 14–year follow-up study. *Journal of the American Academy of Child and Adolescent Psychiatry, 39,* 850–858.

Holmberg, M. S. (1977). *The development of social interchange patterns from 12 to 42 months: Cross-sectional and short-term longitudinal analyses.* Unpublished doctoral dissertation, University of North Carolina at Chapel Hill.

Holmes, G. L. (1987). *Diagnosis and management of seizures in children.* Philadelphia: Saunders.

Hood, K. E. (1996). Intractable tangles of sex and gender in women's aggressive development: An optimistic view. In D. M. Stoff & R. B. Cairns (Eds.), *Aggression and violence: Genetic, neurobiological, and biosocial perspectives* (pp. 309–335). Hillsdale, NJ: Erlbaum.

Horrigan, J. P., & Barnhill, L. J. (1995). Guanfacine for treatment of attention-deficit hyperactivity disorder in boys. *Journal of Child and Adolescent Psychopharmacology, 5,* 215–223.

Hoving, K., Wallace, J., & LaForme, G. (1979). Aggression during competition: Effects of age, sex, and amount and type of provocation. *Genetic Psychology Monographs, 99,* 251–289.

Hoyt, S., & Scherer, D. G. (1998). Female juvenile delinquency: Misunderstood by the juvenile justice system, neglected by social science. *Law and Human Behavior, 22,* 81–107.

Hsu, L. K. G., Wisner, K., Richey, E. T., & Goldstein, C. (1985). Is juvenile delinquency related to an abnormal EEG? *Journal of the American Academy of Child and Adolescent Psychiatry, 24,* 310–315.

Hubbs-Tait, L., Hughes, K. P., Culp, A. M., Osofsky, J. D., Hann, D. M., Eberhart-Wright, A., & Ware, L. M. (1996). Children of adolescent mothers: Attachment representation, maternal depression, and later behavior problems. *American Journal of Orthopsychiatry, 66,* 416–426.

Hudziak, J. J., Rudiger, L. P., Neale, M. C., Heath, A. C., & Todd, R. D. (2000). A twin study of inattentive, aggressive, and anxious/depressed behaviors. *Journal of the American Academy of Child and Adolescent Psychiatry, 39,* 469–476.

Huesmann, L. R., Eron, L. D., Lefkowitz, M. M., & Walder, L. O. (1984). The stability of aggression over time and generations. *Developmental Psychology, 20,* 1120–1134.

Hughes, C. W., Petty, F., Sheikha, S., & Kramer, G. L. (1996). Whole-blood serotonin in children and adolescents with mood and behavior disorders. *Psychiatry Research, 65,* 79–95.

Humphreys, L., Forehand, R., McMahon, R., & Roberts, M. (1978). Parent behavioral training to modify child noncompliance: Effects on untreated siblings. *Journal of Behavior Therapy and Experimental Psychiatry, 9,* 235–238.

Hunt, R. D., Arnsten, A. F. T., & Asbell, M. D. (1995). An open trial of guanfacine in the treatment of attention-deficit hyperactivity disorder. *Journal of the American Academy of Child and Adolescent Psychiatry, 34,* 50–54.

Hunt, R. D., Minderaa, R. B., & Cohen, D. J. (1985). Clonidine benefits children with attention deficit disorder and hyperactivity: Report of a double-blind placebo-crossover therapeutic trial. *Journal of the American Academy of Child and Adolescent Psychiatry, 24,* 617–629.

Hurt, H., Malmud, E., Betancourt, L., Braitman, L. E., Brodsky, N. L., & Giannetta, J. (1997). Children with *in utero* cocaine exposure do not differ from control subjects on intelligence testing. *Archives of Pediatrics and Adolescent Medicine, 151,* 1237–1241.

Huston, A. C., Donnerstein, E., Fairchild, H., Feshbach, N. D., Katz, P. A., Murray, J. P., Rubinstein, E. A., Wilcox, B. L., & Zuckerman, D. (1992). *Big world, small screen: The role of television in American society.* Lincoln: University of Nebraska Press.

Hyde, J. S. (1984). How large are gender differences in aggression?: A developmental meta-analysis. *Developmental Psychology, 20,* 722–736.

Iglehart, J. K. (1996). Health care policy report: Managed care and mental health in children. *New England Journal of Medicine, 334,* 131–135.

Inamdar, S. C., Lewis, D. O., Siomopoulos, G., Shanok, S. S., & Lamela, M. (1982). Violent and suicidal behavior in psychotic adolescents. *American Journal of Psychiatry, 139,* 932–935.

Inoff-Germain, G. E., Arnold, G. S., Nottelmann, E. D., Susman, E. J., Cutler, G. B., Jr., & Chrousos, G. P. (1988). Relations between hormone levels and observational measures of aggressive behavior of young adolescents in family interactions. *Developmental Psychology, 24,* 129–139.

Izard, T. E., Fantauzzo, C. A., Castle, J. M., Haynes, O. M., Rayias, M. R., & Putnam, P. H. (1995). The ontogeny of infants' facial expressions in the first nine months of life. *Developmental Psychology, 31,* 997–1013.

Jacobson, S. W., Jacobson, J. L., Sokol, R. J., Martier, S. S., & Chiodo, L. M. (1996). New evidence for neurobehavioral effects of *in utero* cocaine exposure. *Journal of Pediatrics, 129,* 581–590.

Jansen, L. M. C., Gispen-de Wied, C. C., Jansen, M. A., van der Gaag, R-J., Matthys, W., & van Engeland, H. (1999). Pituitary–adrenal reactivity in a child psychiatric population: Salivary cortisol response to stressors. *European Neuropsychopharmacology, 9,* 67–75.

Jellinek, M., & Little, M. (1998). Supporting child psychiatric services using current managed care approaches: You can't get there from here. *Archives of Pediatrics and Adolescent Medicine, 152,* 321–326.

Jenkins, E. J., & Bell, C. C. (1994). Violence exposure, psychological distress, and high risk behaviors among inner-city high school students. In S. Friedman (Ed.), *Anxiety disorders in African-Americans* (pp. 76–88). New York: Springer.

Jenkins, E. J., & Bell, C. C. (1997). Exposure and response to community violence among children and adolescents. In J. D. Osofsky (Ed.), *Children in a violent society* (pp. 9–31). New York: Guilford Press.

Jenkins, J. M., & Smith, M. A. (1990). Factors protecting children living in disharmonious homes: Maternal reports. *Journal of the American Academy of Child and Adolescent Psychiatry, 29,* 60–69.

Jennett, B. (1976). Assessment of the severity of head injury. *Journal of Neurology, Neurosurgery and Psychiatry, 39,* 647.

Jensen, P. S., & Hoagwood, K. (1997). The book of names: DSM-IV in context. *Development and Psychopathology, 9,* 231–249.

Johnson, B. A., Brent, D. A., Connolly, J., Bridge, J., Matta, J., Constantine, D., Rather, C., & White, T. (1995). Familial aggregation of adolescent personality disorders.

Journal of the American Academy of Child and Adolescent Psychiatry, 34, 798–804.

Johnson, D. L. (1988). Primary prevention of behavior problems in young children: The Houston Parent–Child Development Center. In R. H. Price, E. L. Cohen, R. P. Lorion, & J. Ramos-McKay (Eds.), *14 ounces of prevention: A casebook for practitioners* (pp. 44–52). Washington, DC: American Psychological Association.

Johnson, D. L. (1989, April). *Follow-up of the Houston Parent–Child Development Center: Preliminary analyses.* Paper presented at the biennial meeting of the Society for Research in Child Development, Kansas City, MO.

Johnson, D. L., & Breckenridge, J. N. (1982). The Houston Parent–Child Development Center and the primary prevention of behavior problems in young children. *American Journal of Community Psychology, 10*, 305–316.

Johnson, D. L., & Walker, T. (1987). The primary prevention of behavior problems in Mexican-American children. *American Journal of Community Psychology, 15*, 375–385.

Johnson, E. O., Arria, A. M., Borges, G., Ialongo, N., & Anthony, J. C. (1995). The growth of conduct problem behaviors from middle childhood to early adolescence: Sex differences and the suspected influence of early alcohol use. *Journal of Studies on Alcohol, 56*, 661–671.

Johnson, J. G., Cohen, P., Smailes, E., Kasen, S., Oldham, J. M., Skodol, A. E., & Brook, J. S. (2000). Adolescent personality disorders associated with violence and criminal behavior during adolescence and early adulthood. *American Journal of Psychiatry, 157*, 1406–1412.

Johnston, L. D. (1996, December 19). *The rise in drug use among American teens continues in 1996.* Press release from the Monitoring the Future Study, Ann Arbor, MI.

Jones, M. D., Offord, D. R., & Abrams, N. (1980). Brothers, sisters, and antisocial behavior. *British Journal of Psychiatry, 136*, 139–145.

Joshi, P. T., Capozzoli, J. A., & Coyle, J. T. (1988). Low-dose neuroleptic therapy for children with childhood-onset pervasive developmental disorder. *American Journal of Psychiatry, 145*, 335–338.

Joyce, P. R. (1984). Age of onset in bipolar affective disorder and misdiagnosis as schizophrenia. *Psychological Medicine, 14*, 145–149.

Junger-Tas, J. (1992). Changes in the family and their impact on delinquency. *European Journal of Criminal Policy and Research, 1*, 27–51.

Juon, H.-S., & Ensminger, M. E. (1997). Childhood, adolescent, and young adult predictors of suicidal behaviors: A prospective study of African Americans. *Journal of Child Psychology and Psychiatry, 38*, 553–563.

Kafantaris, V., Campbell, M., Padron-Gayol, M. V., Small, A. M., Locascio, J. J., & Rosenberg, C. R. (1992). Carbamazepine in hospitalized aggressive conduct disorder children: An open pilot study. *Psychopharmacology Bulletin, 26*, 193–199.

Kafantaris, V., Lee, D. O., Magee, H., Winny, G., Samuel, R., Pollack, S., & Campbell, M. (1996). Assessment of children with the Overt Aggression Scale. *Journal of Neuropsychiatry and Clinical Neurosciences, 8*, 186–193.

Kagan, J. (1994). *Galen's prophecy: Temperament in human nature.* New York: Basic Books.

Kagan, J., & Moss, H. A. (1962). *Birth to maturity.* New York: Wiley.

Kalin, N. H. (1997). The neurobiology of fear. *Scientific American, 7*, 76–83.

Kamphaus, R. W., & Frick, P. J. (1996). *The clinical assessment of children's emotion, behavior, and personality.* Boston: Allyn & Bacon.

Kandel, D. B., & Davies, M. (1986). Adult sequelae of adolescent depressive symptoms. *Archives of General Psychiatry, 43*, 255–262.

Kandel, E., Brennan, P. A., Mednick, S. A., & Michelson, N. M. (1989). Minor physical anomalies and recidivistic adult violent criminal behavior. *Acta Psychiatrica Scandinavica, 79*, 103–107.

Kandel, E., Mednick, S. A., Kirkegaard-Sorensen, L., Hutchings, B., Knop, J., Rosenberg, R., & Schulsinger, F. (1988). IQ as a protective factor for subjects at high risk for antisocial behavior. *Journal of Consulting and Clinical Psychology, 56*, 224–226.

Kaplan, S. L., Busner, J., Kupietz, S., Wassermann, E., & Segal, B. (1990). Effects of methylphenidate on adolescents with aggressive conduct disorder and ADDH: A preliminary report. *Journal of the American Academy of Child and Adolescent Psychiatry, 29*, 719–723.

Kasen, S., Cohen, P., Skodol, A. E., Johnson, J. G., Smailes, E., & Brook, J. S. (2001). Childhood depression and adult personality disorder. *Archives of General Psychiatry, 58*, 231–236.

Kashani, J. H., Allan, W. D., Beck, Jr., N. C., Bledsoe, Y., & Reid, J. C. (1997). Dysthymic disorder in clinically referred preschool children. *Journal of the American Academy of Child and Adolescent Psychiatry, 36*, 1426–1433.

Kashani, J. H., Beck, N. C., Hoeper, E. W., Fallahi, C., Corcoran, C. M., McAllister, J. A., Rosenberg, T. K., & Reid, J. C. (1987). Psychiatric disorders in a community sample of adolescents. *American Journal of Psychiatry, 144*, 584–589.

Kashani, J. H., Dahlmeier, J. M., Borduin, C. M., Soltys, S., & Reid, J. C. (1995). Characteristics of anger expression in depressed children. *Journal of the American Academy of Child and Adolescent Psychiatry, 34*, 322–326.

Kaufman, J. (1991). Depressive disorders in maltreated children. *Journal of the American Academy of Child and Adolescent Psychiatry, 30*, 257–265.

Kaufman, J., Birmaher, B., Brent, D., Rao, U., Flynn, C., Moreci, P., Williamson, D., & Ryan, N. (1997). Schedule for Affective Disorders and Schizophrenia for School-Age Children—Present and Lifetime Version (K-SADS-PL): Initial reliability and validity data. *Journal of the American Academy of Child and Adolescent Psychiatry, 36*, 980–988.

Kay, S. R., Wolkenfeld, F., & Murrill, L. M. (1988). Profiles of aggression among psychiatric patients: I. Nature and prevalence. *Journal of Nervous and Mental Disease, 176*, 539–546.

Kazdin, A. E. (1987). Treatment of antisocial behavior in children: Current status and future directions. *Psychological Bulletin, 102*, 187–203.

Kazdin, A. E. (1989). Developmental psychopathology, *American Psychologist, 44*, 180–187.

Kazdin, A. E. (1994). Interventions for aggressive and antisocial children. In L. D. Eron, J. H. Gentry, & P. Schlegel (Eds.), *Reason to hope: A psychosocial perspective on violence and youth* (pp. 341–382). Washington, DC: American Psychological Association.

Kazdin, A. E. (1996). *Conduct disorders in childhood and adolescence* (2nd ed.). Thousand Oaks, CA: Sage.

Kazdin, A. E. (1997). Practitioner review: Psychosocial treatments for conduct disorder in children. *Journal of Child Psychology and Psychiatry, 38*, 161–178.

Kazdin, A. E. (2000). *Psychotherapy for children and adolescents: Directions for research and practice.* New York: Oxford University Press.

Kazdin, A. E., Esveldt-Dawson, K., French, N. H., & Unis, A. S. (1987). Problem-solving skills training and relationship therapy in the treatment of antisocial child behavior. *Journal of Consulting and Clinical Psychology, 55,* 76–85.

Kazdin, A. E., & Wassell, G. (2000). Therapeutic changes in children, parents, and families resulting from treatment of children with conduct problems. *Journal of the American Academy of Child and Adolescent Psychiatry, 39,* 414–420.

Keenan, K., & Shaw, D. (1997). Developmental and social influences on young girls' early problem behavior. *Psychological Bulletin, 121,* 95–113.

Kellam, S. G., Brown, C. H., Rubin, B. R., & Ensminger, M. E. (1983). Paths leading to teenage psychiatric symptoms and substance use. Developmental epidemiological studies in Woodlawn. In S. B. Guze, F. J. Earls, & J. E. Barrett (Eds.), *Childhood psychopathology and development* (pp. 17–51). New York: Raven Press.

Kemph, J. P., DeVane, C. L., Levin, G. M., Jarecke, R., & Miller, R. L. (1993). Treatment of aggressive children with clonidine: Results of an open pilot study. *Journal of the American Academy of Child and Adolescent Psychiatry, 32,* 577–581.

Kendall, P. C. (1985). Toward a cognitive-behavioral model of child psychopathology and a critique of related interventions. *Journal of Abnormal Psychology, 13,* 357–372.

Kendall, P. C., & Braswell, L. (1985). *Cognitive-behavioral therapy for impulsive children.* New York: Guilford Press.

Kendall, P. C., Reber, M., McLeer, S., Epps, J., & Ronan, K. R. (1990). Cognitive-behavioral treatment of conduct-disordered children. *Cognitive Therapy and Research, 14,* 279–297.

Kendall-Tackett, K. A., Williams, L. M., & Finkelhor, D. (1993). Impact of sexual abuse on children: A review and synthesis of recent empirical studies. *Psychological Bulletin, 113,* 164–180.

Kent, M. A., Camfield, C. S., & Camfield, P. R. (1999). Double-blind methylphenidate trials: Practical, useful, and highly endorsed by families. *Archives of Pediatrics and Adolescent Medicine, 153,* 1292–1296.

Kerr, M., Tremblay, R. E., Pagani, L., & Vitaro, F. (1997). Boys' behavioral inhibition and the risk of later delinquency. *Archives of General Psychiatry, 54,* 809–816.

Kim, W. J. (1991). Psychiatric aspects of epileptic children and adolescents. *Journal of the American Academy of Child and Adolescent Psychiatry, 30,* 874–886.

Kindlon, D. J., Tremblay, R. E., Mezzacappa, E., Earls, F., Laurent, D., & Schaal, B. (1995). Longitudinal patterns of heart rate and fighting behavior in 9– through 12–year-old boys. *Journal of the American Academy of Child and Adolescent Psychiatry, 34,* 371–377.

King, J. A., Barkley, R. A., & Barrett, S. (1998). Attention-deficit hyperactivity disorder and the stress response. *Biological Psychiatry, 44,* 72–74.

Kingery, P. M., Pruitt, B. E., & Hurley, R. S. (1992). Violence and illegal drug use among adolescents: Evidence from the U. S. national adolescent student health survey. *International Journal of the Addictions, 27,* 1445–1464.

Kingston, L., & Prior, M. (1995). The development of patterns of stable, transient, and school-age onset aggressive behavior in young children. *Journal of the American Academy of Child and Adolescent Psychiatry, 34,* 348–358.

Klein, N. C., Alexander, J. F., & Parsons, B. V. (1977). Impact of family systems intervention on recidivism and sibling delinquency: A model of primary prevention and program evaluation. *Journal of Consulting and Clinical Psychology, 45,* 469–474.

Klein, R. G. (1991). Preliminary results: Lithium effects in conduct disorders. In *CME syllabus and proceedings summary, Symposium 2* (pp. 119–120). Washington, DC: American Psychiatric Association.

Klein, R. G., Abikoff, H., Barkley, R. A., Campbell, M., Leckman, J. F., Ryan, N. D., Solanto, M. V., & Whalen, C. K. (1994). Clinical trials in children and adolescents. In R. F. Prien & D. S. Robinson (Eds.), *Clinical evaluation of psychotropic drugs: Principles and guidelines* (pp. 501–546). New York: Raven Press.

Klein, R. G., Abikoff, H., Klass, E., Ganeles, D., Seese, L. M., & Pollack, S. (1997). Clinical efficacy of methylphenidate in conduct disorder with and without attention deficit hyperactivity disorder. *Archives of General Psychiatry, 54*, 1073–1080.

Klorman, R., Brumaghim, J. T., Salzman, L. F., Strauss, J., Borgstedt, A. D., McBride, M. C., & Loeb, S. (1988). Effects of methylphenidate on attention-deficit hyperactivity disorder with and without aggressive/noncompliant features. *Journal of Abnormal Psychology, 97*, 413–422.

Knox, M., King, C., Hanna, G. L., Logan, D., & Ghaziuddin, N. (2000). Aggressive behavior in clinically depressed adolescents. *Journal of the American Academy of Child and Adolescent Psychiatry, 39*, 611–618.

Kochanska, G., De Vet, K., Goldman, M., Murray, K., & Putnam, S. P. (1994). Maternal reports of conscience development in young children. *Child Development, 65*, 852–868.

Kolb, L. C. (1987). A neuropsychological hypothesis explaining posttraumatic stress disorders. *American Journal of Psychiatry, 144*, 989–995.

Kolko, D. J., Bukstein, O. G., & Barron, J. (1999). Methylphenidate and behavior modification in children with ADHD and comorbid ODD or CD: Main and incremental effects across settings. *Journal of the American Academy of Child and Adolescent Psychiatry, 38*, 578–586.

Kolvin, I., Miller, F. J., Fleeting, M., & Kolvin, P. A. (1988). Social and parenting factors affecting criminal offense rates: Findings from the Newcastle Thousand Family Study. *British Journal of Psychiatry, 152*, 80–90.

Koren, G., Nulman, I., Rovet, J., Greenbaum, R., Loebstein, M., & Einarson, T. (1998). Long-term neurodevelopmental risks in children exposed *in utero* to cocaine: The Toronto adoption study. *Annals of the New York Academy of Sciences, 846*, 306–313.

Kosson, D. S. (1996). Psychopathy and dual-task performance under focusing conditions. *Journal of Abnormal Psychology, 105*, 391–400.

Kovacs, M. (1985). The Interview Schedule for Children (ISC). *Psychopharmacology Bulletin, 21*, 991–994.

Kovacs, M. (1996). Presentation and course of major depressive disorder during childhood and later years of the life span. *Journal of the American Academy of Child and Adolescent Psychiatry, 35*, 705–715.

Kovacs, M., Akiskal, H. S., Gatsonis, C., & Parrone, P. L. (1994). Childhood-onset dysthymic disorder: Clinical features and prospective naturalistic outcome. *Archives of General Psychiatry, 51*, 365–374.

Kovacs, M., Feinberg, T. L., Crouse-Novak, M. A., Paulauskas, S. L., & Finkelstein, R. (1984). Depressive disorders in childhood. I. A longitudinal prospective study of characteristics and recovery. *Archives of General Psychiatry, 41*, 229–237.

Kovacs, M., Feinberg, T. L., Crouse-Novak, M., Paulauskas, S. L., Pollock, M., & Finkelstein, R. (1984). Depressive disorders in childhood: II. A longitudinal study of the risk for a subsequent major depression. *Archives of General Psychiatry, 41*, 643–649.

Kovacs, M., & Gatsonis, C. (1994). Secular trends in age at onset of major depressive disorder in a clinical sample of children. *Journal of Psychiatric Research, 28,* 319–329.

Kovacs, M., Krol, R. S., & Voti, L. (1994). Early onset psychopathology and the risk for teenage pregnancy among clinically referred girls. *Journal of the American Academy of Child and Adolescent Psychiatry, 33,* 106–113.

Kovacs, M., & Pollock, M. (1995). Bipolar disorder and comorbid conduct disorder in childhood and adolescence. *Journal of the American Academy of Child and Adolescent Psychiatry, 34,* 715–723.

Kowatch, R. A., Suppes, T., Carmody, T. J., Bucci, J. P., Hume, J. H., Kromelis, M., Emslie, G. J., Weinberg, W. A., & Rush, A. J. (2000). Effect size of lithium, divalproex sodium, and carbamazepine in children and adolescents with bipolar disorder. *Journal of the American Academy of Child and Adolescent Psychiatry, 39,* 713–720.

Kowatch, R. A., Suppes, T., Gilfillan, S. K., Fuentes, R. M., Grannemann, B. D., & Emslie, G. J. (1995). Clozapine treatment of children and adolescents with bipolar disorder and schizophrenia: A clinical case series. *Journal of Child and Adolescent Psychopharmacology, 5,* 241–253.

Kraemer, G. W. (1985). Effects of differences in early social experience on primate neurobiological–behavioral development. In M. Reite & T. Field (Eds.), *The psychobiology of attachment* (pp. 135–161). New York: Academic Press.

Kraemer, G. W., & Clarke, S. (1996). Social attachment, brain function, and aggression. *Annals of the New York Academy of Sciences, 794,* 121–135.

Kraepelin, E. (1921). *Manic–depressive insanity and paranoia.* Edinburgh: Livingstone.

Kreutzer, J. S., Marwitz, J. H., & Witol, A. D. (1995). Interrelationships between crime, substance abuse, and aggressive behaviours among persons with traumatic brain injury. *Brain Injury, 9,* 757–768.

Krueger, R. F. (1999). The structure of common mental disorders. *Archives of General Psychiatry, 56,* 921–926.

Kruesi, M. J. P., Hibbs, E. D., Zahn, T. P., Keysor, C. S., Hamburger, S. D., Bartko, J. J., & Rapoport, J. L. (1992). A 2-year prospective follow-up study of children and adolescents with disruptive behavior disorders. *Archives of General Psychiatry, 49,* 429–435.

Kruesi, M. J. P., Rapoport, J. L., Hamburger, S., Hibbs, E., Potter, W. Z., Lenane, M., & Brown, G. L. (1990). Cerebrospinal fluid monoamine metabolites, aggression, and impulsivity in disruptive behavior disorders of children and adolescents. *Archives of General Psychiatry, 47,* 419–426.

Kruesi, M. J. P., Schmidt, M. E., Donnelly, M., Hibbs, E. D., & Hamburger, S. D. (1989). Urinary free cortisol output and disruptive behavior in children. *Journal of the American Academy of Child and Adolescent Psychiatry, 28,* 441–443.

Kumra, S., Frazier, J. A., Jacobsen, L. K., McKenna, K., Gordon, C. T., Lenane, M. C., Hamburger, S. D., Smith, A. K., Albus, K. E., Alaghvand-Rad, J., & Rapoport, J. L. (1996). Childhood onset schizophrenia: A double-blind clozapine–haloperidol comparison. *Archives of General Psychiatry, 53,* 1090–1097.

Kumra, S., Jacobsen, L. K., Lenane, M., Karp, B. I., Frazier, J. A., Smith, A. K., Bedwell, J., Lee, P., Malanga, C. J., Hamburger, S., & Rapoport, J. L. (1998). Childhood-onset schizophrenia: An open-label study of olanzepine in adolescents. *Journal of the American Academy of Child and Adolescent Psychiatry, 37,* 377–385.

Kuperman, S., & Stewart, M. A. (1987). Use of propranolol to decrease aggressive outbursts in younger patients. *Psychosomatics, 28,* 315–319.

Kuperman, S., Schlosser, S. S., Lidral, J., & Reich, W. (1999). Relationship of child psychopathology to parental alcoholism and antisocial personality disorder. *Journal of the American Academy of Child and Adolescent Psychiatry, 38,* 686–692.

Kupersmidt, J. B., Coie, J. D., & Dodge, K. A. (1990). The role of poor peer relationships in the development of disorder. In S. R. Asher & J. D. Coie (Eds.), *Peer rejection in childhood* (pp. 247–308). Cambridge, England: Cambridge University Press.

Kutcher, S. P., Marton, P., & Kornblum, M. (1989). Relationship between psychiatric illness and conduct disorder in adolescents. *Canadian Journal of Psychiatry, 34,* 526–529.

Lachar, D., & Gruber, C. P. (1991). *Manual for Personality Inventory for Children—Revised.* Los Angeles: Western Psychological Services.

Lagerspetz, K. M. J., Bjorkqvist, K., & Peltonen, T. (1988). Is indirect aggression typical of females?: Gender differences in aggressiveness in 11– to 12–year-old children. *Aggressive Behavior, 14,* 403–414.

Lahey, B. B., Applegate, B., Barkley, R. A., Garfinkle, B., McBurnett, K., Kerdyk, L., Greenhill, L. J., Hynd, G. W., Frick, P. J., Newcorn, J., Biederman, J., Ollendick, T., Hart, E. L., Perez, D., Waldman, I., & Shaffer, D. (1994). DSM-IV field trials for oppositional defiant disorder and conduct disorder in children and adolescents. *American Journal of Psychiatry, 151,* 1163–1171.

Lahey, B. B., Applegate, B., McBurnett, K., Biederman, J., Greenhill, L., Hynd, G. W., Barkley, R. A., Newcorn, J., Jensen, P., Richters, J., Garfinkel, B., Kerdyk, L., Frick, P. J., Ollendick, T., Perez, D., Hart, E. L., Waldman, I., & Shaffer, D. (1994). DSM-IV field trials for attention deficit/hyperactivity disorder in children and adolescents. *Journal of the American Academy of Child and Adolescent Psychiatry, 151,* 1673–1685.

Lahey, B. B., Flagg, E. W., Bird, H. R., Schwab-Stone, M. E., Canino, G., Dulcan, M. K., Leaf, P. J., Davies, M., Brogan, D., Bourdon, K., Horwitz, S. M., Rubio-Stipec, M., Freeman, D. H., Lichtman, J. H., Shaffer, D., Goodman, S. H., Narrow, W. E., Weissman, M. M., Kandel, D. B., Jensen, P. S., Richters, J. E., & Regier, D. A. (1996). The NIMH Methods for the Epidemiology of Child and Adolescent Mental Disorders (MECA) study: Background and methodology. *Journal of the American Academy of Child and Adolescent Psychiatry, 35,* 855–864.

Lahey, B. B., Goodman, S. H., Waldman, I. D., Bird, H., Canino, G., Jensen, P., Regier, D., Leaf, P. J., Gordon, R., & Applegate, B. (1999). Relation of age of onset to the type and severity of child and adolescent conduct problems. *Journal of Abnormal Child Psychology, 27,* 247–260.

Lahey, B. B., Hart, E. L., Pliszka, S., Applegate, B., & McBurnett, K. (1993). Neurophysiological correlates of conduct disorder: A rationale and a review of research. *Journal of Clinical Child Psychology, 22,* 141–153.

Lahey, B. B., Loeber, R., Hart, E., Frick, P. J., Applegate, B., Zhang, Q., Green, S. M., & Russo, M. F. (1995). Four-year longitudinal study of conduct disorder in boys: Patterns and predictors of persistence. *Journal of Abnormal Psychology, 104,* 83–93.

Lahey, B. B., Loeber, R., Quay, H. C., Applegate, B., Shaffer, D., Waldman, I., Hart, E. L., McBurnett, K., Frick, P. J., Jensen, P. S., Dulcan, M. K., Canino, G., & Bird, H. R. (1998). Validity of DSM-IV subtypes of conduct disorder based on age of onset. *Journal of the American Academy of Child and Adolescent Psychiatry, 37,* 435–442.

Lahey, B. B., McBurnett, K., Loeber, R., & Hart, E. L. (1995). Psychobiology. In G. P. Sholevar (Ed.), *Conduct disorder in children and adolescents* (pp. 27–44). Washington, DC: American Psychiatric Press.

Lahey, B. B., Waldman, I. D., & McBurnett, K. (1999). Annotation: The development of antisocial behavior. An integrative causal model. *Journal of Child Psychology and Psychiatry, 40,* 669–682.

Lally, R., Mangione, P. L., & Honig, A. S. (1988). The Syracuse University Family Development Research Program: Long-range impact on an early intervention with low-income children and their families. In D. Powell (Ed.), *Parent education as early childhood intervention: Emerging directions in theory, research, and practice* (pp. 79–104). Norwood, NJ: Ablex.

Landry, S. H., & Whitney, J. A. (1996). The impact of prenatal cocaine exposure: Studies of the developing infant. *Seminars in Perinatology, 20,* 99–106.

Lang, P. J., Bradley, M. M., & Cuthbert, B. N. (1998). Emotion, motivation, and anxiety: Brain mechanisms and psychophysiology. *Biological Psychiatry, 44,* 1248–1263.

Langbehn, D. R., Cadoret, R. J., Yates, W. R., Troughton, E. P., & Stewart, M. A. (1998). Distinct contributions of conduct and oppositional defiant symptoms to adult antisocial behavior. *Archives of General Psychiatry, 55,* 821–829.

Lapierre, D., Braun, C. M., & Hodgins, S. (1995). Ventral frontal deficits in psychopathy: Neuropsychological test findings. *Neuropsychologia, 33,* 139–151.

Lappalainen, J., Long, J. C., Eggert, M., Ozaki, N., Robin, R. W., Brown, G. L., Naukkarinen, H., Virkkunen, M., Linnoila, M., & Goldman, D. (1998). Linkage of antisocial alcoholism to the serotonin 5–HT1B receptor gene in 2 populations. *Archives of General Psychiatry, 55,* 989–994.

Lau, M. A., Pihl, R. O., & Peterson, J. B. (1995). Provocation, acute alcohol intoxication, cognitive performance, and aggression. *Journal of Abnormal Psychology, 104,* 150–155.

Laub, J. H., & Vaillant, G. E. (2000). Delinquency and mortality: A 50–year follow-up study of 1,000 delinquent and nondelinquent boys. *American Journal of Psychiatry, 157,* 96–102.

Lavigne, J. V., Binns, H. J., Arend, R., Rosenbaum, D., Christoffel, K. K., Hayford, J. R., & Gibbons, R. D. (1998). Psychopathology and health care use among preschool children: A retrospective analysis. *Journal of the American Academy of Child and Adolescent Psychiatry, 37,* 262–270.

Leckman, J. F., Hardin, M. T., Riddle, M. A., Stevenson, J., Ort, S. I., & Cohen, D. J. (1991). Clonidine treatment of Gilles de la Tourette's syndrome. *Archives of General Psychiatry, 48,* 324–328.

LeDoux, J. (1996). *The emotional brain: The mysterious underpinnings of emotional life.* New York: Simon & Schuster.

LeDoux, J. (1998). Fear and the brain: Where have we been and where are we going? *Biological Psychiatry, 44,* 1229–1238.

LeMarquand, D. G., Pihl, R. O., Young, S. N., Tremblay, R. E., Seguin, J. R., Palmour, R. M., & Benkelfat, C. (1998). Tryptophan depletion, executive functions, and disinhibition in aggressive, adolescent males. *Neuropsychopharmacology, 19,* 333–341.

Lennox, W. G., & Lennox, M. A. (1960). *Epilepsy and related disorders.* Boston: Little, Brown.

Lesch, K.-P., Wolozin, D. L., Murphy, D. L., & Riederer, P. (1993). Primary structure of the human serotonin uptake site: Identity with the brain serotonin transporter. *Journal of Neurochemistry, 60,* 2319–2322.

Lester, D. (1991). Crime as opportunity: A test of the hypothesis with European homicide rates. *British Journal of Criminology, 31,* 186–188.

Lewinsohn, P. M., Hops, H., Roberts, R. E., Seeley, J. R., & Andrews, J. A. (1993). Adolescent psychopathology: I. Prevalence and incidence of depression and other DSM-III-R disorders in high school students. *Journal of Abnormal Psychology, 102,* 133–144.

Lewinsohn, P. M., Klein, D. N., & Seeley, J. R. (1993). Psychosocial characteristics of adolescents with a history of suicide attempt. *Journal of the American Academy of Child and Adolescent Psychiatry, 32,* 60–68.

Lewinsohn, P. M., Klein, D. N., & Seeley, J. R. (1995). Bipolar disorders in a community sample of older adolescents: Prevalence, phenomenology, comorbidity, and course. *Journal of the American Academy of Child and Adolescent Psychiatry, 34,* 454–463.

Lewinsohn, P. M., Rohde, P., Seeley, J. R., & Klein, D. N. (1997). Axis II psychopathology as a function of Axis I disorders in childhood and adolescence. *Journal of the American Academy of Child and Adolescent Psychiatry, 36,* 1752–1759.

Lewis, D. O., Lovely, R., Yeager, C., & Femina, D. D. (1989). Toward a theory of the genesis of violence: A follow-up study of delinquents. *Journal of the American Academy of Child and Adolescent Psychiatry, 28,* 431–436.

Lewis, D. O., Pincus, J. H., Shanok, S. S., & Glaser, G. H. (1982). Psychomotor epilepsy and violence in a group of incarcerated adolescent boys. *American Journal of Psychiatry, 139,* 882–887.

Lewis, D. O., Shanok, S. S., Grant, M., & Ritvo, E. (1983). Homicidally aggressive young children: Neuropsychiatric and experiential correlates. *American Journal of Psychiatry, 140,* 148–153.

Lewis, D. O., Yeager, C. A., Cobham-Portorreal, C. S., Klein, N., Showalter, C., & Anthony, A. (1991). A follow-up of female delinquents: Maternal contributions to the perpetuation of deviance. *Journal of the American Academy of Child and Adolescent Psychiatry, 30,* 197–201.

Liang, S-W, Jemerin, J. M., Tschann, J. M., Irwin, C. E., Wara, D. W., & Boyce, W. T. (1995). Life events, cardiovascular reactivity, and risk behavior in adolescent boys. *Pediatrics, 96,* 1101–1105.

Lichter, R. S., & Amundson, D. (1992). *A day of TV violence.* Washington, DC: Center for Media and Public Affairs.

Lichter, R. S., & Amundson, D. (1994). *A day of TV violence: 1992 vs. 1994.* Washington, DC: Center for Media and Public Affairs.

Liebert, R. M., & Baron, R. A. (1972). Short-term effects of television aggression on children's aggressive behavior. In J. P. Murray, E. A. Rubinstein, & G. A. Comstock (Eds.), *Television and social behavior: Vol. 2. Television and social learning* (pp. 181–201). Washington, DC: U.S. Government Printing Office.

Liebert, R. M., & Sprafkin, J. (1988). *The early window: Effects of television on children and youth* (3rd ed.). Elmsford, NY: Pergamon Press.

Lilienfeld, S. O. (1994). Conceptual problems in the assessment of psychopathy. *Clinical Psychology Review, 14,* 17–38.

Lilienfeld, S. O. (1998). Methodological advances and developments in the assessment of psychopathy. *Behaviour Research and Therapy, 36,* 99–125.

Lincoln, A. J., Bloom, D., Katz, M., & Boksenbaum, N. (1998). Neuropsychological and neurophysiological indices of auditory processing impairment in children with multiple complex developmental disorder. *Journal of the American Academy of Child and Adolescent Psychiatry, 37,* 100–112.

Lindenmayer, J.-P., & Kotsaftis, A. (2000). Use of sodium valproate in violent and aggressive behaviors: A critical review. *Journal of Clinical Psychiatry, 61,* 123–128.

Link, B. G., Andrews, H., & Cullen, F. (1992). The violent and illegal behavior of mental patients reconsidered. *American Sociological Review, 57,* 275–292.

Link, B. G., & Stueve, A. (1998). Commentary: New evidence on the violence risk posed by people with mental illness. *Archives of General Psychiatry, 55,* 403–404.

Linnoila, M., DeJong, J., & Virkkunen, M. (1989). Family history of alcoholism in violent offenders and impulsive firesetters. *Archives of General Psychiatry, 46,* 613–616.

Linnoila, M., Virkkunen, M., Scheinin, M., Nuutila, A., Rimon, R., & Goodwin, F. K. (1983). Low cerebrospinal fluid 5–hydroxyindoleacetic acid concentration differentiates impulsive from nonimpulsive violent behavior. *Life Science, 33,* 2609–2614.

Linz, T. D., Hooper, S. R., Hynd, G. W., Isaac, W., & Gibson, L. J. (1990). Frontal lobe functioning in conduct disordered juveniles: Preliminary findings. *Archives of Clinical Neuropsychology, 5,* 411–416.

Lochman, J. E. (1992). Cognitive-behavioral interventions with aggressive boys: Three year follow-up and preventive effects. *Journal of Consulting and Clinical Psychology, 60,* 426–432.

Lochman, J. E., Burch, P. R., Curry, F. F., & Lampron, L. B. (1984). Treatment and generalization effects of cognitive-behavioral and goal-setting interventions with aggressive boys. *Journal of Consulting and Clinical Psychology, 52,* 915–916.

Lochman, J. E., & Curry, J. F. (1986). Effects of social problem-solving training and self-instruction with aggressive boys. *Journal of Clinical Child Psychology, 15,* 159–164.

Lochman, J. E., & Dodge, K. A. (1994). Social-cognitive processes of severely violent, moderately aggressive, and non-aggressive boys. *Journal of Consulting and Clinical Psychology, 62,* 366–374.

Lochman, J. E., & Lampron, L. B. (1988). Cognitive behavioral interventions for aggressive boys: Seven months follow-up effects. *Journal of Child and Adolescent Psychotherapy, 5,* 15–23.

Lochman, J. E., Lampron, L. B., Gemmer, T. C., & Harris, S. R. (1987). Anger coping intervention with aggressive children: A guide to implementation in school settings. In P. A. Keller & S. R. Heyman (Eds.), *Innovations in clinical practice: A source book* (Vol. 6, pp. 339–356). Sarasota, FL: Professional Resource Exchange.

Lochman, J. E., & Wayland, K. E. (1994). Aggression, social acceptance, and race as predictors of negative adolescent outcomes. *Journal of the American Academy of Child and Adolescent Psychiatry, 33,* 1026–1035.

Lochman, J. E., & Wells, K. C. (1996). A social-cognitive intervention with aggressive children: Prevention effects and contextual implementation issues. In R. D. Peters & R. J. McMahon (Eds.), *Preventing childhood disorders, substance abuse, and delinquency* (pp. 111–143). Thousand Oaks, CA: Sage.

Loeber, R. (1982). The stability of antisocial and delinquent child behavior. *Child Development, 53,* 1431–1446.

Loeber, R. (1988). Natural histories of conduct problems, delinquency, and associated substance use. In B. B. Lahey & A. E. Kazdin (Eds.), *Advances in clinical child psychology* (Vol. 11, pp. 73–124). New York: Plenum Press.

Loeber, R. (1990). Development and risk factors of juvenile antisocial behavior and delinquency. *Clinical Psychology Review, 10,* 1–41.

Loeber, R., & Dishion, T. (1983). Boys who fight at home and school: Family conditions influencing cross-setting consistency. *Journal of Consulting and Clinical Psychology, 52,* 759–768.

Loeber, R., Green, S. M., Keenan, K., & Lahey, B. B. (1995). Which boys will fare worse?: Early predictors of the onset of conduct disorder in a six-year longitudinal study. *Journal of the American Academy of Child and Adolescent Psychiatry, 34,* 499–509.

Loeber, R., Green, S. M., Lahey, B. B., Christ, M. A. G., & Frick, P. J. (1992). Developmental sequences in the age of onset of disruptive child behaviors. *Journal of Child and Family Studies, 1,* 21–41.

Loeber, R., Green, S. M., Lahey, B. B., & Kalb, L. (2000). Physical fighting in childhood as a risk factor for later mental health problems. *Journal of the American Academy of Child and Adolescent Psychiatry, 39,* 421–428.

Loeber, R., Green, S. M., Lahey, B. B., & Stouthamer-Loeber, M. (1991). Differences and similarities between children, mothers, and teachers as informants on disruptive child behavior. *Journal of Abnormal Child Psychology, 19,* 75–95.

Loeber, R., & Hay, D. F. (1994). Developmental approaches to aggression and conduct problems. In M. Rutter & D. F. Hay (Eds.), *Development through life: A handbook for clinicians* (pp. 488–516). Oxford: Blackwell Scientific.

Loeber, R., & Hay, D. F. (1997). Key issues in the development of aggression and violence from childhood to early adulthood. *Annual Review of Psychology, 48,* 371–410.

Loeber, R., Keenan, K., Lahey, B. B., Green, S. M., & Thomas, C. (1993). Evidence for developmentally based diagnoses of oppositional defiant disorder and conduct disorder. *Journal of Abnormal Child Psychology, 21,* 377–410.

Loeber, R., Lahey, B. B., & Thomas, C. (1991). Diagnostic conundrum of oppositional defiant disorder and conduct disorder. *Journal of Abnormal Psychology, 100,* 379–390.

Loeber, R., & Schmaling, K. B. (1985). Empirical evidence for overt and covert patterns of antisocial conduct problems: A metaanalysis. *Journal of Abnormal Child Psychology, 13,* 337–352.

Loeber, R., & Stouthamer-Loeber, M. (1986). Family factors as correlates and predictors of juvenile conduct problems and delinquency. In M. Tonry & N. Morris (Eds.), *Crime and justice* (Vol. 17, pp. 29–149). Chicago: University of Chicago Press.

Loeber, R., & Stouthamer-Loeber, M. (1998). Development of juvenile aggression and violence: Some common misconceptions and controversies. *American Psychologist, 53,* 242–259.

Loeber, R., Wung, P., Keenan, K., Giroux, B., Stouthamer-Loeber, M., Van Kammen, W. B., & Maughan, B. (1993). Developmental pathways in disruptive child behavior. *Development and Psychopathology, 5,* 103–133.

Lofgren, D. P., Bemporad, J., King, J., Lindem, K., & O'Driscoll, G. (1991). A prospective follow-up study of so-called borderline children. *American Journal of Psychiatry, 148,* 1541–1547.

Lombroso, P. J., & Sapolsky, R. (1998). Development of the cerebral cortex: XII. Stress and brain development. I. *Journal of the American Academy of Child and Adolescent Psychiatry, 37,* 1337–1339.

Loney, J., & Milich, R. (1982). Hyperactivity, inattention, and aggression in clinical practice. In M. Wolraich & D. Routh (Eds.), *Advances in developmental and behavioral pediatrics* (Vol. 3, pp. 113–147). Greenwich, CT: JAI Press.

Loranger, A., & Levine, P. (1978). Age at onset of bipolar affective illness. *Archives of General Psychiatry, 35,* 1345–1348.

Losel, F., & Bender, D. (1997). Heart rate and psychosocial correlates of antisocial behavior in high-risk adolescents. In A. Raine, P. A. Brennan, D. P. Farrington, & S. A. Mednick (Eds.), *Biosocial bases of violence* (pp. 321–324). New York: Plenum Press.

Louth, S. M., Williamson, S., Alpert, M., Pouget, E. R., & Hare, R. D. (1998). Acoustic distinctions in the speech of male psychopaths. *Journal of Psycholinguistic Research, 27,* 375–384.

Lundy, M. S., Pfohl, B. M., & Kuperman, S. (1993). Adult criminality among formerly hospitalized child psychiatric patients. *Journal of the American Academy of Child and Adolescent Psychiatry, 32,* 568–576.

Lynam, D. R. (1996). The early identification of chronic offenders: Who is the fledgling psychopath? *Psychological Bulletin, 120,* 209–234.

Lynam, D. R. (1997). Pursuing the psychopath: Capturing the fledgling psychopath in a nomological net. *Journal of Abnormal Psychology, 106,* 425–438.

Lynam, D. R., Caspi, A., Moffitt, T. E., Wikstrom, P. O., Loeber, R., & Novak, S. (2000). The interaction between impulsivity and neighborhood context on offending: The effects of impulsivity are stronger in poorer neighborhoods. *Journal of Abnormal Psychology, 109,* 563–574.

Lynam, D. R., Moffitt, T., & Stouthamer-Loeber, M. (1993). Explaining the relation between IQ and delinquency: Class, race, test motivation, school failure or self-control? *Journal of Abnormal Psychology, 102,* 187–196.

Lyon, G. R., & Rumsey, J. M. (1996). *Neuroimaging: A window to the neurological foundations of learning and behavior in children.* Baltimore: Brookes.

Lyons, M. J., True, W. R., Eisen, S. A., Goldberg, J., Meyer, J. M., Faraone, S. V., Eaves. L. J., & Tsuang, M. T. (1995). Differential heritability of adult and juvenile antisocial traits. *Archives of General Psychiatry, 52,* 906–915.

Lyons-Ruth, K. (1996). Attachment relationships among children with aggressive behavior problems: The role of disorganized early attachment patterns. *Journal of Consulting and Clinical Psychology, 64,* 64–73.

Lyons-Ruth, K., Alpern, L., & Repacholi, B. (1993). Disorganized infant attachment classification and maternal psychosocial problems as predictors of hostile–aggressive behavior in the preschool classroom. *Child Development, 64,* 572–585.

Lytton, H. (1990). Child and parent effects in boys' conduct disorder: A reinterpretation. *Developmental Psychology, 26,* 683–697.

Maccoby, E. E., & Jacklin, C. N. (1974). *The psychology of sex differences.* Stanford, CA: Stanford University Press.

Maccoby, E. E., & Jacklin, C. N. (1980). Sex differences in aggression: A rejoinder and reprise. *Child Development, 51,* 964–980.

MacDonald, V. M., & Achenbach, T. M. (1999). Attention problems versus conduct problems as 6–year predictors of signs of disturbance in a national sample. *Journal of the American Academy of Child and Adolescent Psychiatry, 38,* 1254–1261.

Magnusson, D. (1999). Individual development: Toward a developmental science. *Proceedings of the American Philosophical Society, 143,* 86–96.

Maguire, K., & Pastore, A. L. (Eds.). (1997). *Sourcebook of criminal justice statistics 1996.* Washington, DC: U.S. Government Printing Office.

Maguire, K., & Pastore, A. L. (Eds.). (1999). *Sourcebook of criminal justice statistics 1998.* Washington, DC: U.S. Government Printing Office.

Mailloux, D. L., Forth, A. E., & Kroner, D. G. (1997). Psychopathy and substance use in adolescent male offenders. *Psychological Reports, 81*, 529–530.

Main, M. (1996). Introduction to the special section on attachment and psychopathology: 2. Overview of the field of attachment. *Journal of Consulting and Clinical Psychology, 64*, 237–243.

Maliphant, R., Hume, F., & Furnham, A. (1990). Autonomic nervous system (ANS) activity, personality characteristics and disruptive behaviour in girls. *Journal of Child Psychology and Psychiatry, 31*, 619–628.

Maliphant, R., Watson, S. A., & Daniels, D. (1990). Disruptive behaviour in school, personality characteristics and heart rate (HR) levels in 7–9 year old boys. *Educational Psychology, 10*, 199–205.

Malone, R. P., Bennett, D. S., Luebbert, J. F., Rowan, A. B., Biesecker, K. A., Blaney, B. L., & Delaney, M. A. (1998). Aggression classification and treatment response. *Psychopharmacology Bulletin, 34*, 41–45.

Malone, R. P., Delaney, M. A., Luebbert, J. F., Cater, J., & Campbell, M. (2000). A double-blind placebo-controlled study of lithium in hospitalized aggressive children and adolescents with conduct disorder. *Archives of General Psychiatry, 57*, 649–654.

Malone, R. P., Luebbert, J. F., Delaney, M. A., Biesecker, K. A., Blaney, B. L., Rowan, A. B., & Campbell, M. (1997). Nonpharmacological response in hospitalized children with conduct disorder. *Journal of the American Academy of Child and Adolescent Psychiatry, 36*, 242–247.

Mandoki, M. W. (1995). Risperidone treatment of children and adolescents: Increased risk of extrapyramidal side effects? *Journal of Child and Adolescent Psychopharmacology, 5*, 49–67.

Mann, J. (1994). *The difference: Growing up female in America.* New York: Warner.

Mannuzza, S., Gittelman-Klein, R., Bessler, A., Malloy, P., & LaPadula, M. (1993). Young adult outcome of hyperactive boys almost grown up: Educational achievement, occupational rank, and psychiatric status. *Archives of General Psychiatry, 50*, 565–576.

Mannuzza, S., Klein, R. G., & Addalli, K. A. (1991). Young adult mental status of hyperactive boys and their brothers: A prospective follow-up study. *Journal of the American Academy of Child and Adolescent Psychiatry, 30*, 743–751.

Marmorstein, N. R., & Iacono, W. G. (2001). An investigation of female adolescent twins with both major depression and conduct disorder. *Journal of the American Academy of Child and Adolescent Psychiatry, 40*, 299–306.

Mash, E. J., & Dozois, D. J. A. (1996). Child psychopathology: A developmental–systems perspective. In E. J. Mash & R. A. Barkley (Eds.), *Child psychopathology* (pp. 3–60). New York: Guilford Press.

Mason, D. A., & Frick, P. J. (1994). The heritability of antisocial behavior: A meta-analysis of twin and adoption studies. *Journal of Psychopathology and Behavioral Assessment, 16*, 301–323.

Matier, K., Halperin, J. M., Sharma, V., Newcorn, J. H., & Sathaye, N. (1992). Methylphenidate response in aggressive and nonaggressive ADHD children: Distinctions on laboratory measures of symptoms. *Journal of the American Academy of Child and Adolescent Psychiatry, 31*, 219–225.

Matthys, W., Cuperus, J. M., & Van Engeland, H. (1999). Deficient social problem-solving in boys with ODD/CD, with ADHD, and with both disorders. *Journal of the American Academy of Child and Adolescent Psychiatry, 38*, 311–321.

Mattson, S. N., & Riley, E. P. (1998). A review of the neurobehavioral deficits in children with fetal alcohol syndrome or prenatal exposure to alcohol. *Alcoholism: Clinical and Experimental Research, 22,* 279–294.

Mattsson, A., Schalling, D., Olweus, D., Low, H., & Svensson, J. (1980). Plasma testosterone, aggressive behavior, and personality dimensions in young male delinquents. *Journal of the American Academy of Child Psychiatry, 19,* 476–490.

Max, J. E., & Dunisch, D. L. (1997). Traumatic brain injury in a child psychiatry outpatient clinic: A controlled study. *Journal of the American Academy of Child and Adolescent Psychiatry, 36,* 404–411.

Max, J. E., Robin, D. A., Lindgren, S. D., Smith, Jr., W. L., Sato, Y., Mattheis, P. J., Stierwalt, J. A. G., & Castillo, C. S. (1997). Traumatic brain injury in children and adolescents: Psychiatric disorders at two years. *Journal of the American Academy of Child and Adolescent Psychiatry, 36,* 1278–1285.

Maxfield, M. G., & Widom, C. S. (1996). The cycle of violence revisited 6 years later. *Archives of Pediatrics and Adolescent Medicine, 150,* 390–395.

Maziade, M., Caron, C., Cote, R., Merette, C., Bernier, H., Laplante, B., Boutin, P., & Thivierge, J. (1990). Psychiatric status of adolescents who had extreme temperaments at age 7. *American Journal of Psychiatry, 147,* 1531–1536.

McBurnett, K., Harris, S. M., Swanson, J. M., Pfiffner, L. J., Tamm, L., & Freeland, D. (1993). Neuropsychological and psychophysiological differentiation of inattention/overactivity and aggression/defiance symptom groups. *Journal of Clinical Child Psychology, 22,* 165–171.

McBurnett, K., & Lahey, B. B. (1994). Psychophysiological and neuroendocrine correlates of conduct disorder and antisocial behavior in children and adolescents. In D. C. Fowles, P. Sutker, & S. H. Goodman (Eds.), *Progress in experimental personality and psychopathology research* (pp. 199–231). New York: Springer.

McBurnett, K., Lahey, B. B., Capasso, L., & Loeber, R. (1996). Aggressive symptoms and salivary cortisol in clinic-referred boys with conduct disorder. *Annals of the New York Academy of Sciences, 794,* 169–178.

McBurnett, K., Lahey, B. B., Frick, P. J., Risch, C., Loeber, R., Hart, E. L., Christ, M. A. G., & Hanson, K. S. (1991). Anxiety, inhibition, conduct disorder in children: II. Relation to salivary cortisol. *Journal of the American Academy of Child and Adolescent Psychiatry, 30,* 192–196.

McBurnett, K., Lahey, B. B., Rathouz, P. J., & Loeber, R. (2000). Low salivary cortisol and persistent aggression in boys referred for disruptive behavior. *Archives of General Psychiatry, 57,* 38–43.

McBurnett, K., Pfiffner, L. J., Willcutt, E., Tamm, L., Lerner, M., Ottolini, Y. O., & Furman, M. B. (1999). Experimental cross-validation of DSM-IV types of attention-deficit/hyperactivity disorder. *Journal of the American Academy of Child and Adolescent Psychiatry, 38,* 17–24.

McClellan, J., McCurry, C., Ronnei, M., Adams, J., Eisner, A., & Storck, M. (1996). Age of onset of sexual abuse: Relationship to sexually inappropriate behaviors. *Journal of the American Academy of Child and Adolescent Psychiatry, 35,* 1375–1383.

McClellan, J., & Werry, J. (1994). Practice parameters for the assessment and treatment of children and adolescents with schizophrenia. *Journal of the American Academy of Child and Adolescent Psychiatry, 33,* 616–635.

McConaughy, S. H. (1992). Objective assessment of children's behavioral and emotional problems. In C. H. Walker & M. C. Roberts (Eds.), *Handbook of clinical child psychology* (2nd ed., pp. 163–180). New York: Wiley.

McConville, B. J., Arvanitis, L. A., Thyrum, P. T., Yeh, C., Wilkinson, L. A., Chaney, R. O., Foster, K. D., Sorter, M. T., Friedman, L. M., Brown, K. L., & Heubi, J. E. (2000). Pharmacokinetics, tolerability, and clinical effectiveness of quetiapine fumarate: An open-label trial in adolescents with psychotic disorders. *Journal of Clinical Psychiatry, 61*, 252–260.

McCord, J. (1979). Some child-rearing antecedents of criminal behavior in adult men. *Journal of Personality and Social Psychology, 37*, 1477–1486.

McCord, J. (1988). Parental behavior in the cycle of aggression. *Psychiatry, 51*, 14–23.

McCord, J. (1996). Considerations regarding biosocial foundations of personality and aggression. *Annals of the New York Academy of Sciences, 794*, 253–255.

McCracken, J. T. (1992). The epidemiology of child and adolescent mood disorders. *Child and Adolescent Psychiatric Clinics of North America, 1*, 53–72.

McDougle, C. J., Holmes, J. P., Bronson, M. R., Anderson, G. M., Volkmar, F. R., Price, L. H., & Cohen, D. J. (1997). Risperidone treatment of children and adolescents with pervasive developmental disorders: A prospective, open-label study. *Journal of the American Academy of Child and Adolescent Psychiatry, 36*, 685–693.

McElroy, S. L., Strakowski, S. M., West, S. A., Keck, P. E., & McConville, B. J. (1997). Phenomenology of adolescent and adult mania in hospitalized patients with bipolar disorder. *American Journal of Psychiatry, 154*, 44–49.

McGee, R., Feehan, M., Williams, S., & Anderson, J. (1992). DSM-III disorders from age 11 to age 15 years. *Journal of the American Academy of Child and Adolescent Psychiatry, 31*, 50–59.

McGlashan, T. H. (1988). Adolescent versus adult onset of mania. *American Journal of Psychiatry, 145*, 221–223.

McGuffin, P., & Gottesman, I. I. (1985). Genetic influences on normal and abnormal development. In M. Rutter & L. Hersov (Eds.), *Child and adolescent psychiatry: Modern approaches* (2nd ed., pp. 17–33). Oxford: Blackwell Scientific.

McKenna, K., Gordon, C. T., & Rapoport, J. L. (1994). Childhood-onset schizophrenia: Timely neurobiological research. *Journal of the American Academy of Child and Adolescent Psychiatry, 33*, 771–781.

McLanahan, S., & Bumpass, L. (1988). Intergenerational consequences of family disruption. *American Journal of Sociology, 51*, 557–580.

McLeer, S. V., Callaghan, M., Henry, D., & Wallen, J. (1994). Psychiatric disorders in sexually abused children. *Journal of the American Academy of Child and Adolescent Psychiatry, 33*, 313–319.

McMahon, R. J., & Wells, K. C. (1998). Conduct problems. In E. J. Mash & R. A. Barkley (Eds.), *Treatment of childhood disorders* (2nd ed., pp. 111–207). New York: Guilford Press.

Mednick, S. A., Volavka, J., Gabrielli, W. F., & Itil, T. (1982). EEG as a predictor of antisocial behavior. *Criminology, 19*, 219–231.

Melloni, R. H., Jr., Connor, D. F., Xvan Hang, P. T., Harrison, R. J., & Ferris, C. F. (1997). Anabolic–androgenic steroid exposure during adolescence stimulates aggressive behavior in golden hamsters. *Physiology and Behavior, 61*, 359–364.

Mellor, D. H., Lowit, I., & Hall, D. J. (1974). Are epileptic children behaviourally different from other children? In P. Harris & C. Mawdsley (Eds.), *Proceedings of the Hans Berger Centenary Symposium* (pp. 313–316). Edinburgh: Churchill Livingstone.

Merikangas, K. R., Swendsen, J. D., Preisig, M. A., & Chazan, R. Z. (1998). Psychopathology and temperament in parents and offspring: Results of a family study. *Journal of Affective Disorders, 51,* 63–74.

Merikangas, K. R., Weissman, M. M., Prusoff, B. A., Pauls, D. L., & Leckman, J. F. (1985). Depressives with secondary alcoholism: Psychiatric disorders in offspring. *Journal of Studies on Alcohol, 46,* 199–204.

Mezzacappa, E., Kindlon, D., Saul, J. P., & Earls, F. (1998). Executive and motivational control of performance task behavior, and autonomic heart-rate regulation in children: Physiologic validation of two-factor solution inhibitory control. *Journal of Child Psychology and Psychiatry, 39,* 525–531.

Mezzacappa, E., Tremblay, R. E., Kindlon, D., Saul, J. P., Arseneault, L., Pihl, R. O., & Earls, F. (1996). Relationship of aggression and anxiety to autonomic regulation of heart rate variability in adolescent males. *Annals of the New York Academy of Sciences, 794,* 376–379.

Mezzacappa, E., Tremblay, R. E., Kindlon, D., Saul, J. P., Arseneault, L., Seguin, J., Pihl, R. O., & Earls, F. (1997). Anxiety, antisocial behavior and heart rate regulation in adolescent males. *Journal of Child Psychology and Psychiatry, 38,* 457–469.

Michelson, L., Mannarino, A. P., Marchione, K. E., Stern, M., Figueroa, J., & Beck, S. (1983). A comparative outcome study of behavioural social-skills training, interpersonal-problem-solving and nondirective control treatments with child psychiatric outpatients. *Behaviour Research and Therapy, 21,* 545–556.

Miczek, K. A., & Donat, P. (1989). Brain 5–HT systems and inhibition of aggressive behavior. In P. Bevan, A. R. Cools, & T. Archer (Eds.), *Behavioral pharmacology of 5–HT* (pp. 117–144). Hillsdale, NJ: Erlbaum.

Milich, R., & Loney, J. (1979). The role of hyperactive and aggressive symptomatology in predicting adolescent outcome among hyperactive children. *Journal of Pediatric Psychology, 4,* 93–112.

Miller, B. A., Downs, W. R., & Testa, M. (1993). Interrelationships between victimization experiences and women's alcohol use. *Journal of Studies on Alcohol, 11,* 109–117.

Miller, D., Trapani, C., Fejes-Mendoza, K., Eggleston, C., & Dwiggins, D (1995). Adolescent female offenders: Unique considerations. *Adolescence, 30,* 429–435.

Miller, G. E., & Prinz, R. J. (1990). Enhancement of social learning family interventions for childhood conduct disorder. *Psychological Bulletin, 108,* 291–307.

Miller, L. S., Klein, R. G., Piacentini, J., Abikoff, H., Shah, M. R., Samoilov, A., & Guardino, M. (1995). The New York Teacher Rating Scale for Disruptive and Antisocial Behavior. *Journal of the American Academy of Child and Adolescent Psychiatry, 34,* 359–370.

Milner, B. (1995). Aspects of human frontal lobe function. In H. Jasper, S. Riggio, & P. Goldman-Rakic (Eds.), *Epilepsy and the functional anatomy of the frontal lobe* (pp. 67–84). New York: Raven Press.

Milstein, V. (1988). EEG topography in patients with aggressive violent behavior. In T. E. Moffitt & S. A. Mednick (Eds.), *Biological contributions to crime causation* (pp. 40–52). Dordrecht, The Netherlands: Nijhoff.

Mitchell, J., McCauley, E., Burke, P. M., & Moss, S. J. (1988). Phenomenology of depression in children and adolescents. *Journal of the American Academy of Child and Adolescent Psychiatry, 27,* 12–20.

Modai, I., Apter, A., Meltzer, M., Tyano, S., Walevski, A., & Jerushalmy, Z. (1989). Serotonin uptake by platelets of suicidal and aggressive adolescent psychiatric inpatients. *Neuropsychobiology, 21,* 9–13.

Moffitt, T. E. (1990a). Juvenile delinquency and attention deficit disorder: Boys' developmental trajectories from age 3 to age 15. *Child Development, 61,* 893–910.

Moffitt, T. E. (1990b). The neuropsychology of juvenile delinquency. In M. Tonry & N. Morris (Eds.), *Crime and justice: A review of research* (Vol. 12, pp. 99–169). Chicago: University of Chicago Press.

Moffitt, T. E. (1993a). Adolescence-limited and life-course-persistent antisocial behavior: A developmental taxonomy. *Psychological Review, 100,* 674–701.

Moffitt, T. E. (1993b). The neuropsychology of conduct disorder. *Development and Psychopathology, 5,* 135–151.

Moffitt, T. E., Brammer, G. L., Caspi, A., Fawcett, J. P., Raleigh, M., Yuwiler, A., & Silva, P. (1998). Whole blood serotonin relates to violence in an epidemiological study. *Biological Psychiatry, 43,* 446–457.

Moffitt, T. E., Caspi, A., Belsky, J., & Silva, P. (1992). Childhood experience and the onset of menarche: A test of a sociobiological model. *Child Development, 63,* 47–58.

Moffitt, T. E., & Lynam, D., Jr. (1994). The neuropsychology of conduct disorder and delinquency: Implications for understanding antisocial behavior. In D. C. Fowles, P. Sutker, & S. H. Goodman (Eds.), *Progress in experimental personality and psychopathology research* (pp. 233–262). New York: Springer.

Moffitt, T. E., & Silva, P. A. (1987). WISC-R Verbal and Performance IQ discrepancy in an unselected cohort: Clinical significance and longitudinal stability. *Journal of Consulting and Clinical Psychology, 55,* 768–774.

Moffitt, T. E., & Silva, P. A. (1988a). Neuropsychological deficit and self-reported delinquency in an unselected birth cohort. *Journal of the American Academy of Child and Adolescent Psychiatry, 27,* 233–240.

Moffitt, T. E., & Silva, P. A. (1988b). IQ and delinquency: A direct test of the differential detection hypothesis. *Journal of Abnormal Psychology, 97,* 330–333.

Moffitt, T. E., & Silva, P. A. (1988c). Self-reported delinquency, neuropsychological deficit, and history of attention deficit disorder. *Journal of Abnormal Child Psychology, 16,* 553–569.

Moss, H. B., Vanyukov, M. M., & Martin, C. S. (1995). Salivary cortisol responses and the risk for substance abuse in prepubertal boys. *Biological Psychiatry, 38,* 547–555.

Moss, H. B., & Yao, J. K. (1996). Platelet dense granule secretion in adolescents with conduct disorder and substance abuse: Preliminary evidence for variation in signal transduction. *Biological Psychiatry, 40,* 892–898.

Moss, H. B., Yao, J. K., & Panzak, G. L. (1990). Serotonergic responsivity and behavioral dimensions in antisocial personality disorder with substance abuse. *Biological Psychiatry, 28,* 325–338.

Moyer, K. E. (1968). Kinds of aggression and their physiological basis. *Communications in Behavioral Biology, 2,* 65–87.

Moyer, K. E. (1976). *The psychobiology of aggression.* New York: Harper & Row.

Mulvey, E. (1994). Assessing the evidence of a link between mental illness and violence. *Hospital and Community Psychiatry, 45,* 663–668.

Murphy, D. A., Pelham, W. E., & Lang, A. R. (1992). Aggression in boys with attention deficit-hyperactivity disorder: Methylphenidate effects on naturalistically observed aggression, response to provocation, and social information processing. *Journal of Abnormal Child Psychology, 20,* 451–466.

Murray, J. P. (1997). Media violence and youth. In J. D. Osofsky (Ed.), *Children in a violent society* (pp. 72–96). New York: Guilford Press.

Myers, M. G., Stewart, D. G., & Brown, S. A. (1998). Progression from conduct disorder to antisocial personality disorder following treatment for adolescent substance abuse. *American Journal of Psychiatry, 155,* 479–485.

Myers, W. C., Burket, R. C., & Harris, H. E. (1995). Adolescent psychopathy in relation to delinquent behaviors, conduct disorder, and personality disorders. *Journal of Forensic Sciences, 40,* 436–440.

Nagin, D. S., & Tremblay, R. E. (2001). Parental and early childhood predictors of persistent physical aggression in boys from kindergarten to high school. *Archives of General Psychiatry, 58,* 389–394.

Naglieri, J. A., LeBuffe, P. A., & Pfeiffer, S. I. (1994). *The Devereux Scales of Mental Disorders.* San Antonio, TX: Psychological Corporation.

Najman, J. M., Behrens, B. C., Anderson, M., Bor, W., O'Callaghan, M., & Williams, G. M. (1997). Impact of family type and family quality on child behavior problems: A longitudinal study. *Journal of the American Academy of Child and Adolescent Psychiatry, 36,* 1357–1365.

National Institute of Mental Health (NIMH). (1982). *Television and behavior: Ten years of scientific progress and implications for the eighties. Summary report* (Vol. 1). Washington, DC: U.S. Government Printing Office.

National Institute on Drug Abuse. (1995). 31% of New York murder victims had cocaine in their bodies. *NIDA Notes, 10,* 1.

Needleman, H. L., Riess, J. A., Tobin, M. J., Biesecker, G. E., & Greenhouse, J. B. (1996). Bone lead levels and delinquent behavior. *Journal of the American Medical Association, 275,* 363–369.

Nelson, C. A., & Luciana, M. (1998). Electrophysiological studies: II. Evoked potentials and event-related potentials. In C. E. Coffey & R. A. Brumback (Eds.), *Textbook of pediatric neuropsychiatry* (pp. 331–356). Washington, DC: American Psychiatric Press.

Nemeroff, C. B. (1991). Corticotropin-releasing factor. In C. B. Nemeroff (Ed.), *Neuropeptides and psychiatric disorder* (pp. 75–92). Washington, DC: American Psychiatric Press.

Newacheck, P. W., Brindis, C. D., Cart, C. U., Marchi, K., & Irwin, C. E. (1999). Adolescent health insurance coverage: Recent changes and access to care. *Pediatrics, 104,* 195–202.

Nicolson, R., Awad, G., & Sloman, L. (1998). An open trial of risperidone in young autistic children. *Journal of the American Academy of Child and Adolescent Psychiatry, 37,* 372–376.

Niedermeyer, E. (1998). Frontal lobe functions and dysfunctions. *Clinical Electroencephalography, 29,* 79–90.

Noble, A., Vega, W. A., Kolody, B., Porter, P., Hwang, J., Merk, G. A., II, & Boyle, A. (1997). Prenatal substance abuse in California: Findings from the perinatal substance exposure study. *Journal of Psychoactive Drugs, 29,* 43–53.

Noble, E. P., Ozkaragoz, T. Z., Ritchie, T. L., Zhang, X., Belin, T. R., & Sparkes, R. S. (1998). D2 and D4 dopamine receptor polymorphisms and personality. *American Journal of Medical Genetics, 81,* 257–267.

Nuffield, E. (1961). Neurophysiology and behaviour disorders in epileptic children. *Journal of Mental Science, 107,* 438–458.

Nunes, E. V., Weissman, M. M., Goldstein, R. B., McAvay, G., Seracini, A. M., Verdeli, H., & Wickramaratne, P. J. (1998). Psychopathology in children of parents with opiate dependence and/or major depression. *Journal of the American Academy of Child and Adolescent Psychiatry, 37,* 1142–1151.

O'Brien, B. S., & Frick, P. J. (1996). Reward dominance: Associations with anxiety, conduct problems, and psychopathy in children. *Journal of Abnormal Child Psychology, 24*, 223–240.

O'Connor, T. G., Deater-Deckard, K., Fulker, D., Rutter, M., & Plomin, R. (1998). Genotype–environment correlations in late childhood and early adolescence: Antisocial behavioral problems and coercive parenting. *Developmental Psychology, 34*, 970–981.

O'Donnell, J., Hawkins, J. D., & Abbott, R. D. (1995). Predicting serious delinquency and substance use among aggressive boys. *Journal of Consulting and Clinical Psychology, 63*, 529–537.

O'Donnell, J., Hawkins, J. D., Catalano, R. F., Abbott, R. D., & Day, L. E. (1995). Preventing school failure, drug use, and delinquency among low-income children: Long-term intervention in elementary schools. *American Journal of Orthopsychiatry, 65*, 87–100.

Offord, D. R., Abrams, N., Allen, N., & Poushinsky, M. (1979). Broken homes, parental psychiatric illness, and female delinquency. *American Journal of Orthopsychiatry, 49*, 252–264.

Offord, D. R., Boyle, M. H., Racine, Y. A., Fleming, J. E., Cadman, D. T., Blum, H. M., Byrne, C., Links, P. S., Lipman, E. L., MacMillan, H. L., Rae Grant, N. I., Sanford, M. N., Szatmari, P., Thomas, H., & Woodward C. A. (1992). Outcome, prognosis, and risk in a longitudinal follow-up study. *Journal of the American Academy of Child and Adolescent Psychiatry, 31*, 916–923.

O'Hearn, H. G., Margolin, G., & John, R. S. (1997). Mothers' and fathers' reports of children's reactions to naturalistic marital conflict. *Journal of the American Academy of Child and Adolescent Psychiatry, 36*, 1366–1373.

Olson, H. C., Feldman, J. J., Streissguth, A. P., Sampson, P. D., & Bookstein, F. L. (1998). Neuropsychological deficits in adolescents with fetal alcohol syndrome: Clinical findings. *Alcoholism: Clinical and Experimental Research, 22*, 1998–2012.

Olson, H. C., Streissguth, A. P., Sampson, P. D., Barr, H. M., Bookstein, F. L., & Thiede, K. (1997). Association of prenatal alcohol exposure with behavioral and learning problems in early adolescence. *Journal of the American Academy of Child and Adolescent Psychiatry, 36*, 1187–1194.

Olweus, D. (1979). Stability of aggressive reaction patterns in males: A review. *Psychological Bulletin, 86*, 852–875.

Olweus, D. (1982). Continuity in aggressive and inhibited withdrawn behavior patterns. *Psychiatry and Social Science, 1*, 141–159.

Olweus, D., Mattsson, A., Schalling, D., & Low, H. (1988). Circulating testosterone levels and aggression in adolescent males: A causal analysis. *Psychosomatic Medicine, 50*, 261–272.

Ono, Y., Manki, H., Yoshimura, K., Muramatsu, T., Mizushima, H., Higuchi, S., Yagi, G., Kanba, S., & Asai, M. (1997). Association between dopamine D4 receptor (D4DR) exon III polymorphism and novelty seeking in Japanese subjects. *American Journal of Medical Genetics, 74*, 501–503.

Oosterlaan, J., Logan, G. D., & Sergeant, J. A. (1998). Response inhibition in AD/HD, comorbid AD/HD + CD, anxious, and control children: A meta-analysis of studies with the stop task. *Journal of Child Psychology and Psychiatry, 39*, 411–425.

Oreland, L., Wiberg, A., Asberg, M., Traskman, L., Sjostrand, L., Thoren, P., Bertilsson, L., & Tybring, G. (1981). Platelet MAO activity and monoamine metabolites in cerebrospinal fluid in depressed and suicidal patients and in healthy controls. *Psychiatry Research, 4*, 21–29.

Orrell-Valente, J. K., Pinderhughes, E. E., Valente, E., Jr., Laird, R. D., & Conduct Problems Prevention Research Group. (1999). If it's offered, will they come?: Influences on parents' participation in a community-based conduct problems prevention program. *American Journal of Community Psychology, 27,* 753–783.

Orvaschel, H. (1995). *The K-SADS-E.* Fort Lauderdale, FL: Nova University, Center for Psychological Studies.

Orvaschel, H., Ambrosini, P. J., & Rabinovich, H. (1993). Diagnostic issues in child assessment. In T. H. Ollendick & N. M. Herse (Eds.), *Handbook of child and adolescent assessment* (pp. 26–40). Needham Heights, MA: Allyn & Bacon.

Osofsky, J. D., Hann, D. M., & Peebles, C. (1993). Adolescent parenthood: Risks and opportunities for mothers and infants. In C. H. Zeanah (Ed.), *Handbook of infant mental health* (pp. 106–119). New York: Guilford Press.

Osofsky, J. D., Wewers, S., Hann, D. M., & Fick, A. C. (1993). Chronic community violence: What is happening to our children. *Psychiatry, 56,* 36–45.

Ounsted, C. (1969). Aggression and epileptic rage in children with temporal lobe epilepsy. *Journal of Psychosomatic Research, 13,* 237–242.

Ounsted, C., & Lindsay, J. (1981). The long-term outcome of temporal lobe epilepsy in childhood. In E. H. Reynolds & M. R. Trimble (Eds.), *Epilepsy and psychiatry* (pp. 185–215). Edinburgh: Churchill Livingstone.

Overtoom, C. C. E., Verbaten, M. N., Kemner, C., Kinimans, L. J., van England, H., Buitelaar, J. K., Camfferman, G., & Koelega, H. S. (1998). Associations between event-related potentials and measures of attention and inhibition in the continuous performance task in children with ADHD and normal controls. *Journal of the American Academy of Child and Adolescent Psychiatry, 37,* 977–985.

Pajer, K. A. (1998). What happens to "bad" girls?: A review of the adult outcomes of antisocial adolescent girls. *American Journal of Psychiatry, 155,* 862–870.

Pajer, K. A., Gardner, W., Rubin, R. T., Perel, J., & Neal, S. (2001). Decreased cortisol levels in adolescent girls with conduct disorder. *Archives of General Psychiatry, 58,* 297–302.

Parke, R. D., & Slaby, R. G. (1983). The development of aggression. In P. H. Mussen (Series Ed.) & E. M. Hetherington (Vol. Ed.), *Handbook of child psychology* (4th ed.): *Vol. 4. Socialization, personality, and social development* (pp. 547–641). New York: Wiley.

Parker, J. G., & Asher, S. R. (1987). Peer relations and later personal adjustment: Are low-accepted children at risk? *Psychological Bulletin, 102,* 357–389.

Paternite, C. E., Loney, J., Salisbury, H., & Whaley, M. A. (1999). Childhood inattention–overactivity, aggression, and stimulant medication history as predictors of young adult outcomes. *Journal of Child and Adolescent Psychopharmacology, 9,* 169–184.

Patrick, C. J., Cuthbert, B. N., & Lang, P. J. (1994). Emotion in the criminal psychopath: Fear image processing. *Journal of Abnormal Psychology, 103,* 523–534.

Patrick, C. J., Zempolich, K. A., & Levenston, G. K. (1997). Emotionality and violent behavior in psychopaths. In A. Raine, P. A. Brennan, D. P. Farrington, & S. A. Mednick (Eds.), *Biosocial bases of violence* (pp. 145–161). New York: Plenum Press.

Patterson, G. R. (1975). *Families: Applications of social learning to family life* (rev. ed.). Champaign, IL: Research Press.

Patterson, G. R. (1976). *Living with children: New methods for parents and teachers* (rev. ed.). Champaign, IL: Research Press.

Patterson, G. R. (1982). *Coercive family process.* Eugene, OR: Castalia.

Patterson, G. R. (1986). Performance models for antisocial boys. *American Psychologist,* 41, 432–444.

Patterson, G. R., & Forgatch, M. S. (1987). *Parents and adolescents living together: Part 1. The basics.* Eugene, OR: Castalia.

Patterson, G. R., Reid, J. B., & Dishion, T. J. (1992). *Antisocial boys.* Eugene, OR: Castalia.

Patterson, G. R., & Stouthamer-Loeber, M. (1984). The correlation of family management practices and delinquency. *Child Development,* 55, 1299–1307.

Pattison, E. M., & Kahan, J. (1983). The deliberate self-harm syndrome. *American Journal of Psychiatry, 140,* 867–872.

Pearson, J. L., Ialongo, N. S., Hunter, A. G., & Kellam, S. G. (1994). Family structure and aggressive behavior in a population of urban elementary school children. *Journal of the American Academy of Child and Adolescent Psychiatry, 33,* 540–548.

Pedersen, N. L., Oreland, L., Reynolds, C., & McClearn, G. (1993). Importance of genetic effects from monoamine-activity in thrombocytes in twins reared apart and twins reared together. *Psychiatry Research, 46,* 239–251.

Pelcovitz, D., Kaplan, S., Goldenberg, B., Mandel, F., Lehane, J., & Guarrera, J. (1994). Post-traumatic stress disorder in physically abused adolescents. *Journal of the American Academy of Child and Adolescent Psychiatry, 33,* 305–312.

Pelham, W. E., Jr., Milich, R., Cummings, E. M., Murphy, D. A., Schaughency, E. A., & Greiner, A. R. (1991). Effects of background anger, provocation, and methylphenidate on emotional arousal and aggressive responding in attention-deficit hyperactivity disordered boys with and without concurrent aggressiveness. *Journal of Abnormal Child Psychology, 19,* 407–426.

Pelham, W. E., Jr., Milich, R., Murphy, D. A., & Murphy, H. A. (1989). Normative data on the Iowa Conners Teacher Rating Scale. *Journal of Clinical Child Psychology, 18,* 259–262.

Pennington, B. F., & Ozonoff, S. (1996). Executive functions and developmental psychopathology. *Journal of Child Psychology and Psychiatry, 37,* 51–87.

Pepler, D. J., & Slaby, R. G. (1994). Theoretical and developmental perspectives on youth and violence. In L. D. Eron, J. H. Gentry, & P. Schlegel (Eds.), *Reason to hope: A psychosocial perspective on violence and youth* (pp. 27–58). Washington, DC: American Psychological Association.

Perry, B. D., & Pollard, R. A. (1998). Homeostasis, stress, trauma, and adaptation: A neurodevelopmental view of childhood trauma. *Child and Adolescent Psychiatric Clinics of North America, 7,* 33–51.

Perry, B. D., Pollard, R. A., Blakley, T. L., Baker, W. L., & Vigilante, D. (1995). Childhood trauma, the neurobiology of adaptation, and "use-dependent" development of the brain: How "states" become "traits." *Infant Mental Health Journal, 16,* 271–291.

Perry, R., Campbell, M., Adams, P., Lynch, N., Spencer, E. K., Curren, E. L., & Overall, J. E. (1989). Long-term efficacy of haloperidol in autistic children: Continuous versus discontinuous drug administration. *Journal of the American Academy of Child and Adolescent Psychiatry, 28,* 87–92.

Perry, R., Pataki, C., Munoz-Silva, D. M., Armenteros, J., & Silva, R. R. (1997). Risperidone in children and adolescents with pervasive developmental disorder: Pilot trial and follow-up. *Journal of Child and Adolescent Psychopharmacology, 7,* 167–179.

Petersen, A. C., Sarigiani, P. A., & Kennedy, R. E. (1991). Adolescent depression: Why more girls? *Journal of Youth and Adolescence, 20,* 247–271.

Petersen, K. G. I., Matousek, M., Mednick, S. A., Volavka, J., & Pollock, V. (1982). EEG as antecedents of thievery. *Acta Psychiatrica Scandinavica, 65,* 331–338.

Pfeffer, C. R., Jiang, H., & Domeshek, L. J. (1997). Buspirone treatment of psychiatrically hospitalized prepubertal children with symptoms of anxiety and moderately severe aggression. *Journal of Child and Adolescent Psychopharmacology, 7,* 145–155.

Pfeffer, C. R., Plutchik, R., & Mizruchi, M. S. (1983a). Predictors of assaultiveness in latency age children. *American Journal of Psychiatry, 140,* 31–35.

Pfeffer, C. R., Plutchik, R., & Mizruchi, M. S. (1983b). Suicidal and assaultive behavior in children: Classification, measurement, and interrelations. *American Journal of Psychiatry, 140,* 154–157.

Pfeffer, C. R., Plutchik, R., Mizruchi, M. S., & Lipkins, R. (1987). Assaultive behavior in child psychiatric inpatients, outpatients, and nonpatients. *Journal of the American Academy of Child and Adolescent Psychiatry, 26,* 256–261.

Pfefferbaum, B. (1997). Posttraumatic stress disorder in children: A review of the past 10 years. *Journal of the American Academy of Child and Adolescent Psychiatry, 36,* 1503–1511.

Pham, T. H. (1998). Psychometric evaluation of the Hare psychopathy questionnaire in a Belgian prison population. *Encephale, 24,* 435–441.

Pham, T. H., Remy, S., Dailliet, A., & Lienard, L. (1998). Psychopathy and evaluation of violent behavior in a psychiatric security milieu. *Encephale, 24,* 173–179.

Phillips, B. B., Drake, M. E., Jr., Hietter, S. A., Andrews, J. E., & Bogner, J. E. (1993). Electroencephalography in childhood conduct and behavior disorders. *Clinical Electroencephalography, 24,* 25–30.

Pianta, R. C., & Lothman, D. J. (1994). Predicting behavior problems in children with epilepsy: Child factors, disease factors, family stress, and child–mother interaction. *Child Development, 65,* 1415–1428.

Pickworth, W. B., Brown, B. S., Hickey, J. E., & Muntaner, C. (1990). Effects of self reported drug use and antisocial behavior on evoked potentials in adolescents. *Drug and Alcohol Dependence, 25,* 105–110.

Pietrini, P., Guazzelli, M., Basso, G., Jaffe, K., & Grafman, J. (2000). Neuronal correlates of imaginal aggressive behavior assessed by positron emission tomography in healthy subjects. *American Journal of Psychiatry, 157,* 1772–1781.

Pine, D. S., Bruder, G. E., Wasserman, G. A., Miller, L. S., Musabegovic, A., & Watson, J. B. (1997). Verbal dichotic listening in boys at risk for behavior disorders. *Journal of the American Academy of Child and Adolescent Psychiatry, 36,* 1465–1473.

Pine, D. S., Coplan, J. D., Wasserman, G. A., Miller, L. S., Fried, J. E., Davies, M., Cooper, T. B., Greenhill, L., Shaffer, D., & Parsons, B. (1997). Neuroendocrine response to fenfluramine challenge in boys. *Archives of General Psychiatry, 54,* 839–846.

Pine, D. S., Shaffer, D., Schonfeld, I. S., & Davies, M. (1997). Minor physical anomalies: Modifiers of environmental risks for psychiatric impairment? *Journal of the American Academy of Child and Adolescent Psychiatry, 36,* 395–403.

Pine, D. S., Wasserman, G. A., Coplan, J., Fried, J. A., Huang, Y-Y., Kassir, S., Greenhill, L., Shaffer, D., & Parsons, B. (1996). Platelet serotonin 2A ($5HT_{2A}$) receptor characteristics and parenting factors for boys at risk for delinquency: A preliminary report. *American Journal of Psychiatry, 153,* 538–544.

Pine, D. S., Wasserman, G. A., Miller, L., Coplan, J. D., Bagiella, E., Kovelenku, P., Myers, M. M., & Sloan, R. P. (1998). Heart period variability and psychopathology in urban boys at risk for delinquency, *Psychophysiology, 35*, 521–529.

Pine, D. S., Wasserman, G. A., & Workman, S. B. (1999). Memory and anxiety in prepubertal boys at risk for delinquency. *Journal of the American Academy of Child and Adolescent Psychiatry, 38*, 1024–1031.

Pitts, T. B. (1997). Reduced heart rate levels in aggressive children. In A. Raine, P. A. Brennan, D. P. Farrington, & S. A. Mednick (Eds.), *Biosocial bases of violence* (pp. 317–320). New York: Plenum Press.

Plant, T. M. (1994). Puberty in primates. In E. Knobil & J. D. Neill (Eds.), *The physiology of reproduction* (2nd ed., pp. 453–485). New York: Raven Press.

Pliszka, S. R. (1998). Comorbidity of attention-deficit/hyperactivity disorder with psychiatric disorder: An overview. *Journal of Clinical Psychiatry, 59*(Suppl. 7), 50–58.

Pliszka, S. R., Rogeness, G. A., & Medrano, M. A. (1988). DBH, MHPG, and MAO in children with depressive, anxiety, and conduct disorders: Relationship to diagnosis and symptom ratings. *Psychiatry Research, 24*, 35–44.

Pliszka, S. R., Rogeness, G. A., Renner, P., Sherman, J., & Broussard, T. (1988). Plasma neurochemistry in juvenile offenders. *Journal of the American Academy of Child and Adolescent Psychiatry, 27*, 588–594.

Pliszka, S. R., Sherman, J. O., Barrow, M. V., & Irick, S. (2000). Affective disorder in juvenile offenders: A preliminary study. *American Journal of Psychiatry, 157*, 130–132.

Plomin, R., & Bergeman, C. S. (1991). The nature of nurture: Genetic influence on environmental measures. *Behavioral and Brain Sciences, 14*, 373–427.

Plomin, R., DeFries, J. C., McClearn, G. E., & Rutter, M. (1997). *Behavioral genetics* (3rd ed.). New York: Freeman.

Poe-Yamagata, E., & Butts, J. A. (1996). *Female offenders in the juvenile justice system.* Washington, DC: Office of Juvenile Justice and Delinquency Prevention.

Pollak, O. (1950). *The criminality of women.* Philadelphia: University of Pennsylvania Press.

Pope, H. G., Kouri, E. M., & Hudson, J. I. (2000). Effects of supraphysiologic doses of testosterone on mood and aggression in normal men. *Archives of General Psychiatry, 57*, 133–140.

Pornnoppadol, C., Friesen, D. S., Haussler, T. S., Glaser, P. E. A., & Todd, R. D. (1999). No difference between platelet serotonin 5–HT$_{2A}$ receptors from children with and without ADHD. *Journal of Child and Adolescent Psychopharmacology, 9*, 27–33.

Pottick, K. J., McAlpine, D. D., & Andelman, R. B. (2000). Changing patterns of psychiatric inpatient care for children and adolescents in general hospitals 1988–1995. *American Journal of Psychiatry, 157*, 1267–1273.

Price, J. M., & Dodge, K. A. (1989). Reactive and proactive aggression in childhood: Relations to peer status and social context dimensions. *Journal of Abnormal Child Psychology, 17*, 455–471.

Pride, Inc. (1999). *National summary 1997–98, grades 6 through 12.* Atlanta, GA: Author.

Prinz, R. J., Connor, P. A., & Wilson, C. C. (1981). Hyperactive and aggressive behaviors in childhood: Intertwined dimensions. *Journal of Abnormal Child Psychology, 9*, 191–202.

Prior, M. (1992). Childhood temperament. *Journal of Child Psychology and Psychiatry, 33*, 249–279.

Prior, M., Smart, D., Sanson, A., & Oberklaid, F. (1999). Relationships between learning difficulties and psychological problems in preadolescent children from a longitudinal sample. *Journal of the American Academy of Child and Adolescent Psychiatry, 38*, 429–436.

Provence, S., & Naylor, A. (1983). *Working with disadvantaged parents and children: Scientific issues and practice.* New Haven, CT: Yale University Press.

Puig-Antich, J. (1982). Major depression and conduct disorder in prepuberty. *Journal of the American Academy of Child Psychiatry, 21*, 118–128.

Puig-Antich, J., Goetz, D., Davies, M., Kaplan, T., Davies, S., Ostrow, L., Asnis, L., Twomey, J., Iyengar, S., & Ryan, N. D. (1989). A controlled family history study of prepubertal major depressive disorder. *Archives of General Psychiatry, 46*, 406–418.

Puig-Antich, J., Lukens, E., Davies, M., Goetz, D., Brennan-Quattrock, J., & Todak, G. (1985). Psychosocial functioning in prepubertal major depressive disorders. *Archives of General Psychiatry, 42*, 500–507.

Pulkkinen, L. (1987). Offensive and defensive aggression in humans: A longitudinal perspective. *Aggressive Behavior, 13*, 197–212.

Pulkkinen, L. (1992). The path to adulthood for aggressively inclined girls. In K. Bjorkqvist & P. Niemela (Eds.), *Of mice and women: Aspects of female aggression* (pp. 113–121). San Diego, CA: Academic Press.

Pulkkinen, L. (1996). Proactive and reactive aggression in early adolescence as precursors to anti- and prosocial behaviors in young adults. *Aggressive Behavior, 22*, 241–257.

Quay, H. C. (1986a). Classification. In H. C. Quay & J. S. Werry (Eds.), *Psychopathological disorders of childhood* (3rd ed., pp. 1–34). New York: Wiley.

Quay, H. C. (1986b). Conduct disorders. In H. C. Quay & J. S. Werry (Eds.), *Psychopathological disorders of childhood* (3rd ed., pp. 35–72). New York: Wiley.

Quay, H. C. (1988). The behavioral reward and inhibition system in childhood behavior disorder. In L. M. Bloomingdale (Ed.), *Attention deficit disorder* (Vol. 2, pp. 177–186). Elmsford, NY: Pergamon Press.

Quay, H. C. (1993). The psychobiology of undersocialized aggressive conduct disorder: A theoretical perspective. *Development and Psychopathology, 5*, 165–180.

Rae-Grant, N., Thomas, B. H., Offord, D. R., & Boyle, M. H. (1989). Risk, protective, and the prevalence of behavioral and emotional disorders in children and adolescents. *Journal of the American Academy of Child and Adolescent Psychiatry, 28*, 262–268.

Raine, A. (1989). Evoked potentials and psychopathy. *International Journal of Psychophysiology, 8*, 1–16.

Raine, A. (1993). *The psychopathology of crime.* San Diego, CA: Academic Press.

Raine, A. (1996). Autonomic nervous system factors underlying disinhibited, antisocial, and violent behavior. *Annals of the New York Academy of Sciences, 794*, 46–59.

Raine, A., Brennan, P., & Farrington, D. P. (1997). Biosocial bases of violence: Conceptual and theoretical issues. In A. Raine, P. A. Brennan, D. P. Farrington, & S. A. Mednick (Eds.), *Biosocial bases of violence* (pp. 1–20). New York: Plenum Press.

Raine, A., Brennan, P., & Mednick, S. A. (1994). Birth complications combined with early maternal rejection at age 1 predispose to violent crime at age 18 years. *Archives of General Psychiatry, 51*, 984–988.

Raine, A., Brennan, P., & Mednick, S. A. (1997). Interaction between birth complications and early maternal rejection in predisposing individuals to adult violence:

Specificity to serious, early-onset violence. *American Journal of Psychiatry, 154*, 1265–1271.

Raine, A., Brennan, P., Mednick, B., & Mednick, S. A. (1996). High rates of violence, crime, academic problems, and behavioral problems in males with both early neuromotor deficits and unstable family environments. *Archives of General Psychiatry, 53*, 544–549.

Raine, A., Buchsbaum, M. S., & LaCasse, L. (1997). Brain abnormalities in murderers indicated by positron emission tomography. *Biological Psychiatry, 42*, 495–508.

Raine, A., & Jones, F. (1987). Attention, autonomic arousal, and personality in behaviorally disordered children. *Journal of Abnormal Child Psychology, 15*, 583–599.

Raine, A., Lencz, T., Bihrle, S., LaCasse, L., & Colletti, P. (2000). Reduced prefrontal gray matter volume and reduced autonomic activity in antisocial personality disorder. *Archives of General Psychiatry, 57*, 119–127.

Raine, A., Meloy, J. R., Bihrle, S., Stoddard, J., LaCasse, L., & Bushsbaum, M. S. (1998). Reduced prefrontal and increased subcortical brain functioning assessed using positron emission tomography in predatory and affective murderers. *Behavioral Sciences and the Law, 16*, 319–332.

Raine, A., O'Brien, M., Smiley, N., Scerbo, A., & Chan, C. J. (1990). Reduced lateralization in verbal dichotic listening in adolescent psychopaths. *Journal of Abnormal Psychology, 99*, 272–277.

Raine, A., Reynolds, C., Venables, P. H., Mednick, S. A., & Farrington, D. P. (1998). Fearlessness, stimulation-seeking, and large body size at age 3 years as early predispositions to childhood aggression at age 11 years. *Archives of General Psychiatry, 55*, 745–751.

Raine, A., Reynolds, C., Venables, P. H., & Mednick, S. A. (1997). Resting heart rate, skin conductance orienting, and physique. In A. Raine, P. A. Brennan, D. P. Farrington, & S. A. Mednick (Eds.), *Biosocial bases of violence* (pp. 107–126). New York: Plenum Press.

Raine, A., Reynolds, G. P., & Sheard, C. (1991). Neuroanatomical correlates of skin conductance orienting in normal humans: A magnetic resonance imaging study. *Psychophysiology, 28*, 548–558.

Raine, A., & Venables, P. H. (1981). Classical conditioning and socialization: A biosocial interaction? *Personality and Individual Differences, 2*, 273–283.

Raine, A., & Venables, P. H. (1984a). Electrodermal nonresponding, antisocial behavior, and schizoid tendencies in adolescents. *Psychophysiology, 21*, 424–433.

Raine, A., & Venables, P. H. (1984b). Tonic heart rate level, social class and antisocial behaviour in adolescents. *Biological Psychology, 18*, 123–132.

Raine, A., & Venables, P. H. (1987). Contingent negative variation, P3 evoked potentials, and antisocial behavior. *Psychophysiology, 24*, 191–199.

Raine, A., Venables, P. H., & Mednick, S. A. (1997). Low resting heart rate at age 3 years predisposes to aggression at age 11 years: Evidence from the Mauritius Child Health Project. *Journal of the American Academy of Child and Adolescent Psychiatry, 36*, 1457–1464.

Raine, A., Venables, P. H., & Williams, M. (1990a). Autonomic orienting responses in 15–year-old male subjects and criminal behavior at age 24. *American Journal of Psychiatry, 147*, 933–937.

Raine, A., Venables, P. H., & Williams, M. (1990b). Relationships between central and autonomic measures of arousal at age 15 years and criminality at age 24 years. *Archives of General Psychiatry, 47*, 1003–1007.

Raine, A., Venables, P. H., & Williams, M. (1990c). Relationships between N1, P300, and contingent negative variation recorded at age 15 and criminal behavior at age 24. *Psychophysiology, 27,* 567–574.

Raine, A., Venables, P. H., & Williams, M. (1995). High autonomic arousal and electrodermal orienting at age 15 years as protective factors against criminal behavior at age 29 years. *American Journal of Psychiatry, 152,* 1595–1600.

Randall, J., Henggeler, S. W., Pickrel, S. G., & Brondino, M. J. (1999). Psychiatric comorbidity and the 16–month trajectory of substance-abulsing and substance-dependent juvenile offenders. *Journal of the American Academy of Child and Adolescent Psychiatry, 38,* 1118–1124.

Rantakallio, P., Laara, E., Isohanni, M., & Moilanen, I. (1992). Maternal smoking during pregnancy and delinquency of the offspring: An association without causation? *International Journal of Epidemiology, 21,* 1106–1113.

Rasanen, P., Hakko, H., Isohanni, M., Hodgins, S., Jarvelin, M.-R., & Tiihonen, J. (1999). Maternal smoking during pregnancy and risk of criminal behavior among adult male offspring in the northern Finland 1966 birth cohort. *American Journal of Psychiatry, 156,* 857–862.

Rebok, G. W., Hawkins, W. E., Krener, P., Mayer, L. S., & Kellam, G. (1996). Effect of concentration problems on the malleability of children's aggressive and shy behaviors. *Journal of the American Academy of Child and Adolescent Psychiatry, 35,* 193–203.

Reich, W. (2000). Diagnostic Interview for Children and Adolescents (DICA). *Journal of the American Academy of Child and Adolescent Psychiatry, 39,* 59–66.

Reich, W., Earls, F., Frankel, O., & Shayka, J. J. (1993). Psychopathology in children of alcoholics. *Journal of the American Academy of Child and Adolescent Psychiatry, 32,* 995–1002.

Reinherz, H. Z., Giaconia, R. M., Carmola Hauf, A. M., Wasserman, M. S., & Paradis, A. D. (2000). General and specific hildhood risk factors for depression and drug disorders by early adulthood. *Journal of the American Academy of Child and Adolescent Psychiatry, 39,* 223–231.

Reiss, A. J., & Roth, J. A. (1993). *Understanding and preventing violence.* Washington, DC: National Academy Press.

Remschmidt, H., Schulz, E., & Matthias Martin, P. D. (1994). An open trial of clozapine in thirty-six adolescents with schizophrenia. *Journal of Child and Adolescent Psychopharmacology, 4,* 31–41.

Renken, B., Egeland, B., Marvinney, D., Mangelsdorf, S., & Sroufe, L. A. (1989). Early childhood antecedents of aggression and passive-withdrawal in early elementary school. *Journal of Personality, 57,* 257–281.

Reynolds, C. R., & Kamphaus, R. W. (1992). *The Behavior Assessment System for Children.* Circle Pines, MN: American Guidance Service.

Rice, J., Reich, T., Andreasen, N. C., Endicott, J., Van Eerdewegh, H., Fishman, R., Hirschfeld, R. M., & Klerman, G. L. (1987). The familial transmission of bipolar illness. *Archives of General Psychiatry, 44,* 441–447.

Rich, C. L., Sherman, M., & Fowler, R. C. (1990). San Diego suicide study: The adolescents. *Adolescence, 25,* 856–865.

Richardson, G. A. (1998). Prenatal cocaine exposure: A longitudinal study of development. *Annals of the New York Academy of Sciences, 846,* 144–152.

Richardson, G. A., Conroy, M. L., & Day, N. L. (1996). Prenatal cocaine exposure:

Effects on the development of school-age children. *Neurotoxicology and Teratology, 18,* 627–634.

Richardson, G. A., Hamel, S. C., Goldschmidt, L., & Day, N. L. (1996). The effects of prenatal cocaine use on neonatal neurobehavioral status. *Neurotoxicology and Teratology, 18,* 519–528.

Richman, N., Stevenson, J., & Graham, P. J. (1982). *Preschool to school: A behavioral study.* New York: Academic Press.

Richters, J. E., & Martinez, P. (1993). The NIMH Community Violence Project: I. Children as victims of and witnesses to violence. *Psychiatry, 56,* 7–21.

Rifkin, A., Karajgi, B., Dicker, R., Perl, E., Boppana, V., Hasan, N., & Pollack, S. (1997). Lithium treatment of conduct disorders in adolescents. *American Journal of Psychiatry, 154,* 554–555.

Riggs, P. D., Baker, S., Mikulich, S. K., Young, S. E., & Crowley, T. J. (1995). Depression in substance-dependent delinquents. *Journal of the American Academy of Child and Adolescent Psychiatry, 34,* 764–771.

Riggs, P. D., Leon, S. L., Mikulich, S. K., & Pottle, L. C. (1998). An open trial of bupropion for ADHD in adolescents with substance use disorders and conduct disorder. *Journal of the American Academy of Child and Adolescent Psychiatry, 37,* 1271–1278.

Riley, A. W., Ensminger, M. E., Green, B., & Kang, M. (1998). Social role functioning by adolescents with psychiatric disorders. *Journal of the American Academy of Child and Adolescent Psychiatry, 37,* 620–628.

Riley, W. T., Treiber, F. A., & Woods, M. G. (1989). Anger and hostility in depression. *Journal of Nervous and Mental Disease, 177,* 668–674.

Robins, L. N. (1966). *Deviant children grown up: A sociological and psychiatric study of sociopathic personality.* Baltimore: Williams & Wilkins.

Robins, L. N. (1978). Sturdy childhood predictors of adult antisocial behavior: Replications from longitudinal studies. *Psychological Medicine, 8,* 611–622.

Robins, L. N. (1985). Epidemiology of antisocial personality. In J. O. Cavenar (Ed.), *Psychiatry* (Vol. 3, pp. 1–14). Philadelphia: Lippincott.

Robins, L. N. (1986). The consequences of conduct disorder in girls. In D. Olweus, J. Block, & M. Radke-Yarrow (Eds.), *Development of antisocial and prosocial behavior* (pp. 385–414). Orlando, FL: Academic Press.

Robins, L. N., West, P. A., & Herjanic, B. L. (1975). Arrests and delinquency in two generations: A study of black urban families and their children. *Journal of Child Psychology and Psychiatry, 16,* 125–140.

Robinson, T. N., Wilde, M. L., Navracruz, L. C., Farish Haydel, K., & Varady, A. (2001). Effects of reducing children's television and video game use on aggressive behavior. *Archives of Pediatrics and Adolescent Medicine, 155,* 17–23.

Roebuck, T. M., Mattson, S. N., & Riley, E. P. (1998). A review of the neuroanatomical findings in children with fetal alcohol syndrome or prenatal exposure to alcohol. *Alcoholism: Clinical and Experimental Research, 22,* 339–344.

Rogeness, G. A., Cepeda, C., Macedo, C. A., Fischer, C., & Harris, W. R. (1990). Differences in heart rate and blood pressure in children with conduct disorder, major depression, and separation anxiety. *Psychiatry Research, 33,* 199–206.

Rogeness, G. A., Hernandez, J. M., Macedo, C. A., & Mitchell, E. L. (1982). Biochemical differences in children with conduct disorder socialized and undersocialized. *American Journal of Psychiatry, 139,* 307–311.

Rogeness, G. A., Hernandez, J. M., Macedo, C. A., Mitchell, E. L., Amrung, S. A., & Harris, W. R. (1984). Clinical characteristics of emotionally disturbed boys with very low activities of dopamine-ß-hydroxylase. *Journal of the American Academy of Child Psychiatry, 23,* 203–208.

Rogeness, G. A., Javors, M. A., Maas, J. W., & Macedo, C. A. (1990). Catecholamines and diagnoses in children. *Journal of the American Academy of Child and Adolescent Psychiatry, 29,* 234–241.

Rogeness, G. A., Javors, M. A., Maas, J. W., Macedo, C. A., & Fischer, C. (1987). Plasma dopamine-ß-hydroxylase, HVA, MHPG, and conduct disorder in emotionally disturbed boys. *Biological Psychiatry, 22,* 1158–1162.

Rogeness, G. A., Javors, M. A., & Pliszka, S. R. (1992). Neurochemistry and child and adolescent psychiatry. *Journal of the American Academy of Child and Adolescent Psychiatry, 31,* 765–781.

Rogers, R., Johansen, J., Chang, J. J., & Salekin, R. T. (1997). Predictors of adolescent psychopathy: Oppositional and conduct-disordered symptoms. *Journal of the American Academy of Psychiatry and the Law, 25,* 261–271.

Romig, D. A. (1978). *Justice for our children.* Lexington, MA: Heath.

Rosenbaum, J. F., Fava, M., Pava, J. A., McCarthy, M. K., Steingard, R. J., & Bouffides, E. (1993). Anger attacks in unipolar depression: Part II. Neuroendocrine correlates and changes following fluoxetine treatment. *American Journal of Psychiatry, 150,* 1164–1168.

Rosenbaum, J. L. (1989). Family dysfunction and female delinquency. *Crime and Delinquency, 35,* 31–44.

Rosenstein, D. S., & Horowitz, H. A. (1996). Adolescent attachment and psychopathology. *Journal of Consulting and Clinical Psychology, 64,* 244–253.

Rothbart, M. K., & Ahadi, S. A. (1994). Temperament and the development of personality. *Journal of Abnormal Psychology, 103,* 55–66.

Rothbart, M. K., & Bates, J. E. (1998). Temperament. In W. Damon (Series Ed.) & N. Eisenberg (Vol. Ed.), *Handbook of child psychology (5th ed.): Vol. 3. Social, emotional, and personality development* (pp. 105–176). New York: Wiley.

Rothbaum, F., & Weisz, J. (1994). Parental caregiving and child externalizing behavior in nonclinical samples: A meta-analysis. *Psychological Bulletin, 116,* 55–74.

Rothner, D. (1992). Epilepsy. In D. M. Kaufman, G. E. Solomon, & C. R. Pfeffer (Eds.), *Child and adolescent neurology for psychiatrists* (p. 96–113). Baltimore: Williams & Wilkins.

Rubinow, D. R., & Schmidt, P. J. (1996). Androgens, brain, and behavior. *American Journal of Psychiatry, 153,* 974–984.

Ruchkin, V. V., Eisemann, M., & Cloninger, C. R. (1998). Behaviour/emotional problems in male juvenile delinquents and controls in Russia: The role of personality traits. *Acta Psychiatrica Scandinavica, 98,* 231–236.

Ruchkin, V. V., Eisemann, M., Hagglof, B., & Cloninger, C. R. (1998). Interrelations between temperament, character, and parental rearing in male delinquent adolescents in northern Russia. *Comprehensive Psychiatry, 39,* 225–230.

Rule, B. G. (1974). The hostile and instrumental functions of human aggression. In J. de Wit & W. W. Hartup (Eds.), *Determinants and origins of aggressive behavior* (pp. 125–145). The Hague: Mouton.

Russo, M. F., Stokes, G. S., Lahey, B. B., Christ, M. A. G., McBurnett, K., Loeber, R., Stouthamer-Loeber, M., & Green, S. M. (1993). A sensation seeking scale for children: Further refinement of psychometric development. *Journal of Psychopathology and Behavioral Assessment, 15,* 69–86.

Rutherford, M. J., Alterman, A. I., Cacciola, J. S., & McKay, J. R. (1998). Gender differences in the relationship of antisocial personality disorder criteria to Psychopathy Checklist—Revised scores. *Journal of Personality Disorders, 12,* 69–76.

Rutherford, M. J., Cacciola, J. S., & Alterman, A. I. (1999). Antisocial personality disorder and psychopathy in cocaine-dependent women. *American Journal of Psychiatry, 156,* 849–856.

Rutter, M. (1979). Protective factors in children's responses to stress and disadvantage. In M. W. Kent & S. E. J. E. Rolf (Eds.), *Primary prevention of psychopathology: Vol. 3. Social competence in children* (pp. 49–74). Hanover, NH: University Press of New England.

Rutter, M. (1985). Resilience in the face of adversity. *British Journal of Psychiatry, 147,* 589–611.

Rutter, M. (1986). The developmental psychopathology of depression: Issues and perspectives. In M. Rutter, C. Izard, & P. Read (Eds.), *Depression in young people: Developmental and clinical perspectives.* New York: Guilford Press.

Rutter, M. (1995). Clinical implications of attachment concepts: Retrospect and prospect. *Journal of Child Psychology and Psychiatry, 36,* 549–571.

Rutter, M. L. (1999). Psychosocial adversity and child psychopathology. *British Journal of Psychiatry, 174,* 480–493.

Rutter, M., Dunn, J., Plomin, R., Simonoff, E., Pickles, A., Maughan, B., Ormel, J., Meyer, J., & Eaves, L. (1997). Integrating nature and nurture: Implications of person–environment correlations and interactions for developmental psychopathology. *Development and Psychopathology, 9,* 335–364.

Rutter, M., & Giller, H. (1983). *Juvenile delinquency: Trends and perspectives.* Harmondsworth, England: Penguin.

Rutter, M., Giller, H., & Hagell, A. (1998). *Antisocial behavior by young people.* Cambridge, England: Cambridge University Press.

Rutter, M., Graham, P., & Yule, W. (1970). *Clinics in Developmental Medicine: Nos. 35–36. A neuropsychiatric study in childhood.* London: S.I.M.P./Heinemann.

Rutter, M., MacDonald, H., Le Couteur, A., Harrington, R., Bolton, P., & Bailey, A. (1990). Genetic factors in child psychiatric disorders: II. Empirical findings. *Journal of Child Psychology and Psychiatry, 31,* 39–83.

Rutter, M., Silberg, J., O'Connor, T., & Simonoff, E. (1999). Genetics and child psychiatry: II. Empirical research findings. *Journal of Child Psychology and Psychiatry, 40,* 19–55.

Ryan, N. D., Bhatara, V. S., & Perel, J. M. (1999). Mood stabilizers in children and adolescents. *Journal of the American Academy of Child and Adolescent Psychiatry, 38,* 529–536.

Ryan, N. D., Puig-Antich, J., Ambrosini, P., Rabinovich, J., Robinson, D., Nelson, B., Iyengar, S., & Twomey, J. (1987). The clinical picture of major depression in children and adolescents. *Archives of General Psychiatry, 44,* 854–861.

Rydelius, P. A. (1988). The development of antisocial behavior and sudden death. *Acta Psychiatrica Scandinavica, 77,* 398–403.

Salekin, R. T., Rogers, R., & Sewell, K. W. (1997). Construct validity of psychopathy in a female offender sample: A multitrait–multimethod evaluation. *Journal of Abnormal Psychology, 106,* 576–585.

Salekin, R. T., Rogers, R., Ustad, K. L., & Sewell, K. W. (1998). Psychopathy and recidivism among female inmates. *Law and Human Behavior, 22,* 109–128.

Sampson, R. J., & Lamb, J. H. (1997). Unraveling the social context of physique and delinquency. In A. Raine, P. A. Brennan, D. P. Farrington, & S. A. Mednick (Eds.), *Biosocial bases of violence* (pp. 175–188). New York: Plenum Press.

Sampson, R. J., & Laub, J. H. (1994). Urban poverty and the family context of delinquency: A new look at structure and process in a classic study. *Child Development, 65,* 523–540.

Sampson, R. J., Raudenbush, S. W., & Earls, F. (1997). Neighborhoods and violent crime: A multilevel study of collective efficacy. *Science, 277,* 918–924.

Sanchez, C., & Meier, E. (1997). Behavioral profiles of SSRIs in animal models of depression, anxiety and aggression: Are they all alike? *Psychopharmacology (Berlin), 129,* 197–205.

Sanchez, L. E., Armenteros, J. L., Small, A. M., Campbell, M., & Adams, P. B. (1994). Placebo response in aggressive children with conduct disorder. *Psychopharmacology Bulletin, 30,* 209–213.

Sandberg, S. T., Rutter, M., & Taylor, E. (1978). Hyperkinetic disorder in psychiatric clinic attenders. *Developmental Medicine and Child Neurology, 20,* 279–299.

Sanford, M., Boyle, M. H., Szatmari, P., Offord, D. R., Jamieson, E., & Spinner, M. (1999). Age-of-onset classification of conduct disorder: Reliability and validity in a prospective cohort study. *Journal of the American Academy of Child and Adolescent Psychiatry, 38,* 992–999.

Sanger, D. D., Hux, K., & Ritzman, M. (1999). Female juvenile delinquents' pragmatic awareness of conversational interactions. *Journal of Communication Disorders, 32,* 281–294.

Sanson, A., Smart, D., Prior, M., & Oberklaid, F. (1993). Precursors of hyperactivity and aggression. *Journal of the American Academy of Child and Adolescent Psychiatry, 32,* 1207–1216.

Santa Mina, E. E., & Gallop, R. M. (1998). Childhood sexual and physical abuse and adult self-harm and suicidal behaviour: A literature review. *Canadian Journal of Psychiatry, 43,* 793–800.

Sarrias, M. J., Cabre, P., Martinez, E., & Artigas, F. (1990). Relationship between serotonergic measures in blood and cerebrospinal fluid simultaneously obtained in humans. *Journal of Neurochemistry, 54,* 783–786.

Satcher, D. (2000). *Executive summary of mental health: A report of the surgeon general.* Washington, DC: U.S. Government Printing Office.

Satterfield, J. H., & Schell, A. M. (1984). Childhood brain function differences in delinquent and non-delinquent hyperactive boys. *Electroencephalography and Clinical Neurophysiology, 57,* 199–207.

Satterfield, J. H., Schell, A. M., & Backs, R. W. (1987). Longitudinal study of AERPs in hyperactive and normal children: Relationship to antisocial behavior. *Electroencephalography and Clinical Neurophysiology, 67,* 531–536.

Scahill, L., Chappell, P. B., Kim, Y. S., Schultz, R. T., Katsovich, L., Shepherd, E., Arnsten, A. F. T., Cohen, D. J., & Leckman, J. F. (2001). A placebo-controlled study of guanfacine in the treatment of children with tic disorders and attention deficit hyperactivity disorder. *American Journal of Psychiatry, 158,* 1067–1074.

Scarpa, A., & Raine, A. (1997). Psychophysiology of anger and violent behavior. *Psychiatric Clinics of North America, 20,* 375–394.

Scerbo, A. S., & Kolko, D. J. (1994). Salivary testosterone and cortisol in disruptive children: Relationship to aggressive, hyperactive, and internalizing behaviors. *Journal of the American Academy of Child and Adolescent Psychiatry, 33,* 1174–1184.

Scerbo, A. S., & Kolko, D. J. (1995). Child physical abuse and aggression: Preliminary findings on the role of internalizing problems. *Journal of the American Academy of Child and Adolescent Psychiatry, 34,* 1060–1066.

Schaal, B., Tremblay, R. E., Soussignan, R., & Susman, E. J. (1996). Male testosterone linked to high social dominance but low physical aggression in early adolescence. *Journal of the American Academy of Child and Adolescent Psychiatry, 35,* 1322–1330.

Schachar, R., & Tannock, R. (1995). Test of four hypotheses for the comorbidity of attention-deficit hyperactivity disorder and conduct disorder. *Journal of the American Academy of Child and Adolescent Psychiatry, 34,* 639–648.

Schaffer, S. J., & Campbell, J. R. (1994). The new CDC and AAP lead poisoning prevention recommendations: Consensus versus controversy. *Pediatric Annals, 23,* 592–599.

Schalling, D., Aberg, M., Edman, G., & Levander, S. E. (1984). Impulsivity, nonconformity and sensation seeking as related to biological markers for vulnerability. *Clinical Neuropharmacology, 7*(Suppl. 1), 747–757.

Schlossman, S., & Wallach, S. (1978). The crime of precocious sexuality: Female delinquency in the progressive era. *Harvard Educational Review, 48,* 65–94.

Schmidt, K., Solant, M. V., & Bridger, W. H. (1985). Electrodermal activity of undersocialized aggressive children: A pilot study. *Journal of Child Psychology and Psychiatry, 26,* 653–660.

Schmidt, L. A., & Fox, N. A. (1998). Electophysiological studies: I. Quantitative electroencephalography. In C. E. Coffey & R. A. Brumback (Eds.), *Textbook of pediatric neuropsychiatry* (pp. 315–329). Washington, DC: American Psychiatric Press.

Schneider, B. H. (1992). Didactic methods for enhancing children's peer relations: A quantitative review. *Clinical Psychology Review, 12,* 363–382.

Schulz, K. P., Halperin, J. M., Newcorn, J. H., Sharma, V., & Gabriel, S. (1997). Plasma cortisol and aggression in boys with ADHD. *Journal of the American Academy of Child and Adolescent Psychiatry, 36,* 605–609.

Schvehla, T. J., Mandoki, M. W., & Sumner, G. S. (1994). Clonidine therapy for comorbid attention deficit hyperactivity disorder and conduct disorder. *Southern Medical Journal, 87,* 692–695.

Schwab-Stone, M., Chen, C., Greenberger, E., Silver, D., Lichtman, J., & Voyce, C. (1999). No safe haven: II. The effects of violence exposure on urban youth. *Journal of the American Academy of Child and Adolescent Psychiatry, 38,* 359–367.

Schwab-Stone, M. E., Ayers, T. S., Kasprow, W., Voyce, C., Barone, C., Shriver, T., & Weissberg, R. P. (1995). No safe haven: A study of violence exposure in an urban community. *Journal of the American Academy of Child and Adolescent Psychiatry, 34,* 1343–1352.

Schwartz, D., Dodge, K. A., Coie, J. D., Hubbard, J. A., Cillessen, A. H. N., Lemerise, E. A., & Bateman, H. (1998). Social-cognitive and behavioral correlates of aggression and victimization in boys' play groups. *Journal of Abnormal Child Psychology, 26,* 431–440.

Schwartz, D., McFadyen-Ketchum, S. A., Dodge, K. A., Pettit, G. S., & Bates, J. E. (1998). Peer group victimization as a predictor of children's behavior problems at home and in school. *Development and Psychopathology, 10,* 87–99.

Schweinhart, L. J., Barnes, H. V., & Weikart, D. (Eds.). (1993). *Significant benefits: The High/Scope Perry Preschool study through age 27.* Ypsilanti, MI: High/Scope Press.

Sciarillo, W. G., Alexander, G., & Farrell, K. P. (1992). Lead exposure and child behavior. *American Journal of Public Health, 82,* 1356–1360.

Seguin, J. R., Boulerice, B., Harden, P. W., Tremblay, R. E., & Pihl, R. O. (1999). Executive functions and physical aggression after controlling for attention deficit hyperactivity disorder, general memory, and IQ. *Journal of Child Psychology and Psychiatry, 40,* 1197–1208.

Seguin, J. R., Pihl, R. O., Boulerice, B., Tremblay, R. E., & Harden, P. W. (1996). Low pain sensitivity and stability of physical aggression in boys. *Annals of the New York Academy of Sciences, 794,* 408–410.

Seguin, J. R., Pihl, R. O., Hardern, P. W., Tremblay, R. E., & Boulerice, B. (1995). Cognitive and neuropsychological characteristics of physically aggressive boys. *Journal of Abnormal Psychology, 104,* 614–624.

Seifer, R., Sameroff, A. J., Baldwin, C. P., & Baldwin, A. (1992). Child and family factors that ameliorate risk between 4 and 13 years of age. *Journal of the American Academy of Child and Adolescent Psychiatry, 31,* 893–903.

Seitz, V., Rosenbaum, L. K., & Apfel, N. H. (1985). Effects of family support intervention: A 10–year follow-up. *Child Development, 56,* 376–391.

Semrud-Clikeman, M., Steingard, R. J., Filipek, P., Biederman, J., Bekken, K., & Renshaw, P. F. (2000). Using MRI to examine brain–behavior relationships in males with attention deficit disorder with hyperactivity. *Journal of the American Academy of Child and Adolescent Psychiatry, 39,* 477–484.

Shaffer, D., Fisher, P., Dulcan, M. K., Davies, M., Piacentini, J., Schwab-Stone, M. E., Lahey, B. B., Bourdon, K., Jensen, P. S., Bird, H. R., Canino, G., & Regier, D. A. (1996). The NIMH Diagnostic Interview Schedule for Children Version 2.3 (DISC-2.3): Description, acceptability, prevalence rates, and performance in the MECA study. *Journal of the American Academy of Child and Adolescent Psychiatry, 35,* 865–877.

Shaffer, D., Fisher, P., Lucas, C. P., Dulcan, M. K., & Schwab-Stone, M. E. (2000). NIMH Diagnostic Interview Schedule for Children Version IV (NIMH DISC-IV): Description, differences from previous versions, and reliability of some common diagnoses. *Journal of the American Academy of Child and Adolescent Psychiatry, 39,* 28–38.

Shaffer, D., Gould, M. S., Brasic, J., Ambrosini, P., Fisher, P., Bird, H., & Aluwahlia, S. (1983). A Children's Global Assessment Scale (CGAS). *Archives of General Psychiatry, 40,* 1228–1231.

Shaffer, D., Gould, M. S., Fisher, P., Trautman, P., Moreau, D., Kleinman, M., & Flory, M. (1996). Psychiatric diagnosis in child and adolescent suicide. *Archives of General Psychiatry, 53,* 339–348.

Shamsie, J. (1981). Antisocial adolescents: Our treatments do not work—where do we go from here? *Canadian Journal of Psychiatry, 26,* 357–364.

Shapiro, S. K., Quay, H. C., Hogan, A. E., & Schwartz, K. P. (1988). Response perseveration and delayed responding in undersocialized aggressive conduct disorder. *Journal of Abnormal Psychology, 97,* 371–373.

Shapiro, T. (1989). The psychodynamic formulation in child and adolescent psychiatry. *Journal of the American Academy of Child and Adolescent Psychiatry, 28,* 675–680.

Shaw, D. S., Owens, E. B., Giovannelli, J., & Winslow, E. B. (2001). Infant and toddler pathways leading to early externalizing disorders. *Journal of the American Academy of Child and Adolescent Psychiatry, 40,* 36–43.

Shaw, D. S., & Vondra, J. I. (1993). Chronic family adversity and infant attachment security. *Journal of Child Psychology and Psychiatry, 34,* 1205–1215.

Sheard, M. H., Marini, J. L., Bridges, C. I., & Wagner, E. (1976). The effect of lithium on impulsive aggressive behavior in man. *American Journal of Psychiatry, 133,* 1409–1413.

Sherrill, J. T., & Kovacs, M. (2000). Interview Schedule for Children and Adolescents (ISCA). *Journal of the American Academy of Child and Adolescent Psychiatry, 39,* 67–75.

Siassi, I. (1982). Lithium treatment of impulsive behavior in children. *Journal of Clinical Psychiatry, 43,* 482–484.

Silberg, J. L., Rutter, M. L., Meyer, J., Maes, H., Hewitt, J., Simonoff, E., Pickles, A., Loeber, R., & Eaves, L. (1996). Genetic and environmental influences on the covariation between hyperactivity and conduct disturbance in juvenile twins. *Journal of Child Psychology and Psychiatry, 37,* 803–816.

Silva, R. R., Munoz, D. M., & Alpert, M. (1996). Carbamazepine use in children and adolescents with features of attention-deficit hyperactivity disorder: A meta-analysis. *Journal of the American Academy of Child and Adolescent Psychiatry, 35,* 352–358.

Silver, J. M., Hales, R. E., & Yudofsky, S. C. (1992). Neuropsychiatric aspects of traumatic brain injury. In S. C. Yudofsky & R. E. Hales (Eds.), *The American Psychiatric Press textbook of neuropsychiatry* (2nd ed., pp. 363–395). Washington, DC: American Psychiatric Press.

Silver, J. M., & Yudofsky, S. C. (1994). Aggressive disorders. In J. M. Silver, S. C. Yudofsky, & R. E. Hales (Eds.), *Neuropsychiatry of traumatic brain injury* (pp. 313–353). Washington, DC: American Psychiatric Press.

Silverthorn, P., & Frick, P. J. (1999). Developmental pathways to antisocial behavior: The delayed-onset pathway in girls. *Development and Psychopathology, 11,* 101–126.

Simeon, D., Stanley, B., Frances, A., Mann, J. J., Winchel, R., & Stanley, M. (1992). Self-mutilation in personality disorders: Psychological and biological correlates. *American Journal of Psychiatry, 149,* 221–226.

Simeon, J. G. (1989). Pediatric psychopharmacology. *Canadian Journal of Psychiatry, 34,* 115–121.

Simeon, J. G., Carrey, N. J., Wiggins, D. M., Milin, R. P., & Hosenbocus, S. N. (1995). Risperidone effects in treatment-resistant adolescents: Preliminary case reports. *Journal of Child and Adolescent Psychopharmacology, 5,* 69–79.

Simeon, J. G., Ferguson, H. B., & Van Wyck Fleet, J. (1986). Bupropion effects in attention deficit and conduct disorders. *Canadian Journal of Psychiatry, 31,* 581–585.

Simmons, R. G., & Blyth, D. (1987). *Moving into adolescence: The impact of pubertal change and school context.* New York: Aldine De Gruyter.

Simon, T. R., Crosby, A. E., & Dahlberg, L. L. (1999). Students who carry weapons to high school: Comparison with other weapon-carriers. *Journal of Adolescent Health, 24,* 340–348.

Simson, P. E., & Weiss, J. M. (1988). Altered activity of the locus coeruleus in an animal model of depression. *Neuropsychopharmacology, 1,* 287–295.

Singer, M. I., Anglin, T. M., Song, L. Y., & Lunghofer, L. (1995). Adolescents' exposure to violence and associated symptoms of psychological trauma. *Journal of the American Medical Association, 273*, 477–482.

Singer, M. I., Slovak, K., Frierson, T., & York, P. (1998). Viewing preferences, symptoms of psychological trauma, and violent behaviors among children who watch television. *Journal of the American Academy of Child and Adolescent Psychiatry, 37*, 1041–1048.

Slotkin, T. A. (1998). Fetal nicotine or cocaine exposure: Which one is worse? *Journal of Pharmacology and Experimental Therapeutics, 285*, 931–945.

Smeriglio, V. L., & Wilcox, H. C. (1999). Prenatal drug exposure and child outcome: Past, present, future. *Clinics in Perinatology, 26*, 1–16.

Smith, A. M., Gacono, C. B., & Kaufman, L. (1997). A Rorschach comparison of psychopathic and nonpsychopathic conduct disordered adolescents. *Journal of Clinical Psychology, 53*, 289–300.

Smithmyer, C. M., Hubbard, J. A., & Simons, R. F. (2000). Proactive and reactive aggression in delinquent adolescents: Relations to aggression outcome expectancies. *Journal of Clinical Child Psychology, 29*, 86–93.

Sonuga-Barke, E. J. S. (1998). Categorical models of childhood disorder: A conceptual and empirical analysis. *Journal of Child Psychology and Psychiatry, 39*, 115–133.

Sorgi, P., Ratey, J., Knoedler, D. W., Markert, R. J., & Reichman, M. (1991). Rating aggression in the clinical setting: A retrospective adaptation of the Overt Aggression Scale. Preliminary results. *Journal of Neuropsychiatry and Clinical Neurosciences, 3*(Suppl.), S52–S56.

Southwick, S. M., Krystal, J. H., Bremner, J. D., Morgan, C. A., III, Nicolaou, A. L., Nagy, L. M., Johnson, D. R., Heninger, G. R., & Charney, D. S. (1997). Noradrenergic and serotonergic function in posttraumatic stress disorder. *Archives of General Psychiatry, 54*, 749–758.

Speltz, M. L., DeKlyen, M., Calderon, R., Greenberg, M. T., & Fisher, P. A. (1999). Neuropsychological characteristics and test behaviors of boys with early onset conduct problems. *Journal of Abnormal Psychology, 108*, 315–325.

Spence, S. H., & Marzillier, J. S. (1981). Social skills training with adolescent male offenders: II. Short-term, long-term, and generalized effects. *Behaviour Research and Therapy, 19*, 349–368.

Spencer, E. K., & Campbell, M. (1994). Children with schizophrenia: Diagnosis, phenomenology, and pharmacotherapy. *Schizophrenia Bulletin, 20*, 713–725.

Spencer, T., Biederman, J., Wilens, T., Harding, M., O'Donnell, D., & Griffin, S. (1996). Pharmacotherapy of attention-deficit hyperactivity disorder across the life cycle. *Journal of the American Academy of Child and Adolescent Psychiatry, 35*, 409–432.

Spivak, G., & Shure, M. B. (1974). *Social adjustment of young children: A cognitive approach to solving real-life problems.* San Francisco: Jossey-Bass.

Spoont, M. R. (1992). Modulatory role of serotonin in neural information processing: Implications for human psychopathology. *Psychological Bulletin, 112*, 330–350.

Sroufe, L. A., Carlson, E. A., Levy, A. K., & Egeland, B. (1999). Implications of attachment theory for developmental psychopathology. *Development and Psychopathology, 11*, 1–13.

Sroufe, L. A., & Rutter, M. (1984). The domain of developmental psychopathology. *Child Development, 55*, 17–29.

Stanger, C., Achenbach, T. M., & McConaughy, S. H. (1993). Three-year course of behavioral/emotional problems in a national sample of 4- to 16-year-olds: 3. Predictors of signs of disturbance. *Journal of Consulting and Clinical Psychology, 61,* 839–848.

Stanger, C., Achenbach, T. M., & Verhulst, F. C. (1997). Accelerated longitudinal comparisons of aggressive versus delinquent syndromes. *Development and Psychopathology, 9,* 43–58.

Stanger, C., Higgins, S. T., Bickel, W. K., Elk, R., Grabowski, J., Schmitz, J., Amass, L., Kirby, K. C., & Seracini, A. M. (1999). Behavioral and emotional problems among children of cocaine- and opiate-dependent parents. *Journal of the American Academy of Child and Adolescent Psychiatry, 38,* 421–428.

Stanger, C., McConaughy, S. H., & Achenbach, T. M. (1992). Three-year course of behavioral/emotional problems in a national sample of 4- to 16-year-olds: II. Predictors of syndromes. *Journal of the American Academy of Child and Adolescent Psychiatry, 31,* 941–950.

Stanley, M., Traskman-Bendz, L., & Dorovini-Zis, K. (1985). Correlations between aminergic metabolites simultaneously obtained from human CSF and brain. *Life Sciences, 37,* 1279–1286.

Stattin, H., & Magnusson, D. (1990). *Pubertal maturation in female development.* Hillsdale, NJ: Erlbaum.

Steadman, H. J., Mulvey, E. P., Monahan, J., Robbins, P. C., Appelbaum, P. S., Grisso, T., Roth, L. H., & Silver, E. (1998). Violence by people discharged from acute psychiatric inpatient facilities and by others in the same neighborhoods. *Archives of General Psychiatry, 55,* 393–401.

Stein, D., Apter, A., Ratzoni, G., Har-Even, D., & Avidan, G. (1998). Association between multiple suicide attempts and negative affects in adolescents. *Journal of the American Academy of Child and Adolescent Psychiatry, 37,* 488–494.

Steiner, H., & Cauffman, E. (1998). Juvenile justice, delinquency, and psychiatry. *Child and Adolescent Psychiatric Clinics of North America, 7,* 653–672.

Steiner, H., Cauffman, E., & Duxbury, E. (1999). Personality traits in juvenile delinquents: Relation to criminal behavior and recidivism. *Journal of the American Academy of Child and Adolescent Psychiatry, 38,* 256–262.

Steiner, H., Garcia, I. G., & Matthews, Z. (1997). Posttraumatic stress disorder in incarcerated juvenile delinquents. *Journal of the American Academy of Child and Adolescent Psychiatry, 36,* 357–365.

Steinhausen, H. C. (1995). Children of alcoholic parents: A review. *European Child and Adolescent Psychiatry, 4,* 143–152.

Steinhausen, H. C., & Spohr, H. L. (1998). Long-term outcome of children with fetal alcohol syndrome: Psychopathology, behavior, and intelligence. *Alcoholism: Clinical and Experimental Research, 22,* 334–338.

Stevenson, J. (1999). The treatment of the long-term sequelae of child abuse. *Journal of Child Psychology and Psychiatry, 40,* 89–111.

Stewart, M. A., Cummings, C., Singer, S., & deBlois, C. S. (1981). The overlap between hyperactive and unsocialized aggressive children. *Journal of Child Psychology and Psychiatry, 22,* 35–45.

Stoff, D. M., Friedman, E., Pollock, L., Vitiello, B., Kendall, P. C., & Bridger, W. H. (1989). Elevated platelet MAO is related to impulsivity in disruptive behavior disorders. *Journal of the American Academy of Child and Adolescent Psychiatry, 28,* 754–760.

Stoff, D. M., Ieni, J., Friedman, E., Bridger, W. H., Pollock, L., & Vitiello, B. (1991).

Platelet ³H-imipramine binding, serotonin uptake, and plasma alpha₁ acid glyco-protein in disruptive behavior disorders. *Biological Psychiatry, 29,* 494–498.

Stoff, D. M., Pasatiempo, A. P., Yeung, J., Cooper, T. B., Bridger, W. H., & Rabinovich, H. (1992). Neuroendocrine responses to challenge with *dl*-fenfluramine and aggression in disruptive behavior disorders of children and adolescents. *Psychiatry Research, 43,* 263–276.

Stoff, D. M., Pollock, L., Vitiello, B., Behar, D., & Bridger, W. H. (1987). Reduction of ³H-imipramine binding sites on platelets of conduct-disordered children. *Neuropsychopharmacology, 1,* 55–62.

Streissguth, A. P., Randels, S. P., & Smith, D. F. (1991). A test–retest study of intelligence in patents with fetal alcohol syndrome: Implications for care. *Journal of the American Academy of Child and Adolescent Psychiatry, 30,* 584–587.

Strober, M., & Carlson, G. (1982). Bipolar illness in adolescents with major depression. *Archives of General Psychiatry, 39,* 549–555.

Strober, M., Lampert, C., Schmidt, S., & Morrel, W. (1993). The course of major depressive disorder in adolescents: I. Recovery and risk of manic switching in a follow-up of psychotic and nonpsychotic subtypes. *Journal of the American Academy of Child and Adolescent Psychiatry, 32,* 34–42.

Strober, M., Schmidt-Lackner, S., Freeman, R., Bower, S., Lampert, C., & DeAntonio, M. (1995). Recovery and relapse in adolescents with bipolar affective illness: A five-year naturalistic, prospective follow-up. *Journal of the American Academy of Child and Adolescent Psychiatry, 34,* 724–731.

Suarez, E. C., Kuhn, C. M., Schanberg, S. M., Williams, R. B., & Zimmermann, E. A. (1998). Neuroendocrine, cardiovascular, and emotional responses of hostile men: The role of interpersonal challenge. *Psychosomatic Medicine, 60,* 78–88.

Surgeon General's Scientific Advisory Committee on Television and Social Behavior. (1972). *Television and growing up: The impact of televised violence.* Washington, DC: U.S. Government Printing Office.

Susman, E. J., Dorn, L. D., Inoff-Germain, G., Nottelmann, E. D., & Chrousos, G. P. (1997). Cortisol reactivity, distress behavior, behavior problems, and emotionality in young adolescents: A longitudinal perspective. *Journal of Research on Adolescence, 7,* 81–105.

Susman, E. J., Inoff-Germain, G., Nottelman, E. D., Loriaux, D. L., Cutler, B. G., & Chrousos, G. (1987). Hormones, emotional dispositions, and aggressive attributes in young adolescents. *Child Development, 58,* 1114–1134.

Susman, E. J., & Ponirakis, A. (1997). Hormones–context interactions and antisocial behavior in youth. In A. Raine, P. A. Brennan, D. P. Farrington, & S. A. Mednick (Eds.), *Biosocial bases of violence* (pp. 251–269). New York: Plenum Press.

Susman, E. J., Schmeel, K. H., Worrall, B. K., Granger, D. A., Ponirakis, A., & Chrousos, G. P. (1999). Corticotropin-releasing hormone and cortisol: Longitudinal associations with depression and antisocial behavior in pregnant adolescents. *Journal of the American Academy of Child and Adolescent Psychiatry, 38,* 460–467.

Sussman, N. (1994). The uses of buspirone in psychiatry. *Journal of Clinical Psychiatry Monograph, 12,* 3–19.

Sutker, P. B. (1994). Psychopathy: Traditional and clinical antisocial concepts. In D. C. Fowles, P. Sutker, & S. H. Goodman (Eds.), *Progress in experimental personality and psychopathology research* (pp. 73–120). New York: Springer.

Swanson, J., Holzer, C., Ganju, V., & Jono, R. (1990). Violence and psychiatric disorder in the community: Evidence from the Epidemiologic Catchment Area surveys. *Hospital and Community Psychiatry, 41,* 761–770.

Szabo, C. P., & Magnus, C. (1999). Complex partial seizures in an adolescent psychiatric inpatient setting. *Journal of the American Academy of Child and Adolescent Psychiatry, 38,* 477–479.

Szatmari, P. (1992). The epidemiology of attention-deficit hyperactivity disorders. *Child and Adolescent Psychiatry Clinics of North America, 1,* 361–372.

Szatmari, P., Boyle, M., & Offord, D. R. (1989). ADDH and conduct disorder: Degree of diagnostic overlap and differences among correlates. *Journal of the American Academy of Child and Adolescent Psychiatry, 28,* 865–872.

Szatmari, P., Boyle, M. H., & Offord, D. R. (1993). Familial aggregation of emotional and behavioral problems of childhood in the general population. *American Journal of Psychiatry, 150,* 1398–1403.

Taiminen, T. J., Kallio-Soukainen, K., Nokso-Koivisto, H., Kaljonen, A., & Helenius, H. (1998). Contagion of deliberate self-harm among adolescent inpatients. *Journal of the American Academy of Child and Adolescent Psychiatry, 37,* 211–217.

Tardiff, K., & Sweillam, A. (1980). Assault, suicide, and mental illness. *Archives of General Psychiatry, 37,* 164–169.

Tariot, P. N., Erb, R., Podgorski, C. A., Cox, C., Patel, S., Jakimovich, J., & Irvine, C. (1998). Efficacy and tolerability of carbamazepine for agitation and aggression in dementia. *American Journal of Psychiatry, 155,* 54–61.

Taylor, D. M., & Cameron, P. A. (1998). Deliberate self-inflicted trauma: Population demographics, the nature of injury and a comparison with patients who overdose. *Australian and New Zealand Journal of Public Health, 22,* 120–125.

Taylor, E., Chadwick, O., Heptinstall, E., & Danckaerts, M. (1996). Hyperactivity and conduct problems as risk factors for adolescent development. *Journal of the American Academy of Child and Adolescent Psychiatry, 35,* 1213–1226.

Taylor, P. J., & Gunn, J. (1999). Homicides by people with mental illness: Myth and reality. *British Journal of Psychiatry, 174,* 9–14.

Teicher, M. H., Ito, Y., Glod, C. A., Schiffer, F., & Gelbard, H. A. (1996). Neurophysiological mechanisms of stress response in children. In C. Pfeffer (Ed.), *Intense stress and mental disturbances in children* (pp. 59–84). Washington, DC: American Psychiatric Press.

Tennes, K., & Kreye, M. (1985). Children's adrenocortical responses to classroom activities and tests in elementary school. *Psychosomatic Medicine, 47,* 451–460.

Tennes, K., Kreye, M., Avitable, N., & Wells, R. (1986). Behavioral correlates of excreted catecholamines and cortisol in second-grade children. *Journal of the American Academy of Child and Adolescent Psychiatry, 25,* 764–770.

Terr, L. C. (1985). Children traumatized in small groups. In S. Eth & R. S. Pynoos (Eds.), *Posttraumatic stress disorder in children* (pp. 45–70). Washington, DC: American Psychiatric Press.

Terr, L. C. (1991). Childhood traumas: An outline and overview. *American Journal of Psychiatry, 148,* 10–20.

Thiele, E. A., Gonzalez-Heydrich, J., & Riviello, J. J. (1999). Epilepsy in children and adolescents. *Child and Adolescent Psychiatric Clinics of North America, 8,* 671–694.

Thomas, A., & Chess, S. (1977). *Temperament and development.* New York: Brunner/Mazel.

Thompson, K. M., Wonderlich, S. A., Crosby, R. D., & Mitchell, J. E. (1999). The neglected link between eating disturbances and aggressive behavior in girls. *Journal of the American Academy of Child and Adolescent Psychiatry, 38,* 1277–1284.

Thomson, G. O. B., Raab, G. M., Hepburn, W. S., Hunter, R., Fulton, M., & Laxen, D. P. H. (1989). Blood-lead levels and children's behaviour: Results from the Edinburgh lead study. *Journal of Child Psychology and Psychiatry, 30,* 515–528.

Tiet, Q. Q., Bird, H. R., Davies, M., Hoven, C., Cohen, P., Jensen, P. S., & Goodman, S. (1998). Adverse life events and resilience. *Journal of the American Academy of Child and Adolescent Psychiatry, 37,* 1191–1200.

Tiihonen, J., Isohanni, M., Rasanen, P., Koiranen, M., & Moring, J. (1997). Specific major mental disorders and criminality: A 26–year prospective study of the 1966 northern Finland birth cohort. *American Journal of Psychiatry, 154,* 840–845.

Timmons-Mitchell, J., Brown, C., Schulz, S. C., Webster, S. E., Underwood, L. A., & Semple, W. E. (1997). Comparing the mental health needs of female and male incarcerated juvenile delinquents. *Behavioral Sciences and the Law, 15,* 195–202.

Tomm, K. (1984). One perspective on the Milan systemic approach: Part I. Overview of development, theory, and practice. *Journal of Marital and Family Therapy, 10,* 113–125.

Toren, P., Laor, N., & Weizman, A. (1998). Use of atypical neuroleptics in child and adolescent psychiatry. *Journal of Clinical Psychiatry, 59,* 644–656.

Treiber, F. A., Musante, L., Riley, W., Mabe, P. A., Carr, T., Levy, M., & Strong, W. B. (1989, Winter). The relationship between hostility and blood pressure in children. *Behavioral Medicine,* 173–178.

Treiman, D. M. (1986). Epilepsy and violence: Medical and legal issues. *Epilepsia, 27*(Suppl. 2), S77–S104.

Tremblay, R. E., Masse, B., Perron, D., Leblanc, M., Schwartzman, A. E., & Ledingham, J. E. (1992). Early disruptive behavior, poor school environment, delinquent behavior, and delinquent personality: Longitudinal analyses. *Journal of Consulting and Clinical Psychology, 60,* 64–72.

Tremblay, R. E., Pagani-Kurtz, L., Masse, L. C., Vitaro, F., & Pihl, R. O. (1995). A bimodal preventive intervention for disruptive kindergarten boys: Its impact through mid-adolescence. *Journal of Consulting and Clinical Psychology, 63,* 560–568.

Tremblay, R. E., Pihl, R. O., Vitaro, F., & Dobkin, P. L. (1994). Predicting early onset of male antisocial behavior from preschool behavior. *Archives of General Psychiatry, 51,* 732–739.

Tremblay, R. E., Vitaro, F., Bertrand, L., LeBlanc, M., Beauchesne, H., Boileau, H., & Lucille, D. (1992). Parent and child training to prevent early onset of delinquency: The Montreal Longitudinal Experimental Study. In J. McCord & R. E. Tremblay (Eds.), *Preventing antisocial behavior: Interventions from birth through adolescence* (pp. 117–138). New York: Guilford Press.

Tripp, G., Luk, S. L., Schaughency, E. A., & Singh, R. (1999). DSM-IV and ICD-10: A comparison of the correlates of ADHD and hyperkinetic disorder. *Journal of the American Academy of Child and Adolescent Psychiatry, 38,* 156–164.

Tschann, J. M., Kaiser, P., Chesney, M. A., Alkon, A., & Boyce, W. T. (1996). Resilience and vulnerability among preschool children: Family functioning, temperament, and behavior problems. *Journal of the American Academy of Child and Adolescent Psychiatry, 35,* 184–192.

Tuinier, S., Verhoeven, W., & van Praag, H. (1995). Cerebrospinal fluid 5–

hydroxyindoleacetic acid and aggression: A critical reappraisal of the clinical data. *International Clinical Psychopharmacotherapy, 10,* 147–156.

Turetz, M., Mozes, T., Toren, P., Chernauzan, N., Yoran-Hegesh, R., Mester, R., Wittenberg, N., Tyano, S., & Weizman, A. (1997). An open trial of clozapine in neuroleptic-resistant childhood-onset schizophrenia. *British Journal of Psychiatry, 170,* 507–510.

Twitchell, G. R., Hanna, G. L., Cook, E. H., Fitzgerald, H. E., Little, K. Y., & Zucker, R. A. (1998). Overt behavior problems and serotonergic function in middle childhood among male and female offspring of alcoholic fathers. *Alcoholism: Clinical and Experimental Research, 22,* 1340–1348.

Tygert, C. E. (1991). Juvenile delinquency and number of children in a family: Some empirical and theoretical updates. *Youth and Society, 22,* 525–536.

Unis, A. S., Cook, E. H., Vincent, J. G., Gjerde, D. K., Perry, B. D., Mason, C., & Mitchell, J. (1997). Platelet serotonin measures in adolescents with conduct disorder. *Biological Psychiatry, 42,* 553–559.

Valla, J.-P., Bergeron, L., & Smolla, N. (2000). The Dominic-R: A pictorial interview for 6- to 11-year-old children. *Journal of the American Academy of Child and Adolescent Psychiatry, 39,* 85–93.

Valois, R. F., McKeown, R. E., Garrison, C. Z., & Vincent, M. L. (1995). Correlates of aggressive and violent behaviors among public high school adolescents. *Journal of Adolescent Health, 16,* 26–34.

Van Bellinghen, M., & De Troch, C. (2001). Risperidone in the treatment of behavioral disturbances in children and adolescents with borderline intellectual functioning: A double-blind, placebo-controlled pilot trial. *Journal of Child and Adolescent Psychopharmacology, 11,* 5–13.

van Goozen, S. H. M., Matthys, W., Cohen-Kettenis, P. T., Buitelaar, J. K., & van Engeland, H. (2000). Hypothalamic–pituitary–adrenal axis and autonomic nervous system activity in disruptive children and matched controls. *Journal of the American Academy of Child and Adolescent Psychiatry, 39,* 1438–1445.

van Goozen, S. H. M., Matthys, W., Cohen-Kettenis, P. T., Gispen-de Wied, C., Wiegant, V. M., & van Engeland, H. (1998). Salivary cortisol and cardiovascular activity during stress in oppositional-defiant boys and normal controls. *Biological Psychiatry, 43,* 531–539.

van Goozen, S. H. M., Matthys, W., Cohen-Kettenis, P. T., Thijssen, J. H. H., & van Engeland, H. (1998). Adrenal androgens and aggression in conduct disorder prepubertal boys and normal controls. *Biological Psychiatry, 43,* 156–158.

van Goozen, S. H. M., Matthys, W., Cohen-Kettenis, P. T., Westenberg, H., & van Engeland, H. (1999). Plasma monoamine metabolites and aggression: Two studies of normal and oppositional defiant disorder children. *European Neuropsychopharmacology, 9,* 141–147.

van Goozen, S. H. M., van den Ban, E., Matthys, W., Cohen-Kettenis, P. T., Thijssen, J. H. H., & van Engeland, H. (2000). Increased adrenal androgen functioning in children with oppositional defiant disorder: A comparison with psychiatric and normal controls. *Journal of the American Academy of Child and Adolescent Psychiatry, 39,* 1446–1451.

van Honk, J., Tuiten, A., Verbaten, R., van den Hout, M., Koppeschaar, H., Thijssen, J. H. H., & de Haan, E. (1999). Correlations among salivary testosterone, mood, and selective attention to threat in humans. *Hormones and Behavior, 36,* 17–24.

Van Hulle, C. A., Corely, R., Zahn-Waxler, C., Kagan, J., & Hewitt, J. K. (2000). Early childhood heart rate does not predict externalizing behavior problems at age 7 years. *Journal of the American Academy of Child and Adolescent Psychiatry, 39*, 1238–1244.

van IJzendoorn, M. H. (1995). Adult attachment representations, parental responsiveness, and infant attachment: A meta-analysis on the predictive validity of the Adult Attachment Interview. *Psychological Bulletin, 117*, 387–403.

van IJzendoorn, M. H., Goldberg, S., Kroonenberg, P. M., & Frenkel, O. J. (1992). The relative effects of maternal and child problems on the quality of attachment: A meta-analysis of attachment in clinical samples. *Child Development, 63*, 840–858.

van Praag, H. M. (1986). Affective disorders and aggression disorders: Evidence for a common biological mechanism. *Suicide and Life-Threatening Behavior, 162*, 103–132.

Vanyukov, M. M., Moss, H. B., Plail, J. A., Blackson, T., Mezzich, A. C., & Tarter, R. E. (1993). Antisocial symptoms in preadolescent boys and in their parents: Associations with cortisol. *Psychiatry Research, 46*, 9–17.

Varanka, T. M., Weller, R. A., Weller, E. B., & Fristad, M. A. (1988). Lithium treatment of manic episodes with psychotic features in prepubertal children. *American Journal of Psychiatry, 145*, 1557–1559.

Varma, V. K., Basu, D., Malhotra, A., Sharma, A., & Mattoo, S. K. (1994). Correlates of early- and late-onset alcohol dependence. *Addictive Behaviors, 19*, 609–619.

Velhurst, F. C., Eussen, M. L. J. M., Berden, G. F. M. G., Sanders-Woudstra, J., & Van Der Ende, J. (1993). Pathways of problem behaviors from childhood to adolescence. *Journal of the American Academy of Child and Adolescent Psychiatry, 32*, 388–396.

Venables, P. H. (1989). The Emanuel Miller Memorial Lecture 1987: Childhood markers for adult disorders. *Journal of Child Psychology and Psychiatry, 30*, 347–364.

Verhulst, F. C., & van der Ende, J. (1992). Six-year developmental course of internalizing and externalizing problem behaviors. *Journal of the American Academy of Child and Adolescent Psychiatry, 31*, 924–931.

Vetro, A., Szentistvanyi, I., Pallag, L., Vargha, M., & Szilard, J. (1985). Therapeutic experience with lithium in childhood aggressivity. *Neuropsychobiology, 14*, 121–127.

Viesselman, J. O. (1999). Antidepressant and antimanic drugs. In J. S. Werry & M. G. Aman (Eds.), *Practitioner's guide to psychoactive drugs for children and adolescents* (2nd ed., pp. 249–296). New York: Plenum Press.

Villani, S. (2001). Impact of media on children and adolescents: A 10-year review of the research. *Journal of the American Academy of Child and Adolescent Psychiatry, 40*, 392–401.

Virkkunen, M. (1976). Self-mutilation and anti-social personality disorder. *Acta Psychiatrica Scandinavica, 54*, 347–352.

Virkkunen, M. (1985). Urinary free cortisol secretion in habitually violent offenders. *Acta Psychiatrica Scandinavica, 72*, 40–44.

Visser, J. H., van der Ende, J., Koot, H. M., & Verhulst, F. C. (1999). Continuity of psychopathology in youths referred to mental health services. *Journal of the American Academy of Child and Adolescent Psychiatry, 38*, 1560–1568.

Vitaro, F., Gendreau, P. L., Tremblay, R. E., & Oligny, P. (1998). Reactive and proactive aggression differentially predict later conduct problems. *Journal of Child Psychology and Psychiatry, 39*, 377–385.

Vitiello, B., Behar, D., Hunt, J., Stoff, D., & Ricciuti, A. (1990). Subtyping aggression in children and adolescents. *Journal of Neuropsychiatry and Clinical Neurosciences, 2*, 189–192.

Vitiello, B., Hill, J. L., Elia, J., Cunningham, E., McLeer, S. V., & Behar, D. (1991). P. R. N. medications in child psychiatric patients: A pilot placebo-controlled study. *Journal of Clinical Psychiatry, 52*, 499–501.

Vitiello, B., Ricciuti, A. J., & Behar, D. (1987). P. R. N. medications in child state hospital inpatients. *Journal of Clinical Psychiatry, 48*, 351–354.

Vivona, J. M., Ecker, B., Halgin, R. P., Cates, D., Garrison, W. T., & Friedman, M. (1995). Self- and other-directed aggression in child and adolescent psychiatric inpatients. *Journal of the American Academy of Child and Adolescent Psychiatry, 34*, 434–444.

Volkmar, F. R. (1996). Childhood and adolescent psychosis: A review of the past 10 years. *Journal of the American Academy of Child and Adolescent Psychiatry, 35*, 843–851.

Wadsworth, M. E. J. (1976). Delinquency, pulse rate, and early emotional deprivation. *British Journal of Criminology, 16*, 245–256.

Wakefield, J. C. (1992a). Disorder as harmful dysfunction: A conceptual critique of DSM-III-R's definition of mental disorder. *Psychological Review, 99*, 232–247.

Wakefield, J. C. (1992b). The concept of mental disorder: On the boundary between biological facts and social values. *American Psychologist, 47*, 373–388.

Wakefield, J. C. (1996). DSM-IV: Are we making diagnostic progress? *Contemporary Psychology, 41*, 646–652.

Wakefield, J. C. (1997). Normal inability versus pathological disability: Why Ossorio's definition of mental disorder is not sufficient. *Clinical Psychology: Science and Practice, 4*, 249–258.

Wakschlag, L. S., Lahey, B. B., Loeber, R., Green, S. M., Gordon, R., & Leventhal, B. L. (1997). Maternal smoking during pregnancy and the risk of conduct disorder in boys. *Archives of General Psychiatry, 54*, 670–676.

Walker, J. L., Lahey, B. B., Russo, M. F., Frick, P. J., Christ, M. A. G., McBurnett, K., Loeber, R., Stouthamer-Loeber, M., & Green, S. M. (1991). Anxiety, inhibition, and conduct disorder in children: I. Relations to social impairment. *Journal of the American Academy of Child and Adolescent Psychiatry, 30*, 187–191.

Walker, R. (1991). PRN psychotropic drug use on a psychiatry unit. *Psychiatric Quarterly, 62*, 1–8.

Walsh, B. W., & Rosen, P. (1988). *Self-mutilation: Theory, research, and treatment.* New York: Guilford Press.

Walsh, K. (1987). *Neuropsychology: A clinical approach* (2nd ed.). New York: Churchill Livingstone.

Walsh, R. (1997). Trends in health care coverage and financing and their implications for policy. *New England Journal of Medicine, 337*, 1000–1003.

Wannan, G., & Fombonne, E. (1998). Gender differences in rates and correlates of suicidal behaviour amongst child psychiatric outpatients. *Journal of Adolescence, 21*, 371–381.

Warner, V., Weissman, M. M., Mufson, L., & Wickramaratne, P. J. (1999). Grandparents, parents, and grandchildren at high risk for depression: A three-generation study. *Journal of the American Academy of Child and Adolescent Psychiatry, 38*, 289–296.

Waschbusch, D. A., Willoughby, M. T., & Pelham, W. E., Jr. (1998). Criterion validity and the utility of reactive and proactive aggression: Comparisons to attention deficit hyperactivity disorder, oppositional defiant disorder, conduct disorder, and other measures of functioning. *Journal of Clinical Child Psychology, 27,* 396–405.

Wasserman, G. A., Kline, J. K., Bateman, D. A., Chiriboga, C., Lumey, L. H., Friedlander, H., Melton, L., & Heagarty, M. C. (1998). Prenatal cocaine exposure and school-age intelligence. *Drug and Alcohol Dependence, 50,* 203–210.

Wasserman, G. A., Miller, L. S., Pinner, E., & Jaramillo, B. (1996). Parenting predictors of early conduct problems in urban, high-risk boys. *Journal of the American Academy of Child and Adolescent Psychiatry, 35,* 1227–1236.

Wasserman, G. A., Staghezza-Jaramillo, B., Shrout, P., Popovac, D., & Graziano, J. (1998). The effect of lead exposure on behavior problems in preschool children. *American Journal of Public Health, 88,* 481–486.

Webster's ninth new collegiate dictionary. (1989). Springfield, MA: Merriam-Webster.

Webster-Stratton, C. (1996a). Early intervention with videotape modeling: Programs for families of children with oppositional defiant disorder or conduct disorder. In E. S. Hibbs & P. S. Jensen (Eds.), *Psychosocial treatments for child and adolescent disorders: Empirically based strategies for clinical practice* (pp. 435–474). Washington, DC: American Psychological Association.

Webster-Stratton, C. (1996b). Early-onset conduct problems: Does gender make a difference? *Journal of Consulting and Clinical Psychology, 64,* 540–551.

Webster-Stratton, C., Hollinsworth, T., & Kolpacoff, M. (1989). The long-term effectiveness and clinical significance of three cost-effective training programs for families with conduct-problem children. *Journal of Consulting and Clinical Psychology, 57,* 550–553.

Webster-Stratton, C., Kolpacoff, M., & Hollinsworth, T. (1988). Self-administered videotape therapy for families with conduct-problem children: Comparison with two cost-effective treatments and a control group. *Journal of Consulting and Clinical Psychology, 56,* 558–566.

Weinberg, N. Z. (1997). Cognitive and behavioral deficits associated with parental alcohol use. *Journal of the American Academy of Child and Adolescent Psychiatry, 36,* 1177–1186.

Weinberg, N. Z., Rahdert, E., Colliver, J. D., & Glantz, M. D. (1998). Adolescent substance abuse: A review of the past 10 years. *Journal of the American Academy of Child and Adolescent Psychiatry, 37,* 252–261.

Weinshilboum, R. M. (1983). Biochemical genetics of catecholamines in man. *Mayo Clinic Proceedings, 58,* 319–330.

Weiss, G., & Hechtman, L. (1993). *Hyperactive children grown up* (2nd ed.). New York: Guilford Press.

Weissman, M. M., Warner, V., Wickramaratne, P. J., & Kandel, D. B. (1999). Maternal smoking during pregnancy and psychopathology in offspring followed to adulthood. *Journal of the American Academy of Child and Adolescent Psychiatry, 38,* 892–899.

Weissman, M. M., Wolk, S., Wickramaratne, P., Goldstein, R. B., Adams, P., Greenwald, S., Ryan, N. D., Dahl, R. E., & Steinberg, D. (1999). Children with prepubertal-onset major depressive disorder and anxiety grown up. *Archives of General Psychiatry, 56,* 794–801.

Weist, M. D., Paskewitz, D. A., Jackson, C. Y., & Jones, D. (1998). Self-reported delinquent behavior and psychosocial functioning in inner-city teenagers: A brief report. *Child Psychiatry and Human Development, 28,* 241–248.

Weitzman, M., Gortmaker, S., & Sobol, A. (1992). Maternal smoking and behavioral problems in children. *Pediatrics, 90,* 342–349.

Weller, E. B., Weller, R. A., & Fristad, M. A. (1995). Bipolar disorder in children: Misdiagnosis, underdiagnosis, and future directions. *Journal of the American Academy of Child and Adolescent Psychiatry, 34,* 709–714.

Weller, E. B., Weller, R. A., Fristad, M. A., Rooney, M. T., & Schecter, J. (2000). Children's Interview for Psychiatric Syndromes (ChIPS). *Journal of the American Academy of Child and Adolescent Psychiatry, 39,* 76–84.

Wells, K. C., Forehand, R., & Griest, D. L. (1980). Generality of treatment effects from treated to untreated behaviors resulting from a parent training program. *Journal of Clinical Child Psychology, 9,* 217–219.

Werner, E. E. (1986). Resilient offspring of alcoholics: A longitudinal study from birth to age 18. *Journal of Studies on Alcohol, 47,* 34–40.

Werner, E. E. (1987). Vulnerability and resiliency in children at risk for delinquency: A longitudinal study from birth to young adulthood. In J. D. Burchard & S. N. Burchard (Eds.), *Prevention of delinquent behavior: Vol. 10. Primary prevention of psychopathology* (pp. 16–43). Newbury Park, CA: Sage.

Werner, E. E. (1994). Overcoming the odds. *Journal of Developmental and Behavioral Pediatrics, 15,* 131–136.

Werner, E. E., & Smith, R. S. (1982). *Vulnerable but invincible: A longitudinal study of resilient children and youth.* New York: McGraw-Hill.

Werner, E. E., & Smith, R. S. (1992). *Overcoming the odds: High risk children from birth to adulthood.* Ithaca, NY: Cornell University Press.

Wessely, S. (1993). Violence and psychosis. In C. Thompson & P. Cowen (Eds.), *Violence: Basic and clinical science* (pp. 119–134). London: Butterworth–Heinemann.

West, S. A., McElroy, S. L., Strakowski, S. M., Keck, P. E., & McConville, B. J. (1995). Attention deficit hyperactivity disorder in adolescent mania. *American Journal of Psychiatry, 152,* 271–273.

White, J. L., Moffitt, T. E., & Silva, P. A. (1989). A prospective replication of the protective effects of IQ in subjects at high risk for juvenile delinquency. *Journal of Consulting and Clinical Psychology, 57,* 719–724.

White, J. L., Moffitt, T. E., Caspi, A., Bartusch, D. J., Needles, D. J., & Stouthamer-Loeber, M. (1994). Measuring impulsivity and examining its relationship to delinquency. *Journal of Abnormal Psychology, 103,* 192–205.

Whitman, S., Hermann, B. P., Black, R. B., & Chhabria, S. (1982). Psychopathology and seizure type in children with epilepsy. *Psychological Medicine, 12,* 843–853.

Widom, C. S. (1989a). The cycle of violence. *Science, 244,* 160–166.

Widom, C. S. (1989b). Does violence beget violence?: A critical examination of the literature. *Psychological Bulletin, 106,* 3–28.

Wilens, T. E., Biederman, J., Abrantes, A. M., & Spencer, T. J. (1997). Clinical characteristics of psychiatrically referred adolescent outpatients with substance use disorder. *Journal of the American Academy of Child and Adolescent Psychiatry, 36,* 941–947.

Wilens, T. E., Biederman, J., Geist, D. E., Steingard, R., & Spencer, T. (1993). Nortriptyline in the treatment of ADHD: A chart review of 58 cases. *Journal of the American Academy of Child and Adolescent Psychiatry, 32,* 343–349.

Wilens, T. E., Biederman, J., Kiely, K., Bredin, E., & Spencer, T. J. (1995). Pilot study of behavioral and emotional disturbances in the high-risk children of parents with opioid dependence. *Journal of the American Academy of Child and Adolescent Psychiatry, 34,* 779–785.

Williams, D. T., Mehl, R., Yudofsky, S., Adams, D., & Roseman, B. (1982). The effect of propranolol on uncontrolled rage outbursts in children and adolescents with organic brain dysfunction. *Journal of the American Academy of Child and Adolescent Psychiatry, 21,* 129–135.

Willis, L. M., & Foster, S. L. (1990). Differences in children's peer sociometric and attribution ratings due to context and type of aggressive behavior. *Journal of Abnormal Child Psychology, 18,* 199–215.

Winchel, R. M., & Stanley, M. (1991). Self-injurious behavior: A review of the behavior and biology of self-mutilation. *American Journal of Psychiatry, 148,* 306–317.

Winokur, G., Coryell, W., Endicott, J., Keller, M. B., Akiskal, H. S., & Solomon, D. (1996). Familial alcoholism in manic–depressive (bipolar) disease. *American Journal of Medical Genetics, 67,* 197–201.

Wolfgang, M. E., Figho, R. M., & Sellin, T. (1927). *Delinquency in a birth cohort.* Chicago: University of Chicago Press.

Wonderlich, S. A., & Mitchell, J. E. (1997). Eating disorders and comorbidity: Empirical, conceptual, and clinical implications. *Psychopharmacology Bulletin, 33,* 381–390.

Wonderlich, S. A., & Swift, W. J. (1990). Borderline versus other personality disorders in the eating disorders: Clinical description. *International Journal of Eating Disorders, 9,* 629–638.

Wootton, J. M., Frick, P. J., Shelton, K. K., & Silverthorn, P. (1997). Ineffective parenting and childhood conduct problems: The moderating role of callous–unemotional traits. *Journal of Consulting and Clinical Psychology, 65,* 301–308.

World Health Organization (WHO). (1978). *International classification of diseases* (9th rev.). Geneva: Author.

World Health Organization (WHO). (1992). *International statistical classification of diseases and related health problems* (10th rev.). Geneva: Author.

Wozniak, J., Biederman, J., Kiely, K., Ablon, J. S., Faraone, S. V., Mundy, E., & Mennin, D. (1995). Mania-like symptoms suggestive of childhood-onset bipolar disorder in clinically referred children. *Journal of the American Academy of Child and Adolescent Psychiatry, 34,* 867–876.

Wyman, P. A., Cowen, E. L., Work, W. C., Raoof, A., Gribble, P. A., Parker, G. R., & Wannon, M. (1992). Interviews with children who experienced major life stress: Family and child attributes that predict resilient outcomes. *Journal of the American Academy of Child and Adolescent Psychiatry, 31,* 904–910.

Yoshikawa, H. (1994). Prevention as cumulative protection: Effects of early family support and education on chronic delinquency and its risks. *Psychological Bulletin, 115,* 28–54.

Yoshikawa, H. (1995). Long-term effects of early childhood programs on social outcomes and delinquency. *The Future of Children: Long-Term Outcomes of Early Childhood Programs, 5,* 51–75.

Young, N. K. (1997). Effects of alcohol and other drugs on children. *Journal of Psychoactive Drugs, 29,* 23–42.

Young Women's Christian Association (YWCA). (1996). *Families taking action: A YWCA survey about making homes and communities safer.* New York: Louis Harris and Associates.

Yudofsky, S. C., Silver, J. M., Jackson, W., Endicott, J., & Williams, D. (1986). The Overt Aggression Scale for the objective rating of verbal and physical aggression. *American Journal of Psychiatry, 143,* 35–39.

Zagar, R., Arbit, J., Hughes, J. R., Busnell, R. E., & Busch, K. (1989). Developmental and disruptive behavior disorders among delinquents. *Journal of the American Academy of Child and Adolescent Psychiatry, 28,* 437–440.

Zahn-Waxler, C. (1993). Warriors and worriers: Gender and psychopathology. *Development and Psychopathology, 5,* 79–89.

Zeanah, C. H., Boris, N. W., & Larrieu, J. A. (1997). Infant development and developmental risk: A review of the past 10 years. *Journal of the American Academy of Child and Adolescent Psychiatry, 36,* 165–178.

Zigler, E., Taussig, C., & Black, K. (1992). Early childhood intervention: A promising preventative for juvenile delinquency. *American Psychologist, 47,* 997–1006.

Zillmann, D. (1983). Arousal and aggression. In R. G. Green & E. I. Donnerstein (Eds.), *Aggression: Theoretical and empirical reviews* (Vol. 1, pp. 75–101). New York: Academic Press.

Zito, J. M., & Riddle, M. A. (1995). Psychiatric pharmacoepidemiology for children. *Child and Adolescent Psychiatric Clinics of North America, 4,* 77–95.

Zito, J. M., Safer, D. J., dosReis, S., Gardner, J. F., Boles, M., & Lynch, F. (2000). Trends in the prescribing of psychotropic medications to preschoolers. *Journal of the American Medical Association, 283,* 1025–1030.

Zlotnick, C., Mattia, J. I., & Zimmerman, M. (1999). Clinical correlates of self-mutilation in a sample of general psychiatric patients. *Journal of Nervous and Mental Disease, 187,* 296–301.

Zlotnick, C., Shea, M. T., Recupero, P., Bidadi, K., Pearlstein, T., & Brown, P. (1997). Trauma, dissociation, impulsivity, and self-mutilation among substance abuse patients. *American Journal of Orthopsychiatry, 67,* 650–654.

Zoccolillo, M. (1992). Co-occurrence of conduct disorder and its adult outcomes with depressive and anxiety disorders: A review. *Journal of the American Academy of Child and Adolescent Psychiatry, 31,* 547–556.

Zoccolillo, M. (1993). Gender and the development of conduct disorder. *Development and Psychopathology, 5,* 65–78.

Zoccolillo, M., Pickles, A., Quinton, D., & Rutter, M. (1992). The outcome of childhood conduct disorder: Implications for defining adult personality disorder and conduct disorder. *Psychological Medicine, 22,* 971–986.

Zoccolillo, M., & Rogers, K. (1991). Characteristics and outcome of hospitalized adolescent girls with conduct disorder. *Journal of the American Academy of Child and Adolescent Psychiatry, 30,* 973–981.

Zoccolillo, M., Tremblay, R., & Vitaro, F. (1996). DSM-III-R and DSM-III criteria for conduct disorder in preadolescent girls: Specific but insensitive. *Journal of the American Academy of Child and Adolescent Psychiatry, 35,* 461–470.

Zubieta, J. K., & Alessi, N. E. (1992). Acute and chronic administration of trazodone in the treatment of disruptive behavior disorders in children. *Journal of Clinical Psychopharmacology, 12,* 346–351.

Zuckerman, M. (1991). *Psychobiology of personality.* Cambridge, England: Cambridge University Press.

Index